MEDICINE MEETS VIRTUAL REALITY 2001

Studies in Health Technology and Informatics

Editors

Jens Pihlkjaer Christensen, European Commission, Luxembourg; Arie Hasman, EFMI and University of Maastricht; Ilias Iakovidis, European Commission, Brussels; Zoi Kolitsi, University of Patras; Olivier Le Dour, European Commission DG Research, Brussels; Antonio Pedotti, Politecnico di Milan; Otto Rienhoff, Georg-August-Universität Göttingen; Francis H. Roger France, Centre for Medical Informatics, UCL, Brussels; Niels Rossing, National University Hospital, Copenhagen; Faina Shtern, National Institutes of Health, Bethesda, MD

Volume 81

Earlier published in this series

ISSN: 0926-9630

Medicine Meets Virtual Reality 2001

Outer Space, Inner Space, Virtual Space

Edited by

James D. Westwood
Program Coordinator MMVR2001
Aligned Management Associates, Inc., New London, CT, USA

Helene Miller Hoffman, PhD
Assistant Dean, Curriculum & Educational Computing
Associate Adjunct Professor of Medicine
Director, Learning Resources Center
University of California, San Diego, School of Medicine, La Jolla, CA, USA

Greg T. Mogel, MD
Assistant Professor of Radiology
Children's Hospital Los Angeles / University of Southern California
Los Angeles, CA, USA

Don Stredney
Director, Interface Laboratory
Research Scientist, Biomedical Applications
Ohio Supercomputer Center, Columbus, OH, USA

Richard A. Robb, PhD
Scheller Professor in Medical Research
Professor of Biophysics and Computer Science
Director, Biomedical Imaging Resource
Director, Biomedical Engineering Program
Associate Dean for Academic Affairs, MGS
Mayo Clinic & Foundation, Rochester, MN, USA

IOS
Press

OHM
Ohmsha

Amsterdam • Berlin • Oxford • Tokyo • Washington, DC

ISBN 1 58603 143 0 (IOS Press)
ISBN 4 274 90419 9 C3047 (Ohmsha)
Library of Congress Catalog Card Number: 00-111495

Publisher
IOS Press
Nieuwe Hemweg 6B
1013 BG Amsterdam
The Netherlands
fax: +31 20 620 3419
e-mail: order@iospress.nl

Distributor in the UK and Ireland
IOS Press/Lavis Marketing
73 Lime Walk
Headington
Oxford OX3 7AD
England
fax: +44 1865 75 0079

Distributor in the USA and Canada
IOS Press, Inc.
5795-G Burke Centre Parkway
Burke, VA 22015
USA
fax: +1 703 323 3668
e-mail: iosbooks@iospress.com

Distributor in Germany, Austria and Switzerland
IOS Press/LSL.de
Gerichtsweg 28
D-04103 Leipzig
Germany
fax: +49 341.9954255

Distributor in Japan
Ohmsha, Ltd.
3-1 Kanda Nishiki-cho
Chiyoda-ku, Tokyo 101
Japan
fax: +81 3 3233 2426

LEGAL NOTICE
The publisher is not responsible for the use which might be made of the following information.

PRINTED IN THE NETHERLANDS

Preface

James D. Westwood
Aligned Management Associates, Inc.

The theme of the 2001 *Medicine Meets Virtual Reality* conference is "Outer Space, Inner Space, Virtual Space." (How could we resist the cinematic reference?) These three different ideas, or domains, are linked by their use of interactive, computer-based, image-producing technology: *virtual reality*. And while they aren't automatically associated with medicine, they significantly affect health care practice — now and certainly in the future.

Outer Space. While space programs seem to be experiencing a reality check after their initial glory, our species' fascination with the moon, the planets, and the stars is unflagging. We won't soon travel to Mars with today's jetliner nonchalance (including frequent flier miles and seating upgrades), but every step in that direction develops valuable tools for use now. Aerospace ambition nurtures simulation, visualization, robotics, telemedicine, and other technologies integral to *MMVR*.

Inner Space. The human body is also a "final frontier," perhaps the most important one. We no longer want to see a surgeon with an obsidian blade, nor a barber's pole advertising trimmed hair and opened veins on the same premises. The efforts of *MMVR* researchers will some day result in tools that will make today's operating rooms look primitive. Satisfied by the integration of microscopic, information-fed devices into their bodies, our descendents may think of us as well-intentioned but naïve. A future child may be astonished to learn that doctors once operated on problems from the outside of the body instead of from within.

Virtual Space. Cultural commentators have noted that the image is usurping the supreme position of the word. Fortunately, for *MMVR* participants, this image-based world isn't about marketing and brand recognition, but about creating new drawing boards on which to solve health problems and plan new extensions to human capability. At its best, this new image-world is an interactive domain where solutions can be envisioned and tested faster and safer than in real life. It is a catalytic environment that uses data from wide-ranging disciplines to create something entirely new.

2001. Many scenes in Stanley Kubrick's *Space Odyssey* seem silly in comparison to how electronic technology has evolved since 1968. (Rows of blinking lights are impressive, but what's on the monitor?) And Kubrick's monolith heralding revolutions in human behavior is dramatic, but not emblematic of how progress typically occurs. Progress comes not as a towering and inescapable revelation upon a boulder-strewn landscape, but as gradual understanding that, more likely than not, takes place at a paper-strewn desk.

We have borrowed Kubrick's infant as an icon of the future. While we may not know that future child who is baffled by the ancient healing methods of the year 2001, we hope this child lives in a world that has been improved by the ideas and knowledge shared here.

Medicine Meets Virtual Reality 2001
J.D. Westwood et al. (Eds.)
IOS Press, 2001

vii

BioIntelligence Age: Implications for the Future of Medicine

Richard M. Satava, MD FACS

Professor of Surgery, Yale University School of Medicine,
40 Temple Street, New Haven, Connecticut 06510 &
Telemedicine and Advanced Technology Research Center (TATRC), US Army Military
Research and Materiel Command (USAMRMC)*, Ft. Detrick, Maryland, USA

Scientists have begun to wonder about the direction of the future of scientific research. The Information Age is not the future; the Information Age is the present. Information has achieved the status of a dimension, similar to space and time. It is a function of one's perception, it influences action or changes in the real world, and it results in practical applications, products or services. Like the Agricultural Age and the Industrial Age, the Information Age is reaching a plateau (Figure 1). There are a number of interesting concepts embedded in figure 1, which depicts the development of a scientific era over time. The first and most obvious is that the rate of development (slope) is becoming steeper, a fact that is repeatedly emphasized. However, there are other important implications that can be derived from this figure. First and foremost, there are long periods of discovery, testing and evaluation before the age begins the accelerated growth. This phenomenon is painfully obvious to all researchers as they try to move their discoveries from laboratory to commercial success. Although the Industrial Age is usually considered a nineteenth century event, the inception of this era clearly has its roots as far back as the Renaissance when innovators such as Leonard DaVinci envisioned machines that eventually came to fruition when the technology had finally matured. Another insight that can be derived from figure 1 is that the plateau of scientific discovery within an Age seems to occur at the time when there is public and consumer acceptance of the discoveries. It is at this point where research is focused upon iterative and evolutionary discovery, not on revolutionary and disruptive discovery. This is as true today as always, as manifest by the life cycle of the many information technologies that are emerging. The Internet is also following that pathway, and may signal the inflection point for the Information Age. If this figure is to have any value it must be able to provide insight into the future. The key factor is that during the inflection point, revolutionary discoveries will be coming from a new Age, not from the existing field of science.

There is an arbitrarily drawn curve labeled the BioIntelligence Age (this is a place holder name until the true nature of the change is understood). Like the prior Ages, it has a "tail" that begins before the rapid acceleration phase of the preceding Age and represents the scientific discipline in which the revolutionary discoveries are occurring in the laboratory. Until recently research was focused within a single discipline. The BioIntelligence Age has its roots in interdisciplinary research, the combination of scientific disciplines. The Venn diagram (Figure 2) is a visualization of the nature of the new direction of scientific research. The three circles represent the traditional "stovepipe" areas of research – Biologic, Physical and Information Sciences. Research usually occurred within one of these disciplines, with little if any contribution from another science. What is

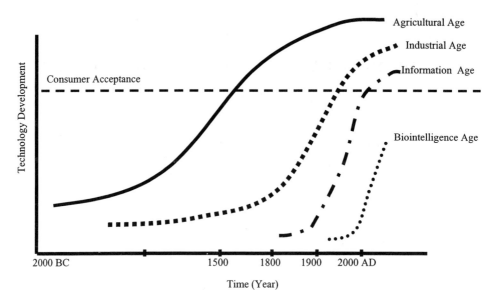

Figure 1. Bio Intelligence Age

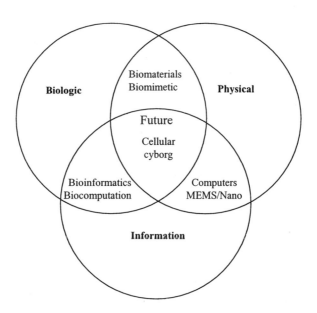

Figure 2.

emerging now is interdisciplinary research that is occurring at the intersection of two of the sciences – this is the hallmark of the BioIntelligence Age. The evidence for this premise is that throughout academia, industry and government laboratories there is the creation of new departments and divisions, such as bioinformatics or biorobotics. Thus between Biology and Physical sciences we see biosensors, DNA chips, biomaterials and biomimetic systems. Between Biology and Information sciences there are drug design and genomics, bioinformatics and biocomputation. Between Physical and Information Sciences there are intelligent micro-robots, microelectromechanical systems (MEMS) and nanotechnology. If the diagram has validity, then the power of the future will be occurring where all three circles intersect, taking advantage of the biologic (flexible, adaptable, self assembly, self repair, etc) world, the physical (precision, robust, predictable, etc) world and the information (communication, networking, intelligent, etc) world. What makes the integration of the three worlds possible is that at the micro and nano levels, the energy requirements from the different fields are comparable. For example, the membrane potential of a cell changes from 20 to more than 100 millivolts during excitation, and some MEMS devices require 50 millivolts for actuation, demonstrating that cells (living systems) can "communicate" directly with MEMS (machines). Currently cell based sensors on a silicon MEMS are being demonstrated for biosensing. One theoretical example of a combination of all three worlds would be a "cellular cyborg", a MEMS chip with a stem cell programmed for glucose detection on the surface, a decision support system, and a micro-well MEMS with insulin. The stem cell detects hyperglycemia, which changes the cellular membrane potential, which is detected by the MEMS device, interpreted by the decision support software, and allows one of the thousands of microwells containing insulin to release the insulin. Such a system, an artificial pancreas, could be embedded or injected subcutaneously and provide months of autoregulation for a diabetic patient. Another example is the field of tissue engineering. Using computational mathematics, a 3 dimensional branching scaffold representing the vascular tree is designed and then produced by stereolithographic techniques using a bioresorbable polymer in which vascular endothelial growth factor, angiogenesis factor, etc is embedded. This is coated by endothelial stem cells and then smooth muscle stem cells to form a vascular tree, followed by immersion into hepatic, renal or other cells to form the appropriate organs. While this is admittedly a simplified hypothesis, the significance is that the technologies mentioned exist today and illustrate how the interdisciplinary approach can be the pathway to the next generation of scientific research. The fields of complexity and chaos theory have helped elucidate the processes whereby seemingly random or incomprehensibly complex systems can be reduced to understandable, inter-related systems through an interdisciplinary approach. The preceding Ages have been dominated by the Physical and Information sciences, however the coming era will have a large component of the Biologic sciences, with their strength in self assembly and adaptability. Thus the arbitrary name BioIntelligence Age to signify the importance of the contribution of biotechnology, and the fact that the systems that will be built will create a world that is networked and "smarter" than today.

Even as the struggle continues to understand the vortex of change around us, there are words of caution. Ray Kurzweiler, in his Age of Spiritual Machines, and Eric Drexler, in his Engines of Creation, caution about the ability to control the new technologies which are unleashed. Bill Joy has raised the specter of a future where our creations, nanobots, intelligent robots and genetically designed foods or organisms, will take on a life of their. Concerned scientists are beginning to seriously deliberate these questions, wondering if the new directions of research are a Faustian bargain. While it is extrapolated from current growth of computer science that by 2030 to 2040 AD computers will have the same computational power of a human brain, will such systems be intelligent, have emotions or even be controllable by humans? For the first time, a species (homo sapiens) is able to control the evolution of species or create new life forms. Unlike any time in history, scientists are proactively considering the long-term social consequences for mankind of their scientific inquiry. The success of cloning in animals has forced the world to address its implications for humans and put in place regulatory barriers; will such regulation be necessary for the technologies of the BioIntelligence Age?

In a world enamored by technology and exhilarated by the accelerated rate of change, how can we proceed prudently without slowing the rate of progress? Many of our national agencies already have exploratory programs in many of these interdisciplinary areas. The Defense Advanced Research Projects Agency (DARPA) has initiated its Bio Futures program, National Aeronautics and Space Administration (NASA) has begun programs in Astrobiology and Bioastronautics, the National Cancer Institute (NCI) of the National Institutes of Health (NIH) has the Unconventional Innovations Program, and the National Science Foundation (NSF) is proceeding with the Nanotechnology initiative. It is therefore contingent upon the scientific community to squarely face these issues and participate in their evaluation and, if necessary, their regulation before external forces take the decisions out of the hands of scientists. Technology has provided an opportunity for a future that is bright, but we must walk into the BioIntelligence Age with our eyes wide open.

* The opinions or assertions contained herein are the private views of the author and are not to be construed as official, or as reflecting the views of the Department of the Army, Department of the Navy, the Advanced Research Projects Agency, or the Department of Defense.

Medicine Meets Virtual Reality 2001
Program Committee

Michael J. Ackerman PhD
Office of High Performance Computing &
Communications
National Library of Medicine
Bethesda, MD

Ian Alger MD
New York Presbyterian Hospital/
Weill Medical College of Cornell University
New York, NY

David C. Balch
The Telemedicine Center
East Carolina University
Greenville, NC

Steven T. Charles MD
MicroDexterity Systems &
University of Tennessee
Memphis, TN

Terence M. Davidson MD
Continuing Medical Education
University of California, San Diego, School of
Medicine
La Jolla, CA

Henry Fuchs PhD
Dept. of Computer Science
University of North Carolina
Chapel Hill, NC

Walter J. Greenleaf PhD
Greenleaf Medical Systems
Palo Alto, CA

Wm. LeRoy Heinrichs MD PhD
Medical Media & Information Technologies &
Dept. of Gynecology & Obstetrics
Stanford University
Stanford, CA

Helene M. Hoffman PhD
Learning Resources Center
University of California, San Diego, School of
Medicine
La Jolla, CA

Christoph Kaufmann MD MPH FACS
National Capital Area Medical Simulation Center
Uniformed Services University of the Health
Sciences
Bethesda, MD

Heinz U. Lemke PhD
Institute for Technical Informatics
Technical University Berlin
Berlin, Germany

John D. McBrayer PhD
SAMPLES Program
Sandia National Laboratories
Albuquerque, NM

Greg T. Mogel MD
Childrens Hospital Los Angeles/
University of Southern California
Los Angeles, CA

Kevin Montgomery PhD
National Biocomputation Center
Stanford University
Palo Alto, CA

Lutz-P. Nolte PhD
M. E. Muller Institute for Biomechanics
University of Bern
Bern, Switzerland

Makoto Nonaka MD PhD
Foundation for International Scientific Advancement
La Jolla, CA

Roger Phillips PhD MBCS
Dept. of Computer Science
University of Hull
Hull, United Kingdom

Richard A. Robb PhD
Biomedical Imaging Resource
Mayo Clinic & Foundation
Rochester, MN

Jannick P. Rolland PhD
O.D.A. Laboratory
University of Central Florida
Orlando, FL

Gerald M. Roth MD
Continuing Medical Education &
Dept. of Radiological Sciences
University of California, Irvine, College of Medicine
Irvine, CA

Richard M. Satava MD FACS
Department of Surgery,
Yale University School of Medicine
New Haven, CT

Rainer M.M. Seibel MD
Institute of Diagnostic & Interventional Radiology,
University of Witten/Herdecke
Mulheim a.d. Ruhr, Germany

Ramin Shahidi PhD
Image Guidance Laboratories / Neurosurgery
Stanford University Medical Center
Stanford, CA

Faina Shtern MD
Office of Research Affairs & Dept. of Radiology
Beth Israel Deaconess Medical Center &
AdMeTech
Boston, MA

Don Stredney
Interface Laboratory
Ohio Supercomputer Center
Columbus, OH

Kirby G. Vosburgh PhD
CIMIT/Center for Innovative Minimally Invasive
Therapy
Boston, MA

Dave Warner MD PhD
MindTel LLC &
Institute for Interventional Informatics
Syracuse, NY & San Diego, CA

Suzanne J. Weghorst
Human Interface Technology Lab
University of Washington
Seattle, WA

Brenda Wiederhold MBA PhD BCIA-C
Center for Advanced Multimedia Psychotherapy
CSPP Research & Service Foundation
San Diego, CA

Contents

Medicine Meets Virtual Reality 2001
J.D. Westwood et al. (Eds.)
IOS Press, 2001

Clinical Fluoroscopic Fiducial-Based Registration of the Vertebral Body in Spinal Neuronavigation

Hamid R. Abbasi[1], Robert Grzeszczuk[1], Shao Chin[1], Rebecca Fahrig[2], Hilary Holz[1], Sanaz Hariri[1], Daniel Kim[1], John Adler[1], Ramin Shahidi[1]

[1]*Image Guidance Laboratories, Stanford University*
[2]*Department of Radiology, Stanford University*

Abstract. We present a system involving a computer-instrumented fluoroscope for the purpose of 3D navigation and guidance using pre-operative diagnostic scans as a reference. The goal of the project is to devise a computer-assisted tool that will improve the accuracy, reduce risk, minimize the invasiveness, and shorten the time it takes to perform a variety of neurosurgical and orthopedic procedures of the spine. For this purpose we propose an apparatus that will track surgical tools and localize them with respect to the patient's 3D anatomy and pre-operative 3D diagnostic scans using intraoperative fluoroscopy for *in situ* registration and embedded fiducials. Preliminary studies have found a fiducial registration error (FRE) of 1.41 mm and a Target Localization Error (TLE) of 0.48 mm. The resulting system leverages equipment already commonly available in the operating room (OR), providing an important new functionality that is free of many current limitations, while keeping costs contained.

1. Introduction

Computer-assisted spine surgery is an active area, and numerous systems, both commercial and research, have been described in the literature. Most of these currently available systems provide similar functionality and methodology. The majority employs optical trackers for the purpose of registration and localization.

Typically, the vertebral body of interest is fully exposed intra-operatively and a small number of distinct anatomical landmarks are digitized for the purpose of coarse registration. Subsequently, a larger number of points are digitized on the surface of the vertebrae to refine the registration with a surface matching technique. The procedure is often cumbersome, time consuming, and of limited accuracy. This is mainly due to difficulties in identifying characteristic anatomical landmarks in a reproducible fashion and inherent inaccuracies of surface matching techniques. While dynamic reference frames (DRFs) are commonly used to monitor target movement, any safeguarding against DRF misregistration requires the entire process, including the laborious manual digitization part, to be repeated. This gets even more cumbersome in procedures involving multiple vertebrae (e.g., cage placements) that require multiple DRFs to be maintained. Finally, aforementioned techniques cannot be applied in the context of percutaneous procedures because they rely on the target structure being directly visible to the optical tracking device.

Recently, several academic researchers [1] and commercial vendors (e.g., FluoroNav, Medtronic, Minneapolis, MN, USA) began experimenting with fluoroscopy as an intra-operative imaging modality. The relative low cost and pervasiveness of C-Arm devices in modern ORs can explain this increased interest. Most of these attempts focus on improving conventional 2D navigation techniques via tracking of the C-Arm and re-projecting pre-operative CT data onto multiple planes. Such techniques are helpful in lowering the amount of ionizing radiation delivered to the patient and the OR staff during free-hand navigation and also in providing more information to the surgeon about the relative position of the surgical tools with respect to the patient's anatomy. However, they essentially automate and streamline the current workflow and rely on the surgeon's ability to create a complex spatial model mentally. In contrast, our approach employs stereoscopic registration in order to relate patient's anatomy to pre-operative diagnostic scans in 3D.

2. Materials and Methods

2.1. Overview

A mobile fluoroscopic device (C-Arm, GE, Milwaukee, WI, USA) is used for instrumented intra-operative free hand imaging of skeletal anatomy. The position and orientation of the camera are tracked by an optoelectronic device (Optotrack, Northern Digital, Waterloo, Ontario, Canada). NTSC video output of the X-ray camera as well as its position and orientation are processed by an SGI 320 (SGI, Mountain View, CA, USA) NT workstation. The image data is used by the system to register a pre-operative CT data set (512x512 130 slices, 1.0 mm thick) to the patient's reference frame. Tracking data is used to monitor the relative position changes of the camera with respect to the patient during free-hand navigation.

Three to four internal markers are used for registration. These markers are stainless steel spheres (diameter = 2 mm) covered with a hard plastic shell in the form of a cone with a sharp tip. A silk string attached to the marker is used to extract the marker after the surgery. A T-shaped needle is used to insert the markers (Fig. 1). The string on the marker is threaded through the hollow needle and holds the marker at the end of the needle. After insertion of the marker close to bony structure of the vertebral body, the string is released and allowed to come out of the needle.

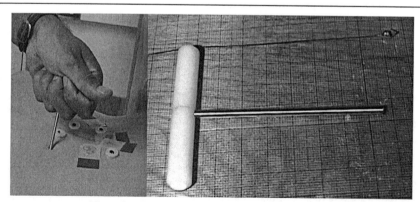

Figure 1. A T-shaped needle is used to insert the markers.

During the procedure, after a CT has been performed, the system operator performs an initial registration of the patient's anatomy to the pre-operative CT study by taking two fluoroscopic views of the target vertebrae with at least a 45 degree between the two fluoroscopic images. These images are used to compute the C-Arm-to-CT registration using a fully automatic technique described in detail below. As a result, we obtain the position and orientation of the C-Arm's camera in the reference frame of the CT study. We can then use this information, together with the position and orientation of the camera in the tracker reference frame, to follow the future relative motions of the camera, assuming a static system. Misregistration, due to either patient movement or system error, can be detected at any time by comparing the predicted digitally reconstructed radiograph (DRR) to the actual fluoroscopic image, at which point the objects can be re-registered within 30 second.

2.2. Intrinsic Camera Calibration

Before the system can be used effectively, it needs to be calibrated to eliminate imaging distortions and extract parameters required to characterize the imaging system. During the process of intrinsic camera calibration, we determine the set of parameters that characterize the internal geometry of our imaging system. All of these parameters are well documented in the computer vision literature [2]: effective focal length (i.e., the exact distance from the X-ray source to the image plane), focal spot (i.e., the exact place where the optical axis pierces the image plane), magnification factors, and pincushion distortions. It is also well understood that many of C-Arm's intrinsic parameters vary with orientation. For example, the focal length and focal spot will be different for vertical and horizontal positioning, due to mechanical sag of the arm. Similarly, the pincushion distortion depends on the orientation of the device with respect to the Earth's magnetic field and external sources of EMFs [7]. For these reasons, a calibration jig is attached to the face of the image intensifier to adaptively calibrate the system every time an image is acquired. The intrinsic parameters thus produced are used during the registration phase.

2.3. Extrinsic Camera Calibration and Registration

Once the intrinsic camera parameters are measured, registration of the imaging system to the patient can be preformed. The problem can be posed as follows: given a CT study of the relevant anatomy and two fluoroscopic images of the same internal fiducial marker configuration, one must find the position and orientation of the camera in the reference frame of the CT study that produced the image. In this approach, the system hypothesizes about the camera's actual six degrees of freedom (DOF) position by introducing a virtual camera and computing a simulated radiograph (a digitally reconstructed radiograph, or DRR). The radiograph represents the actual patient position.

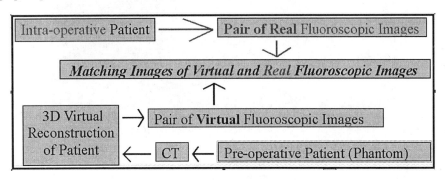

If the DRR matches the radiograph exactly, the virtual camera position identifies the actual camera position and thus the registration is found, otherwise another hypothesis is formed. In practice, the accuracy of such basic radiograph-to-DRR registration method can be substantially improved if more views of the same anatomy can be used. In this scenario, it is assumed that the relative positions of the cameras are known (e.g., from an optical tracking device), so instead of finding two or more independent camera positions [4], the problem can be reformulate to that of finding the pose of the CT study with respect to the rigid configuration of multiple cameras.

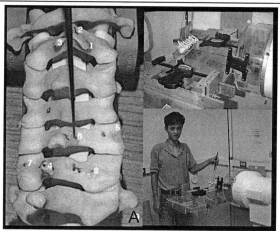

Figure 2. *Left:* Anatomic spine phantom; all fiducials are used as targets in accuracy testing; fiducials 5-8 are also used in course and fine registration. *Right:* Experimental setup showing the C-arm registration apparatus with phantom vertebrae (top) and the registration procedure (bottom).

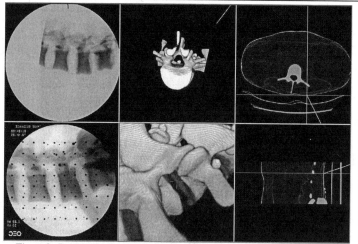

Figure 3. Registration in progress for a rigid torso phantom. *Top left:* Virtual fluoroscopic view. *Bottom left:* Real flouroscopic view. *Top middle:* 3D reconstruction of the vertebral body, which can be rotated freely in space. *Bottom middle:* The probe eye view. *Right:* Standard axial (top) and coronal (bottom) views. The position of the probe can be tracked in all windows.

To reduce the processing time, the approximate position in space around phantom where the best results are expected is described to the system. This is done in a process of external registration comparable to cranial neuronavigation. Once the algorithm is running, the computer stochastically searches for the position of the virtual fluoroscope around the CT data, where it can get the best match between the real and virtual fluoroscope images. In essence, this registration process can be viewed as an extrinsic calibration of an abstract imaging system consisting of multiple, rigidly mounted cameras.

2.4. Assessment of System Accuracy

Eight stainless steel BB's are glued onto the anatomical phantom to be used as targets for system accuracy assement. Four BB's (numbers 5-8) are also used for course registration, as described above. After course registration, the phantom is translated (maximal translation = 1 cm) and rotated (maximal rotation = 10°).

After movement of the phantom, two flouroscopic images (lateral and AP) are captured and the registration algorithm is run. After the registration algorithm has positioned the CT data in the reference frame of the camera, a standard neuronavigation probe is used to digitize the positions of the anatomical targets, yielding the position of these targets in the tracker referencing frame and also tranfering them to the reference frame of the CT which was positioned in the tracker frame. The positions of the targets according to the algorithm are compared to their real positions according to the DICOM data.

3. Results

3.1 Target Localization Error (TLE)

The process of accuracy assessment requires that the experimenter touch the probe tip to the BBs. The human error in accurately localizing the BB with the probe tip is called Target Localization Error (TLE) [6]. To find the TLE, the operator digitized the eight targets, ten times each, yielding 80 spatial values for the BB locations in the x-, y-, and z-axes. Assuming the average of x-, y-, and z-values as the true spatial value of each BB, each BB localization value (80 values total) was compared to the true spatial value for each BB to determine TLE. TLE was found to be 0.48 mm.

3.2 System Accuracy

We repeated the procedure for accuracy testing described above 20 times, resulting in 160 measurments (20 x 8 targets). The overally accuracy of the algorithm, with TLE (human error) subtracted, is 1.44 mm [7] (Fig. 4). Of that 1.44 mm error, the camera error alone is approximatly 0.5 mm [8].

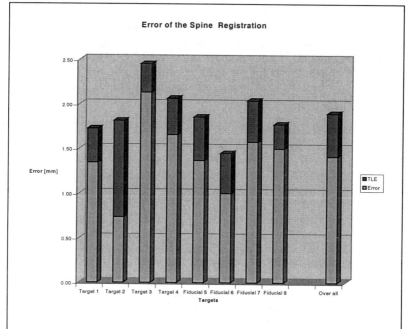

Figure 4. Overall error for each target determined by comparing the algorithm spatial value with the measured position of the target in DICOM images. The overall result includes a "Target Localization Error" (TLE) of 0.48 mm, verified in another set of measurements under standard conditions.

4. Discussion

The main factors differentiating our solution from that of others include: selecting fluoroscopy for the *in situ* imaging technique, using stereo photogrammetry to extract 3D information from projective images, as well as using a robust and accurate registration method. Unlike most currently available 3D spinal navigation packages, which require full exposure of the vertebral body for the sake of registration and real-time optical tracking, our method employs fluoroscopic imaging and registration using percutaneously implanted markers or skeletal anatomy as a minimally invasive approach.

A surgical tool visible in at least two fluoroscopic views can be back-projected into the CT reference frame using standard stereoscopic techniques well known in the computer vision community. Alternatively, we can track a surgical tool externally (e.g., using the optical tracking device already employed, or a robotic interface) to facilitate a variety of procedure types.

While our method does not permit a real-time DRF for the sake of target movement monitoring, periodic re-registration is much more practical than in conventional approaches: misregistration can be detected and eliminated by simply re-acquiring two new fluoroscopic images and running a fairly automatic procedure that requires little or no intervention by the operator. Additional proprietary improvements in digital re-projection techniques using off-the-shelf computer graphics hardware will further enhance the robustness, accuracy, and performance of the registration method.

Similarly, our registration method coupled with more sophisticated visualization and biomechanical modeling techniques can potentially be generalized to handle non-rigid deformations resulting from inter-vertebral displacement. This would allow us to apply our methodology in clinical scenarios that involve more than a single vertebral body, without cumbersome patient fixation or making assumptions about unchanged pose between the time of the scan and intra-operative positioning. The ability to intra-operatively register articulated, deformable spinal anatomy in near real-time and with high accuracy would be a critical improvement over existing systems. For the future, we are working on fiducial-less registration of the vertebral body, similar to a technique used by a commercial frameless image-guided radiosurgery system (Cyberknife, Accuracy Inc., Sunnyvale, CA, USA) [3].

5. References

1. Hofstetter R, Slomczynski M, Sati M, Nolte L. *CAS*. 1999: 4:65-76.
2. Murphy MJ. "An automatic six-degree-of-freedom image registration algorithm form image-guided frameless stereotaxic radiosurgery." *Medical Physics*. June 1997: 24(6).
3. Roth M, Brack C, Burgkart R, Zcopf A, Gotte H, Schwiekard A. "Multi-view contourless registration of bone structures using single calibrated X-ray fluoroscope." *CARS*. 1999: 756-761.
4. Tsai RY. "An Efficient and Accurate Camera Calibration Technique for 3D Machine Vision." *Proceedings of IEEE Conference on Computer Vision and Pattern Recognition*. 1986: 364-374.
5. Weese J, Penny GP, Buzug TM, Fassnacht C, Lorenz C. "2D/3D registration of pre-operative CT images and intra-operative X-ray projections for image guided surgery." *CARS*. Lemke HU, Vannier MW, InamuraK. [Editorial]. *CARS*. 1997: 833-838.
6. Fitzpatrick JM, West JB, Maurer CR, "Predicting Error in, Rigid-Body Point Based Registration," *IEEE Trans. on Medical Imaging*. 1998: 17(5), 694-702.
7. Fahrig R, Moreau M, Holdsworth DW. "Three-dimensional computed tomographic reconstruction using a C-arm mounted XRII: Correction of image intensifier distortion." *Medical Physics*. July 1997: 24(7).
8. Khadem R, Yeh C, Sadeghi-Tehrani M, Bax M, Johnson J, Welch J, Wilkinson E, Shahidi R. "Comparative Tracking Error Analysis of Five Different Optical Tracking Systems." *Computer Aided Surgery*. 2000: (5) 98-107.

Medicine Meets Virtual Reality 2001
J.D. Westwood et al. (Eds.)
IOS Press, 2001

Neuronavigational Epilepsy Focus Mapping

Hamid Reza Abbasi, Sanaz Hariri, David Martin, Michael Risinger, Gary Heit
Department of Neurosurgery, Stanford University Medical Center

Abstract. The localization of a seizure focus for resective surgery often requires invasive monitoring for precise localization of the target as well as structures to avoid. We report on the use of intra-operative surgical navigation to precisely localize and co-register subdural electrodes to regions of know radiographic pathology. Additionally, the navigation system was used to develop intra-operative electrode maps. These maps were subsequently used in the sub-acute recording phase to assign electrographic pathology and function (e.g. speech) to a specific cortical surface anatomy. This permitted for more precise planning of surgery and better assessment of potential risk, based on functional as well as anatomical criterion.

1. Introduction

Epilepsy occurs with a prevalence of about 0.5 percent and a cumulative lifetime incidence of 3 percent. [4] Approximately one quarter of these patients eventually become refractory to pharmacotherapy despite the introduction of a number of new and relatively improved drugs. [1,6] For medically intractable patients, resective surgery represents the next therapeutic intervention.

Noninvasive attempts to localize the epileptogenic focus consist of anatomical imaging (CT/MRI), functional imaging (PET fMRI), neuropsychological testing, and, most importantly, electroencephalography (EEG) involving prolonged recording and video monitoring. In many cases of medial temporal lobe sclerosis it is possible to obtain enough convergent evidence from these studies to be able to proceed straight to a resective surgery. However, in extratemporal epilepsy an exact localization of the resection target with this Phase I data alone is often not possible. [3,7] In these cases, subdural recordings are employed to better define the location of the seizure focus as well as surrounding areas of eloquent cortex. [2,5]

Oftentimes the seizure focus is associated with an anatomical defect that can be visualized on scans (e.g. cortical dysgenesis or a cicatrix). In many cases, however, no such landmarks exist and the seizure focus resides in a grossly normal appearing brain. We have been using a surgical navigation system (SNS) in both cases of absent structural abnormalities as well as in cases of "normal" cortex to determine the precise relation between the subdural electrodes and the underlying anatomy. This correlation is achieved by co-registering the "electrographic map" generated during sub-acute intracranial recordings to the images of the three-dimensional MRI patient gyral anatomy, allowing a priori surgical resection planning.

2.　Materials and Methods

Six patients were selected for intracranial recordings based on convergent evidence consisting of scalp EEG, seizure semiology, structural and metabolic imaging studies, and neuropsychometrics. On the day of the surgery, 6 to 8 skin MR-compatible registration markers were placed on the patient's head. These fiducials were clustered such that they centered around the hypothesized site of seizures to maximize their accuracy with respect to the proposed implant site. A T1 weighted axial MR was performed (FOV = 30 cm, TE = 13, TR = 800, NEX = 256 x 256, 2.0 mm slices, 0 skip interleaved). The data was sent via DICOMM transfer protocols to the navigation system (Radionics Maynard MA, software OTS version 2.2).

The patient was given a general anesthesia and placed in a Mayfield head holder, with care being taken not to displace the MR fiducials. A dynamic reference frame (DRF) was attached to the Mayfield adapter, and the fiducials were registered in the SNS system by touching the probe to the center of each fiducial (telling the system where in space each marker was). A standard craniotomy was performed using the SNS to define important structures to incorporate in the exposure. Upon dual opening, a photograph of the operational field was taken supplementing the radiographic constructs with an optical view of the gyral anatomy. The SNS was then used to center the subdural electrodes over an area of known pathology and/or to co-register the electrode to the gyral anatomy (Fig. 1). With the SNS probe touching a representative contact on an electrode, a display screen capture was performed. This precisely localized each electrode in the axial, sagital, and coronal planes of the MR (Fig. 2). After complete documentation with the SNS of the electrode localization, a post-implant photograph of the operational field was taken.

The operative field was secured in the standard fashion, and the patient was taken to the telemetry unit after an appropriate post-operative recovery interval. During the sub-acute phase, continuous intracranial EEG and simultaneous video were recorded. Two functional maps were generated: one based on inter-ictal and ictal events recorded from specific electrode pairs and the other identifying which electrodes, if any, overlie the eloquent cortex. These maps were co-registered via common electrode contacts to the SNS maps.

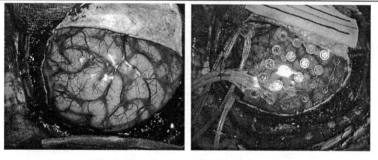

Fig. 1. Operative views of subdural electrodes.

The combined data was then used to preplan the resection boundaries. Landmarks consisted of the spatial relation of the subdural grid to gyral/sulcal anatomy and/or structural abnormalities as defined by the SNS maps and the photographic record of the electrode's relation to surface vascular markers. At the time of resection these landmarks were used to identify the pre-planned boundaries. The primary orientation of the resection was based on the geography of the subdural electrodes, followed by the regional anatomy as defined in the pre-planning session.

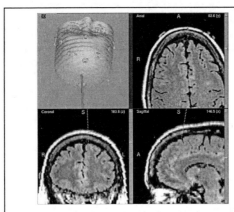

Fig. 2. Cross-sections as displayed on the neuronavigation
monitor. Dashed lines indicate the probe's approach.

3.   Discussion

Resections in extratemporal cortex require definition of a seizure focus that often lacks anatomical boundaries. In contrast, the resection site for medial temporal sclerosis is clearly demarcated as the pes hippocampi, amygala, and lateral temporal cortices. Further complicating the definition of an extratemporal resection site are structural lesions that may have a complex spatial relationship to the actual ictal focus. Additionally the potential presence of cortex involved in language, primary sensory processing, motor control or cognition can provide further constraints on the extent of tissue to extirpate. These constraints can demand a precision of seizure focus localization that prompted this technical development of SNS during the intracranial electrode implant. This technique allows for a direct mapping of the functional data to the relevant anatomy.

As more sophisticated mapping technologies are developed, this technique can be used to integrate those additional data sets to the resection plan. For example, interictal spike triggered functional magnetic resonance images could be fused with the navigation scan to ensure that subdural electrode coverage encompasses all regions of functional pathology. Likewise, a variety of image sets could be brought to the OR to assist in localization of the electrode over identified structural lesions.

4.   References

1. Blaise FD, Bourgeois BF: Clinical aspects of epilepsy including diagnosis, management, pharmacotherapy, and surgery. *Current Opinion in Neurology & Neurosurgery.* 6(2):233-9, April 1993.
2. Cross JH: Update on surgery for epilepsy. *Archives of Disease in Childhood.* 81(4):356-9, Oct. 1999.
3. Gates JR, Dunn ME: Presurgical assessment and surgical treatment for epilepsy. *Acta Neurologica Belgica.* 99(4):281-94, Dec 1999.
4. Marks WJ Jr, Garcia PA: Management of seizures and epilepsy. *American Family Physician.* 57(7):1589-600, 1603-4, April 1, 1998.
5. Munari C, Giallonardo AT, Brunet P, Broglin D, Bancaud J: Stereotactic investigations in frontal lobe epilepsies. *Acta Neurochirurgica: Supplementum.* 46:9-12, 1989.
6. McLaughlin D: Epilepsy. Key management issues. *Australian Family Physician.* 28(9):889-91, 896, Sep 1999.
7. Worthington C: Surgical management of epilepsy: invasive monitoring and temporal lobectomy. *Journal of the South Carolina Medical Association.* 88(5):241-4, May 1992.

Medicine Meets Virtual Reality 2001
J.D. Westwood et al. (Eds.)
IOS Press, 2001

A Comparative Statistical Analysis of Neuronavigation Systems in a Clinical Setting

Hamid Reza Abbasi, Sanaz Hariri, David Martin, Ramin Shahidi

Department of Neurosurgery – Stanford University, Pasteur Dr. 300 - R S008,
Stanford CA, 94305 USA 300

Abstract. The use of neuronavigation (NN) in neurosurgery has become ubiquitous. A growing number of neurosurgeons are utilizing NN for a wide variety of purposes, including optimizing the surgical approach (macrosurgery) and locating small areas of interest (microsurgery). The goal of our team is to apply rapid advances in hardware and software technology to the field of NN, challenging and ultimately updating current NN assumptions. To identify possible areas in which new technology may improve the surgical applications of NN, we have assessed the accuracy of neuronavigational measurements in the Radionics™ and BrainLab™ systems. Using a phantom skull, we measured how accurate the visualization of a navigational probe's tip was in these systems, taking a total of 2180 measurements. We found that, despite current NN tenets, error is maximal at the six marker count and minimal in the spreaded marker setting; that is, placing less markers around the area of interest maximizes accuracy and active tracking does not necessarily increase accuracy. Comparing the two systems, we also found that accuracy of NN machines differs both overall and in different axes. As researchers continue to apply technological advances to the NN field, an increasing number of currently held tenets will be revised, making NN an even more useful tool in neurosurgery.

1. Introduction

Neuronavigation (NN) has emerged as an essential tool in neurosurgery. A growing number of neurosurgeons are utilizing NN for a wide variety of purposes. In the early stages of their development, NN machines were very expensive and thus predominantly used only to locate hard-to-find areas of interest (e.g. tumors, aneurysms, abscesses, etc.) in vital regions (e.g. the brainstem, cerebellum, etc). Today, as systems have become less expensive, NN is routinely used to optimize the craniotomy and the neurosurgical approach to the region of interest (ROI).

In macroneurosurgery, neurosurgeons use NN to optimize their approach, minimizing disturbances to surrounding anatomical structures such as the ventricular system. Five mm of accuracy is sufficient for macrosurgery. Microneurosurgery, in contrast, requires much greater accuracy; neurosurgeons must be able to localize extremely small areas of interest in vital regions. All current NN systems have enough accuracy to optimize the approach to the ROI. However, to date, no system has achieved the submillimeter precision truly needed for free-hand stereotaxy and for the location of small areas of interest.

Certain experimental and methodological assumptions have been retained in the use of NN over its development. Current conventional tenets of NN include:

1. Using more markers increases accuracy.
2. Putting more markers around the area of interest increases accuracy.
3. Using 6 markers yields greatest accuracy.
4. Using active tracking [e.g. an active DRF (dynamic reference frame) and probe which emit infrared beams rather than passively reflecting them] increases accuracy.
5. Minimizing the distance from the marker or marker group to the area of interest increases accuracy.

While rapid advances in hardware and software have emerged in the last few of years, there have been only some attempts at challenging the old NN tenets and applying new technology to update these systems. To identify possible areas in which new technology may improve the surgical applications of NN, we conducted accuracy tests of neuronavigational measurements in two currently used systems: Radionics and BrainLab.

The ultimate goal of this project is to give surgeons confidence in the NN machines. Surgeons should be able to trust the image generated by the system to optimize their surgical accuracy within a 1 mm range. To effectively apply NN to microsurgery, the following questions must be systematically addressed:

1. How many markers efficiently maximize accuracy?
2. What pattern of marker localization maximizes accuracy?
3. Are there significant accuracy differences between various marker arrangements?
4. Are systems significantly different in their level of accuracy?
5. Is accuracy different in the x-, y- and z-axis?

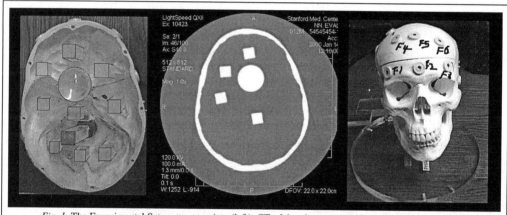

Fig. 1. The Experimental Setup: target points (left); CT of the phantom (middle); the phantom (right).

2. Materials and Methods

We built a phantom skull to most realistically simulate the surgical setting. (Had we used a geometric object instead of reproducing the curvature of the skull, our results would not have been applicable to the surgical setting.) We obtained a standard plastic skull, removed the calvaria, and installed three Plexiglas square rods of different heights in each of the three anatomical fossae (anterior, middle and posterior). We used the edges of these rods as our targets. We installed a Plexiglas ball of known diameter on the phantom's sella turcica (Fig. 1). Replacing the calvaria, we placed a total of 12 markers bilaterally on the exterior of the skull in the following regions: 6 frontal, 2 mastoid, 2 occipital and 2 high parietal. We performed a CT of the skull in 1.25 mm slices and sent the data over the network to the two NN machines evaluated in this study. The systems utilize different registration and tracking systems to localize the probe's tip in 3D:

BrainLab VectorVision version 2.3: Passive registration and tracking system: the DRF and probe merely reflect the infrared signal shot out by emitters around the cameras.

Radionics OTS version 2.2: Active registration and tracking system: the DRF and probe contain diodes emitting infrared signals that are collected by two cameras. The DRF and probe are connected to the tracking box that supplies both with electricity.

When the probe tip was placed at the edge of a rod, the NN systems visualized the probe's position on their screens in the original axial plane of the CT scans and in the sagital and coronal planes reconstructed from the CT scans (Fig. 2). The exact edge of the rod as displayed on each monitor cross-section was assigned the coordinate values x=0 and y=0. The x and y coordinates assigned to each cross-sectional view on the monitor were translated as the "real" coordinate axes of the skull (Fig. 2) using Table 1.

Table 1: Relation of the measurements on the monitor to the actual coordinates of the skull as illustrated in *Fig. 2*

Screen Coordinate	Skull Coordinate	Screen Coordinate	Skull Coordinate
Axial X	+X	Axial Y	+Y
Sagital X	-Y	Sagital Y	+Z
Coronal X	+X	Coronal Y	+Z

In each of the three cross-sections, we measured how far from the actual edge of the rod (x=0, y=0) the monitor was representing the probe tip. Zooming in and out on the monitor to find the largest diameter of the Plexiglas sphere, we used the known diameter of the sphere to establish a system-independent scale for measurements. These measurements were acquired for both the Radionics and BrainLab NN systems. The Radionics system was analyzed when using local and spreaded marker settings with 4, 6, and 8 markers. The BrainLab system was analyzed when using local and spreaded marker settings with 4 and 6 markers. Table 2 defines the marker locations in these different setups. Thus, we obtained 10 series of measurements, each series consisting of 218 separate measurements.

Table 2: Placement of the markers

Marker count	Local Setting	Spreaded Setting
4	F1, F3, F4, F6	F1, F3, O1, O6
6	F1, F2, F3, F4, F5, F6,	F1, F3, O1,O3, O4, O6
8 (Radionics only)	F1, F2, F3, F4, F5, F6, O1, O6	F1, F3, O1, O2, O3, O4, O5, O6

F1: Frontolateral right below calvaria line   F2: Frontomedian below calvaria line
F3: Frontolateral left below calvaria line   F4: Frontolateral right above calvaria line
F5: Frontomedian above calvaria line   F6: Frontolateral left above calvaria line
O1: Above right mastoid process   O2: Right occipital
O3: High parietal right   O4: High parietal left
O5: Left occipital   O6: Above left mastoid process

The absolute distance between the edge of the rod and the NN representation of the probe tip was calculated as SQR $(X^2 + Y^2)$ in each plane. The 3D absolute distance was calculated as SQR $(X^2 + Y^2 + Z^2)$. Because the numbers were squared, the sign of the measurements on each axis was unimportant in these calculations.

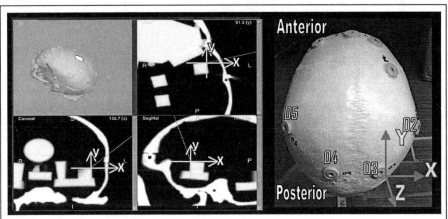

Fig. 2. Phantom cross-sections as displayed on the NN monitor, dashed lines indicate the probe's approach (left); skull coordinate axes (right).

3. Results

Radionics: In the local marker setting, the Radionics system was highly sensitive to the number of markers. Specifically, the range of error increased in the z-axis when fewer markers were used. Also, increasing the distance of the probe tip from the marker groups augmented z-axis error. We found that error in reconstructed planes (sagital and coronal) increased rapidly with decreasing marker numbers while error in the original plane (axial) was not very sensitive to the number of markers.

The findings for the spreaded marker setting were similar to the local marker setting, with a few exceptions. In the spreaded marker setting, there were fewer differences in accuracy between the three anatomical fossae. Localization of the probe tip in the occipital area was most accurate, even though the markers were clustered more frontally.

BrainLab: In the local marker setting, increasing the distance of the probe tip from the marker groups augmented z-axis error. Increasing the marker count from 4 to 6 decreased accuracy, particularly in the z-axis. The error increased in both the original (axial) and the reconstructed (sagital and coronal) planes, but error in the reconstructed images was greater. Perhaps the algorithm in the procedure registering the various markers can account for this discrepancy.

In contrast to the Radionics system, in which greatest error was observed in the z-axis, the BrainLab spreaded marker setting demonstrated greatest error in the y-axis. Also in contrast to the Radionics system, where we could improve accuracy by increasing marker counts, accuracy for BrainLab's spreaded marker settings deteriorated when the marker count was increased from 4 to 6. The SD and variance of 4 versus 6 markers were not significantly different. This data discounts bias in data collection. Again, we observed the greatest degree of overall accuracy in the occipital region although most of the markers were placed more anteriorly.

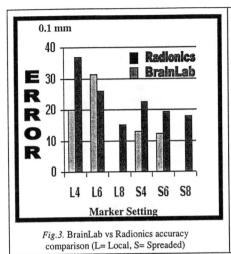

Fig.3. BrainLab vs Radionics accuracy comparison (L= Local, S= Spreaded)

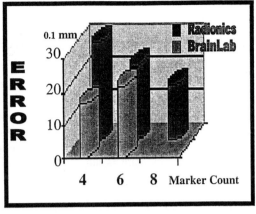

Fig.4. BrainLab vs Radionics Overall accuracy comparison

4. Discussion

4.1 Accuracy in Different Axes

The CT images of the patient's head are usually gathered in axial slices of 1.25 or 2.5 mm thickness (resolution = 512x512). The NN machine then uses the 2D data to recreate a 3D image of the brain. Therefore, the x- and y-axis, as defined by this study (Fig. 2), are obtained from original data while the z-axis is visualized only from reconstructed data, resulting in an image accuracy in the x- and y-axis 5 times greater than in the z-axis. Most NN machines use algorithms for interpolation of original data to reduce this source of error, but there is a compromise between errors in different axes (tradeoff in accuracy between x-/y-axes and z axis). We found poorer accuracy in the Radionics z-axis, but, as expected, we observed an increase in accuracy in this axis when we used more markers. However, in the BrainLab system, the x- and y-axes were the sources of greater inaccuracy. Accuracy escalated as the probe tip was placed at increased distances from the marker group.

4.2 Comparing the Two Systems

The BrainLab system has a better overall accuracy, especially when using fewer markers (Figs. 3 & 4). This finding is contrary to a currently accepted NN assumption: that systems with active registration and tracking are more accurate than the passive models. We considered the possibility that the newer NDI camera used by BrainLab (versus the older IGT camera used by Radionics) could account for this finding. However, another study conducted in our lab showed that the IGT camera was more accurate than the NDI camera. Therefore, we concluded that the registration algorithm accounted for BrainLab's better accuracy.

4.3 Accuracy Using Different Marker Counts

Except for 8 markers, 6 frontal markers and a marker above each mastoid process, the spreaded marker setting yielded greater accuracy than the local marker setting. In the local marker setting, the Radionics system yielded unique data in this experiment -- increasing the number of markers and placing the tip closer to the marker groups increased accuracy. However, in every other situation, increasing the marker count from 4 to 6, especially in the local marker setting, decreased overall accuracy. Also, placing the tip further from the marker groups increased accuracy.

We believe that the quality of the markers themselves account for the decreased accuracy when the number of markers are increased. In the early stages of NN, surgeons attached bone screw markers directly to the skull. The registration area in these markers (i.e. where the probe tip is placed when the surgeon is telling the NN machine where each marker is located) was very small. With the advent of better registration algorithms and faster, more reliable hardware, particularly improvements in camera technology, surgeons found that they could obtain sufficient accuracy with less invasive skin markers. The skin marker, however, has a larger registration area (~ 4 mm) and moves in relation to the skull because it is only attached to the skin (Fig. 5). Using the improved registration algorithm, we obtained a visualization of the skull's geometry within ~2-5 mm. While this degree of accuracy is suitable for macroneurosurgery, more delicate microneurosurgery procedures demand much greater accuracy.

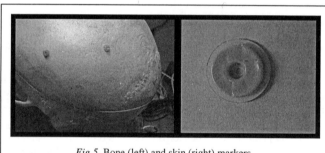

Fig.5. Bone (left) and skin (right) markers

To isolate sources of error, we found that:

Overall Error = Registration Error + System Error

Registration error is the error generated during the process of telling the NN system where each marker is located. The surgeon attempts to place the probe's tip as close to the center of the marker as possible, registering each marker in the system. However, the diameter of the skin marker's center is relatively large, resulting in part of this registration error as finding the exact center of each marker is virtually impossible. Registration error probably accounts for this experiment's finding that placing fewer markers near the area of interest maximizes accuracy. System error is defined as mechanical, engineering, and software errors, such as machine or camera error.

Having more markers can decrease system accuracy. However, at some point, the marginal increase in error associated with registering an additional marker surpasses the marginal decrease in system error due to more markers (Fig. 6). Using our phantom, we discovered that, given today's registration and system technology, maximal error is found at the 6 marker count. The registration error found in surgeries is probably greater than the registration error found in our phantom model because skin markers used for patients are applied to the skin while the skin markers used for the phantom were applied directly to the skull.

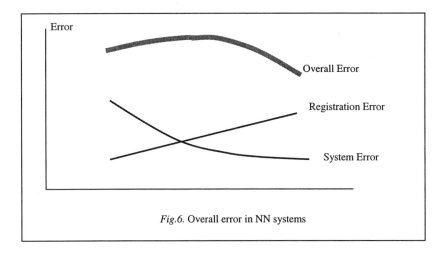

Fig.6. Overall error in NN systems

5. Conclusion

This study scrutinized conventional assumptions of neuronavigation and found many of them to be invalid. The new NN tenets supported by our findings are:

1. 4 or 8, but not 6, markers maximize accuracy. The counterintuitive nature of this finding is not fully understood and our lab is currently investigating this result. Additionally, the movement of skin on the skull is not included in this study and may influence the clinical results.
2. Placing fewer markers around the area of interest maximizes accuracy.
3. Active tracking does not necessarily increase accuracy.
4. The spreaded marker setting increases accuracy.
5. Accuracy of the NN machines differs both overall and in different axes.

As researchers continue to apply recent developments in hardware and software technology to the NN field, an increasing number of currently held tenets will be challenged and revised, rapidly and dramatically changing the field.

6. References

1. Germano, IM; Villalobos, H; Silvers, A; Post, KD. "Clinical use of the optical digitizer for intracranial NN." *Neurosurgery.* Aug 1999, 45(2): 261-9, discussion 269-70.
2. Gumprecht, HK; Widenka, DC; Lumenta, CB. "BrainLab VectorVision NN System: technology and clinical experiences in 131 cases." *Neurosurgery.* Jan. 1999, 44(1): 97-104, discussion 104-5.
3. Ostertag, CB; Warnke, PC. "NN. Computerassistierte Neurochirurgie. [NN. Computer-assisted neurosurgery]." *Nervenarzt.* June 1999, 70(6): 517-21.
4. Schmieder, K; Hardenack, M; Harders, A. "NN in daily clinical routine of a neurosurgical department." *Computer Aided Surgery.* 1998, 3(4): 159-61.
5. Spetzger, U; Laborde, G; Gilsbach, JM. "Frameless NN in modern neurosurgery." *Minimally Invasive Neurosurgery.* Dec. 1995, 38(4): 163-6.
6. Wirtz, CR; Knauth, M; Hassfeld, S; Tronnier, VM; Albert, FK; Bonsanto, MM; Kunze, S. "NN--first experiences with three different commercially available systems." *Zentralblatt fur Neurochirurgie.* 1998, 59(1): 14-22.
7. Wirtz, CR; Tronnier, VM; Bonsanto, MM; Hassfeld, S; Knauth, M; Kunze, S. "NN. Methoden und Ausblick. [NN. Methods and prospects]." *Nervenarzt.* Dec. 1998, 69(12): 1029-36.

Medicine Meets Virtual Reality 2001
J.D. Westwood et al. (Eds.)
IOS Press, 2001

Real-time Anatomical 3D Image Extraction for Laparoscopic Surgery

Jeremy D. Ackerman[a], Kurtis Keller[b], Henry Fuchs[c]

University of North Carolina at Chapel Hill, Department of Computer Science, Campus Box #3175, Chapel Hill, NC 27599 USA
[a] *ackerman@cs.unc.edu*
[b] *keller@cs.unc.edu*
[c] *fuchs@cs.unc.edu*

Abstract

Progress in the application of augmented reality to laparoscopic surgery has been limited by the difficulty associated with generating geometric information about the current patient in real time. Structured light techniques are well known methods for generating range images using a camera and projector, but typically fail when faced with biological specimens. We describe techniques and equipment that have shown promise for acquisition of range images for use in a real-time augmented reality system for laparoscopic surgery.

1. Introduction

Augmented reality, fusing synthetic imagery with the user's view of the real world, is likely to be beneficial when applied to laparoscopic surgery because it may provide a view of the operative site similar to open surgery while using a minimally invasive approach.

Laparoscopic surgery faces one technological challenge that other augmented reality applications do not face. In augmented reality systems where a physician's view is augmented with radiological data (such as pre-operative or intra-operative CT, MR, or tracked ultrasound) three-dimensional information is inherent, or at least strongly implied, by the method of acquisition and the data itself. For example, in our augmented reality ultrasound guided breast biopsy application, a pixel of ultrasound data is three-dimensionally registered to the patient, and correctly rendered from the perspective of the physician using the a calibration of the ultrasound probe and the probe's current position. This is possible because the ultrasound slice roughly corresponds to a plane emanating from the tip of the probe. By accurately estimating the position of this plane, we can determine where in three-dimensional space the two dimensional pixel data originated. Likewise, MR and CT images correspond to slices in three-dimensional space relative to the imaging system's internal coordinate system.

Images acquired through a tracked laparoscope have insufficient information to correctly render them in augmented reality because the three dimensional source of the data seen in the image may be any point along a specific ray emanating from the tip of the laparoscope. Correctly incorporating laparoscopic information into an augmented reality environment requires that the distance from the laparoscope is known for each pixel or at least a significant sampling of pixels [1]. An image where both appearance (color) and distance information is known is frequently called a range image.

The problem of finding range images is widely addressed in the field of computer vision. Unfortunately, many of these techniques are not easily applied to laparoscopic surgery because they frequently do not work on curved surfaces, on shiny surfaces, or are too slow for use in a real-time system [4]. An ideal system for use in laparoscopic surgery would meet the following requirements: generate a minimum of twenty range images per second, work on curved surfaces, work on shiny surfaces, be fairly tolerant to movement, and be small enough to integrate into the operating room.

2. Proposed Methods

Structured light was selected as the basis for our method because it has been demonstrated to work on curved surfaces and because the computations can be done very rapidly. Structured light techniques work by projecting a known light pattern into a scene. A camera records the scene and a range image is calculated based on the distortion of the known light pattern, and the position and characteristics of the camera and projector [3] A schematic drawing of this set-up is shown in Figure 1.

Early experiments demonstrated that use of structured light is feasible in the abdominal cavity by showing the light patterns projected onto abdominal organs of animal cadavers could be recognized and recovered. Using images with different patterns of illumination was also demonstrated to be useful in reducing specular effects.

Our method uses projection of a structured light pattern and its negative to reduce specular effects. When the image containing the structured light pattern are subtracted from those where the structured light pattern's negative is projected, the resulting image shows the structured light pattern strongly enhanced, while specular and non-illuminated regions converge to a narrow intensity range. The structured patterns, as well as regions of the image that contain no structured information (shadows, specular spots) can be easily segmented by thresholding. Once structure patterns are identified in the images, standard methods may be applied to generate range information. All of this processing takes

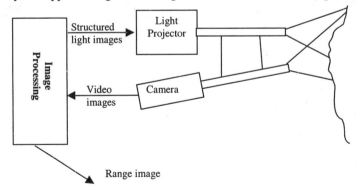

Figure 1 A schematic diagram of a structured light range image acquisition system. A light projector projects light patterns (often stripes onto a surface. A camera captures images of the light pattern and the image processing system generates range images.

approximately 20ms for six pairs of images on a PC with a Matrox Genesis card once the images are in the card's memory.

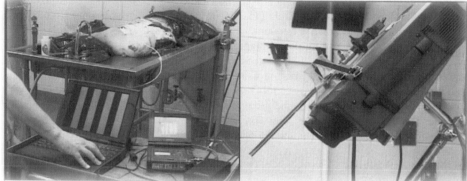

Figure 2 The lab setup of for test image acquisition. The image on the left shows the pig cadaver, the laptop generating structured light patterns, and the image recording system. The image on the right shows the video projector with a laparoscope and camera mounted to it.

These methods were tested on the abdominal organs of a pig cadaver. A large video projector with a zoom lens was used to project the light patterns onto the surface of the open abdomen. Images were captured with a black and white camera through a standard laparoscope. This images were digitally recorded and processed offline. Because the artifacts introduced by biological surfaces are known to disrupt many computer vision techniques, we also repeated the data capture after coating the abdominal organs with a substance that makes the surface less shiny. The capture set-up is shown in Figure 2. Two images of structure patterns being projected on abdominal organs are shown in Figure 3. The resulting estimated range images are shown in Figure 4. Neither the camera nor the projector was calibrated in this experiment so the calculated range images are only estimates.

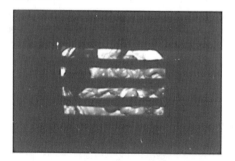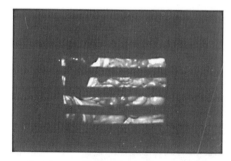

Figure 3 Two coarse resolution raw images of stripe patterns (a pattern and its inverse) are shown in these two images. The fact that the acquired images do not contain stripes that appear as straight lines can be analyzed to determine the distance from the camera and projector to the objects seen in the images.

3. New Equipment

Previous work done locally has used a variety of equipment to attempt laparoscopic range acquisition. Our initial attempts have made use of large LCD or DLP based video projectors to provide the structured light patterns. Our first system had such a projector, weighing nearly 10kg, rigidly mounted to a laparoscope. This large and unwieldy contraption was clearly not suitable for the operating room. We have tried projecting light patterns with the large projectors by transmitting the light through flexible endoscopes. These systems suffered from poor light transmission and blurry structured light patterns due to the low resolution of the flexible scope. All of these systems also suffered because the structured light pattern had to be changed at video rates (30-80Hz), making them unusable for real-time range image acquisition.

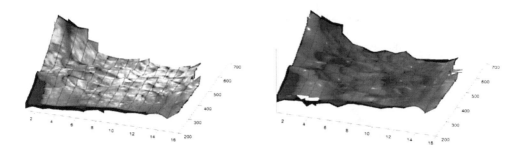

Figure 4 Two range images acquired and calculated with our system. The Image on the left was constructed after coating tissues to reduce potential artifacts. The image on the right shows the results from raw tissue.

We have now built a miniaturized high-speed projector [2]. This projector is approximately the same size as a laparoscope camera. The projector uses a standard laparoscope light source for illumination, and provides black and white images at 180Hz. The core of this projector is a ferro-reflective LCD. A schematic exploded view of the projector is shown in Figure 5.

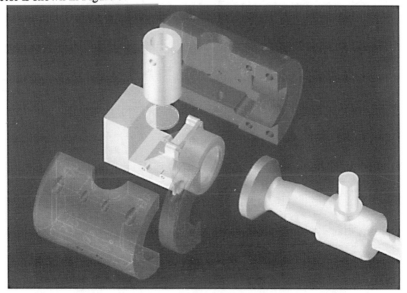

Figure 5 Exploded view of miniature laparoscopic projector. A standard laparoscope is shown in the bottom right corner for scale.

4. Future Work

Much work is still needed to build a working real-time laparoscopic range image acquisition system. Remaining tasks include high-speed image capture combined with high-speed processing, calibration, and validation.

The applications of a real-time laparoscopic range image acquisition system are not limited to the augmented reality environment for which we are developing it. The are many other potential applications areas including education and teleproctoring which this technology has potential to enable or improve new methods.

After our range image acquisition system is complete, we will still need to incorporate it into an augmented reality system. Significant effort will be needed to optimally display the acquired data in order to maximize the utility and usability of such a system to clinicians.

5. References

1. Henry Fuchs, Mark A. Livingston, Ramesh Raskar, D'nardo Colucci, Kurtis Keller, Andrei State, Jessica R. Crawford, Paul Rademacher, Samuel H. Drake, and Anthony A. Meyer, "Augmented Reality Visualization for Laparoscopic Surgery", MICCAI (Proceedings of First International Conference on Medical Image Computing and Computer-Assisted Intervention) 1998.

2. Kurtis Keller and Jeremy Ackerman "Real-time Structured Light Depth Extraction", SPIE EI 2000, Photonics West - Electronic Imaging 2000.

3. P. Levoie, D. Ionescue, & E.M. Petriu, " 3-D Object Model Recovery from 2-D Images Using Structured Light", IEEE Instrument Measurement Technology Conference, pp. 377-382.

4. M. Oren and S. Nayar, A Theory of Specular Surface Geometry, The Int. J. Computer Vision, Vol 24:2 September 1997

Medicine Meets Virtual Reality 2001
J.D. Westwood et al. (Eds.)
IOS Press, 2001

An Integrated Environment for Stereoscopic Acquisition, Off-line 3D Elaboration, and Visual Presentation of Biological Actions

Marco Agus, Fabio Bettio, Enrico Gobbetti

CRS4, Visualization and Virtual Reality Group, Cagliari, Italy

{magus,fabio,gobbetti}@crs4.it, http://www.crs4.it/vvr

Luciano Fadiga

Institute of Human Physiology, University of Parma, Italy

lfadiga@ipruniv.cce.unipr.it

Abstract. We present an integrated environment for stereoscopic acquisition, off-line 3D elaboration, and visual presentation of biological hand actions. The system is used in neurophysiological experiments aimed at the investigation of the parameters of the external stimuli that mirror neurons visually extract and match on their movement related activity.

1 Introduction

In spite of its fundamental role for human/animal behavior, very little is known on how individuals recognize actions performed by others. It has been often proposed that a common code should exist between the observed events and an internally produced motor activity. Neurophysiological evidence in favor of this putative common code was, however, until recently lacking. Recent experiments have shown that neurons located in a monkey premotor area (F5, [1, 2]) are very likely involved in this process [3]. These neurons discharge both when the monkey actively performs goal-directed hand/mouth actions and when it observes them performed by others. Typically, however, there is no discharge when similar actions, identical in terms of goal, are made by manipulated mechanical tools, or when the actions are mimicked without the target object [4]. Such data suggests that actions made by others are represented in those same areas of the premotor cortex where motor primitives for active execution are stored. If one admits that an individual, when making an action, may predict its outcome, it appears likely that she will recognize an action made by others because it evokes a discharge in those same neurons that fire when she makes the identical action. It remains unclear which are the visual features used to match a given seen action on the internal repertoire of motor primitives normally used for action execution. A Human Frontiers Science Program project that brings together a consortium of European, American, and Japanese researchers is investigating this subject in detail. The planned neurophysiological experiments will require the presentation of visual stimuli of different types. To simplify the creation and handling of a catalog of digitized stimuli, we are creating a specialized animation system that enables animators to create short animation sequences which closely follow a video-recorded action, and to later modify the sequences to obtain all the required variations. This paper briefly describes the current system prototype.

The rest of the paper is organized as follows. Section 2 provides a general overview of the system, section 3 concentrates on video acquisition and playback, section 4 details the

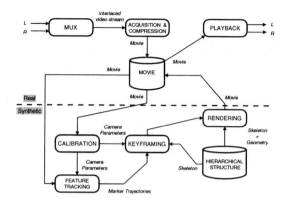

Figure 1: **System overview.** Main data processing components and flow of data among them.

video analysis and animation synthesis subsystem. The paper concludes with a discussion of the results obtained and a view of future work.

2 System Overview

In order to study the encoding of visual stimulus parameters for hand action recognition in monkeys, single neurons will be recorded from premotor area F5 and from the inferior parietal lobule of monkeys trained to fixate a spot of light on a projection screen and to detect its dimming by pressing a lever. During fixation, digitized stimuli showing goal-directed actions will be stereoscopically presented on the same screen by means of polarized light projection.

Two different kinds of stimuli will be presented: direct reproductions of "real" sequences, and elaborations of those sequences, both in terms of modification of visual appearance and/or behavior (i.e. same action with variations in the kinematics and/or in the geometry and material of the performing object). The first situation is handled by components that support recording, storage, and playback of stereoscopic movies, while the second requires components that create artificial sequences starting from the acquired stereo movies. Since the type of operations required (variations in kinematics and/or hand shape) are not easily obtainable by image manipulation, the system needs to work directly in 3D space. In our approach, the original sequence is first reconstructed by animating the degrees of freedom (DOFs) of a virtual 3D hand model. The resulting 3D animation, interactively constructed exploiting a combination of artificial vision and standard key-framing techniques, is then refined, modified, and rendered to produce all the desired variations. Figure 1 provides a general overview of the system, depicting the main data processing components and the flow of data among them.

3 Stereoscopic Video Acquisition and Video Playback

The acquisition part of the system, built using off-the-shelf components, deals with the procedures for the acquisition of a stereoscopic video and its storage on a disk. The selected technical solution uses two video cameras placed on a tripod for stereo recording. The two

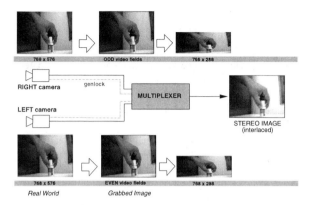

Figure 2: **Stereo acquisition.** The two inputs are synchronized and multiplexed in a single PAL or NTSC stream, which is then fed to the graphics workstation for recording or real-time display.

inputs are synchronized and multiplexed in a single PAL or NTSC stream, which is then fed to a graphics workstation for recording or real-time display (see figure 2). A digital compression card is used for real-time signal compression, enabling direct-to-disk recording. Using M-JPEG compression, a typical stereoscopic sequence of 10 s requires about 20 Mb of storage (PAL format, 50 fields per second, 768x288 pixels per eye). We have successfully run our applications on a Silicon Graphics IMPACT connected to a VREX Cam3C system and on a Silicon Graphics Octane connected to a TD003 3D Multiplexer with two CCD cameras for input.

The playback part of the system deals with the decoding of compressed stereoscopic movies and the stereo visualization of the video acquired. In order to reach high-level performances for stereo visualization, we have decided to completely load and decompress video sequences in memory prior to visualization. During visualization, left and right images are copied to the frame buffer in the format needed for stereo presentation and the graphics card is suitably configured. Shutter or polarized glasses are used for image presentation. Both stereo-in-a-window and full-screen presentations are possible.

4 Video Analysis and Animation Synthesis

The video analysis and animation synthesis subsystem provides tools for creating animations of articulated 3D models that closely follow the actions of a real hand depicted in a stereoscopic movie. In order to reach this goal, we have combined in a single interactive environment the basic features of artificial vision systems, to extract meaningful information from the stereo movie, with the concept of key-framed animation. In our approach, the original sequence is reconstructed by estimating the projection and viewing matrices of the cameras, tracking the 3D trajectory of interesting hand features, and animating the DOFs of a virtual 3D hand model so as to obtain the best match with the recorded movie. The resulting 3D animation is then refined, modified, and rendered using standard editing features to produce all the desired variations. The system has been implemented on a PC platform running Windows NT and requires consumer-level graphics boards (e.g. NVIDIA GeForce based systems).

4.1 Camera Registration

The camera transformation matrices contain all the geometric information (intrinsic and extrinsic camera parameters) which is necessary to calculate 3D coordinates from correspondences between two stereo perspective images of a scene. Since a metric reconstruction of the environment is required, we have implemented a strong calibration system that estimates camera parameters by observing a calibration object whose geometry is known. We currently use a semi-automatic approach in which the user selects a set of at least seven matching points on a camera view and associates them with their known 3D coordinates. The process is applied independently for the left and right camera. Given a set of 2D points $\mathcal{U} = \{u_1, u_2, \cdots, u_n\}$ and a set of corresponding 3D points $\mathcal{X} = \{x_1, x_2, \cdots, x_n\}$, the camera projection matrix $P(\theta, x_s, y_s, x_c, y_c)$ and the camera viewing matrix $V(r_x, r_y, r_z, t_x, t_y, t_z)$ are estimated by minimizing the following functional:

$$\sum_{i=1}^{n} \left\| \begin{bmatrix} \frac{t_1 \cdot x_i}{t_3 \cdot x_i} \\ \frac{t_2 \cdot x_i}{t_3 \cdot x_i} \end{bmatrix} - u_i \right\|^2 \tag{1}$$

where t_1, t_2, t_3 are the rows of $T = P(\theta, x_s, y_s, x_c, y_c) V(r_x, r_y, r_z, t_x, t_y, t_z)$, θ is the horizontal field of view, x_s, y_s are the dimensions of the image in pixels, x_c, y_c are the pixel coordinates of the center of projection, r_x, r_y, r_z are the Euler angles specifying the camera orientation and t_x, t_y, t_z are the coordinates of the camera position. In our implementation, we use a conjugate gradient algorithm to search for the optimal solution. A series of different starting points for the viewing parameters are generated on the sphere containing the bounding box of the 3D data set. The minimization algorithm is applied for each starting point and the minimum error solution is chosen as the optimal one.

4.2 Feature Tracking

Once the camera transformation matrices are known, the system has all the information to calculate the 3D coordinates of a point from point matches on the left and right images. This is used to help users track interesting features (e.g. finger tips) over time and use them to guide the keyframing process. Reconstructing the 3D position of a point x from its two projections $u^{(l)}$ and $u^{(r)}$ requires the solution of an homogeneous system. Let $T^{(l)}$ be the left camera transformation matrix and let $T^{(r)}$ be the right camera transformation matrix. The 3D coordinates of the point x are the solution of the linear equation $Ax = 0$ where A is the 4x4 matrix given by: $A = \left[t_1^{(l)} - u_1^{(l)} t_3^{(l)}, t_2^{(l)} - u_2^{(l)} t_3^{(l)}, t_1^{(r)} - u_1^{(r)} t_3^{(r)}, t_2^{(r)} - u_2^{(r)} t_3^{(r)} \right]^T$.

This problem is solved using an iterative linear least-squares method [5]. To construct the 3D trajectory of a feature during the animation, the user determines its position in a small set of interesting frames and lets the system build an interpolating 3D spline that provides the position of the feature as a function of time (see figure 3).

4.3 Virtual Hand Positioning and Key-Framing

The key-framing animation system aims at generating synthetic animations by positioning a virtual hand model, specifying the joint values (DOFs) for some time values and interpolating for the others. The appearance and structure of the virtual hand are fixed for a single animation sequence. The model is encoded using a VRML node graph [6]. The structure of the standard hand used for creating the reference animation that matches the video recorded one is based on the one described in the MPEG4 Version 2 (PDAM1) specification [7]. The system, however, is not restricted to this model and is able to animate objects with arbitrary structure. The model position at a key frame is specified with a 6 DOF input device (Magellan SpaceMouse), and it is also possible to specify each joint angle using both direct and inverse techniques. Our inverse specification module takes as input the marker trajectories and computes the optimal DOF values that permit to reach these goal positions, helping the animator in modeling the key-frames and obtaining more realistic animations. The approach that we used is to let animators freely manipulate the root position using the 6 DOF input device, while the system concurrently selects the optimal joint values by minimizing a cost function. This very general approach has proven very helpful in a number of animation contexts [8]. Reducing the number of DOFs under direct animator control in the generation of hand animations is also motivated by the fact that the mechanical structure of the hand introduces constraints that reduce the ability to control hand joints independently (see [9] for a task-level computer animation application). We currently use the following cost function:

$$Cost(\varphi) = \sum_i \|\mathbf{P}^i_{tip}(\varphi) - \mathbf{P}^i_{goal}\|^2 + \sum_j barrier(\varphi_j) + \sum_j \frac{1}{\sigma_j^2}\|\varphi_j - \hat{\varphi}_j\|^2 \qquad (2)$$

where $\varphi = \{\varphi_1, \varphi_2, ..., \varphi_n\}$ is the joint value vector to determinate, P^i_{goal} is the goal position for the i-th finger tip and $P^i_{tip}(\varphi)$ is the current position of the i-th finger tip, function of DOF vector φ. The first component drives the tips of the hand fingers (or other selected points in the local reference frame of the hand) towards the associated goal positions. The second component implements joint value constraints by summing the penalty functions associated to joint limits. The limit function increases as joint angle φ_j approaches either its maximum or minimum limit and is zero otherwise. This strongly inhibits each joint from bending beyond its prescribed limits. One such function which enforces joint limits is the following:

$$barrier(\varphi_j) = \begin{cases} -\frac{\varphi_j - (\varphi_j^{min}+\alpha)}{\alpha} + \ln\left(\frac{\delta}{\alpha}\right), & \varphi_j < \varphi_j^{min} + \alpha \\ \ln\left(\frac{\delta}{\varphi_j - \varphi_j^{min}}\right), & \varphi_j^{min} + \alpha < \varphi_j < \varphi_j^{min} + \delta \\ 0, & \varphi_j^{min} + \delta < \varphi_j < \varphi_j^{max} - \delta \\ \ln\left(\frac{\delta}{\varphi_j^{max} - \varphi_j}\right), & \varphi_j^{max} - \delta < \varphi_j < \varphi_j^{max} - \alpha \\ \frac{\varphi_j - (\varphi_j^{max} - \alpha)}{\alpha} + \ln\left(\frac{\delta}{\alpha}\right), & \varphi_j > \varphi_j^{max} - \alpha \end{cases} \qquad (3)$$

where φ_j is the angle of the current j-th joint , δ is the angular distance from the limits at which the limit function becomes non-zero, and α is the angular distance at which the logarithmic barrier is substituted with a linear barrier for numerical reasons. The third component drives each joint value φ_j towards a rest position $\hat{\varphi}_j$ and is weighted by a sensitivity parameter σ_j. This parameter approximates how much the j-th joint variation influences the correspondent tip position changes. A gradient descent algorithm is used to modify the joint angles of the model in order to drive the equation 2 to a minimum. The algorithm used is adaptive in the sense that it computes each descent steps using golden search bracketing and line search algorithms [10]. Figure 3 illustrates key-frame editing using constrained manipulation. Direct and inverse (constrained) techniques are usually iteratively applied until the animator judges the matching between the pose and the original movie sufficiently precise. Once the desired pose is found, all the joint values are stored in the key-framing system so as to participate as control points in the animation. This is repeated for a number of key-frames, until the animator is satisfied with the resulting animation.

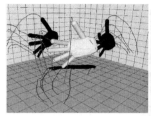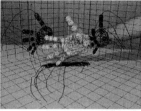

Figure 3: **Tracking features over time with constrained manipulation.** Lines represent the trajectories of selected features for the duration of the movie, while dots represent the position of the markers in this particular frame. The optimization algorithm computes optimal values for joint angles, while the user controls the hand wrist using the SpaceMouse. In the left image, orthogonal projections are used to guide interactive positioning, while in the right image the movie frame is also displayed in the background.

4.4 Animation Editing

In order to get meaningful modifications of sequences, the system makes it possible to interactively manipulate the animation. These manipulations involve geometry and appearance modifications (i.e. the system is able to apply the same animation data to various models, that differ in geometry and appearance) and time warping (i.e. the system provides tools that enable the animator to modify the animations by applying different time functions to joint angles). Currently, geometry and appearance modification is obtained by re-using the same animation tracks with different articulated structures (i.e. different VRML files) containing the same DOFs, while time warping features are limited to global scaling. More sophisticated motion retargeting techniques (e.g. those presented in [11, 12]) will be explored in the future.

5   Conclusions and Future Work

Our integrated system combines stereoscopic acquisition and presentation of biological actions in an experimental environment with the possibility to manipulate the acquired data for generating pictorial and/or kinematics modifications of the original action. The modified actions, successively presented in discrimination tasks in humans or during single neurons recording experiments in monkeys, will allow neurophysiology researchers to better understand how the brain works in understanding actions made by others. The first movies to be used as digital stimuli in the neurophysiological experiments are in the production phase. Figure 4 shows selected frames of three different versions of a grasping sequence. The future work will concentrate on improving the animation manipulation and motion warping features, and in producing higher-quality renderings.

Acknowledgments

This work is carried out within the research project "MIRRORS: Mirror Neurons and the Execution/Matching System in Humans", sponsored by the Human Frontiers Science Program Foundation. The project partners are: Università di Parma, Italy (Coord.); CRS4, Cagliari, Italy; Helsinki University of Technology, Espoo, Finland; Kyoto University, Inuyama, Japan; Dept. of Basic Sciences, University of Crete Medical School and IACM FORTH, Heraklion, Greece; University of California School of Medicine, Los Angeles, USA. We also acknowledge the contribution of Sardinian regional authorities.

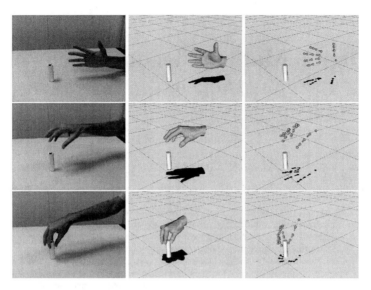

Figure 4: **Animation results.** The left images show selected frames of a video-taped grasping sequence. The middle images shows a synthesized animation replicating the same motion. The right images shows the same animation applied to a different geometric structure.

References

[1] M.Matelli, G. Rizzolatti, and G.Luppino. Patterns of cytochrome oxidase activity in the frontal agranular cortex of the macaque monkey. *Behav. Brain Res.*, 18:125–136, 1985.

[2] G. Di Pellegrino, L. Fadiga, L. Fogassi, V. Gallese, and G. Rizzolatti. Understanding motor events: a neurophysiological study. *Exp. Brain Res.*, 91:176–180, 1992.

[3] G. Rizzolatti, L. Fadiga, V. Gallese, and L. Fogassi. Premotor cortex and the recognition of motor actions. *Behav. Brain Res.*, 3:131–141, 1996.

[4] V. Gallese, L. Fadiga, L. Fogassi, and G. Rizzolatti. Action recognition in the premotor cortex. *Brain*, 119:593–609, 1996.

[5] Zhengyou Zhang. Determining the epipolar geometry and its uncertainty: A review. Technical Report 2927, Institut National de Recherche en Informatique et en Automatique, Sophia-Antipolis Cedex, France, July 1996.

[6] Rikk Carey and Gavin Bell. *The VRML 2.0 Annotated Reference Manual*. Addison-Wesley, Reading, MA, USA, January 1997. Includes CD-ROM.

[7] ISO/IEC 14496-1:   MPEG-4 PDAM1.   Available on the web at the address http://www.cslet.stet.it/mpeg.

[8] David E. Breen. Cost minimization for animated geometric models in computer graphics. *The Journal of Visualization and Computer Animation*, 8(4):201–220, 1997. ISSN 1049-9807.

[9] Hans Rijpkema and Michael Girard. Computer animation of knowledge-based human grasping. *Computer Graphics*, 25(4):339–348, July 1991.

[10] W. H. Press, B. P. Flannery, S. A. Teukolsky, and W. T. Vetterling. *Numerical Recipes in C: The Art of Scientific Computing*. Cambridge University Press, Cambridge, UK, second edition, 1992.

[11] Andrew Witkin and Zoran Popović. Motion warping. *Computer Graphics*, 29(Annual Conference Series):105–108, November 1995.

[12] Kwangjin Choi and Hyeongseok Ko. On-line motion retargetting. In *Proceedings of the International Pacific Graphics '99*, 1999.

30

Medicine Meets Virtual Reality 2001
J.D. Westwood et al. (Eds.)
IOS Press, 2001

Digital Motion Phenomenology of Depression

Norman E. Alessi, M.D.
Milton P. Huang, M.D.
Psychiatric Informatics Program, Department of Psychiatry, University of Michigan,
48109

Abstract.   The long-term objective of our project is to use motion capture technology to identify and characterize body alterations in motion associated with depression that have not been previously recognized or characterizable. These motion phenomena will be studied to determine their utility in the nosology and subtyping of depression. Quantitatively, they may have a significant impact in the areas of research, education and the clinical management of depression; and allow the creation of "virtual humans" which manifest depressive digital motion phenomena that can be used to train researchers, trainees and clinicians.

1. Phenomenology of Depression

There has been a consistency in the phenomenology used to describe depression for a number of centuries [1]. Sleep, appetite alterations, mood, anhedonia, disturbances in concentration, poor self-concept, hopelessness and alterations in motor functioning have been noted. During the 20th century there have been few advances in either our use of these phenomenon or in our ability to describe or characterize these disturbances. Most of the rating scales and diagnostic criteria (DSM-IV) have favored the primacy of mood, with less emphasis placed on motion alterations. Further, they have relied primarily on reported symptoms such as "How one feels?" "If one feels sad or depressed?", and "Does one feel motivated and have a sense of the future?" Rating scales, such as the Hamilton Depression Rating Scale (HDRS) and self-rating scales, such as the Zung, provide a methodology to quantify reported symptoms. The HDRS has only 2 items that are used to characterize motor alterations associated with depression; the remaining items are dependent on the gathering of symptoms reported by the patient. There have been too few attempts to develop techniques to characterize the phenomenology or signs of the depression, in particular the alteration in motor functioning that presents itself as slowing in gait, stooping and in the most severe forms an inability to move or catatonia.

The following section reviews the relevance of psychomotor alterations to depression, critiques previous technologies and studies that have attempted to characterize psychomotor alterations among the depressed and presents the current use of motion capture applications in various industries and the potential value of such a technology in the study of depression.

2. Psychomotor Retardation in Depression

Psychomotor alterations have long been noted to be an essential component of mood disorders. Reports by Burton, Kraepelin and Bleuler, noted the presence of psychomotor slowing among depressed and speeding up among manic patients [2, 3]. It has been noted to be present in the trunk and the limbs; The patient rarely moves his/her limbs, preferring to use his hands instead of the upper limb; The trunk barely moves and it appears as if the body is suspended and immobile; There is a paucity of all movement of the face, trunk or the limbs; and, The patient appears to be weakened and often moves by shuffling his/her feet and with a stooped posture. The face is immobile and there is no modulation of affect; there is no happiness and there is no sadness. There appears to be a vacuum that once contained human movement. There is an abundance of descriptive data that has characterized the clinical presence of psychomotor slowing in depression, yet these data have lacked objectivity and quantitation.

Many studies have reported on the significance of motor alterations in depression. In a study of 391 psychotic versus 250 neurotic depressed patients discriminant function analysis indicated that among 60 symptoms, psychomotor symptoms were the most robust discriminator [4]. In a review of factor analytic studies, 11 of the 12 reports found that psychomotor retardation loaded on the endogenous factor at 0.5 or higher [5]. Of 20 depressive symptoms, psychomotor retardation had the highest loading on the endogenous factor. Recent reviews have supported this finding [6, 7]. As noted, psychomotor signs occur with a high rate of frequency, yet it is rarely evaluated except by clinical observation [8]. Motion alterations have been noted to occur in subtypes of depression with greater frequency. These have included: marked slowing among those with bipolar depressive disorders versus unipolar depression; endogenous versus non-endogenous depression; psychotic versus non-psychotic depression; and, vascular versus non-vascular depressive disorders [9-13]. Gender and age also correlate with the degree of motion alteration with males and those over 40 being at increased risk for more retardation [14, 15]. Psychomotor retardation has been correlated with the potential response to ECT and medications among those with endogenous depression [16]. Based on these and many other studies, some have argued that the motor component of depression is the central deficit in depressive illnesses rather than mood [17, 18]. This fact has only been exploited by one group clinically, using an observer based rating scale.

Parker and his colleagues have pursued the psychomotor alterations methodologically in an attempt to understand their significance. Their efforts have led to the development of the CORE, an observation based instrument that codifies the presence of psychomotor alterations among patients [19-22]. Based on observations of the patient, the CORE allows one to quantify the severity of psychomotor phenomena present among patients with any motor alteration into three groups regardless of etiology: retardation, agitation and non – interactiveness. Using the CORE, Parker and colleagues have been able to predict response to treatment intervention and track treatment outcome [20, 23]. Further, correlation with severity of the depression has been shown to be consistent with elevated CORE scores. The development and application of the CORE strongly supports the significance of motor alterations among those with mood disorders. Despite the contribution that the CORE makes it does little to characterize the actual motion alterations in depressed patients. It is a gross measure of psychomotor retardation based on clinical observations, still lacking in objectivity. It does not provide objective descriptions of motion patterns that could be used for either clinical or research purposes.

If there was an objective and quantitative method to characterize alterations in motion associated with depression, there are a number of questions that could be asked? Do depression motion alterations involve the entire body or are there instances where they affect only the upper or the lower body, as in the case of Parkinson's where "lower half" disturbances can occur [24]? Do depression motion alterations affect speed or the ability to initiate motion? Do depression motion alterations change or develop with age? Do depression motion alterations decrease uniformly with treatment across all body areas? Do we know what the significance of the motion alteration is in the daily living of our patients or in the work setting of our patients who make their living by lifting and moving objects? To my knowledge there are no examples in the study of motion alterations associated with depression that have used motion capture techniques that would allow this level of study and understanding.

3. Pathophysiology of Motion Alterations

The two different conceptualizations of the pathophysiology of motion alterations are structural or neurotransmission pathway disruption. Based on imaging studies of disorders with basal ganglia abnormalities, the structural lesions have been suggested to involve the disruption of the circuits that connect the basal ganglia to the prefrontal and anterior cingulated cortex resulting in apathy, dystonia, and depression [25-29]. Perfusion studies of depressives have shown reduced levels of CBF in paralimbic regions, including the inferior frontal, anterior cingulated and anterior temporal cortex [30-32]. These findings are paralleled by similar findings among schizophrenics with psychomotor poverty; reductions are noted in CBF in the dorsolateral prefrontal cortex, an area suggested to be involved in volitional willful behavior [33, 34].

Despite most biological studies concentrating on serotonin and noradrenaline, a select number involve the potential role of dopamine. A number of theories have suggested a potential role for dopamine. These are based on: 80 % of dopamine is produced in the basal ganglia; levels of dopamine, CSF homovanillic acid (HVA), a dopamine metabolite are abnormal in depressed patients; and, decreased plasma HVA in depressed patients [35-38]. Based on this premise, studies using antidepressants with dopamimetic specificity have been shown to be effective in treating patients with psychomotor-retardation [39-41]. These studies have all used the most rudimentary characterization of motion alterations of the body in their hypothesis development and testing. What might detailed and refined motion characterization demonstrate? It might allow the development of more specific imaging paradigms, neurotransmitter and intervention studies.

4. Previous Instrumentation Monitoring Techniques

Given the significance, prominence and consistency of psychomotor alterations in mood disorders, a number of attempts have been made to use them as a means to characterize mood disorders using objective instrumentation monitoring techniques. They have been used in a number of investigations of mood disorders including: the relationship between motor activity and mood states, mood switches, clinical improvement, sleep criteria, diagnostic categories, biochemical measures, therapeutic medication regiments and various circadian rhythms [12]. A review in 1981 by Greden, emphasized electromyographic (EMG) determinations of facial expression of emotion, measurement of speech phonation and pause times, and movement activated recording monitors to quantify motility [42]. Facial EMG were shown to differentiate depressed from normal individuals, especially when the groups were asked to "think and feel" positive thoughts. It was suggested that this technique might be used to identify those who were hedonic moving, with a lack of pleasure. Speech alterations, slowing in depression and speeding up in mania, have a tradition in clinical psychiatry as being a predictable observation. Speech pause time varies less than speed of spoken word and quantity of utterance with the occurrence of depression and severity [42-44]. Although facial EMG and speech pause characteristics were objective measures that demonstrated the slowing found in depression, they do not provide detailed information concerning body motion alterations, as this project will do.

Movement in depressed patients has been assessed using two approaches: gross motor activity and fine motor analysis. Gross motor activity has been accessed using telemetric electronic devices worn by patients [11, 12, 45, 46]. These devices are usually worn on the wrist and measure the amount of movement of that limb during a designated period. Studies using this technology showed that psychomotor retardation was worse among those with bipolar depressive disorders vs. unipolar; that levels of activity varied within manic depressives according to their affective state; and motor levels approached normal after successful treatment. In one case video was used as a means to record "non-verbal behavior of depressed patients" [47]. The video did not provide a means for analysis, only a method to record movements for subsequent qualitative observation analysis. Attempts to characterize specific movement during motor activity such as gait has been reported as well [48, 49]. Sloman used a "frame-by-frame" technique using film as the medium of record to study gait among depressed patients. The study showed that not only were depressed subjects slower, but they also had a different gait pattern than normals. The ability to study many subjects was hindered by the work required for a frame-by-frame analysis. Sabbe tracked the ability of depressed patients to draw a figure. Not only were movements slowing but the interaction between concentration and movement time had slowed. A recent review added the use of video taped interviews to document motion alterations, and reaction times [8]. As in the case of the facial EMG and speech pause time, these objective measures demonstrate that slowing is found in these disorders, but they do not provide the quantitative data needed for comprehensive total body analysis or potential reconstruction.

No matter what technical method is used when assessing motor functioning, we know that psychomotor slowing is present among depressed subjects; the degree of retardation correlates with the severity of the depression and the state of the disorder; and, it appears to persist in a subset of patients even after treatment. Despite the significance of motion alteration, it is rare that objective measures of body motion have been pursued. This was noted by Greden in a recent editorial entitled "Psychomotor Monitoring: A Promise Being Fulfilled?" [50] The findings to date such as gross delay in speech pause time, slowing motion within a 24-hour period, delayed reaction time, nor clinical observation, add little to our understanding of the disorder and does not provide the information necessary to answer fundamental questions about the motion alterations.

5. Digital Motion Capture Technology

Digital motion capture technology refers to: *digital*, data captured in a native computerized versus analog state, thereby allowing the data to be easily used in a number of computer applications; *motion*, the movement of any body in space, such as the trunk and limbs of a human; *capture technology*, technologies developed to facilitate the gathering of data from objects that are in motion. The first attempts at motion capture technology took place in the late 19th century, used multiple cameras that took a sequence of photos as an object moved to trip the shutter of each camera [51]. These images were then reconstructed to demonstrate the motion of the object in space and time. Techniques have evolved since that time using either electromagnetic or passive/active markers that allow the tracking of objects. Some systems can allow the capture of over 1000 data points per second, thereby allowing for the capture of motion that would be beyond the temporal resolution of human perception.

These digital data can be used for a broad range of applications. In medicine and kinesiology, the data can be used to study gait alterations among those with different diseases. In engineering, they can be used to study interior design of automobiles, tanks or airplanes, where humans have to reach and sit and stand. The data can also be used to reconstruct the configuration of the original object, as well as, its motion. The most frequent use of motion capture technology for this purpose is in the field of animation, where the motion, body and faces of actors serve as the starting point of the creation of animated figures.

6. Why Use Digital Capture Technology in Psychiatry?

One can question the use of motion capture technology in this population. Hasn't the slowing associated with motional alterations been demonstrated in each research paradigm using various technologies? Can't the slowing adequately be characterized using clinical observation as exemplified by the CORE? Yes, the motion alteration has been demonstrated and it can be seen and qualitatively characterized, but the degree to which it has been studied and can be seen and documented has been quite limited. An understanding of the potential data that can be captured and characterized requires a rudimentary understanding of the body, not as a biological entity but as a biomechanical entity. As such, the body has enormous complexity and must be understood not only as muscles that act to move limbs and the body, but also as a machine where movements and the forces needed to move the body can be studied to determine if and when, it is exceeding limits that might prove to be injurious. Occupational ergonomics is a field that studies the impact of motions and forces on the body in the work environment; kinesiology is a field that studies these factors or exercise in clinical areas [52]. To date, most of the technical measures used to study the motions of depressed patients have been extremely minimal and at best, limited potential value. Further, the quantitative basis of the CORE, although much more than the HDRS, provides little detail about motion alterations, and it certainly does not produce any objective measures. Is the detail needed? Certainly, the value of the detail will not be known until it is systematically studied and organized to allow its use to be evaluated. Potential benefits include: an appreciation of other subtypes of depression; the development of tools that can monitor depression independent of patient reporting for patients incapable of reporting their depression or who have limited communication skills, aptitude, or insight into motion alterations that have different biological substrates, i.e. neurotransmitter, serotonin versus dopamine motion alterations, and/or structural, cortical versus subcortical origins [53].

7. Significance of Digital Motion Phenomenology

The significance of the proposed research project is as follows: 1. It will create a new methodology for the characterization of mood disorders using objective measurement of body motion alterations as the principal component of digital motion phenomena. To my knowledge this is the first study that has used motion capture technology for this purpose. 2. It will create new paradigms of motion sampling, shorter in duration and specific per body segment, limb, or joint within an array of sampling protocols. This technology will allow the collection and recording of data about motion alterations associated with depression that would have otherwise been unobtainable, and uncharacterizable. 3. It will allow the study of known subtypes of depression, endogenous, psychotic, and vascular and possibly lead to the identification of other subtypes based on motion alteration patterns; 4. It will allow the identification of depression in populations known to have difficulties in reporting the presence of depressive symptoms, e.g., aged, demented, developmental disabilities, mental retarded and children/ adolescents [53]. 5. It will allow a more precise manner to study the interface of neuropsychiatric conditions where motor disturbances are prevalent with depression i.e. Parkinson's, Huntington Chorea, and Alzheimer's. 6. It will provide a more exacting technology that will allow the study of different pathophysiological models of depression. The impact of proposed different structural alterations have been difficult to assess since they deal with global alterations in motion. The proposed project will provide greater detail in almost every dimension, i.e. tempo, anatomical distribution, torques and force. In pharmacotherapeutic studies the potential differences between serotonin and dopamimetic agents can be evaluated and motional alterations can be used in the choice of therapeutic agents. 7. It will extend our sampling beyond one-dimensional or two-dimensional data sets; it will allow the creation of three-dimensional data sets that can be used both for morphometric analysis and the recreation of the "motion" of the subject as a virtual human to be used for training, patient education, and potential clinical tracking of refractory depressive conditions. 8. It will allow the development of "patient digital models or avatars" that can be experienced as a human being with expressive emotions, whether normal or abnormal. This has enormous potential in regard to how we see patients, characterize psychiatric disorders, recall their disturbances, or compare their response to treatment.

References

[1]   S. W. Jackson, *Melancholia and Depression: From Hippocratic Times to Modern Times*. New Haven and London: Yale University Press, 1986.

[2]   M. G. Evans B, *The Psychiatry of Robert Burton*. New York: Columbia University Press, 1944.

[3]   E. Kraepelin, *Manic-Depressive Insanity and Paranoia*. Edinburgh: Livingstone, 1921.

[4]   K. RE, *The Classification of Depressive Illness: Maudsley Monograph 18*. London: Oxford University Press, 1968.

[5]   J. C. Nelson, and Charney, D. S., "The Symptoms of Major Depressive Illness," *The American Journal of Psychiatry*, vol. 138, pp. 1-13, 1981.

[6]   A. J. Rush and J. E. Weissenburger, "Melancholic symptom features and DSM-IV [see comments]," *Am J Psychiatry*, vol. 151, pp. 489-98, 1994.

[7]   G. Parker, and Hadzi-Pavlovic, "Melancholia: A Disorder of Movement and Mood," . New York: Cambridge Press, 1996.

[8]   C. a. S. Sobin, H, "Psychomotor Symptoms of Depression," *American Journal of Psychiatry*, vol. 154, pp. 4-17, 1997.

[9]   G. S. Alexopoulos, B. S. Meyers, R. C. Young, T. Kakuma, D. Silbersweig, and M. Charlson, "Clinically defined vascular depression," *Am J Psychiatry*, vol. 154, pp. 562-5, 1997.

[10]   M. N. Bhrolchain, G. W. Brown, and T. O. Harris, "Psychotic and neurotic depression: 2. Clinical characteristics," *Br J Psychiatry*, vol. 134, pp. 94-107, 1979.

[11]   M. D. Kupfer, David J., Weiss, M.D., Brian L., Foster, M.D., Gordon, Detre, M.D., Thomas P., Delgado, M.D.; Jose, McPartland, Richard, and MEE, Pittsburgh, "Psychomotor Activity in Affective States," *Arch Gen Psychiatry*, vol. 30, pp. 765-768, 1974.

[12]   E. A. Wolff III, Putnam, M.D., Frank W., and Robert M. Post, M.D., "Motor Activity and Affective Illness: The Relationship of Amplitude and Temporal Distribution to Changes in Affective State.," *Arch Gen Psychiatry*, vol. 42, pp. 288-294, 1985.

[13]   J. L. Fleiss, "Classification of the Depressive Disorders by Numerical Typology," *Journal of Psychiat. Res.*, vol. 9, pp. 141-153, 1972.

[14]   D. Avery, and Judy Silverman, "Psychomotor Retardation and Agitation in Depression: Relationship to Age, Sex, and Response to Treatment.," *Journal of Affective Disorders*, vol. 7, pp. 67-76, 1984.

[15]   G. Winokur, J. Morrison, J. Clancy, and R. Crowe, "The Iowa 500: familial and clinical findings favor two kinds of depressive illness," *Compr Psychiatry*, vol. 14, pp. 99-106, 1973.

[16]   S. Brandon, P. Cowley, C. McDonald, P. Neville, R. Palmer, and S. Wellstood-Eason, "Electroconvulsive therapy: results in depressive illness from the Leicestershire trial," *Br Med J (Clin Res Ed)*, vol. 288, pp. 22-5, 1984.

[17]   M. D. Widlocher, Daniel J., "Psychomotor Retardation: Clinical, Theoretical, and Psychometric Aspects.," *Psychiatric Clinics of North America*, vol. 6, pp. 27-40, 1983.

[18]   G. P. D. Hadzi-Pavlovic, "Prediction of Response to Antidepressant Medication by a Sign-based Index of Melancholia," *Australian and New Zealand Journal of Psychiatry*, vol. 27, pp. 56-61, 1993.

[19]   I. H. B. P. a. G. Parker, "Prediction of Response to Electroconvulsive Therapy," *British Journal of Psychiatry*, vol. 157, pp. 65-71, 1990.

[20]   G. Parker, Hadzi-Pavlovic, Dusan, Brodaty, Henry, Boyce, Philip, Mitchell, Philip, Wilhelm, Kay, Hickie, Ian, and Kerrie Eyers, "Psychomotor disturbance in depression: defining the constructs.," *Journal of Affective Disorders*, vol. 27, pp. 255-265, 1993.

[21]   G. Parker, Hadzi-Pavlovic, Dusan, Brodaty, Wilhelm, Kay, Hickie, Ian, Henry, Boyce, Philip, Mitchell, Philip, and Kerrie Eyers, "Defining Melancholia: Properties of a Refined Sign-Based Measure.," *British Journal of Psychiatry*, vol. 164, pp. 316-326, 1994.

[22]   G. Parker, Hadzi-Pavlovic, D., Austin, M.-P., Mitchell, P., Wilhelm, K., Hickie, I., Boyce, P., and
        Kerrie Eyers, "Sub-typing depression, I. Is psychomotor disturbance necessary and sufficient to the
        definition of melancholia?," *Psychological Medicine*, vol. 25, pp. 815-823, 1995.
[23]   I. Hickie, Mason, Catherine, and Gordon Parker, "Comparative validity of two measures of
        psychomotor function in patients with severe depression.," *Journal of Affective Disorders*, vol. 37,
        pp. 143-149, 1996.
[24]   R. J. Elble, R. Cousins, K. Leffler, and L. Hughes, "Gait initiation by patients with lower-half
        parkinsonism," *Brain*, vol. 119, pp. 1705-16, 1996.
[25]   G. E. Alexander, M. R. DeLong, and P. L. Strick, "Parallel organization of functionally segregated
        circuits linking basal ganglia and cortex," *Annu Rev Neurosci*, vol. 9, pp. 357-81, 1986.
[26]   J. L. Cummings, "Frontal-subcortical circuits and human behavior," *Arch Neurol*, vol. 50, pp. 873-
        80, 1993.
[27]   C. E. Peyser and S. E. Folstein, "Huntington's disease as a model for mood disorders. Clues from
        neuropathology and neurochemistry," *Mol Chem Neuropathol*, vol. 12, pp. 99-119, 1990.
[28]   S. E. Starkstein, R. G. Robinson, M. L. Berthier, R. M. Parikh, and T. R. Price, "Differential mood
        changes following basal ganglia vs thalamic lesions," *Arch Neurol*, vol. 45, pp. 725-30, 1988.
[29]   D. Laplane, M. Levasseur, B. Pillon, B. Dubois, M. Baulac, B. Mazoyer, S. Tran Dinh, G. Sette, F.
        Danze, and J. C. Baron, "Obsessive-compulsive and other behavioural changes with bilateral basal
        ganglia lesions. A neuropsychological, magnetic resonance imaging and positron tomography
        study," *Brain*, vol. 112, pp. 699-725, 1989.
[30]   R. J. Dolan, C. J. Bench, R. G. Brown, L. C. Scott, K. J. Friston, and R. S. Frackowiak, "Regional
        cerebral blood flow abnormalities in depressed patients with cognitive impairment," *J Neurol
        Neurosurg Psychiatry*, vol. 55, pp. 768-73, 1992.
[31]   C. J. Bench, K. J. Friston, R. G. Brown, R. S. Frackowiak, and R. J. Dolan, "Regional cerebral
        blood flow in depression measured by positron emission tomography: the relationship with clinical
        dimensions," *Psychol Med*, vol. 23, pp. 579-90, 1993.
[32]   H. S. Mayberg, P. J. Lewis, W. Regenold, and H. N. Wagner, Jr., "Paralimbic hypoperfusion in
        unipolar depression," *J Nucl Med*, vol. 35, pp. 929-34, 1994.
[33]   P. F. Liddle, K. J. Friston, C. D. Frith, and R. S. Frackowiak, "Cerebral blood flow and mental
        processes in schizophrenia," *J R Soc Med*, vol. 85, pp. 224-7, 1992.
[34]   P. S. Goldman-Rakic, "Motor control function of the prefrontal cortex," *Ciba Found Symp*, vol. 132,
        pp. 187-200, 1987.
[35]   A. Roy, D. Pickar, M. Linnoila, A. R. Doran, P. Ninan, and S. M. Paul, "Cerebrospinal fluid
        monoamine and monoamine metabolite concentrations in melancholia," *Psychiatry Res*, vol. 15, pp.
        281-92, 1985.
[36]   P. L. Reddy, S. Khanna, M. N. Subhash, S. M. Channabasavanna, and B. S. Rao, "CSF amine
        metabolites in depression," *Biol Psychiatry*, vol. 31, pp. 112-8, 1992.
[37]   A. Gjerris, L. Werdelin, O. J. Rafaelsen, C. Alling, and N. J. Christensen, "CSF dopamine increased
        in depression: CSF dopamine, noradrenaline and their metabolites in depressed patients and in
        controls," *J Affect Disord*, vol. 13, pp. 279-86, 1987.
[38]   a. G. S. Brown AS, "Dopamine and Depression," *J Neural Transm*, vol. 91, pp. 75-109, 1993.
[39]   B. J. Goldstein, B. Brauzer, D. Kentsmith, S. Rosenthal, and K. D. Charalampous, "Double-blind
        placebo-controlled multicenter evaluation of the efficacy and safety of nomifensine in depressed
        outpatients," *J Clin Psychiatry*, vol. 45, pp. 52-5, 1984.
[40]   L. Rampello, G. Nicoletti, and R. Raffaele, "Dopaminergic hypothesis for retarded depression: a
        symptom profile for predicting therapeutical responses," *Acta Psychiatr Scand*, vol. 84, pp. 552-4,
        1991.
[41]   M. V. Rudorfer, R. N. Golden, and W. Z. Potter, "Second-generation antidepressants," *Psychiatr
        Clin North Am*, vol. 7, pp. 519-34, 1984.
[42]   J. F. Greden, Albala, A. Ariav, Smokler, Irving A., Gardner, Robert, and Bernard J. Carroll,
        "Speech Pause Time: A Marker of Psychomotor Retardation Among Endogenous Depressives,"
        Biological Psychiatry, vol. 16, pp. 851-859, 1981.
[43]   A. Flint, J., Black, Sandra E., Campbell-Taylor, Irene, Gailey, Gillian F., and Carey Levinton,
        "Abnormal Speech Articulation, Psychomotor Retardation, and Subcortical Dysfunction in Major
        Depression.," *J. Psychiat Res.*, vol. 27, pp. 309-319, 1993.
[44]   G. M. A. Hoffmann, Gonze, J.C., and J. Mendlewicz, "Speech Pause Time as a Method for the
        Evaluation of Psychomotor Retardation in Depressive Illness.," *British Journal of Psychiatry*, vol.
        146, pp. 535-538, 1985.
[45]   D. J. Kupfer, Detre, Thomas P., Foster, Gordon, Tucker, Gary J., and Jose Delgado, "The
        Application of Delgado's Telemetric Mobility Recorder for Human Studies.," *Behavioral Biology*,
        vol. 7, pp. 585-590, 1972.

[46]   M. D. Post, Robert M., Stoddard, M.D., Frederick J., Gillin, M.D., J. Christian, Buchsbaum, M.D., Monte S., Runkle, Deborah C., Black, Katherine E., and William E. Bunney, Jr., M.D., "Alterations in Motor Activity, Sleep, and Biochemistry in a Cycling Manic-Depressive Patient.," *Arch Gen Psychiatry*, vol. 34, pp. 470-477, 1977.

[47]   U. G. a. K. Harms, "A Video Analysis of the Non-Verbal Behaviour of Depressed Patients Before and After Treatment," *Affective Disorders*, vol. 9, pp. 63-67, 1985.

[48]   B. Sabbe, Hulstijn, Wouter, Van Hoof, Jacques, and Frans Zitman, "Fine Motor Retardation and Depression.," *J. psychiat. Res.*, vol. 30, pp. 295-306, 1996.

[49]   M. D. Sloman, Leon, Berridge, M.S., Mavis, Homatidis, M.A., S., Hunter, C.C.W., D., and T. Duck, Ph.D., "Gait Patterns of Depressed Patients and Normal Subjects," *Am J Psychiatry*, vol. 139, pp. 94-96, 1982.

[50]   J. F. Greden, "Psychomotor Monitoring: A Promise Being Fulfilled?," *J psychiat. Res.*, vol. 27, pp. 285-287, 1993.

[51]   E. Muybridge, *The Human Figure in Motion, An Electro-Photographic Investigation of Consecutive Phases of Muscular Actions*. London: Chapman &Hall, 1901.

[52]   D. B. Chaffin, G. B. J. Andersson, and B. J. Martin, *Occupational Biomechanics*, Third ed. New York: John Wiley & Sons, Inc., 1999.

[53]   P. Wiener, G. S. Alexopoulos, T. Kakuma, B. S. Meyers, E. Rosenthal, and J. Chester, "The limits of history-taking in geriatric depression," *Am J Geriatr Psychiatry*, vol. 5, pp. 116-25, 1997.

Medicine Meets Virtual Reality 2001
J.D. Westwood et al. (Eds.)
IOS Press, 2001

Internet as an "Honest" Management Tool First Experience in a National Institute of Health and Social Services in Argentina

Rodolfo Altrudi, MD; Ricardo Herrero, MD; Ariel Melamud, MD; Eduardo Rodas, MD
Department of Medical Informatics
The National Institute of Social Services for Retired and Pensioned

Abstract. The PAMI's website creation (www.pami.org.ar) has had the purpose of spreading its activities, the standards of medical care and administrative management, offering - at the same time - a honest channel of interaction with the community.

1. Introduction

The National Institute of Social Services for Retired and Pensioned (Instituto de Servicios Sociales para Jubilados y Pensionados [INSSJP]), was created in 1971. The goal of this agency was to cover all senior citizens under a single universal and mandatory health plan. The medical branch of this coverage became official with the creation of the Program of Integral Medical Assistance (Programa de Asistencia Médica Integral [PAMI]).

Currently the PAMI offers its services to approximately 3.376.000 individuals (the most extensive public medical coverage in Latin America), with a budget in 1999 of $ 2.845 million. This amount is originated from contributions of senior citizens, the active workers and the Argentinean Government.

Due to previous financial miss-management, the INSSJP was taken under direct governmental control by the current government administration.

The purpose of this paper is to present the authors' experience in using, for the first time, the Internet as the main tool to improve and monitor the quality of health care services in Argentina provided by the PAMI.

2. Material y methods

In order to accomplish the project, a workgroup integrated by web programmers, graphic designers, net analysts, physicians and system analysts was created, under supervision of the Division of Medical Informatics. The accomplished tasks were:
1) Analysis of the current situation about IPS, broadband, telecommunication providers, etc.
2) Analysis of the current situation about website.
3) Analysis of the projected site.
4) Redesign of the site

3. Results

In the image below the new appearance of the website (http://www.pami.org.ar) can be appreciated.

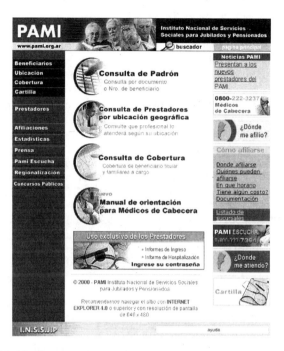

Website is divided in four areas:
1) Consultation area: affiliates data, assistance resources, pharmacies, geriatrics and optical institutes.
2) Professional area: orientation handbook of prevalent diseases for first level physicians. Future plans include offering to professional customers useful working tools, such us diagnostic and therapeutic guidelines of common diseases of the elderly, telemedicine and continuing medical education among others.
3) Services area: here the affiliation regulations can be consulted (users can print PAMI's affiliation form), PAMI's statistics, regionally reports, institutional press reports and the PAMI's telephonic service of listeners designated "PAMI ESCUCHA Y RESPONDE" (PAMI listeners and answers).
5) Public contest area: here it can be consulted preliminary contest and bid versions, then final versions and in a near future, the information on the results of the contests and bids.

In following table we can see a monthly visits report to the site (from 09/212000 to 10/21/2000):

09/21/00 – 10/21/00	
Page view:	14225
Sessions:	4176
Visitors:	2320

4. Discussion

The lNSSJP′s population consists mainly by senior citizens with their families, handicapped and veterans of war.

The medical system is divided in three levels of health services:

- Level I: consists of radiology services, regular consultation, access to a family practice physician and laboratory studies.
- Level II: consists of hospital admissions, specialist consultation and median complexity treatments.
- Level III: consists of high complexity treatments.

In addition to these 3 levels, the PAMI provides with other medical and social services such as dialysis, renal transplantation, ambulances, optical devices, headphones, transportation, burial services, free food and medical drugs.

After a reiterate poor administration history, the INSSJP was intervened by the government with the objective of transforming the PAMI into a much more responsible organization. Improved quality of their services was achieved by employing a better monitoring policy resulting in a much more efficient administration of its resources.

As a part of this transformation process, the "Honest Management Program" was created with the support of Anti-corruption Office of the Ministry of Justice and Human Rights.

An essential component of this program was the design of a communication channel via the World Wide Web for those interested in improving the quality of services.

The Public Contest Area is, with no doubt, one of the most valuable strategies to achieve an honest management of the health care plan, fighting against corruption. Not only does it provide all citizens with the opportunity of expressing their thoughts and recommendations regarding all PAMI business but also it makes every commerce decision universally accessible.

Since its creation, the INSSJP has been an example to the others social health systems of the country, those which have made the procedures established by the Institute for the effective development of the health care their own.

The backbone of the organization is the Program of Integral Medical Assistance (PAMI), to such point that it has become synonymous of the INSSJP. For this reason the creation of this communication channel between the PAMI and the community represents a transcendental step in the honesty process suggested by the current political authorities of our country.

Medicine Meets Virtual Reality 2001
J.D. Westwood et al. (Eds.)
IOS Press, 2001

Telemedicine Used in a Simulated Disaster Response

David C. Balch and Vivian L. West
East Carolina University, Telemedicine Center, The Brody School of Medicine
Greenville, NC

Abstract: *In June 2000, the Telemedicine Center at the Brody School of Medicine, East Carolina University in Greenville, NC participated in a simulated disaster response in Pu'u Paa, Hawaii, a lava plain without running water, electricity, or human habitation. During the five-day exercise we evaluated the ability to establish telecommunications and the effectiveness of the infrastructure, services, and applications implemented for an operational global emergency response. Scaleable technologies were configured and systematically tested to determine the ability to provide medical and health care in an austere environment. A medical communications matrix was constructed and used throughout the evaluation. Results show that telemedicine can be an important contribution to humanitarian relief efforts and medical support following disasters. Additional research is needed to build upon the lessons learned from participation in this exercise.*

1. Introduction

East Carolina University's (ECU) Telemedicine Center at the Brody School of Medicine in Greenville, NC participated in a mock disaster response with a code name "Strong Angel". Organized by the United States Navy Third Fleet, Strong Angel was part of the Rim of the Pacific (RIMPAC) exercise, a biennial month-long exercise in the Asia-Pacific region involving the maritime forces of seven countries: Australia, Canada, Chile, Great Britain, Korea, Japan, and the United States. This was the first time in a thirty-year history of RIMPAC that a humanitarian assistance exercise was conducted [1]. Participants included: the Office for the Coalition of Human Affairs, the United Nations High Commissioner for Refugees, the World Food Program, the United Nations Children's Fund, the American Red Cross, and several other government and non-government participants. A refugee camp was constructed and staffed by the United States Marines and Navy at the base of an 800-foot volcanic hill, Pu'u Paa, in a remote northwestern corner of the big island of Hawaii. The camp was run by the United Nations. One hundred twenty-five volunteers, selected and trained by the American Red Cross, simulated victims of a natural disaster.

Testing new technologies for telemedicine in the kind of austere environment and the conditions in which this exercise occurred has never been possible before. Strong Angel provided us with a unique testing environment for our research for biomedical applications over the Next Generation Internet, and enabled us to evaluate some of the technological configurations for telemedicine applications for the Next Generation Internet that we are currently studying in fulfilling requirements of a contract with the National Library of Medicine. Therefore, this large-scale civilian-military exercise was of special interest to us. We planned and constructed a medical communications matrix with global connectivity and scaleable technologies, and then configured and systematically tested these links. The purpose of the study was to evaluate the ability to establish telecommunications configured in a simulated disaster, and the ability to effectively deliver health and medical care through telemedicine designed and implemented for an operational global emergency response.

2. Methods

All of the telecommunications equipment we used in Hawaii was configured and tested in Greenville, NC in the weeks prior to the exercise at Pu'u Paa. In addition to IP video via satellite, we also planned several experiments using ham radio communications. Tests were conducted using a satellite dish mounted on the roof of the medical school. A non-operating Voice of America site in Greenville was used for the ham radio experiments.

Because of the volcanic hill, our configuration used wireless Ethernet components located at the refuge camp, and a repeater at the top of the hill to the Civilian Military Operations Center (CMOC) on the other side of the hill. This provided data transmission to the Naval ships and the Internet. Video traffic and data were transmitted via the satellite uplink from the camp at Pu'u Paa to a geostationary satellite 22,300 feet above California, and from the satellite to a transceiver in Greenville, NC. Transmissions from ECU to other participants included the use of T1, ISDN, or IP over Internet 2.

Experiments were designed, implemented, and assessed by the ECU Telemedicine Center staff. Video models were developed to test the technical feasibility and parameters for utilizing real-time and store and forward transmissions through Internet Protocols in several clinical specialties (dermatology, cardiology, pathology, psychiatry, trauma, obstetrics, pulmonology, endocrinology, and rehabilitation medicine). The speed and quality of transmissions through ham radio were also tested.

Throughout the five days of our participation in Strong Angel, we used distributed medical intelligence (DMI), a model of care currently used by ECU's Telemedicine Center (see Figure 1). The DMI model consists of care portals, the ECU bridge, and docking stations. The ECU bridge is the communications site linking the points of need (Care Portals) to the points of expert services [2].

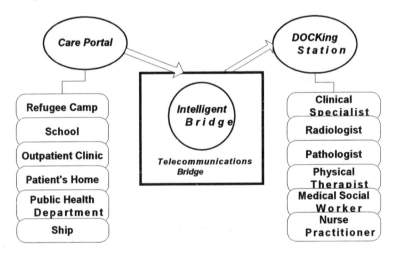

Figure 1. The Distributed Medical Intelligence (DMI) model used at East Carolina University and throughout Strong Angel. Care Portal was the refugee camp; docking stations were the clinical specialists.

Other telemedicine organizations around the world also agreed to evaluate transmissions and telemedicine delivered by the telecommunications established between Hawaii and Greenville. The data and video connectivity from refugee camp to the ECU bridge were via a satellite 512kbps IP link. Connectivity using ISDN, Internet 2, or T1 was used by the participating sites. These sites included: NASA: Houston, Texas; Ohio Supercomputer Center: Columbus, Ohio; Health Sciences University of Transkei, Umtata: Eastern Cape, South Africa; Denver Health Telemedicine Program: Denver, Colorado; Small World Foundation, International Craniofacial Institute: Dallas, Texas; St. Francis Hospital: Kona, Hawaii; Hawaii Health Systems Corporation (HHSC) — (Hilo); University of Hawaii; NASA Medical Informatics & Technology Applications Consortium (MITAC), Virginia Commonwealth University/MCV: Richmond, VA; Consortium for Worker Education: New York City, NY and the Greater New York Hospital Association; Catholic University of America: National Rehabilitation Hospital; and CRNR in Syracuse, New York and Loma Linda, California.

3. Results

We had planned on setting up a 1.2-meter satellite dish at the refugee camp, but found that the dish was too small for IP connectivity between Hawaii and ECU, providing only 64 kbps. Fortunately, we found a 1.8-meter dish on the island that provided adequate coverage, although it was not large enough for T1 transmissions and only operated reliably at 512 kbps. Once we obtained adequate equipment, it took 12 hours to operationalize the telemedicine system.

To establish connectivity using the ham radio, we needed to erect a 40-foot tower. Stabilizing the tower was a challenge due to the winds we encountered. We needed additional guy wire before we were confident in the stability of the tower. We realized as we were assembling the equipment for ham radio transmissions that the equipment for an austere environment was too large and bulky, and would not be an easy solution for telemedicine in most humanitarian responses. The technology must be scaled down before it is useful in austere environments. A possible solution might be the use of VHF instead of HF frequencies if the desired connection site could be reached. This type of local or regional transmission would provide higher bandwidth with a smaller antenna.

We used the Alicube software on the CyberMDx Telemedicine Instrumentation Pack (TIP) to create simulated patient encounters. Medical history data was used to establish 14 patient medical records, then images of dermatologic lesions, retinal scans, or pathology were stored with each patient record as a bundled file. Average file size was 175 Kb. A total of 2.45 megabytes of data were transmitted using IP via satellite at 512 kbps. Average transfer time was 39 seconds. The quality of the files did not differ when compared to transmission through a land based T1 line.

We were unable to use ham radio to transfer the same files. We experienced software problems at our receiving site, and were not prepared to make adjustments necessary to complete this experiment with ham radio.

The use of high frequency (HF) packet using ham radios is frequency dependent, but because of federal regulations, we could not go above 300 baud. We took a non-military approach and did not obtain any special permission for operating at reserved frequencies or higher bandwidth. While better performance over ham is possible with special permission during real disasters, our tests were designed to determine what the capabilities were in a non-military civilian environment.

Using slow scan analog audio, we were able to transmit three still images: one of a dermatologic lesion, one of an eardrum, and one of a patient's uvula. We also transmitted images of the refugee tents and one from inside the ham tent. It took an average of 29 minutes to transfer a file; files ranged from 35-55 Kb when transmitted, but 56-76 Kb when received. Average file size when transmitted was 37.4 Kb, and 65.3 Kb upon receipt. There was significant data interference due to sunspots and propagation errors, rendering some of the files useless upon receipt.

We found ham radios for file transfer unreliable, not only because it took about a half hour to transmit 65 Kb, but also because of the environmental conditions. The difficulty in erecting a radio tower in one day, a major solar flare the first day of operations, and the difficulty obtaining bandwidth, sometimes limited to 100 baud, prevented use of ham radio for most of the experiments we had planned. Ham radio was reliable for voice communications; we did communicate with 125 ham radio operators around the world throughout the four days of the exercise. Voice communication alone has tremendous value during disasters, and the usefulness of ham radio should not be underestimated because of its low cost and portability.

To evaluate interactive consultations, several simulations of traumatic injury (blunt facial trauma, blunt cardiac contusion, and chest injury with tension pneumothorax) and psychiatric conditions (depression, drug withdrawal, and anxiety) were enacted by the refugees at the camp. Consultations were provided by the ECU clinical staff, the Denver Health Authority, and the New York City Consortium for Worker Education and greater New York Hospital Association. Due to limited bandwidth and environmental factors, the only codec used was the Polycom. We experienced power problems that created artifacts and unsatisfactory audio signals, noticeable during windstorms. A 30-pound transceiver was mounted on the satellite dish at the refuge camp, with two aluminum rods holding it in place. There were artifacts and unsatisfactory audio signals with transmissions via IP video using 384 kbps and 512 kbps during these windstorms. We believe that the feed horn was being deflected from its axis, reducing the maximum bandwidth we were getting that resulted in perceived motion artifacts. Color was affected below 384 kbps, but was acceptable above this bandwidth. The lighting in the tent where the telemedicine consultations were conducted was poor, and contributed significantly to the low amplitude color level.

Accuracy of diagnosis was not affected, in spite of the slight but noticeable time delay. Participants were able to communicate without difficulty; they quickly developed listening skills that allowed for delays in the audio, and were patient when talking to one another. In one scenario, a clinical specialist provided guidance to a medic simulating the insertion a chest tube for a patient with a pneumothorax. Both the medic and consultant stated that the ability to communicate for this medical intervention was not affected by the telecommunications, and the medic's abilities were enhanced by the telecommunications and the knowledgeable resource at the docking station.

The ability to hear was evaluated with fetal heart tones previously recorded as digital audiotapes (DAT) played through a Polycom using a DAT machine. The consulting physician at ECU found the sounds to be clearly audible, stating that there was no difference between those sent through IP and those heard in person. We had intended to use the AMD 3200 stethoscope to assess pulmonary sounds. Technical problems at the remote site prevented the consultant at ECU from hearing anything further. Additional testing is planned for a later date.

The ability to transmit the digital measurements of knee flexion and extension from a goniometer was evaluated. Ten angles were measured and then transmitted to ECU, where readings were compared to actual measurements in Hawaii. The data was transferred without corruption, and measurements were consistent with each other.

We also expanded the use of our DMI model of care, adding a nurse to the bridge as a human component of the Intelligent Bridge. During this pilot study, a registered nurse who had never seen or used telemedicine talked to a non-clinical responder at the care portal. Five problems were discussed: lack of potable water, diarrhea in several small children, lack of formula for several infants, infestation of mosquitoes and their risk, and two term pregnancies that were breech presentations. The nurse had had over 15 years of experience, including experience in public health. She adapted to telemedicine equipment and real-time consultation immediately, providing knowledgeable and appropriate information for the concerns of the responder at the Care Portal in Hawaii, and also reassured the responder that help was forthcoming. To arrange for possible transfer of the two pregnant women, she then triaged the call to a clinical specialist on the nearest Hawaiian island.

During a second scenario, the bridge nurse talked to a medic evaluating a patient simulating a crushing blow to the chest. The nurse noted the need for emergency insertion of a chest tube due to tension pneumothorax, and triaged the call to a trauma physician in New York City who directed the medic. Adding a human component to the distributed medical intelligence model, in this case in humanitarian response, is a valuable part of the DMI model and deserves further exploration.

4. Conclusion

Telemedicine can be used in disaster situations and can be an important contribution to humanitarian relief efforts, but further research is needed to streamline the mission and develop a critical list of the appropriate equipment, supplies, and clinical personnel. As Garshnek and Burkle state, "the main challenge is to match the right communication and contingency systems with a given disaster medicine plan or scenario." [3] We found that even in a simulated disaster, simple things such as relief from the heat and wind, protecting equipment, and maintaining--at minimum--voice communication, were simple problems that became complex problems when not dealt with immediately. It was a challenge to configure the telecommunications, but once established we were able to use telemedicine to respond to the health and medical needs at the refugee camp.

Acknowledgements

This project has been funded in whole or in part with Federal funds from the National Library of Medicine, National Institutes of Health, under Contract No. N01-LM-9-3541, the National Aeronautic Space Administration, and the Brody School of Medicine at East Carolina University. Companies providing assistance / equipment during the study includes: Cisco Systems, Polycom, Inc., VBrick Systems, Inc., ViTel Net, American Medical Development, Prodelin Corporation, CyberMDx, MedWeb, Ball Aerospace and Technologies Corporation, and MindTel L.L.C. We would like to thank the Telemedicine Center staff who assisted in this study: Ron Rouse, Lori Maiolo, Tony Cook, Billy Igoe, Gloria Jones, and Chad Waters.

References

[1]   United States Navy, Learning lessons in RIMPAC 2000's "Strong Angel", http://www.cpf.navy.mil/rimpac2000/news/rimpac021.html, accessed June 23, 2000.
[2]   D.J. Warner, J.M. Tichenor, and D.C. Balch, Perspective: Telemedicine and distributed medical intelligence, *Telemedicine Journal* **2** (1996) 295-301.
[3]   V. Garshnek and F.M. Burkle, Applications of telemedicine and telecommunications to disaster medicine: Historical and future perspectives, *Journal of the American Medical Informatics Association* **6** (1999) 26-37.

Medicine Meets Virtual Reality 2001
J.D. Westwood et al. (Eds.)
IOS Press, 2001

REAL-TIME SIMULATION OF DYNAMICALLY DEFORMABLE
FINITE ELEMENT MODELS
USING MODAL ANALYSIS and SPECTRAL LANCZOS DECOMPOSITION
METHODS

Cagatay Basdogan, Ph.D.

Jet Propulsion Laboratory
California Institute of Technology
Pasadena, CA, 91109
Cagatay.Basdogan@jpl.nasa.gov

Real-time simulation of deformable objects using finite element models is a challenge in medical simulation. We present two efficient methods for simulating real-time behavior of a *dynamically* deformable 3D object modeled by finite element equations. The first method is based on modal analysis, which utilizes the most significant vibration modes of the object to compute the deformation field in real-time for applied forces. The second method uses the spectral Lanczos decomposition to obtain the explicit solutions of the finite element equations that govern the dynamics of deformations. Both methods rely on modeling approximations, but generate solutions that are computationally faster than the ones obtained through direct numerical integration techniques. In both methods, the errors introduced through approximations were insignificant compare to the computational advantage gained for achieving real-time update rates.

1. Physically-based modeling of deformable objects for medical simulation
Simulation of soft tissue behavior in real-time is a challenging problem. Once the contact between an instrument and tissue is determined, the problem centers on tool-tissue interactions. This involves a realistic haptic feedback to the user and a realistic graphical display of tissue behavior depending on what surgical task (e.g. suturing, grasping, cutting, etc.) the user chooses to perform on the tissue. This is a nontrivial problem which calls for prudence in the application of mechanistic and computer graphics techniques in an endeavor to create a make-believe world that is realistic enough to mimic reality but efficient enough to be executable in real time. Soft-tissue mechanics is complicated not only due to non-linearities, rate and time dependence in material behavior, but also because the tissues are layered and non-homogeneous. The finite element methods (FEM), though they demand more CPU time and memory, seem promising in integrating tissue characteristics into the organ models. Although mechanics community has developed sophisticated tissue models based on FEM, their integration with medical simulators has been difficult due to real-time requirements. Simulating the real-time deformable dynamics of a 3D object using FEM is increasingly more difficult as the total number of nodes/degrees of freedom (dof) increase. With the addition of haptic displays, this has been even more challenging since a haptic loop typically requires a much higher update rate than a visual loop for stable force interactions. Although fast finite element models have been developed for medical applications (Bro-Nielsen and Cotin, 1996; Berkley et al., 2000), less attention has been paid to displaying *time dependent* deformations of large size models in real-time. This paper introduces two numerically fast techniques for real-time simulation of *dynamically* deformable (i.e. time-dependent deformations) 3D objects modeled by FEM: (a) Modal analysis (Basdogan, 1999; Basdogan et al., 2000) and (b) spectral Lanczos Decomposition.

2. Our Finite Element Model
The finite element formulation: The 3D models of organs used in our simulations were constructed from discrete triangular surface elements interconnected to each other through nodal points. The coordinates of vertices (nodal points), the polygon indexing, and the connectivity of vertices were derived from the geometric model of each organ. In order to analyze the deformations of the organs

under various loading conditions, we considered a combination of membrane and bending elements in our finite element model. This facilitated the continuity in the formulation and enabled us to compute the displacements of nodal points in X, Y, Z directions for both inplane and bending loads. For each node of the triangular element subjected to inplane loads, the displacements in the local x and y directions were taken as the degrees of freedom. The resulting system equations were expressed in local coordinate system as

$$F_m = \left[k^e_m \right] U_m$$

(Eq. 1)

where, m represents the membrane action. Similarly, for each node of the triangular element subjected to bending loads, the displacement in local direction and rotations about the local x and y axes were considered. The relation between the vertex displacements and forces were written as

$$F_b = \left[k^e_b \right] U_b$$

(Eq. 2)

where, b represents the bending action. In order to obtain the local stiffness matrix for each triangular element, the inplane and bending stiffness matrices were combined. Since 6 degrees of freedom were assumed for each of the vertices, the resulting combined local stiffness matrix ($\left[k^e \right]$) became 18x18 for each triangular element.

Transformations: The stiffness matrix derived in the previous section utilizes a system of local coordinates. However, the geometric model of each organ was generated based on the global coordinate system. In order to apply the computations described in the previous section, a transformation from the global coordinates to local coordinate system was required (Zienkiewicz, 1990). It was also necessary to transform the results back to the global reference frame to display the deformations following the solution of finite element equations. The new positions of each nodal point for a given force were computed using system equations in the local coordinate system. Then, these new coordinates were transformed to the global coordinate system in order to update the graphics.

Assembly of Element Stiffness Matrices: The element stiffness matrices (K^e) were put together to construct the overall stiffness matrix (K). This process can be symbolically written as

$$K = \sum_{e=1}^{p} K^e$$

(Eq. 3)

where, p represents the number of triangles (Rao, 1988).

Implementation of Boundary Conditions: In order to obtain a unique solution for finite element equations, at least one boundary condition must be supplied. The boundary conditions modify the stiffness matrix K and make it nonsingular. There are multiple ways of implementing boundary conditions (Huebner et al., 1995). The easiest way to implement the boundary conditions is to modify the diagonal elements of the K matrix and the rows of the force vector F at which the boundary conditions will be applied. In our model, at least one end of the organ was always fixed, which implied zero displacements for the associated fixed nodes. To implement this boundary condition, diagonal elements of the K matrix and the rows of the F vector associated with those fixed nodes were multiplied by a large number. This procedure makes the unmodified terms of K very small compared to the modified ones.

<u>Eliminating the Rotational Degrees of Freedom (Condensation):</u> The global stiffness matrix was assembled as a symmetric square matrix and its length was six times the number of nodes of the object (recall that we defined 6-dof, 3 translations and 3 rotations, for each node of the object). Although the rotational dof were necessary for the continuity of the solution, their computation was not required for our simulations. Since our main interest was to obtain the translational displacements of each node, the overall stiffness matrix K was condensed such that the rotational dof were eliminated from the formulation. In addition, the condensation of K matrix automatically reduced the number of computations to half, which was helpful for achieving real-time rendering rates. To condense the K matrix, we first partitioned the displacement and load vectors of the static problem as

$$\begin{bmatrix} K_{tt} & K_{tr} \\ K_{rt} & Krr \end{bmatrix} \begin{bmatrix} U_t \\ U_r \end{bmatrix} = \begin{bmatrix} F_t \\ F_r \end{bmatrix}$$

(Eq. 4)

where, subscripts t and r represent the translational and rotational dof respectively. Then, we set the forces acting on the rotational degrees of freedom to zero, and condensed the stiffness matrix as

$$K_{condensed} = K_{tt} - K_{tr}(K_{rr})^{-1}K_{rt} \qquad \text{(Eq. 5)}$$

The condensed stiffness matrix was a full square matrix and its length was three times the number of nodes of the object.

3. Modal Analysis Method
The dynamic equilibrium equations for a deformable body modeled by FEM can be written as

$$M\ddot{U} + B\dot{U} + KU = F \qquad \text{(Eq. 6)}$$

where, M and B represent the mass and the damping matrices respectively. Once the equations of motion for deformable body are derived, the solution is typically obtained using numerical techniques. The real-time display of FEM becomes increasingly more difficult as the number of elements is increased. However, a particular choice of the mass and damping matrices reduces the number of computations significantly. If the mass matrix is assumed to be diagonal (mass is concentrated at the nodes) and the damping matrix is assumed to be linearly proportional with the mass matrix ($B = \alpha M$), the equations are greatly simplified. A further modeling simplification can be implemented if we assume that high frequency vibration modes contribute very little to the computation of deformations and forces. If dynamic equilibrium equations are transformed into a more effective form, known as modal analysis, fast real-time solutions can be obtained with very reasonable accuracy. Pentland and Williams (1989) demonstrated the implementation of this technique in graphical animation of 3D objects. In modal analysis, global coordinates are transferred to modal coordinates to decouple the differential equations. Then, one can either obtain the explicit solution for each decoupled equation as a function of time or integrate the set of decoupled equations in time to obtain the displacements and forces. Moreover, we can also reduce the dimension of the system, as well as the number of computations, by picking the most significant vibration modes of the object and re-arranging the mass, damping, and stiffness matrices. This procedure is also known as modal reduction.

3.1. Modal Transformation
We defined the following transformation to transform our differential system into a modal system:

$$U(t)_{nx1} = \Phi_{nxn} X(t)_{nx1} \qquad \text{(Eq. 7)}$$

where, Φ is the modal matrix, U and X represent the original and modal coordinates respectively. The modal matrix was obtained by solving the eigen problem for free undamped equilibrium equations:

$$K\phi = \omega^2 M\phi \qquad\qquad\qquad \text{(Eq. 8)}$$

where, ω and ϕ represent the eigenvalues (i.e. vibration frequencies) and eigenvectors (i.e. mode shapes) of the matrix ($M^{-1}K$) respectively. The modal matrix was constructed by first sorting the frequencies in ascending order and then placing the corresponding eigenvectors into the modal matrix in column-wise format ($0 \leq \omega_1 \leq \omega_2 \leq \omega_3 ... \leq \omega_n$, $\Phi = [\phi_1, \phi_2, \phi_3, ..., \phi_n]$). Finally, a set of decoupled differential equations (i.e. modal system) was obtained using the modal matrix and the transformation defined by Eq. 7:

$$\ddot{X}_i + \alpha_i \dot{X}_i + \omega_i^2 X = f_i \qquad\qquad i = 1, ..., n \qquad\qquad \text{(Eq. 9)}$$

where, n is the degrees of freedom (dof) of the system, $\alpha_i = 2\omega_i \zeta_i$, and $f_i = \phi_i^T F$ are the modal damping and force respectively. Note that ζ is known as the damping ratio or modal damping factor.

3.2. Modal Reduction

Once the equations for modal system are derived, the explicit solutions can be obtained using the Duhamel integral (see Bathe 1996). Alternatively, one can use numerical integration techniques to obtain the modal solution. At this stage, we can also implement the modal reduction approach to significantly reduce the number of computations. For a deformable body under external loading, the high frequency modes do not significantly contribute to the displacements. Hence, the final, deformed shape of the object can be approximated by "r" number of low frequency modes. To implement the modal reduction, we picked the most significant vibration modes of the object (i.e. the first "r" columns of the modal matrix). As a result, our differential system was reduced to "r" number of equations, which were solved using the Newmark numerical integration technique:

$$\ddot{X}^R_i + \alpha \dot{X}^R_i + \omega_i^2 X^R = f^R_i \qquad\qquad i = 1, ..., r \qquad\qquad \text{(Eq. 10)}$$

where, the superscript R represents the reduced system. We then transferred the modal solutions back to the original coordinate frame using the following transformation:

$$U(t)_{nx1} = \Phi^R_{nxr} X^R(t)_{rx1} \qquad\qquad\qquad \text{(Eq. 11)}$$

3.3. Numerical Integration

Numerical integration techniques are typically used to solve the differential equations that arise from finite element models. Various integration schemes based on finite difference techniques have been suggested in the literature for the dynamic analysis of FEM (Bittnar and Sejnoha, 1996; Bathe 1996). In surgical simulation, real-time performance and the stability of solutions for various loading, initial, and boundary conditions are equally important. For example, the central difference method appears to be fast and simple to implement, but the solutions become unstable if the integration step (Δt) is greater than (T_n / π), where T_n is the shortest period of vibration. Bathe (1996) suggests Newmark numerical integration procedure due to its favorable stability and accuracy characteristics. Using the Newmark method, we first formulated the displacement and velocity of each reduced modal coordinate at $t + \Delta t$ as

$$^{t+\Delta t}\dot{X}^R = {}^t\dot{X}^R + [(1-\delta){}^t\ddot{X}^R + \delta\,{}^{t+\Delta t}\ddot{X}^R]\Delta t \qquad \text{(Eq. 12)}$$

$$^{t+\Delta t}X^R = {}^tX^R + {}^t\dot{X}^R\,\Delta t + [(\frac{1}{2}-\eta){}^t\ddot{X}^R + \eta\,{}^{t+\Delta t}\ddot{X}^R]\Delta t^2 \qquad \text{(Eq. 13)}$$

where, η and δ are parameters that can be determined to obtain integration accuracy and stability (solutions become unconditionally stable for $\eta = 1/4$ and $\delta = 1/2$). Then, the equilibrium equation for each reduced modal coordinate was formulated at $t + \Delta t$ as

$$^{t+\Delta t}\ddot{X}^R + \alpha\,{}^{t+\Delta t}\dot{X}^R + \omega^2\,{}^{t+\Delta t}X^R = {}^{t+\Delta t}f^R \qquad \text{(Eq. 14)}$$

Finally, we substituted the displacement and velocity formulations into the equilibrium equation derived for $t + \Delta t$ and obtained a system that looks quite similar to the static analysis:

$$\hat{F}\hat{U} = \hat{K} \qquad \text{(Eq. 15)}$$

where, $\hat{F}, \hat{U}, \hat{K}$ are modified force and displacement vectors and modified stiffness matrix.

4. The Spectral Lanczos Decomposition Method (SLDM)

Druskin and Knizhnerman (1994) have recently introduced a new technique, called Spectral Lanczos Decomposition method (SLDM), to solve the Maxwell's diffusion equations for multiple frequencies with negligible additional computation. Zunoubi (1998) have demonstrated the efficiency of this technique by studying the resonant frequencies of various microwave cavities. We have followed their approach with some modifications to find the explicit solutions of our finite element equations. In order to solve the finite element equations using the SLDM, we first rearrange the terms of the finite element equations as:

$$\left[\frac{\partial}{\partial t^2}I + \alpha\frac{\partial}{\partial t}I + K'\right]E' = F' \qquad \text{(Eq. 16)}$$

where, $K' = M^{-1/2}KM^{-1/2}$, $E' = M^{1/2}U$, $F' = M^{-1/2}F$. If we transfer the equations to Laplace domain and assume that the applied force is constant for a short period of time with a magnitude of F_o, we obtain $E'(s) = F_o/(s(s^2I + \alpha s + K'))$. Using the separation of variables:

$$E'(s) = A/s + (Bs + C)/(s^2I + \alpha s + K') \qquad \text{(Eq. 17)}$$

where, $A = F_o/K'$, $B = -F_o/K'$ and $C = -(\alpha F_o)/K'$. Then, if we apply the inverse Laplace transform, we obtain:

$$E'(t) = F_o\frac{1}{K'}(1 - e^{\frac{-\alpha t}{2}}Cos(\sqrt{K' - (\alpha^2/4)I}\,t) + \frac{\alpha}{2}\frac{1}{\sqrt{K' - (\alpha^2/4)I}}e^{\frac{-\alpha t}{2}}Sin(\sqrt{K' - (\alpha^2/4)I}\,t)$$

$$\text{(Eq. 18)}$$

Now, if K' matrix is approximated as a diagonal matrix, we can easily obtain the time domain solutions. To achieve our goal, we implement the classical Lanczos scheme (Datta, 1994) with complete reorthogonalization using Householder transformations (Golub, 1996). For this purpose, we first compute the tridiagonal Ritz approximation (T) of the matrix K':

$$Q^T K'Q = T \qquad \text{(Eq. 19)}$$

where, $Q = [q_1, q_2, ..., q_M]$ is an orthogonal matrix (The vectors $q_1, q_2, ..., q_M$ are called Lancsoz vectors), M is the size of the square K' matrix (also the number of equations) and T is the tridiagonal matrix which is determined using the complete reorthogonalization Lanczos scheme that relies on repetitive Householder transformations (Golub, 1996). If we define the Λ and V are the eigen-values and -vectors of the matrix T, one can then write matrix T as:

$$T = V\Lambda V^T \qquad \text{(Eq. 20)}$$

where, $\Lambda = diag[\lambda_1, \lambda_2, \cdots, \lambda_M]$. Finally, $E'(t)$ can be approximated as:

$$E'(t) = F_o QV \left[\frac{1}{\Lambda}(1 - e^{\frac{-\alpha}{2}} Cos(\sqrt{\Lambda - (\alpha^2/4)}\, t)) + \frac{\alpha}{2} \frac{1}{\sqrt{\Lambda - (\alpha^2/4)}} e^{\frac{-\alpha}{2}} Sin(\sqrt{\Lambda - (\alpha^2/4)}\, t) \right] V^T e_1$$

$$\text{(Eq. 21)}$$

where, $e_1 = (1,0,0,\cdots,0)^T$ is a unit vector.

4.1. Superposition

After obtaining the explicit solutions of the finite element equations, we generate, an *"impedance map"* of the 3D object. This involves the pre-computation of displacement fields (i.e. a look-up table) by applying unit loads along each nodal degrees of freedom, while assuring the positive definiteness of the structure. Such a look-up table can be pre-computed well ahead of the actual interactions. We used this look-up table in conjunction with the "superposition" technique to calculate the deformations of the object for applied loads. The superposition approach calculates the response of the complete system by superimposing (i.e., adding together) the individual responses of the nodes. To calculate the response of a certain node, only the responses of neighboring nodes were used (i.e. define a *radius of influence* and consider the contribution of nodes which are within the radius of influence). The superposition approach provides a solution, which is an approximation to the exact solution, but this approximation is reasonably accurate (please note that we use a linear finite element model for simulating the behavior of tissues and this approximation will not work well with a nonlinear model).

5. Discussion

In this study, a modal analysis and the Spectral Lanczos Decomposition method were proposed to simulate the *dynamic* deformations of a 3D object modeled using finite elements. Although the proposed methods can simulate the real-time dynamics of a deformable object, our finite element model only approximates the characteristics of living tissues with a certain degree due to the stringent requirements of real-time simulation. However, we should point out that both methods are computationally faster than the direct numerical integration methods. For example, we have observed that the direct numerical integration of the original differential system results in $O(n^2)$ floating point operations (flops) where n is the degrees of freedom or the number of nodes of the object. However, the solutions generated using modal analysis lead to $O(n \log n)$ flops. Therefore, the real-time simulation of finite element models using the direct integration techniques will be increasingly more difficult as n increases. While the proposed modal approach enables to compute real-time solutions numerically, the SLDM can easily return the explicit solutions of the finite element equations for various frequencies. The SLDM, when combined with the superposition technique, is very efficient in simulating real-time deformations of objects. A pre-computed *"impedance* map" of an object using the SLDM enables us to estimate the deformation field of the object easily at the contact point during the real-time interactions.

References

1. Basdogan C., 2000, Course Name: Simulating Minimally Invasive Surgical Procedures in Virtual Environments: from Tissue Mechanics to Simulation and Training, Medicine Meets Virtual Reality (MMVR'2000), Jan. 27-30, Irvine, CA,
   http://www.amainc.com/MMVR/MMVR2000pro.html
   http://eis.jpl.nasa.gov/~basdogan/Tutorials/alltutorials.html (tutorial notes)
1. Basdogan, C., Ho, C., Srinivasan, M.A., 2000, "Virtual Environments for Medical Training: Graphical and Haptic Simulation of Laparoscopic Common Bile Duct Exploration", submitted to IEEE/ASME Transactions on Mechatronics.
2. Datta, B. N., 1994, "Numerical Linear Algebra and Applications", (Chapter 8: Numerical Matrix Eigenvalue Problems).
3. Druskin, V., Knizhnerman, L., 1994, "Spectral Approach to Solving Three-Dimensional Maxwell's Diffusion Equations in the Time and Frequency Domains", Radio Science, Vol. 29, No. 4, pp. 937-953.
4. Zunoubi, M., Donepudi, K.C., Jin, J.M., Chew W.C., 1998, "Efficient Time-Domain and Frequency-Domain Finite-Element Solution of Maxwell's Equations Using Spectral Lanczos Decomposition Method", IEEE Transactions on Microwave Theory and Techniques", Vol. 46, No.8, 1141-1149.
5. Golub, G.H., Van Loan C., 1996, "Matrix Computations", The Johns Hopkins University Press, Baltimore (see Chapters 5.1 and 9.2)
6. Rao, S.S., (1988), "The finite element method in engineering", Pergamon Press, New York.
7. Zienkiewicz, O.C., (1979), "The finite element method", McGraw-Hill, New Delhi.
8. Bathe, K., (1996), "Finite Element Procedures", Prentice Hall, New Jersey.
9. Bittnar, Z., Sejnoha, J., 1996, "Numerical Methods in Structural Mechanics", ASCE Press, New York.
10. Huebner, K.H., Thornton, E.A., Byrom, T.G., 1995, "The finite element method for engineers", John Wiley & Sons, Inc., New York.
11. Pentland, A., Williams, J., 1989, "Good Vibrations: Modal Dyanmics for Graphics and Animation", SIGGRAPH Proceedings, Vol. 23, No. 3, pp.215-222.
12. Bro-Nielsen, M., Cotin, S., 1996, "Real-time Volumetric Deformable Models for Surgery Simulation using Finite Elements and Condensation", EUROGRAPHICS'96, Vol. 15, No. 3, pp. 57-66.
13. Berkley, J., et al., 2000, "Creating Fast Finite Element Models from Medical Images", Proceedings of Medicine Meets Virtual Reality 2000, pp. 26-32.

Medicine Meets Virtual Reality 2001
J.D. Westwood et al. (Eds.)
IOS Press, 2001

Stereoscopic x-ray image processing

Alexander BERESTOV

Canon R&D Center Americas, Inc., 3300 N. First St., San Jose, CA 95134

Abstract. A three-step stereoscopic image-processing algorithm is proposed in order to improve image quality and depth perception of stereoscopic radiographs taken with C-arm equipment. The steps include illumination correction, geometry conversion and screen parallax adjustment. Flipping of stereoscopic radiographs is also discussed.

1. Introduction

Stereoscopic x-ray imaging can be an effective method for obtaining three-dimensional (3D) spatial information from two-dimensional (2D) projection x-ray images without the need for tomographic reconstruction. This much-needed information is missed in many x-ray diagnostic and interventional procedures, for example in orthopedic or chest x-ray imaging. New digital equipment such as the Canon Digital Radiography System CXDI-22 can obtain stereoscopic image pairs in digital format, which are ready for fast image processing and display.

A related problem is that of binocular stereo. The application of binocular stereo to x-ray imaging is not easy because there are no visible surfaces on the radiograph and information about different objects can be located at the same area of the x-ray image.

One of the problems with stereoscopic imaging is image distortion in stereoscopic video systems. Various image distortions include depth plane curvature, depth non-linearity, depth and size magnification, shearing distortions and keystone distortions. These problems were addressed in the papers [1] and [2].

Another source of errors in stereo image processing is illumination. When images of the same scene are taken by two different cameras or by one camera shifted horizontally or temporally, illumination of the scene changes depending on the conditions. This illumination change results in different brightness and contrast of the same area in two images. These errors lead to difficulties in observing images in stereo, in visual comparison of two images taken at different times, and in mathematical analysis such as stereo matching or image subtraction. This problem is important for both projective and reflective photography, and was addressed in the paper [3].

Here we propose a three-step stereoscopic image-processing algorithm in order to improve image quality and depth perception of stereoscopic radiographs taken with C-arm equipment. The first step is to adjust the illumination of x-ray stereo pairs. We propose to adjust the vertical columns of the images by equalizing the mean and standard deviation of grayscale pixel values in the vertical columns. The mean and standard deviation must be calculated, and then the histograms have to be adjusted to equalize them. Prior algorithms adjust histograms for the whole images and neglect illumination changes from left to right due to the rotation of the x-ray source.

The second step is to convert the toed-in stereoscopic system into a parallel one. A toed-in configuration has a big disadvantage. The problem lies in the inherent depth plane curvature. This curvature leads to incorrect depth perception and wrong calculations of relative object distances. This distortion can be eliminated. In order to do that the algorithm rotates the images in three-dimensional space. More specifically, the first image rotates clockwise and the second image rotates counter-clockwise for the same angle. This transformation places the images in the same plane, which is parallel to the base line between the two locations used to capture the images. During this procedure the keystone distortion is eliminated as well.

The final step is to change the screen parallax so that as many people as possible may view the stereoscopic image. It was suggested in [1] that the depth range should be minimized and the primary area of interest should be located near the surface of the monitor.

In chest radiography doctors always observe images with the heart located at the right side of the picture even if the radiograph was taken from the back. It is easy to flip regular film or a 2D digital radiograph and introduce no depth distortion because there is no depth in 2D images. The flipping of the stereoscopic x-ray images is different. The algorithm for flipping stereoscopic radiographs will be also presented.

2. Stochastic illumination adjustment

Usually digital stereo radiographs are taken with C-arm type equipment when the x-ray tube and sensor plate rotate in synchrony around the object for some angle. In this case the difference in contrast and brightness between stereo images depends on the position of the x-ray source, which illuminates the sensor plate at different angles, and varies in the direction perpendicular to the rotation axis.

It is possible to adjust brightness and contrast of two images using histogram adjustment [4]. In this paper the authors propose a color-matching algorithm, which equalizes the mean and standard deviation of grayscale values. The mean and standard deviation were calculated, and then the histogram was adjusted to equalize them. The problem with this adjustment is that the matching is made for the whole image, so the differences in illumination within the images remain unchanged. It is also not clear what algorithm the authors use for equalization.

In the present paper we suggest to utilize *a priori* known information about the illumination changes within the image and propose the algorithm for brightness, contrast, and color correction to eliminate the distinctions between images. Adjustments proposed in the above-mentioned paper do not change the horizontal variations in color and brightness. In order to correct them one needs to take into account the longitudinal trajectory of the x-ray tube.

Let X_1 and X_2 be discrete random variables with values $\{x_i^1\}$ and $\{x_i^2\}$. Then the expected or mean values of $X_{1,2}$ are defined by

$$EX_{1,2} = \mu_{1,2} = \sum_i x_i^{1,2} p(x_i^{1,2}) \qquad , \qquad (1)$$

where p is the probability function. The quantities

$$EX_{1,2}^2 - \mu_{1,2}^2 = \sigma_{1,2}^2 \qquad (2)$$

are the variances of $X_{1,2}$ or the expected values of the square of the deviations of $X_{1,2}$ from their expected values. We would like to adjust variables $X_{1,2}$ so that the expected values $\mu_{1,2}$ and variances $\sigma_{1,2}^2$ would be the same for both variables. In the simplest case we can use the linear transformation:

$$X_2 = aX_1 + b \qquad , \qquad (3)$$

where a and b are constant parameters. Substitution of (3) into (1) and (2) gives:

$$b = \mu_2 - a\mu_1 \; ,$$

$$a = \sqrt{\frac{\sigma_2^2}{\sigma_1^2}} . \qquad (4)$$

We propose to adjust the stochastic parameters of the images along the corresponding longitudes of the C-arm path. If the sensor plate rows are parallel to the plane of rotation, the adjustment has to be done for every column of pixels in the images.

Let us consider the pixel brightness level in the column of pixels in one image as X_1 and in another as X_2. This consideration gives as the mechanism of image adjustment. First we calculate expected values and variances for both columns using probability function. In the simplest case of the uniform distribution $p=1/H$, where H is the number of rows in the image, but it could be also any other reasonable distribution (exponential, normal, or derived from the data). The second step is pixel brightness recalculation in one or both images using equation (3). We can adjust one image to another, or adjust both images to some values μ and σ^2 (for example, to average values $\mu = (\mu_1 + \mu_2)/2$, $\sigma^2 = (\sigma_1^2 + \sigma_2^2)/2$, or to some other desirable values). Here we adjusted columns with the same number in both images, but it is possible to estimate the average disparity and equalize expected value and variance in the shifted columns.

3. Geometry conversion

C-arm configuration of an x-ray system is convenient for fast and accurate stereo pair acquisition. From the geometric point of view it is similar to a toed-in binocular stereo system. The toed-in configuration of the cameras in stereoscopic systems has two significant problems. The first problem is the depth plane curvature, which could lead to incorrect calculations of relative object distances (see [1], [2]).

Another well-known effect of the toed-in stereo system is keystone distortion. Keystone distortion causes vertical parallax in the stereoscopic radiograph due to the baseline of the two x-ray sources not being parallel to the surface of the screen. This is also the case when the stereo radiographs are obtained by the rotation of the object. In one of the radiographs, the image of the square appears larger at one side than at the other. In the other radiograph, this effect is reversed. This results in a vertical difference between homologous points, which is called vertical parallax. The amount of vertical parallax is greatest in the corners of the image and it causes difficulties in stereoscopic analysis and image perception.

Making the stereo system parallel can eliminate these distortions. In order to make it parallel, the proposed algorithm first rotates the images in three-dimensional virtual space as shown in Figure 1, and second eliminates vertical parallax.

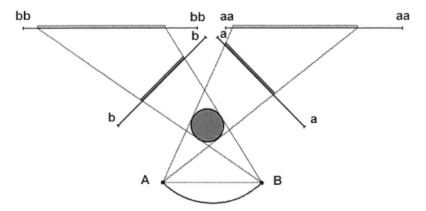

Figure 1. Conversion of toed-in geometry into parallel geometry

Here A and B represent the x-ray source location; b-b and a-a are the physical locations of the corresponding digital sensor plates; bb-bb and aa-aa are the new virtual locations of the corrected images. For every pixel of the converted image we locate the corresponding position on the physical sensor plate and assign to it the weighted data from the closest sensors. This transformation places the images in the same plane, which is parallel to the base line between the two locations used to capture the images.

In order to eliminate vertical parallax caused by keystone distortion and other factors two different approaches can be used. The first one is described in [3] and based on the fast correction algorithm, which adjusts the pixels in the images and sets them along the same rows. The algorithm estimates the epipolar geometry in the left and right parts of the images using a correlation matching technique and adjusts the rows if pixel line-by-line. Another approach is to use physical pointers in order to recover epipolar geometry. Those pointers can be located anywhere around the object, but must be present in the images.

The step of line-to-line row adjustment is the same as in the previous approach and is based on the assumption that the vertical parallax is a linear function of both the column and row number. Then, for every pixel in every row in the second image we have its own vertical parallax, which is not an integer value. Finally every pixel in the second image has to be recalculated at the new shifted position. The new grayscale value of the pixel is calculated by the linear interpolation between the values of the nearest pixels. For example, in Figure 2 the resultant shift is minus 3.3 pixels, so we take the forth and the third pixel above the point to be corrected, calculate a new weighted value, and make a substitution. The resulting pair of images has matching pixels lying on the same row, which is ideal for stereoscopic perception and helps in image analysis.

One of the advantages of the proposed algorithm is simultaneous correction of the keystone distortion along with any other linear distortions, which cause vertical parallax. For example, such distortions occur when the axis of c-arm rotation is not parallel to the columns of sensors on the digital plate. In these cases part of the image or the whole image could be shifted vertically and the effect of such a distortion could be even severe than keystone distortion.

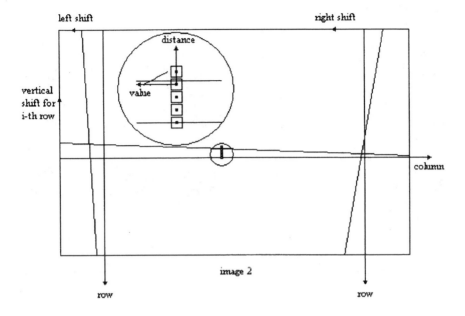

Figure 2. Epipolar adjustment scheme

4. Screen parallax adjustment

The final step is to change the screen parallax so that as many people as possible may view the stereoscopic image. It was suggested in [1] that the depth range should be minimized and the primary area of interest should be located near the surface of the monitor. This step can be performed manually or automatically. Physical or artificial pointers can be used during this process. We used the fiducial point located at the surface of the phantom and adjusted screen parallax, so that this point was at the level of the screen and the phantom appeared behind the screen.

Figure 4 illustrates the process with side-by-side images. In Figure 4a the original radiograph of the pelvis phantom is presented. One can see that four fiducial points at the corners are horizontally shifted due to the keystone distortion, illumination of the images is different and the stereo image appears in front of the screen.

5. Flip of stereo radiographs

In chest radiography doctors always observe images with the heart located at the right side of the picture even if the radiograph was taken form the back. It easy to flip regular film or 2D digital radiographs and no depth distortion will be introduced because there is no depth in 2D images. Flipping of stereoscopic radiographs is different. The curvature of the depth plane as the result of the toed-in camera configuration will cause undesirable effects after the flip.

For example, an object, which is parallel to the screen may transform into a curved one. In contrast the parallel camera configuration results in depth planes, which are parallel to the surface of the monitor and the mentioned distortions due to flipping do not exist. That is why the first step in flipping should be the conversion of toed-in camera geometry into parallel camera geometry described above.

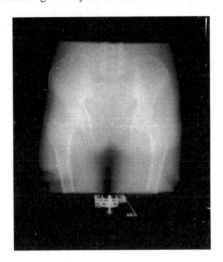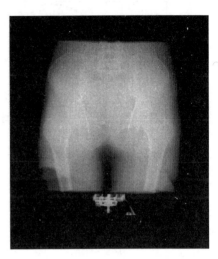

Figure 3a. Original stereo image of the pelvis phantom

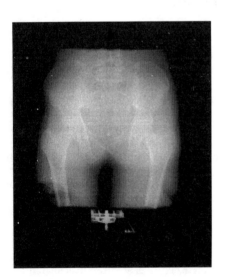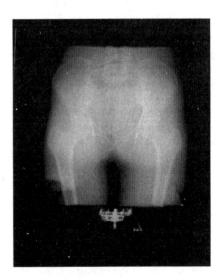

Figure 3b. Processed stereo image of the pelvis phantom

But even after conversion simple flip of both left and right images does not give the result anticipated by doctores. Figure 4 illustrates the problem.

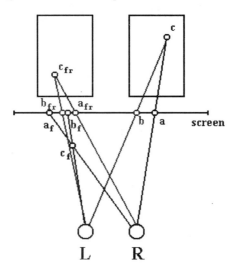

Figure 4. Geometry of the stereoscopic flips

Let us suppose that after adjustment the doctor sees a stereo radiograph of the black box with an object "c" behind the screen. In order to see the object "c" in 3D the left eye "L" and the right eye "R" must see the images of the object "c" on display in points "b" and "a" respectively. A simple flip of the left and right stereo images will put points "a" and "b" in different places "a_f" and "b_f", so that the object "c" will be seen at the new location "c_f". What is really needed is to look at the box from behind. Then, the images of the object "c" will be seen in the new locations "a_{fr}" and "b_{fr}", and the flipped box will appear behind the screen with the correct location of the object "c_{fr}".

This new screen parallax could be easily estimated from the geometry of the system. There are several ways to do that. The first is to locate the area of interest (object "c") and use it as a center of symmetry for display "rotation". The other way is to use the center of the body (black box in figure 3) as a center of symmetry. The third way is to always place the area of interest (object "c") or the surface of the body (black box) at the level of the display.

References

[1] A. Woods, T Docherty, and R. Koch, Image Distortions in Stereoscopic Video Systems, *Proceedings of the SPIE* **1915**, (1993) 36-48.
[2] A. Talukdar, and D. Wilson, Modeling and Optimization of Rotational C-Arm Stereoscopic X-Ray Angiography, *IEEE Transactions on Medical Imaging*, **18** (1999) 604-616.
[3] A. Berestov, Stereo Fundus Photography: Automatic Evaluation of Retinal Topography, *Proceedings of the SPIE* **3957**, (2000) 50-59.
[4] R. H. Eikelboom *et al.*, Development of stereo flicker chronometry and chronoscopy for serial retinal images, and correcting for color changes, *Technical Abstracts, SPIE's International Symposium on Medical Imaging*, (1999) p. 375.

Medicine Meets Virtual Reality 2001
J.D. Westwood et al. (Eds.)
IOS Press, 2001

Issues in Validation of a Dermatologic

Surgery Simulator

Daniel Berg, Jeff Berkley, Suzanne Weghorst, Gregory Raugi, George
Turkiyyah, Mark Ganter, Fernando Quintanilla, Peter Oppenheimer
*University of Washington Division of Dermatology, Department of
Engineering and Human Interface Technology Laboratory, Seattle,
Washington*

Abstract. At the University of Washington, we have been developing a suturing
simulator using novel finite element model techniques which allow real-time
haptic feedback. The issues involved in measuring validity in a suturing model
have not been examined in a systematic way. Very few studies exist on the
surgical factors that lead to good sutures. We have examined published data on
these factors as well as previously studied metrics in suture training. This
information has been combined with a review of types of validity (e.g., face,
construct, predictive and concurrent) and reliability that must be considered in
assessing any surgical simulator.

1. Introduction

Surgical simulation is increasingly being considered for training, testing and possibly
credentialing in surgery. Surgery on the skin ranges from simple suturing of lacerations to
complex tissue movements such as flaps. Simple suturing of lacerations may be
performed by many health care providers, including nurse practitioners, primary care
physicians, dermatologists and plastic surgeons. Training in cutaneous surgery uses the
traditional surgical apprenticeship model aided by tools such as suturing boards, pig's foot
training courses, or use of live animals. For a variety of reasons, these methods are not
ideal. At the University of Washington we have been developing a suturing simulator
based on finite element modeling methods that allow for real-time haptic interaction and
soft tissue deformation (Figure 1)[1-3]. Our model, as with all new technologies, should
be proven effective and reliable before its incorporation into medical training or
assessment programs. There can be pitfalls, as evidenced by previous virtual reality
simulators, which have failed tests of validity or reliability[4-7].

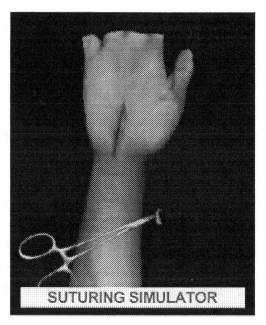

Figure 1. University of Washington Skin Surgery Simulator

2. Concepts in Validation

The key question that needs to be answered is, "Does proficiency in the simulator correlate with (in the case of surgical skill assessment) or lead to (in the case of surgical training) proficiency in reality"? This is a difficult question and requires assessment of multiple variables, often with multiple studies over time. The educational literature describes measurable definitions of validity and reliability, which can be used to assess an educational or assessment tool. These are summarized by Neufeld to include credibility, comprehensiveness, reliability, validity and feasibility[8].

Prior to any other test being performed, a simulator must first show *face validity* (credibility) for the task or subtask it is simulating. This means that the simulator must subjectively look and feel real enough to model the skills being tested. The absence of face validity means that operators of the simulator will not "buy into" the task. Surgeons will not use a simulator without face validity. Once the simulator demonstrates credibility, it should also be tested for *reliability* (precision, consistency). This means that the simulator, if tested, should return similar results under different conditions (e.g., at different times). *Content validity* measures the extent to which the simulator samples all possible aspects of the area of competence being looked at. For example, a test of technical competence has low content validity for global surgical competence because it does not test surgical judgment. To test *concurrent validity*, performance on the simulator is compared concurrently with performance on an external measure. For example, those who perform better in real-life arthroscopy should also perform better on the arthroscopy simulator. *Predictive validity* is demonstrated by showing that performance on the simulator correlates with performance on a future testable variable. For example, good dexterity on the suture simulator should correlate with subsequent evaluations by surgical training supervisors on trainees' dexterity. Finally, *construct validity* is shown when performance on the simulator is better in the hands of better-trained personnel. Orthopedic surgeons, for example, should perform better on an arthroscopy simulator than undergraduate students. Lack of construct validity calls into question the tasks that the simulator is testing. Particularly with respect to teaching, a simulator should also show *instructional effectiveness* which implies that repeated use of the model will improve user's performance[9].

Studies of validity and reliability may help to improve already useful simulations. A recent study of reliability and construct validity of an anesthesia patient simulation suggested areas of the simulation environment that showed poor reliability and needed further attention[5].

3. Reasons for Simulation Failure in Tests of Validation

There are many reasons a specific simulator may fail some of the tests of validation above. The simulator may be actually testing one or more confounding factors rather than surgical skill. For example, performance on a simulator may reflect differences in eye-hand coordination, eyesight or gamesmanship more than the skill being tested. This can lead to poor construct validity in testing. It is known that manual dexterity does not coordinate necessarily with experience or surgical skill. In one study looking at standardized tests of hand function, staff surgeons performed worse than staff internists, medical and surgical residents[10]. Many other factors can lead to poor results in validity testing. For example, if the task is not complex enough, a novice can do well, making it difficult to separate scores from those of an expert. An experienced surgeon knows what the real thing is like and may not suspend disbelief, focusing on the difference between the simulation and reality rather than on completing the task. Factors related to the validity testing itself may be a source of error. For example, if involved in the performance as well as evaluation of the test, an evaluator may influence or show bias in rating the subjects' performance[11]. Ultimately, true validity will only be determined if performance or training on a simulator can be shown to positively influence patient outcomes.

4. Possible Metrics in Evaluation of a Suture Simulator

In trying to evaluate what makes a good suturing model we must first define what makes good suture technique. Considering that this is a fundamental tool of all surgery, there has been surprisingly little attention paid to this issue. Seki has studied the factors involved in obtaining good sutures and he has shown that suture placement is less precise than many surgeons have predicted[12-18]. He has pointed out that there are no objective good data to allow gauging of the forces on the tissue that are appropriate for any organ such as skin[12]. In one study he measured distance deviated and force (expressed as torque on the needle driver – not tissue) used when placing sutures into predetermined entry and exit points on a foam model[12]. He found that a short grip on the needle and inclination of the tissue model generally enhanced accuracy and reduced force needed. There was considerable variation in results between the six surgeons tested. In this study, the ideal result was assumed to be precisely placed sutures producing minimal distortions of the tissue. He found also that precision of suturing as measured by distance away from a predetermined exit point showed that a grip in which all fingers are placed around the holder is more accurate than if the 1st and 4th fingers are placed in the holder.

Given the lack of quantitative data, it is not obvious which metrics to employ when evaluating any VR suture simulator. To date, several measures have been examined in validation studies of VR and mechanical suturing models. In one study of laparoscopic bowel suturing in a pig[19], subjects were asked to suture as quickly as possible 3 to 5mm from enterotomy edge and at 3 to 5 mm intervals. Vertical/horizontal deviations from desired entry/exit point of suture, execution time and failure to complete sutures were recorded. In a laparoscopic simulator [9,20], time to complete a task was measured. In addition, for each task a penalty was calculated for a predetermined measure of inaccuracy. Construct validity was examined by determining the correlation of score on the simulator with level of training[9]. Interestingly, the correlation was significant only for four out of seven tasks. One study comparing knot tying of medical students following either a lecture and seminar or a computer demonstration videotaped the students doing two knots[7]. Blinded surgeons reviewed the tapes and rated whether the knot was square.

They also measured time and used a rating scale identifying actions necessary for optimal performance. Interestingly, there was no difference in performance between the two groups. A more recent study looking at knot tying in a vascular VR model measured the skills of 8 experienced vascular surgeons and 12 medical students performing a virtual reality suturing task. Eight parameters of the suturing task were measured: total tissue damage, accuracy of needle puncture, peak tissue tearing force, time to complete the task, damage to the surface of the tissue, angular error in needle technique, total distance traveled by the tool tip, and a measure of overall error[21]. Construct validity was shown in this model.

At present we are considering the measurement of several parameters in future validation of our simulator. The simulator can easily track time taken per suture, symmetry of entry and exit points and spacing of sutures. Whether these parameters or others chosen will ultimately be useful at demonstrating simulator validity remains to be seen. Ultimately, it will need to be shown that performance or training on a simulator can be shown to positively influence patient outcomes.

References

[1]   Berkley, J., Oppenheimer, P., Weghorst, S., Berg, D., Raugi, G., Ganter, M., Brooking, C. and Turkiyyah, G. (2000) Creating fast finite element models from medical images. In: Medicine Meets Virtual Reality 2000 (Westwood, J. et al., eds.), pp. 26-32, IOS Press, Newport Beach.

[2]   Berkley, J., Weghorst, S., Gladstone, H., Raugi, G., Berg, D. and Ganter, M. (1999) Fast finite element modeling for surgical simulation. Stud Health Technol Inform 62, 55-61.

[3]   Gladstone, H.B., Raugi, G.J., Berg, D., Berkley, J., Weghorst, S. and Ganter, M. (2000) Virtual reality for dermatologic surgery: virtually a reality in the 21st century. J Am Acad Dermatol 42, 106-12.

[4]   Beckmann, C.R., Lipscomb, G.H., Ling, F.W., Beckmann, C.A., Johnson, H. and Barton, L. (1995) Computer-assisted video evaluation of surgical skills. Obstet Gynecol 85, 1039-41.

[5]   Devitt, J.H., Kurrek, M.M., Cohen, M.M., Fish, K., Fish, P., Noel, A.G. and Szalai, J.P. (1998) Testing internal consistency and construct validity during evaluation of performance in a patient simulator [see comments]. Anesth Analg 86, 1160-4.

[6]   Prystowsky, J.B., Regehr, G., Rogers, D.A., Loan, J.P., Hiemenz, L.L. and Smith, K.M. (1999) A virtual reality module for intravenous catheter placement. Am J Surg 177, 171-5.

[7]   Rogers, D.A., Regehr, G., Yeh, K.A. and Howdieshell, T.R. (1998) Computer-assisted learning versus a lecture and feedback seminar for teaching a basic surgical technical skill. Am J Surg 175, 508-10.

[8]   Neufeld, V. (1985) An introduction to measurement properties. In: Assessing Clinical Competence (Neufeld, V. and Norman, G., eds.), pp. 39-50, Springer, New York.

[9]   Derossis, A.M., Bothwell, J., Sigman, H.H. and Fried, G.M. (1998) The effect of practice on performance in a laparoscopic simulator. Surg Endosc 12, 1117-20.

[10]   Squire, D., Giachino, A.A., Profitt, A.W. and Heaney, C. (1989) Objective comparison of manual dexterity in physicians and surgeons. Can J Surg 32, 467-70.

[11]   Kapur, P.A. and Steadman, R.H. (1998) Patient simulator competency testing: ready for takeoff? [editorial; comment]. Anesth Analg 86, 1157-9.

[12]   Seki, S. (1988) Suturing techniques of surgeons utilizing two different needle-holder grips. Am J Surg 155, 250-2.

[13]   Seki, S. (1988) Techniques for better suturing. Br J Surg 75, 1181-4.
[14]   Seki, S. (1989) Suturing techniques of individual surgeons--differences in accuracy and
         mechanics. Jpn J Surg 19, 425-31.
[15]   Seki, S., Iwamoto, H. and Osaki, H. (1993) Suturing techniques for a restricted operating
         space. Int Surg 78, 86-90.
[16]   Seki, S., Iwamoto, H., Osaki, H. and Komoto, Y. (1993) The surgeon's technical skill in
         suturing: an analysis of the actual suture tracks. Surg Today 23, 800-6.
[17]   Seki, S. (1987) Accuracy of suture techniques of surgeons with different surgical
         experience. Jpn J Surg 17, 465-9.
[18]   Seki, S. (1987) Accuracy of suture placement. Br J Surg 74, 195-7.
[19]   Joice, P., Hanna, G.B. and Cuschieri, A. (1998) Ergonomic evaluation of laparoscopic
         bowel suturing. Am J Surg 176, 373-8.
[20]   Derossis, A.M., Fried, G.M., Abrahamowicz, M., Sigman, H.H., Barkun, J.S. and
         Meakins, J.L. (1998) Development of a model for training and evaluation of
         laparoscopic skills. Am J Surg 175, 482-7.
[21]   O'Toole, R.V., Playter, R.R., Krummel, T.M., Blank, W.C., Cornelius, N.H., Roberts,
         W.R., Bell, W.J. and Raibert, M. (1999) Measuring and developing suturing technique
         with a virtual reality surgical simulator [see comments]. J Am Coll Surg 189, 114-27.

Medicine Meets Virtual Reality 2001
J.D. Westwood et al. (Eds.)
IOS Press, 2001

Software Framework for a Surgical Guidance System using Magnetic Markers

Ankur Bhargava[2], C. Sean Hundtofte[1,2], Mark Thober[2], A. Bzostek[1,2], R.H. Taylor[1,2]

[1] *Computer Integrated Surgical Systems and Technology ERC*
[2] *Department of Computer Science, Johns Hopkins University*

Use of active, optical tracking Surgical Guidance systems provides line of sight problems to the surgeon. We plan to use a new magnetic system, 'Aurora' from Northern Digital Inc. (Canada) and Mednetix AG (Switzerland), in intra-operative fluoroscopy to develop an integrated system for surgical guidance. Here we outline the modules developed for use with this system, including a novel registration method.

1. Summary

Intra-operative fluoroscopy is useful in many percutaneous procedures and spinal surgeries, such as bone biopsy and vertebroplasty. Drawbacks, however, include exposing the surgeon to repeated doses of radiation, obstructing access with the C-arm in the operating area, and the limited number of views available.

A possible solution to these problems is 'virtual fluoroscopy', where an initial fluoroscopic image is captured and a representation of a (tracked) instrument is projected onto the image. This reduces the amount of exposure to radiation during the procedure, allows multiple views and reduces the amount of obstruction from the C-arm during surgery.

2. Previous work

Existing 2D-3D point registration algorithms rely on the availability of a large number of data points; Iterative Closest Point (ICP) and other statistical approaches do not work well with small data sets owing to local minima. Our system is intended to be used with 4 to 6 markers. A recent, and similar, alternative to ICP is 3PLFLS[1] - we will discuss the differences in our approach later.

3. Workflow

The markers will be in view of the C-arm whenever calibration/registration is performed or updated, they could be on the instrument to be artificially rendered itself, or a separate calibration object.

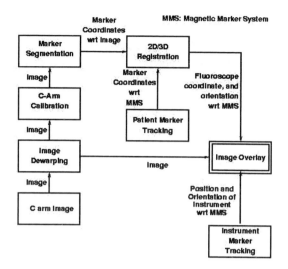

Figure 1. System Diagram of envisioned Virtual Fluoroscopy System

- C-arm image acquisition - A C-arm image is acquired with a frame grabber card.
- Image Dewarping - A patterned aluminum plate is imaged by the C-Arm and the two-pass scan line strategy as shown in [2] is used for building an LUT for dewarping.
- C-arm Calibration - A helix of beads is imaged in the C-Arm and calibration methods shown by Schreiner in [3] are used to determine the intrinsic parameters of the C-Arm.
- Segmentation of markers - Magnetic markers are segmented from the C-Arm images using a generalized Hough Transform and interpolation. The segmented markers are used to compute their 2D coordinates on the image (geometric centers).
- 2D/3D registration - The set of 3D marker coordinates and their corresponding set of 2D image coordinates are used to compute the orientation and position of the camera (C-arm) with respect to the marker coordinate system. The algorithm assumes knowledge of the focal length and image scale. It selects three points out of the set segmented in the image, then cycles through all possible permutations of triangles in

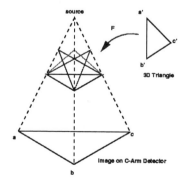

Figure 2. Four poses of a triangle

3D, each of which give 4 different poses (Figure 2), using constraints[4] for a closed-form solution to select the pose with least error. A gradient descent approach is used to refine this pose. Our approach here avoids the use of optimization methods to find point-to-point correspondence[1].

- Marker tracking - As the magnetic marker system is not yet available, we have used the Polaris optical tracking system from Northern Digital Inc. (NDI). The tracking device supplies the 3D coordinates of the markers in its coordinate system.
- Image Overlay - Slicer[5] was extended to take fluoroscope input and project a 3D representation of an instrument onto the image using the previously obtained transformation from tracking system to C-arm space. This stage provides the real-time surgical guidance.

4. Results

The software framework has been tested on real and simulated data sets. Preliminary registration results with artificial data sets (4 and 6 points) and white noise (magnitude 1 mm): average time 7.9s, residual RMS error of 0.5, 4 degree maximum error in the rotation matrix, L2 error in translation of 1.1 mm.

5. Conclusions

The Registration algorithm as developed so far provides quick and accurate solutions. Further degrees of information from the markers should provide us with more opportunities than the existing point-to-point correspondence. We hope to extend this using the orientation and length(in image space) of identified markers.

The final system is envisioned to be a part of a larger surgical aid which can present a surgeon with visualizations of different data sets (fluoroscope, CT data, MRI data) embedded with rendered surgical tools in real time. Further work is required: integration of the system, experimentation in more realistic conditions (animal, cadaver experiments); testing the segmentation algorithm in more cluttered images, and the monitoring of deformations that occur during surgery. Effects on surgical efficiency and operative time will also be examined.

Acknowledgements

The authors greatly acknowledge the support of the National Science Foundation under Engineering Research Center grant #EEC9731478.

References

[1] T.S.Y.Tang, R.E.Ellis, G.Fichtinger, `Fiducial Registration from a Single X-Ray Image: A New Technique for Fluoroscopic Guidance and Radiotherapy', MICCAI conference proceedings, 2000.

[2] J.Yao, R.H.Taylor et al, `A progressive Cut Refinement Scheme for Revision Total Hip Replacement Surgery using C-arm Fluoroscopy', MICCAI conference proceedings, 1999.

[3] S.Schreiner et al, `A System for Percutaneous Delivery of Treatment with a Fluoroscopically-guided Robot', Joint Conf. Of Computer Vision, Virtual Reality and Robotics in Medicine and Medical Robotics and Computer Surgery, Grenoble, France, 1997.

[4] Haralick, Lee, Ottenburg, Noelle, `Analysis and solutions of the three point perspective pose estimation problem', Computer Vision and Pattern Recognition, 1991. Proceedings CVPR '91., IEEE Computer Society Conference on , 1991.

[5] D.Gering et al, `An Integrated Visualization System for Surgical Planning and Guidance Using Image Fusion and Interventional Imaging', MICCAI conference proceedings, 1998.

Medicine Meets Virtual Reality 2001
J.D. Westwood et al. (Eds.)
IOS Press, 2001

Measuring In Vivo Animal Soft Tissue Properties for Haptic Modeling in Surgical Simulation

Iman Brouwer, Jeffrey Ustin, Loren Bentley, Alana Sherman, Neel Dhruv
and Frank Tendick
Department of Surgery, University of California, San Francisco, CA 94143-0475, and
Robotics and Intelligent Machines Laboratory, University of California, Berkeley
frankt@itsa.ucsf.edu

Abstract. To provide data for the design of virtual environments and teleoperated systems for surgery, it is necessary to measure tissue properties under both in vivo and ex vivo conditions. The former provides information about tissue behavior in its physiological state, while the latter can provide better control over experimental conditions. We have developed devices to measure tissue properties under extension and indentation, as well as to record instrument-tissue interaction forces. We are creating a web database of data recorded from porcine abdominal tissues.

1. Introduction

To produce realistic behavior in virtual environment simulations for surgical training, it is important to have good models of tissue behavior and instrument-tissue interaction. Although much of the research in modeling the mechanical behavior of tissue has emphasized load-bearing tissues for biomechanics, there has been work on measuring and modeling the behavior of soft tissues as well [1,2]. This work has relied on ex vivo tissue samples from animals and human cadavers. More recently, devices were developed to test tissue behavior in vivo under limited conditions [3–5]. Several devices have also been created to measure interaction forces between instruments and tissue [6,7].

Each of these types of measurements has advantages and limitations. Ex vivo tissue allows precise control of sample shape for modeling. In vivo measurements give data on tissue in its natural state (i.e., perfused with blood, in a typical stress state, and with muscle activation). Mounting surgical instruments with force sensors can measure interaction forces that are too complex to model, but direct tissue measurements are necessary to augment this data. Our research group has developed devices for each of these types of measurements, allowing us to produce a database of properties and integrate models based on data from different types of measurements.

2. Methods

2.1 Tissue Extension

To measure in vivo and ex vivo properties of tissues in extension we designed a device with interchangeable jaws to grasp tissue (Figure 1). A stepper motor-driven linear stage

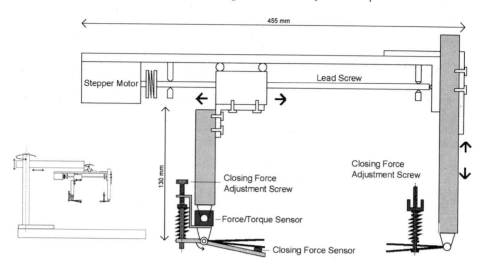

Figure 1. The instrument used for unixial stretching experiments in-vivo and ex-vivo. Inset shows how the device mounts on the operating table.

allows one of the jaws to be moved with specified velocity and acceleration until a certain position or force is reached. The closing force of this jaw is recorded by a button force sensor. The forces that the tissue exerts on the jaws are recorded by a 6-axis force-torque sensor. The jaws can be rotated to grip the tissue at an angle. Dimensions of the device are such that it can be used in the abdomen of a pig. The device can be mounted on an operating table.

The button sensor that measures the closing force is a miniature load cell (Sensotec model 13, www.sensotec.com). This sensor is read by a 12 bit A/D converter. The 6-axis force-torque sensor is a nano-17 transducer from ATI Industrial Automation (www.ati-ia.com) with a resolution of 0.0125 N. Custom software on a PC records the force/torque data from the two sensors, the position from the stepper motor, and the time with a frequency of 40 Hz.

For the in vivo measurements, jaws from laparoscopic Babcock graspers (U.S. Surgical, www.ussurg.com) are placed on both sides on the instrument. The distance between the jaws is marked on the tissue before clamping the tissue in the instrument. Soft tissues have very low resistance to deformation in their physiological rest state and even careful handling of the tissue can cause it to deform and change the perceived initial length. The viscoelastic behavior of the tissues requires all measurements to be performed on a new stretch of tissue.

Different organs required different techniques. For example, the small intestine was grasped as a double layer of tissue. The stomach was emptied and incisions were made in the stomach wall to insert the grasper jaws to grasp a single wall. Measurements on the intestine and stomach were carried out in both longitudinal and transverse directions. The gall bladder was first drained and than removed from the liver to avoid the mechanical properties of the liver interfering with the measurement.

For ex vivo measurements, custom clamps are used that minimize local stress concentrations. Ex vivo data is often presented on tissues in the preconditioned state. This state is reached by stretching and relaxing the tissue until the obtained stress-strain loop no longer changes over each cycle. Preconditioning of tissue makes it easier to compare results because repeatable measurements can be obtained. Since information about the original state of the tissue is lost in this process, we also obtain first-stretch measurements of the tissues. To minimize the change of properties during removal of the tissue, the time between removal and measurement needs to be kept as short as possible. To minimize stretching of tissue in the plane of measurement while preparing the samples, the samples were cut with a 'cookie cutter' that only exerted vertical forces while cutting. To trace the change in geometry of the tissue while being cut out of the organ and cut into a sample, the tissue was marked at certain points before removal and compared to the distances between the marks afterward. For the measurements on the stomach, the mucosa was detached from the muscularis and serosa.

For analysis, the data can be curve-fitted to the function $F(\lambda) = \alpha e^{\beta\lambda}$ in which λ is the Lagrangian stretch ratio l/l_0 and F is the measured force [8]. Taking the derivative $dF/d\lambda = \beta F$ results in parameter β as a measure of the stiffness of the tissue.

2.2 Tissue Indentation

Some tissues are too fragile to be tested under tension. For these, a system was designed for indenting abdominal tissues in vivo. The system consisted of a position- and velocity-sensitive indentation device and a force sensor mounted at the end of the device. The indentor used was a Phantom 1.5 haptic device from Sensable Technologies (www.sensable.com) while the force sensor was a six-axis force/torque sensor (described in section 2.1). The nominal position resolution of the Phantom was 30 microns. The sensor was mounted between the Phantom and a 2 cm diameter hemispherical plastic indentor. Computer control was provided by a Silicon Graphics workstation, which sampled position and force at a rate of 30 Hz. The Phantom can be used in a controlled mode so that indentation occurs at a constant velocity to determine viscoelastic effects, or contact force increased up to a set level.

A platform rigidly attached to the Phantom was arranged to lie over the abdominal cavity so that tissues could be pulled out of the abdominal cavity and placed on the platform. The sample tissues were not separated from their anatomical connections ensuring that the tissue properties were gathered in a physiological state. After a tissue was placed on the platform, the Phantom indentor and ATI sensor were used to measure displacement and contact force information. So far, we have gathered data for porcine stomach, liver, spleen, and skin.

2.3 Instrument-Tissue Interaction Forces

The third set of measurement devices were designed to record interaction forces between instruments and tissue. Force and torque data was collected while driving a needle through a variety of tissue types while applying tension to the tissue. A standard laparoscopic grasper with a 5 mm diameter shaft was modified to incorporate a force-torque sensor in the shaft (Figure 2, top). The shaft was cut approximately 5.5 cm from the handle and 4 cm from the grasper tip. Two aluminum mounting fixtures consisting of a tube fitted to the shaft and an end plate for attachment to the mounting plates of the sensor were used. The cylinder was attached to the instrument shaft with set screws while the end plate was attached with fasteners to the sensor mounting surfaces. The inside diameter of the fixture on the grasper side was drafted to allow the jaws to be opened, while two additional set screws were used to clamp the jaws. The sensor used was the six-axis ATI sensor described in section 2.1. A curved tapered needle was clamped into the jaws such that the plane of curvature was normal to the instrument shaft. The tip of the needle was offset

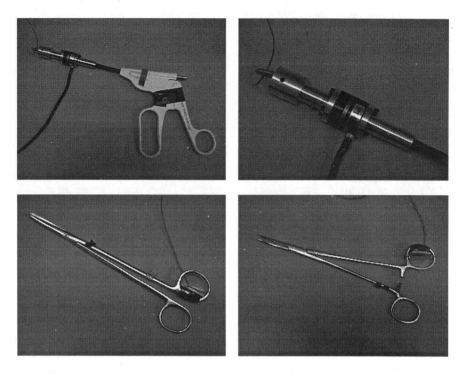

Figure 2. Force sensors mounted on surgical instruments. Top: 6-axis force/torque sensor on adapted grasper (left); close-up of sensor attachment (right). Bottom: load cell mounted on scissors (left) and clamp (right) to measure cutting and spreading forces, respectively.

from the sensor origin by 10 mm along the x-axis, 8 mm along the y axis, and 42.7 mm along the z axis. Force data was recorded at a rate of about 30 Hz.

In the needle-driving task, the needle was driven through a bite of the tissue, as in suturing, while an uninstrumented grasper was used in the opposite hand to put the tissue in tension. The 'traction' task measured the amount of force on the instrument being used to apply the tension. The needle was first driven through the tissue as a means of holding the tissue, then the appropriate amount of tension was applied. All of the tasks were performed by a surgical resident, whose judgment determined the size of the bite of tissue used and the amount of tension necessary for putting in a suture. For each task and tissue combination, five sets of data were collected. A continuous stream of data was collected during the performance of the task. Trials were performed on both a 20 kg pig and an immature 10 kg pig. There were eight tissue and activity combinations: driving a 3.0 suture through anterior stomach wall tissue, driving a 3.0 suture through the abdominal wall, putting the anterior stomach wall in tension, driving a 3.0 suture through bladder, putting the bladder in tension, driving a 3.0 suture through the esophagus tissue, driving a 4.0 suture through small intestine tissue, and driving a 4.0 suture through the common bile duct.

The second set of data was collected using a 1-axis force sensor to measure the forces involved in cutting and spreading tissue. The one axis sensor was mounted on the handle of standard open surgical instruments used for cutting and spreading tissues (Figure 2, bottom). The instruments used were curved Metzenbaum scissors and a curved Kelly clamp. A fixture was built such that the forces applied between the surgeon's thumb and the handle were collected. Five tissue and task combinations were investigated using the immature pig: dissecting peritoneum near the common bile duct, spreading mesentery,

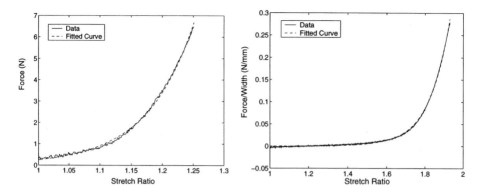

Figure 3. Plots of in-vivo (left) and ex-vivo (right) measurements of porcine small intestine. The width of the ex-vivo sample is 15mm. The in-vivo measurement is performed with an 8mm wide babcock gripper.

cutting anterior stomach wall, cutting abdominal wall, and cutting skin. Each task was repeated five times.

3. Results

Measurements were obtained in the Experimental Surgery Laboratory at UCSF from pigs used immediately prior to the experiments for other research. The animals were anesthetized and supervised under appropriate animal care protocols. An incision was introduced in the belly to allow access to the abdominal cavity.

Both in-vivo and ex-vivo uniaxial stretching experiments were been performed on porcine abdominal tissue. We have performed measurements on the gallbladder, stomach (muscularis and mucosal layers), and large and small intestine, and achieved excellent exponential fits to obtain curve parameters. Two typical examples of preliminary results with exponential fits are presented in Figure 3.

Curve fitting the datasets to the function $\alpha e^{\beta \lambda}$ gives the following values for α and β:

in-vivo: $\quad \alpha = 4.3E-7 \quad \beta = 13$

ex-vivo: $\quad \alpha = 3.7E-9 \quad \beta = 9.4$

Differences in boundary conditions between the in-vivo measurements and ex vivo measurements cause the curves to have a different shape. The slope of the in vivo curve increases at lower stretch ratios than the ex vivo curve. The effect of preconditioning of ex vivo tissue is shown in Figure 4. With the increase in the number of cycles, the hysteresis decreases while the curve shifts. The differences between the cycles become smaller with increasing number of cycles.

In the instrument-tissue experiments, the data of interest included the maximum forces and torques on the instrument and any differences between the adult and immature pigs. For both the large and small animals, the maximum forces in most trials were between 1.5 and 3 N. There were isolated instances in which forces above this range, between 6 and 12.5 N, were recorded. These cases occurred in situations in which the instrument was being used to lift the weight of the tissue being investigated, so that the force on the instrument was a combination of forces due to the tissue properties and those due to gravity. Over all the trials, the forces and torques in the adult were slightly higher, but not by a significant amount. The maximum forces recorded on a given trial in the cutting and spreading experiments ranged between 3–6 N.

Additional data from these trials and results from the indentation measurements are available on our web page, http://robotics.eecs.berkeley.edu/~tendick/tissue.html.

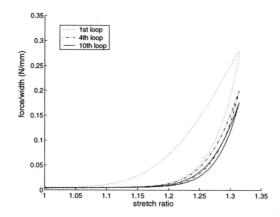

Figure 4. Ex vivo preconditioning of stomach mucosal tissue, showing first, fourth, and tenth stretch-relax cycles of the same tissue sample.

4. Future Work

The project is proceeding in several directions. We are gathering a database of properties that will be made public on the web site as a resource for other researchers. We are attempting to develop finite element models to relate in vivo tissue and instrument-tissue interaction data to the more accurate ex vivo data to estimate the result of tissue behavior local to contact. In particular, we are interested in estimating when tissue damage will occur as a function of instrument type, contact, and tissue type. Finally, we are using the data to establish design parameters for teleoperative surgical systems as well as simulation.

5. Acknowledgments

This research was supported by the National Science Foundation under grants IRI-9531837 and CDA-9726362.   We thank Mark Fighera of U.S. Surgical for donating the laparoscopic instruments used.

References

[1] Fung, Y.C. (1990). Biomechanics: Motion, Flow, Stress, and Growth. Springer-Verlag, New York.
[2] Yamada, H. (1970). Strength of Biological Materials. Edited by F. Gaynor Evans. Williams & Wilkins, Baltimore, MD.
[3] Carter, F.J. (1998). "Biomechanical testing of intra-abdominal soft tissue," Intl Workshop on Soft Tissue Deformation and Tissue Palpation, Cambridge, MA.
[4] Hoeg, H.D., A.B. Slatkin, J.W. Burdick, and W.S. Grundfest (2000). "Biomechanical modeling of the small intestine as required for the design and operation of a robotic endoscope," Proc. IEEE Intl. Conf. Robotics and Automation, San Francisco, CA, pp 1599-1606.
[5] Vuskovic, V. M. Kauer, G. Szekely, and M. Reidy (2000). "Realistic force feedback for virtual reality based diagnostic surgery simulators," Proc. IEEE Intl. Conf. Robotics and Automation, San Francisco, CA, pp 1592-8.
[6] Hannaford B., J. Trujillo, M. Sinanan, et al. (1998). "Computerized endoscopic surgical grasper," Medicine Meets Virtual Reality, J.D. Westwood et al., eds., IOS Press, Amsterdam, pp. 265-71.
[7] Morimoto A.K., R.D. Foral, J.L. Kuhlman, et al. (1997). "Force sensor for laparoscopic Babcock," Medicine Meets Virtual Reality, K.S. Morgan et al., eds., IOS Press, Amsterdam, pp. 354-61.
[8] Fung, Y.C. (1993). Biomechanics: Mechanical properties of living tissues. Springer-Verlag, New York.

Medicine Meets Virtual Reality 2001
J.D. Westwood et al. (Eds.)
IOS Press, 2001

A Virtual Environment
for Simulated Rat Dissection

Cynthia Bruyns[1] Kevin Montgomery[2] Simon Wildermuth [2]

[1] *Lockheed Martin Space Operations, Mail Stop 239-11, Moffett Field, CA, 94035*
[2] *National Biocomputation Center, 701 Welch Road, Suite 1128, Palo Alto, CA 94304*

Abstract Animal dissection for the scientific examination of organ subsystems is a delicate procedure. Performing this procedure under the complex environment of microgravity presents additional challenges because of the limited training opportunities available that can recreate the altered gravity environment. Traditional crew training often occurs several months in advance of experimentation, provides limited realism, and involves complicated logistics. We have developed an interactive virtual environment that can simulate several common tasks performed during animal dissection. In this paper, we describe the imaging modality used to reconstruct the rat in virtual space, provide an overview of the simulation environment and briefly discuss some of the techniques used to manipulate the virtual rat.

1. Introduction

The International Space Station will be expanding its research capabilities over a number of years to support a wide variety of scientific and technological experiments. The biological experiments performed within this facility will investigate the effects of near weightlessness on successive generations of organisms of various complexities. These experiments will allow scientists to analyze the physiological processes that are modified during space flight without exposing living tissue of the organism to the biological modifications what would occur during re-entry to a 1g environment. Both on-orbit and subsequent terrestrial evaluation will require the tissues to be of the highest quality in order to increase the scientific return from each mission [1].

Some of the constraints on the amount of Life Sciences training crew members receive are the access to high fidelity physical mockups (which can simulate only the physical, not gravitational environment within an experiment module), and by the limited time the crew members are given with the Life Science crew trainers. In addition, there will be at least a 6-month lag in-between training completion and performance of the experiment, which will impact the success of the research.

Within a *virtual* environment however, many scenarios can be presented to the user and allow for training in any remote environment both before launch and during flight. Scenarios, such as changes to the original protocol, emergency procedures and experimental countermeasures can be simulated in such an environment. Moreover, specific animal characteristics such as species, strain, gender, age and pathologies can be varied and presented within the simulation without requiring the actual specimen. An evaluation mode can also be added to the simulation so that the user can review their performance within the training system and track their progress during the space mission. A virtual environment can also help crew trainers plan scientific protocols and investigate the time and resources that will be required during the difficult process of retrieving bio-specimens in the unusual environment of space.

The principal concept of this project has been to create a flexible, multi-user, remote-capable system in order to provide Science Payloads Operations with an advanced way to train crew on performing life science experiments in space. This paper will discuss the technologies required to create a virtual environment for the simulation of a rat dissection procedure incorporating simulated weightlessness and mention the issues that arise when trying to provide an interactive semi-immersive, haptic interface to the user.

2. Methods

Acquisition and Segmentation

In order to achieve narrow beam collimations thereby increasing the spatial resolution of detail along the slice axis, the multi-detector computed tomography (MDCT) technique was performed using a Siemens SOMATOM Plus 4 Volume Zoom (Erlangen, Germany). A 218g 44-day old male Norway rat (rattus norvegicus) was chosen for the animal model. Data was acquired under 'in vivo' conditions in a fully anesthetized animal however Ionidated intravenous contrast media was not injected. The animal was scanned in the supine position and embedded in foam material to prevent motion during imaging. 240 axial slices were obtained with the following parameters: slice collimation 2x0.5mm, slice width 0.5mm, rotation time 0.8s, field of view 11x11cm, 512x512 matrix, 120.0 kV and 150.0 mA. The segmentation was performed using Amira 2.0 (Template Graphics Software Inc., San Diego, CA). Amira provides a component for 3D-image segmentation with several special-purpose features, ranging from purely manual to fully automatic ones. In our reconstruction process, we found the automatic thresholding function along with manual region selection functions provided reasonable segmentation for both skeletal and soft organ systems.

Once the interesting organs in a 3D-image volume have been segmented, Amira is able to create a corresponding polygonal surface model by extracting isosurfaces using the Generalized Marching Cubes module. The resulting mesh of the skin, internal organs and bones consisted of over 6 million triangles. This mesh was then simplified using the mesh simplification module, resulting in a mesh of under 100,000 polygons, which is more reasonable for interactive simulations. Figure 1 demonstrates the segmentation and mesh generation process. Frame A illustrates the segmentation of the skin, bones, and internal organs with the raw data projected on the x-y, y-z and x-z planes. Frame B shows a close-up of the high-resolution mesh around the skull and Frame C illustrates the entire high-resolution mesh.

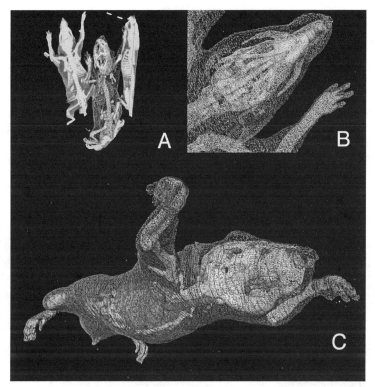

Figure 1 Segmentation and mesh generation: projection onto orthogonal planes (A), close-up on skull (B) and entire reconstruction rendered in wireframe (C).

Soft-tissue deformation

The reconstructed anatomy of the rat is represented as deformable objects within physically-based modeling simulation system [2]. In order to provide real-time, haptic-compatible update rates of truly arbitrary deformations, a simplified mass-spring system is currently the only modeling paradigm capable of providing adequate performance. Although some researchers have described advances in the use of finite element models to model localized soft-tissue deformations [3], this simulation not only requires coupling regions with varying stiffness but also performs interactive mesh manipulation via cutting [4].

This system models an object as a collection of point masses connected by linear springs in a mesh structure. The behavior of each tissue is modeled by modulating these stiffness coefficients and additional springs are placed between adjacent internal organs in order to propagate the effects of grasping connected components. Bones are modeled as rigid objects that are used primarily for constraining the deformable geometry in space. Solution of the deformation equations is done using a localized semi-static solver, which is a simplification of the traditional Euler method that ignores inertial and damping forces but provides a significant increase in performance. In order to speed up the simulation further, we have chosen to solve the deformation equations asynchronously, using a multithreaded model on multi-processor Sun (Mountain View, CA) E3500 8x400 MHz UltraSparc workstation. The simulation system is written in C++ using the OpenGL, GLUT, and POSIX libraries.

Interaction

Along with the common rendering options, such as coloring, lighting, solid/wire drawing and view control, several virtual tools for grasping, cutting and probing were developed. Figure 2 demonstrates four frames of the simulation. Frame A shows the creation of an incision along the midline of the abdomen. Frame B demonstrates the user grasping one side of the incision with the virtual forceps, exposing the underlying anatomy. Frame C illustrates pulling on the other side of the cut to further expose the internal organs of the animal. Frame D further depicts the deformation when the user releases the skin in order to remove an internal organ.

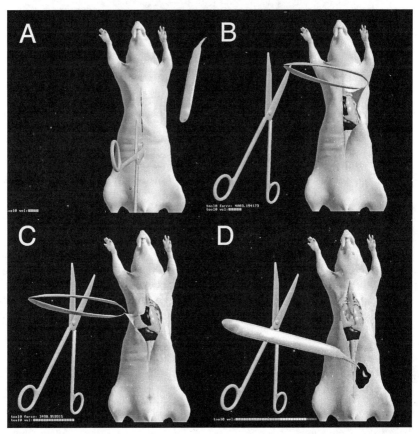

Figure 2 User interaction: Creating an incision (A), pulling it open (B-C) and removing the heart (D).

Non-force Feedback Devices
In order to allow the user to interact with the environment using actual dissection tools, an Ascension Technologies (Burlington, VT) Flock-of-Birds electromagnetic tracker is attached to real surgical forceps, scalpels and scissors. By mapping the actual three-dimensional position and orientation of the tools to their counterpart in the virtual space, the user can easily interact with the tissue of the virtual rat.

Haptic Devices
Probing the virtual rat can be used to extend the grasping or cutting procedures by adding force-feedback in order to give an impression of the compliance of each tissue. The haptic interface is achieved by using devices such as a SensAble Technologies (Woburn, MA) Phantom or an Immersion (San Jose, CA) 3GM or Laparoscopic Impulse Engine. This device is connected to an embedded processor (Intel Pentium-based dedicated PC) and communicates via 100Mbps Ethernet to the Sun server running the simulation. In this way, the update of the haptic device can be decoupled from the simulator in order to reduce the computation load on the machine controlling the stability of the haptics device.

Display Devices

Desktop Displays
Stereoscopic viewing of the system is achieved by using StereoGraphics (San Ramon, CA) CrystalEyes stereo glasses and a workstation monitor (Figure 3).

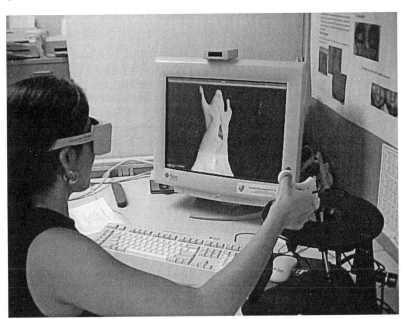

Figure 3 Interactive session with the dissection simulator.

Head-Mounted Displays

We can also view the simulation using a Sony (USA) PLM-S700 Glasstron head mounted display with an attached electromagnetic tracking device. The use of a tracked head-mounted display allows us to superimpose the image of the rat at the same location as the origin of the haptics space and thereby increase the level of realism within the simulation.

3. Results

We have assembled a preliminary environment for simulating tasks that are performed in animal dissection. By integrating components for imaging, segmentation, mesh generation and reduction, we can import a very high-quality geometry into a system that models objects with different physical properties. This system provides for interaction with both non-force-feedback and haptic devices and for display with a stereo workstation monitor or tracked head-mounted display. The next phase of this project will focus on increasing the visual and haptic realism presented to the user.

Future directions

Highly realistic visualization of the rat anatomy is essential in providing a meaningful learning experience. To address this issue, we will incorporate additional organ systems as well as investigate the benefits of photorealistic effects such as texture mapping and modeling complex components such as connective tissue, blood and fur. In addition, we are acquiring supplementary datasets, providing models of rats with various anatomical and pathological conditions. We are also combining CT and various Magnetic Resonance Imaging modalities for greater soft-tissue differentiation.

Extending visual realism will require research into the nature of organ movement. More exploration needs to be done in order to determine the proper method for capturing the dynamics of tissue motion. Currently we are connecting organs and bones to one another by using simplified virtual muscles and ligaments. However, the exact placement and behavior of these virtual structures requires further research.

In order to provide an effective learning environment, additional operational realism may be also be necessary. This realism could be provided by using multi-model interaction, incorporating additional auditory or visual cues, or by employing novel haptic interfaces. One obvious need is to provide a haptic interface that allows the user to manipulate the rat with two hands facilitating the dissection procedure.

As features are added to the system, there will be an obvious need to evaluate the effectiveness of the environment as a learning tool. Other researchers have characterized the benefit of various systems for the performance of complex tasks [5], this system could benefit from similar user studies.

4. Conclusion

We have developed a virtual reality system for simulating animal dissection that can facilitate the learning process both before launch and during space flight. This system can be used to simulate diverse procedures on a variety of specimens in a novel physical environment and can reduce the need to transport personnel and equipment to specific training locations.

5. Acknowledgements

The authors would like to thank Richard Boyle and Jeff Smith of the Center for Bioinformatics at the NASA Ames Research Center and the Science Payloads Operations personnel including Carol Eland, Chris Maese, Marianne Steele for their discussions and Marilyn Vasquez for her dissection instruction. Furthermore, we wish to thank Joel Brown, Benjamin Lerman and Jean-Claude Latombe of the National Biocomputation Center at Stanford University for their support of this research.

6. References

[1] Improving Life on Earth and in Space, The NASA Research Plan, An Overview, http://www.hq.nasa.gov/office/olmsa/ISS/cover.htm
[2] D. Terzopoulous and A. Witkin, Deformable Models, *IEEE Comp Graph and Appl*, Vol. 8, Nov 1988, No. 6, pp.41-51.
[3] J. Berkley, P. Oppenheimer, S. Weghorst, D. Berg, G. Raugi, D. Haynor, M. Gaunter, C. Brooking, G. Turkiyyah, Creating Fast Finite Element Models from Medical Images, In J.D. Westwood et al. (ed.) *Medicine Meets Virtual Reality 2000*, IOS Press, 2000, pp. 55-61.
[4] C. Bruyns and S. Senger, Interactive Cutting of 3D Surface Meshes, *Computer and Graphics (accepted)*.
[5] N. Taffinder, C. Sutton, R.J. Fishwick, I.C. Manus, and A. Darzi, Validation of Virtual Reality to Teach and Assess Psychomotor Skills in Laparoscopic Surgery: Results from Randomized Controlled Studies Using the MIST VR Laparoscopic Simulator, *Stud Health Technol Inform*, Vol. 50, 1998, pp. 124-130.

Medicine Meets Virtual Reality 2001
J.D. Westwood et al. (Eds.)
IOS Press, 2001

Safety in Computer Assisted Surgery

Catherina R. Burghart*, Stefan Hassfeld#, Luc Soler°, Heinz Woern*
*Institute of Process Control and Robotics, University of Karlsruhe, 76128 Karlsruhe,
Germany, e_mail: burghart@ira.uka.de
#Clinic of Maxillofacial Surgery, University of Heidelberg, 69120 Heidelberg,
Germany, e_mail: stefan.hassfeld@med.uni-heidelberg.de
°Digestive Cancer Research Institute (IRCAD-EITS), Hôpital Civil, University of Strasbourg,
67091 Strasbourg, France, e_mail: luc.soler@ircad.u-strasbg.fr

Abstract Today, surgeons accept computer assisted technologies as important tools to enhance the treatment of a patient. The positive impact and acceptance of computer assisted technologies could be increased to a great extent, if all methods and devices used for diagnosis and treatment of a patient are better co-ordinated and more finely tuned. Often computer assisted treatments cannot be performed due to a lack of communication between hospital departments, useless patient data, deficient interfaces, etc. Risks for the patient and potential errors within the treatment are often unrecognised, as up to now the safety of computer integrated surgery is only product-, device and security oriented. We have developed a new approach for a safety architecture, which includes safety aspects considering patients, users, interdependencies and interactions of computer assisted methods and apparatuses.

1. Introduction

Within the last two decades, computer and computer operated apparatuses have become very important tools to improve medical skills. The incorporation of digital technology into medical devices and procedures is a subject of high priority in many industrialised countries. It is expected that this technology will greatly effect the quality of medical services rendered and will provide more accurate and efficient support to physicians and other medical personnel. Newly developed computer supported methods and procedures will challenge many hitherto used practices and will fundamentally improve the way physicians carry out their diagnostics, planning, surgery and therapy.

An important issue when using computers in medicine is the consideration of adequate safety aspects. Up to now safety in computer integrated surgery (CIS) is product-, device- and security oriented, which implies high safety standards for individual devices and high security standards for data transfer. The engineers of the Universities of Karlsruhe and Strasbourg and the surgeons of the Universities of Heidelberg and Strasbourg have conceived a new concept to enhance safety in computer integrated surgery. Our research aims at reducing risks and errors, which are due to the interdependencies and interactions of computer assisted methods and apparatuses, humans, departments and co-operating hospitals. Up to now these risks and errors are not explicitly considered in CIS (i.e. deficient interfaces, unrecognised transformations of data, useless patient data).

In current research mainly the safety aspects of surgical robotic systems and of secure patient image data transfer are considered. Davies [1] postulates the principle of the surgeon being the "last link" of a surgical robot and thus being responsible for the robot's actions. A mathematical evaluation of safety of a surgical robotic intervention is presented by Masamune [2]. Security aspects and image data transfer are already realised by various PACS systems [3]; first works modelling data workflows in radiology are also presented [4].

2. Workflow design and classification

When performing computer integrated surgery many aspects are involved in a typical workflow for CIS treatments (Fig. 1). A workflow comprises the registration of the patient in the hospital, anamnesis, data acquisition, processing of image data, 3D modelling, diagnosis, surgical planning, the actual surgical intervention, and the hospitalisation and monitoring in a ward. At each step of the workflow the performed actions have a bearing on later steps. The single steps of the workflow often do not concern just one hospital or clinic but are spread over a variety of co-operating clinics, departments and hospitals connected via intranet and internet.

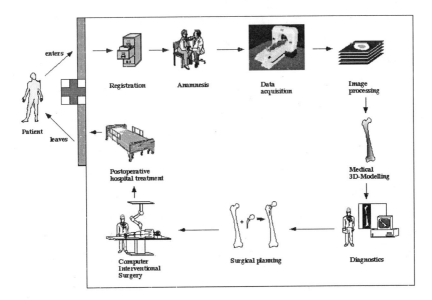

Figure 1: Typical workflow of a computer assisted surgical treatment

The risks and errors are classified according to their order and their character; i.e. risks due to an applied surgical robot are of first order, errors due to a wrong planning are of higher order. Risks and errors in CIS can depend on the characteristics of the patient, an applied apparatus, device or method (i.e. segmentation method). The safety is also influenced by organisation, management, communication, all data accesses, transfers, transformations and processes as well as interdependencies between data, devices, departments and co-operating hospitals. Hereby special stress is laid on the human element within a workflow.

3. Modelling

All relations, risks, errors, characteristics, interactions and interdependencies are formally described. The formal description serves as a basis for theoretical models of designated workflows for computer assisted surgery. Specific characteristics of new CIS technologies and surgical robots are considered, classified and integrated into the formal description.

4. Control agents and architecture

Structured control agents are generated on the basis of the model and integrated into each step of a CIS workflow within a hospital network. Their main task is to control potential risks, to give out checklists and warnings, to monitor CIS actions and to communicate with other control agents. Specific control agents consider the human machine interface and the co-operation via Internet.

A prototype of a control system architecture will integrate the structured control agents at all the stations of CIS workflows. This implies the design of specific control set-ups for different CIS treatments within a knowledge base. The control architecture as well as formal descriptions and models will help to enhance the safety of CIS treatments. They are easily applicable to further medical areas and other safety critical fields.

5. Conclusion

The ultimate goal of our concept is to develop a safety control architecture and software for computer assisted surgery, which is to be integrated into hospital networks. Special stress is laid on safety aspects considering the specific applications applied, the user of a computer assisted surgical device and the patient's characteristics. Device and security oriented safety aspects are included as well, but are not subject to further research within this project.

Acknowledgement

This research is performed at the Institute of Process Control and Robotics headed by Prof.. H.Woern at the University of Karlsruhe, at the Clinic of Maxillofacial Surgery of the University of Heidelberg headed by Prof. J. Muehling and at the Digestive Cancer Research Institute of the University of Strasbourg headed by Prof. Marescaux.

References

[1]   Davies B. (1995). A Discussion of Safety Critical Issues for Medical Robots, Computer Integrated Surgery, pp. 287-294.
[2]   Masamune K. et al. (1999). Safety of Medical Mechatronics-Mechanical and Medical Aspects of Safety, In Proceedings of Computer Assisted Radiology and Surgery (CARS'99), Paris.
[3]   Wendl U. et al. (1999). The Reality of Implementing a PACS, In Proceedings of Computer Assisted Radiology and Surgery (CARS'99), Paris.
[4]   von Berg J. et al. (2000). Organizational Modeling to support Workflow Management in Radiology. In Proceedings of Computer Assisted Radiology and Surgery (CARS'2000), San Francisco.

Medicine Meets Virtual Reality 2001
J.D. Westwood et al. (Eds.)
IOS Press, 2001

The Virtual Anatomy Lab: A Hands-on Anatomy Learning Environment

Bruce Campbell   Cornelius Rosse   J.F. Brinkley

{bdc@hitl|rosse@u|brinkley@u}.washington.edu   *University of Washington*

Abstract. This paper introduces the Virtual Anatomy Lab software platform for coordinating on-line gross anatomy learning sessions over time.

1. Introduction

Over 24 million health professionals rely on their knowledge of anatomy to effectively perform their work. Yet, successful anatomy knowledge acquisition techniques vary by individual. Many anatomy learning tools exist on the Web. For example, The University of Washington's Structural Informatics Group creates symbolic (text-based), semantic (text-based), and spatial (2-D and 3-D image-based) anatomy learning tools all of which are Web-accessible. In this paper we describe the Virtual Anatomy Lab (VAL), a collaborative environment that allows students to coordinate their learning process across available on-line tools by providing a dynamic, persistent 3-D online lab space that students modify to represent their understanding or focus on a particular area of study. From those spaces, students can continue to investigate gross anatomy from anywhere they have Web access.

2. The Virtual Playground

The VAL is based on the Virtual Playground architecture, developed in 1997 by the Human Interface Technology Laboratory at the University of Washington (UW) [1]. The VP in turn was based on the success of previous GreenSpace software development done between 1993 and 1996 [2]. Both platforms investigated the use of on-line, 3D cyberspace as a medium for overcoming geographical distance in visual and aural communication. While GreenSpace made its reputation as an early proof of concept platform demonstrating Trans-Pacific feasibility using expensive SGI computers and multiple ISDN lines, the Virtual Playground demonstrated Trans-Pacific feasibility using $1000 Pentium-based computers, $100 graphics accelerator cards, and inexpensive Internet communications. Before its use as an underlying architecture for the Virtual Anatomy Lab, the VP provided infrastructure for the Netgate Mall, Adjective World, and Virtual Big Beef Creek projects at the UW HIT Lab.

3. The Virtual Anatomy Lab

The Virtual Anatomy Lab (VAL), a Java-based software application using the Java 2 SDK [3] and Java 3D API [4], focuses students' personal learning through an interactive interface that lets them build their own 3D anatomy study space on-line. They modify their spaces by moving their viewpoint in six degrees of freedom, clicking on available tools, and dragging objects to change object position and orientation. Text and images available via Web URLs (such as UW's Digital Anatomist Interactive Atlas [5]) can be imported into their space and moved to appropriate locations. 3-D models are provided for import onto a virtual cadaver table using cadaver mesh data maintained by the Digital Anatomist Project, but just as well could come from imported VRML files made available elsewhere on the Web. An in-world blackboard, connected to the UW's Foundational Model Server (FMS) [6], allows students to mouse click up and down multiple hierarchies that define relationships among body parts (part of, is a, adjacent to, tributary of, branch of, etc.). Students can also collect URL's to sites with study aids and interactive quizzes, take their own screenshots, and leave personalized push-pin messages anywhere within the room. Students can leave their spaces and return at a later date to find them exactly as they left them, facilitating repetitive and iterative use at work, home, or other location. Over time, their persistent lab space helps them document their knowledge acquisition progress while providing their memory with a highly visual memory aid.

By coordinating their use of 3-D body part meshes, students can dissect and rebuild the body as if in a physical cadaver lab. Although realism lacks currently in both the fidelity of model appearance and the methods for dissection, the VAL demonstrates a blueprint for a viable future in cadaver lab simulation, important for a world where access to cadavers becomes increasingly cost prohibitive.

4. Illustrative Use

Figure 1 shows a VAL session where a beginning anatomy student has loaded the vertebrae as a yardstick for study of the main veins and arteries of the thorax. The student has moved the heart to the side to better see the tributaries of blood flow. After loading the desired models, the student can move around the cadaver table to see from any angle, or click on a specific mesh to confirm the body part name and its relationship to others on the FMS blackboard.

Figure 2 shows the same VAL user focusing on the semantic tools. The student has clicked down the is-a hierarchy to find all body parts that are classified as parenchymatous organs. The student will study the list and then select each item to load a model mesh on the cadaver table. Inspection of the meshes provides a reaffirming reminder of tubular characteristics.

Figure 3 shows a health care professional brushing up on visualizations of the left recurrent laryngeal nerve. Since the user's learning is highly specific, illustrations from Web sites have been imported to provide a wider range of renderings. A link to the best found on-line reference has been saved on the blackboard.

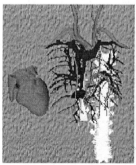 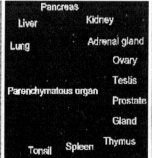 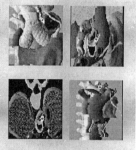

Figure 1 The Cadaver Table   **Figure 2** The FMS Blackboard   **Figure 3** Importing Images

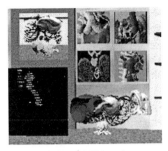

Figure 4 The VAL in action

Figure 4 shows the level of complexity that is possible by using all of the available VAL tools at once. The student is focusing on the lower thorax and has taken a snapshot of the cadaver table earlier as the process unfolded.

The cadaver table is below, the FMS blackboard is at lower left, a cadaver table screenshot hangs on the door, other images hang on the wall and a bookshelf at right holds links to on-line references.

5. Conclusions

The VAL prototype effectively integrates components of a personal anatomy-learning journey into a 3D space, navigable by students in six degrees of freedom. 3D virtual environments are interactive places for organizing knowledge acquisition journeys of complex subject matter. With the VAL, the student can take control of the camera instead of relying solely upon those who create pre-rendered illustrations. Or, the student can hang an expert's rendered illustration on the wall and annotate it with his or her own words. Although no formal use studies have been made of the VAL, four UW anatomists suggest that the approach is very promising and in line with their views on appropriate web-based instructional methods. Negative comments typically refer to the lack of fidelity in the rendered 3D space, overcome in the near future by more powerful computers and better graphics subsystems.

Users can build rooms that attempt to externalize their own unique cognitive maps. Since the VAL is built on top of the VP architecture that emphasizes meeting spaces over geographical distance, rooms can be shared on-line allowing for student-tutor or student-student VAL sessions. Informal discussions with anatomy students have found that most students prefer to have their own personalized space, but perhaps that reflects on the past history of traditional study methods. Like the many successful Web pages that index other sites and organize cyberspace around a topic for learning, VALs could be built over time that get updated with the best resources on Earth for common anatomical learning objectives. Curricula could be organized by knowledgeable instructors to provide VAL spaces that come with pre-defined learning exercises. Instructors could assist in doing the exercises within the VAL.

Acknowledgements

This work was funded by NIH grants LM06316 and LM06822. The rapid prototyping of the VAL would not be possible without the availability of the Java 3D API developed at Sun Microsystems and the enthusiastic vision of Dr. Tom Furness of the UW HIT Lab.

References

[1] Mandeville, Jon et al, GreenSpace: Creating a Distributed Virtual Environment for Global Applications, http://www.hitl.washington.edu/publications/p-95-17/
[2] Schwartz, Paul et al, Virtual Playground: Architectures for a Shared Virtual World, http://www.hitl.washington.edu/publications/r-98-12/
[3] Sun Microsystems, Java 2 SDK, http://www.javasoft.com/products/jdk/1.2/
[4] Sun Microsystems, Java 3D 1.2 API, http://www.javasoft.com/products/java-media/3D/
[5] The Digital Anatomist Project, http://sig.biostr.washington.edu/projects/da/
[6] Rosse, C et al, 'The Digital Anatomist foundational model: principles for defining and structuring its concept domain,' in *Proceedings, American Medical Informatics Association Fall Symposium* pp. 820-824, 1998.

Medicine Meets Virtual Reality 2001
J.D. Westwood et al. (Eds.)
IOS Press, 2001

Telesonography: Technical Problems, Solutions And Results In The Routine Utilization From Remote Areas

E. Cavina, O. Goletti, P. V. Lippolis, G. Zocco
Department of Surgery- University of Pisa - Via Roma 67, 56100 Pisa – Italy
e.mail: o.goletti@dc.med.unipi.it

TeleSonography can be considered a new diagnostic procedure based on the possibility to perform in remote areas ultrasound exams which, after a real-time transmission or as static-like images, allow experts to diagnose pathologies. The aims of this present study are: assessment of the use of a software dedicated to ultrasound consult managed by a personnel with no ultrasound expertise; feasibility of ultrasound consult with not dedicated connection systems (ISDN lines, Internet); assessment of responses' time and of the actual possibilities of the clinical impact in critical emergencies cases [1-2-3].

In the period between 24th July and 8th August 2000, at the clinical ambulatory of Tilos island (Dodecanesum Greece) 30 ultrasound exams have been performed and transmitted to the Department of Surgery of Pisa University.(Italy). All of them have been performed on patients coming to the clinical ambulatory of the island routinely, with no planning at all, and have been performed by medic and paramedic staff with no expertise in ultrasound diagnosis, guided at distance via videoconference in order to perform the most suitable scans for an organ's study: the remote personnel had as only didactic device a table with the ultrasound scans to perform. There were on the spot a physician expert in ultrasound diagnosis as supervisor who, by the way, did not interfere with the performance of ultrasound scans. The role of the supervisor physician was also to confirm the diagnosis performed at distance. The transmission was made from the remote area by an expert in telematics and software. The devices used were: a) Ultrasound System SonoSite 180 apparatus with a convex 3.5-5 MHz. Probe; b) 2 twin computers, 1 in Tilos and 1 in Pisa; c) 2 standard computers to perform teleconference in Netmeeting (Microsoft); d) InVIVO Teleconsult Software developed and produced by MedCom GmbH distributed in Italy by EBIT; e) ISDN Line.

All ultrasound exams have been performed with standard scans used usually and generally accepted for an ultrasound exam performed both routinely and in emergency. The images' assessment has been considered sufficient for a correct diagnosis considered that both scans and selection have been performed by untrained personnel; moreover, in all cases, it was possible to make a diagnosis of both positive and negative exam, confirmed by the medical trained personnel on the spot and by the transmission to Pisa of the selected images. The diagnosis' conformity between the exam performed in telesonography and the one performed on the spot by the expert has been of 100 %. It was possible, thanks to the results, to consider both the diagnosis's reliability together with the exam's feasibility, and the assessment of the "random" working from the remote area and connection 's time. The working's average of the whole system has been of about 5,43 minutes (range 1,45-20,45 min.) for the direct TeleConsult connection, and of about 12,30 minutes (range 5,35-32,40 min.) for NetMeeting's working for the VideoConference. The TeleConsult connection included static images and dynamic loops' transmission with transmission of scans' size and ISDN line's quality [4,5]. The mean time of procedure's working, after the arrival of the images fit for diagnosis, has been of 9.53 min. including 2 cases of colour images requiring a longer time. The mean times from working to diagnosis' conclusion have been of 11.06 min. For the interpretation at distance of transmitted images, main clinical data must be considered besides simple clinical findings' record of what has been received and transmitted. This means that there must be a basic medical knowledge and a basic ultrasound diagnosis training for the main scans. This preliminary experience has allowed the assessment of ultrasound methodology's actual use as instrumental procedure in remote areas and the "on field" evaluation of technical problems and their solutions. It is important indeed: a) assemblage in central and peripheral seat by qualified expert personnel; b) conformity of ISDN lines to ECC rules; c) improvement of TeleConsult Software with the possibility to use a Webcam on the same computer for remote control of untrained personnel; d) technical and technological basic improvement (like professional Webcam); e) a proper personnel training to the use of ultrasound apparatus. TeleSonography could be applied to: 1) routine remote diagnoses; 2) emergency remote diagnoses; 3) 3rd level consult for peripheral centres; 4) training in remote areas. It is essential to define the use's modalities, the applications with clear algorithms and the training procedure of the personnel properly chosen for this task. The personnel devoted to ultrasound study can be simply divided into: personnel performing ultrasound scans, personnel transmitting images and personnel interpreting the transmitted images. It must be possible to make a precise diagnosis in relation to the patient's clinical picture: therefore, it is necessary to standardise the diagnostic protocols and the scans to be acquired [6]. Personnel performing in remote area must be able to interpret the images, but above all must be able to get the scans in agreement with the reference centre and to have some basic informatic knowledge. This is the reason why a one-month training, at least, is necessary for the technical informatic side and for the performance of an ultrasound exam with essential elements for the organs' assessment.

References

[1] Cavina E., Zocco G., Goletti O., Lippolis P.V.
Islands: Experiences on the field and practical problems.
Abstract book Expo 2000 Telemedicine Present and Future. Hannover 29 September 2000

[2] Cavina E., Aliferis A., Goletti O., Balestri R., Lippolis P.V., Zocco G., Franceschi M., Cotrozzi A., Economu S., Christofidis E.
TIM-TEM: A telemedicine project on a Greek Island. Preliminary results.
The European Journal of Emergency Surgery and Intensive Care, Vol. XXI n° 2- June 1998

[3] Balestri R, Cavina E, Aliferis A, Goletti O, Rocci R, Lippolis PV, Zocco G., Franceschi M, Cotrozzi A, Economou S, Christofidis E.
Telemedicine on a small island.
J Telemed Telecare. 1999;5 Suppl 1:S50-52.

[4] Malone FD, Athanassiou A, Nores J, D'Alton ME. Effect of ISDN bandwith on image quality for telemedicine transmission of obstetric Ultrasonography. Telemed J 1998 Summer;4(23):161-165

[5] Li X, Hu G, Gao S. Design and implementation of a novel compression method in a tele-ultrasound system. IEEE Trans Inf Technol Biomed 1999 Sep; 3(3) 205-213

[6] Johnson MA, Davis P, McEwan Aj, Jhangri GS, Warshawski R, Gargun A, Either J, Anderson WW. Preliminary Findings from a teleultrasound study in Alberta. Telemed J 1998 Fall; 4(3) 267-276.

Medicine Meets Virtual Reality 2001
J.D. Westwood et al. (Eds.)
IOS Press, 2001

90

Autocolorization of Three-dimensional Radiological Data

Ankur Chhadia, Fred Dech, Zhuming Ai and Jonathan C. Silverstein

University of Illinois at Chicago
VRMedLab, HHSB M/C 530
Chicago, IL 60612-7249
achhad1@uic.edu, fdech@uic.edu, zai@uic.edu, jsilver@uic.edu

Abstract. It requires skill, effort, and time to visualize desired anatomic structures from radiological data in three-dimensions. There have been many attempts at automating this process and making it less labor intensive. The technique we have developed is based on mutual information for automatic multi-modality image fusion (MIAMI Fuse, University of Michigan). The initial development of our technique has focused on the autocolorization of the liver, portal vein, and hepatic vein. A standard dataset in which these structures had been segmented and assigned colors was created from the full color Visible Human Female (VHF) and then optimally fused to the fresh CT Visible Human Female. This semi-automatic segmentation and coloring of the CT dataset was subjectively evaluated to be reasonably accurate. The transformation could be viewed interactively on the ImmersaDesk, in an immersive Virtual Reality (VR) environment. This 3D segmentation and visualization method marks the first step to a broader, standardized automatic structure visualization method for radiological data. Such a method, would permit segmentation of radiological data by canonical structure information and not just from the data's intrinsic dynamic range.

1. Introduction

Radiological data, including Computed Tomography (CT), provides the clinician with layers of 2D cross sections in which structure segmentation is typically performed based on the data's dynamic range (tissue type or density). In order to perceive the 3D structure of interest, the clinician has to add to this segmentation his or her own intrinsic knowledge of anatomic structure and mentally stack the data. This process is often difficult and requires radiological expertise. For example, the hepatic and portal veins often contrast similarly and cannot be distinguished in the substance of the liver without knowing their expected normal courses. Furthermore, tracing their course and branching from slice to slice can be difficult. In typical segmentation methods today, the tissue type of interest is segmented by the data's dynamic range and then the structure of interest is separated by hand. In the method we describe, we select the structure of interest first in a standard dataset, use anatomic similarity to place this information into the radiological data, and then use the resulting fused data for real-time segmentation and visualization.

There have been many attempts at automating these processes. Automatic liver segmentation techniques and 3D visualization have been developed but still require significant user modification [1]. Automatic color labeling and 3D visualization have also been developed. There has been success with highly conserved areas such as the brain [2]. Automatic 3D reconstruction of abdominal CT datasets based on deformable modeling and thresholding algorithms have been developed [3]. The technique we have developed is based on mutual information for automatic multi-modality image fusion (MIAMI Fuse, University of Michigan) [4]. It operates at very high fidelity even for datasets of differing resolutions and color tables (different modalities).

By generating a canonical atlas including three-dimensional and symbolic (term) information from the Visible Human [5] and then fusing this to instances of radiological data, we create a method for structure autocolorization that can be applied to any radiological data. This technique assigns specific colors to specific normal structures in radiological data and then permits visualization of them along with the radiological data in a VR environment. Our long-term goal is to create a standard method that can be applied to any radiological data from any person to any region of the body.

2. Methods

A standard dataset was created from the full color Visible Human Female by segmenting the liver, portal vein, and hepatic vein and coloring them red, green, and blue respectively. The portal vein segmentation includes the splenic vein from which the portal vein arises and the spleen from which the splenic vein arises. The hepatic vein segmentation includes the inferior vena cava and renal veins. The CT dataset used was the fresh CT VHF. The autocolorization is done using MIAMI Fuse. MIAMI Fuse empirically aligns two datasets by maximizing the mutual information between them and calculating the three-dimensional transformation required to move from one to the other. It is capable of accurately fusing two datasets of different modalities at high fidelity. We register the two datasets by transforming the standard data into the three-dimensional space of the CT. Therefore, the patient CT data remains unchanged while it is augmented by the standard anatomic segmentations scaled to fit.

MIAMI Fuse requires that the two datasets that will be fused be in 8-bit Advanced Visual Systems (AVS) [6] field format. The 32-bit RGB format VHF dataset was converted to 8-bit using the NTSC standard (0.299 R + 0.587 G + 0.114 B). The 12-bit DICOM format CT dataset was converted to 8-bit using a linear contrast function with an input range of negative 800 to positive 1000 Hounsfield Units.

Various combinations of control points and parameters were selected when running MIAMI Fuse. The first three control points were selected along the border of the liver in an axial section at the tenth thoracic vertebrae. Two of them were placed between the liver and the lateral borders of the right and left rectus abdominis muscles. One was placed between the liver and the body of the vertebrae. A fourth control point was selected in a mid-sagital section at the inferior margin of the liver. Parameters include degrees of freedom (rotate, translate, scale, and shear), interpolation x, y, and z scale, and number of control points (3 or 4). The optimized transform function of the standard dataset to the CT dataset was then applied to each structure dataset (corresponding to the liver, portal vein, and hepatic vein). Accuracy in terms of the optimized mutual information was compared to the computational time.

The three transformed structure datasets were combined such that the liver dataset was put into the red channel, the portal vein into the green channel, and the hepatic vein into the blue channel. This resulted in 8 possible colors. The pure red, green, and blue correspond to the liver, portal vein, and hepatic vein and combinations of these pure colors correspond to regions of overlap. This 32-bit combined version of the transformed structure datasets was converted to an 8-bit file in which each of 8 values code for the 8 possible colors.

The segmentations and fusions were evaluated subjectively using an image compare module in AVS. It allows display of alternating checkers of the same user selected slice of the two datasets being compared. The segmentations were evaluated by overlaying them on the VHF data after conversion to 8-bit by the NTSC method. The fusions were evaluated by comparing the 8-bit CT dataset to the transformed structure datasets.

In order to generate a color LUT that could render either one of the resulting datasets correctly, the entire 8-bit standard volume was sampled to find data values occupying the least number of voxels. The eight least-used data values had their gray-scale value replaced in a new lookup table that combined grayscale and the 8-color fused dataset.

The resulting transformed 8-bit AVS datasets were converted into groups of individual RAW images and then converted to DICOM file format using the dicom3tools library [7]. Once this was done, the DICOM files of an individual volume could be read into a volume rendering application with the correct 8-bit color LUT applied to the data. This was viewed and evaluated interactively on an ImmersaDesk [8] in an immersive Virtual Reality (VR) volume-rendering environment separately described in these proceedings.

3. Results

The flow of data involved decreasing the dynamic range of both datasets significantly in order to fuse them. We evaluated four methods to convert the full color data (VHF) to 8-bit. We measured the entropy after each conversion using a module in AVS. The NTSC standard retained the highest average information, highest entropy, compared to other conversion methods (Table 1). This suggests that NTSC standard is the most promising method of reducing the dynamic range for data fusion.

Table 1: Comparison of different conversion methods

Method	Formula			Entropy
NTSC	0.299 R + 0.587 G + 0.114 B			-4.38870
Rec 709	0.2126 R + 0.7152 G + 0.0722 B			-4.35729
332	R=(0 to 7)	G=(0 to 7)	B=(0 to 3)	-4.31976
216 Index	R=(0 to 5)	G=(0 to 5)	B=(0 to 5)	-3.71359

The processing time versus accuracy trade-off is dependent on the selected control points and parameters used to run MIAMI Fuse. Empiric usage revealed "optimal" fusion was performed when permitting the algorithm to rotate, translate, and scale the standard data using four control points. Using fixed set parameters, computational times ranged from 5 to 45 minutes on our SGI Onyx2 Deskside. Selection of control points in the CT dataset corresponding to those pre-selected in the standard dataset is anticipated as the major interaction that will ultimately be required by the user when the method is in practical use.

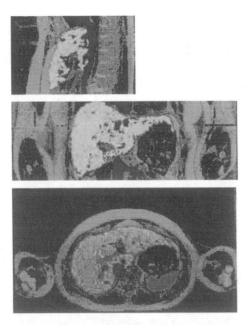

Figure 1: Automatic segmentations of Visible Human Data demonstrated by overlaying NTSC slice images with segmentations. (top = sagital section) (middle = coronal section) (bottom = axial section)

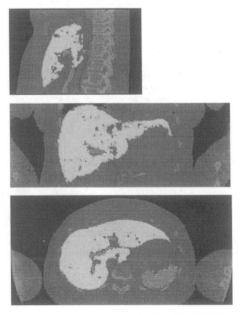

Figure 2: Transformed structure segmentations compared with original CT dataset by overlaying images. (top = sagital section) (middle = coronal section) (bottom = axial section)

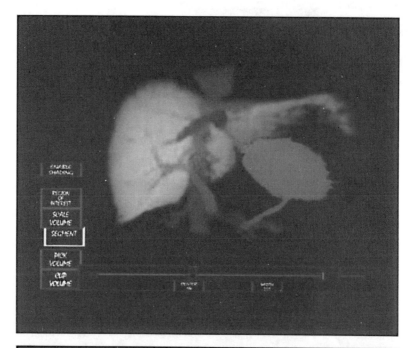

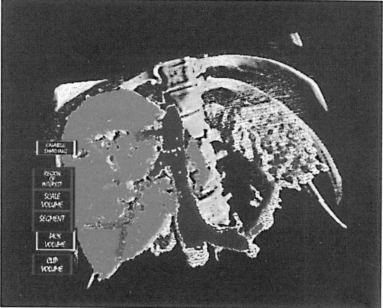

Figure 3: Visualization on ImmersaDesk of transformed liver (red), portal vein (green), and hepatic vein (blue) data alone (top image), and combined with original CT in arbitrarily windowed, clipped, and shaded display (bottom image).

The automatic segmentation and coloring of the CT dataset was subjectively evaluated to be highly accurate (Figures 1 and 2). The segmentation data alone and the autocolorized CT dataset were each visualized in interactive VR on the ImmersaDesk (Figure 3). The resulting volumes could be viewed in their entirety at interactive rates (approximately 18 frames per second).

Since the fusion is done using an 8-bit file, the issue of color limitations arises. There can only be a maximum of 256 colors in the final visualization. This includes original structure colors and different combinations of overlap colors. Overlap is an artifact of segmentation and fusion that defines the transition between two neighboring structures. There can be a maximum of eight different colors assigned as original structure colors, but each color may be used for multiple structures that do not overlap. Any structure in the transformed and combined structure datasets can be identified by its original color and one point of its location. A maximum of eight structures can converge at one point and still accommodate the number of colors available. Thus, we suspect color limitation will not ultimately be a problem.

4. Conclusions

We have developed a technique that colors the liver, portal vein, and hepatic vein in abdominal CT data red, green, and blue respectively. This technique is nearly automatic, reasonably quick, and applicable to different modality datasets at high fidelity. This 3D visualization technique marks the first step to a broader, standardized automatic structure colorization method for radiological data.

Although this initial technique was applied to only three anatomic structures, each individual lobe or branch can be assigned its own color. Other structures and their individual segments could also be included. The process simply requires segmentation of the desired structure in the standard dataset. It is then assigned its own color and can be transformed to the radiological data using MIAMI Fuse. Obtaining reasonably quick and accurate fusions between standard datasets and radiological data from arbitrary patients should be possible by using parameters that allow for warping and more control points. The only step that we anticipate will require user intervention is selection of control points in the CT dataset corresponding to those pre-selected in the standard dataset.

The method described here, if it can be broadly applied, promises to make the process of interpreting radiological data easier for clinicians by identifying normal structures automatically. It is anticipated that major branches of the vasculature and solid organs will be matched sufficiently, but highly variable structure such as finer vascular detail and hollow organs will be matched insufficiently. The images themselves would be able to answer questions about what a certain structure on the image is or where on the image a specific structure is. A similar method may ultimately provide a foundation for advances in visualization, simulation, education, diagnostics, and treatment planning.

5. Acknowledgments

This project has been funded in whole or in part with Federal funds from the National Library of Medicine, National Institutes of Health, under Contract No. N01-LM-9-3543 and under Grant No. R01-LM-06756-01.

References

1. L. Gao, D.G. Heath, B.S. Kuszyk, and E.K. Fishman. Automatic liver segmentation technique for three-dimensional visualization of CT data. *Radiology* 1996, 201, 359-64.

2. W.L. Nowinski, A. Fang, B.T. Nguyen, J.K. Raphel, L. Jagannathan, R. Raghavan, R.N. Bryan, and G.A. Miller. Multiple brain atlas database and atlas-based neuroimaging system. *Computer Aided Surgery* 1997, 2, 42-66.

3. L. Soler, H. Delingette, G. Malandain, N. Ayache, C. Koehl, J.M. Clement, O. Dourthe, and J. Marescaux. An automatic Virtual Patient Reconstruction from CT-scans for Hepatic Surgical Planning. *Stud Health Technol Inform 2000*;70, 2000, pp. 316-322.

4. C.R. Meyer, J.L. Boes, B. Kim, P. Bland, K.R. Zasadny, P.V. Kison, K. Koral, K.A. Frey, and R.L. Whal. Demonstration of accuracy and clinical versatility of mutual information for automatic multimodality image fusion using affine and thin plate spline warped geometric deformations. *Medical Image Analysis* 1997, 3, 195-206.

5. http://www.nlm.nih.gov/research/visible/visible_human.html

6. Advanced Visual Systems, release 5.3. Advanced Visual Systems Inc., Waltham MA, 1996.

7. http://idt.net/~dclunie/dicom3tools.html

8. M. Czernuszenko, D. Pape, D. Sandin, T. DeFanti, G.L. Dawe, and M.D. Brown. The ImmersaDesk and Infinity Wall Projection-Based Virtual Reality Displays, *Computer Graphics*, Vol. 31 Number 2, May 1997 pp 46-49.

Medicine Meets Virtual Reality 2001
J.D. Westwood et al. (Eds.)
IOS Press, 2001

Development and Evaluation of an Epidural Injection Simulator with Force Feedback for Medical Training

Thao Dang[1], Thiru M. Annaswamy[2], Mandayam A. Srinivasan[1]

[1]*Laboratory for Human and Machine Haptics*
Massachusetts Institute of Technology
Cambridge, MA 02139

[2]*Department of Physical Medicine & Rehabilitation*
UT Southwestern Medical Center
Dallas, TX 75390-9055

Abstract. Performing epidural injections is a complex task that demands a high level of skill and precision from the physician, since an improperly performed procedure can result in serious complications for the patient. The objective of our project is to create an epidural injection simulator for medical training and education that provides the user with realistic feel encountered during an actual procedure. We have used a Phantom haptic interface by SensAble Technologies, which is capable of three-dimensional force feedback, to simulate interactions between the needle and bones or tissues. An additional degree-of-freedom through an actual syringe was incorporated to simulate the "loss of resistance" effect, commonly considered to be the most reliable method for identifying the epidural space during an injection procedure. The simulator also includes a new training feature called "Haptic Guidance" that allows the user to follow a previously recorded expert procedure and feel the encountered forces. Evaluations of the simulator by experienced professionals indicate that the simulation system has considerable potential to become a useful aid in medical training.

1. Introduction

An epidural injection is a commonly performed procedure for pain relief. For example, it is used to reduce pain during labor and delivery, and to reduce pain in the lower back and legs from nerve irritation such as from a herniated disc. Epidural injections require a high level of precision and skill from the administering physician. While inserting the needle into the epidural space, one must be careful so as to not perforate the dura matter, a tough fibrous layer that covers and protects the spinal cord and its nerves, as this would result in complications such as spinal headache and CSF leak that can lead to life threatening infections on rare occasions.

When guiding the needle into the epidural space, physicians depend on one or more of several feedback cues, such as the resisting forces occurring at the needle or x-ray imaging (fluoroscopy). Another important method to identify the epidural space is the so-called "loss of resistance" effect. After the needle tip has entered the supraspinous ligament, a syringe filled with a small amount of air or fluid is attached to the needle. While the needlepoint is still in the dense ligaments, fluid or air injection is not possible.

However, as soon as the needle enters the epidural space, a relatively low pressure environment, a significant drop in resistance is encountered and the fluid or gas can easily be injected.

Currently, residents in post-graduate medical training and other trainees learn to administer epidural injections by performing supervised procedures on real patients or less frequently on cadaver specimens. Several attempts have been made to create a computer-based simulator for training in this procedure, typically using one-dimensional haptic feedback devices [1-5]. At Millersville University, Pennsylvania, a three-dimensional simulation of a similar medical procedure, lumbar puncture to obtain cerebro-spinal fluid, has been developed [6]. A training program developed at the Manchester Visualization Center that uses a Logitech Wingman Force Feedback Mouse can be downloaded from the World Wide Web [7].

We have created an epidural injection simulator for medical training that is capable of three-dimensional force feedback and incorporates an additional degree-of-freedom through an actual syringe to simulate the "loss-of-resistance". As a new training feature, we have developed a method of recording the forces used by an expert, which can be played back to the trainee for haptic guidance. Experienced physicians in pain management and anesthesia rated the accuracy of our simulation and its utility as a training tool. Our paper concludes with preliminary results of these assessments.

2. Methods and Tools

Needle-Tissue Interaction
Our simulator uses a Phantom haptic interface by SensAble Technologies and its software toolkit GHOST. The lower vertebrae L4 and L5 have been modeled as well as the important soft tissues for an epidural injection, namely skin, subcutaneous tissue, supraspinous ligament, interspinous ligament, ligamentum flavum, epidural space, dura mater and subdural space. The geometrical models of the virtual objects are stored as Open Inventor files.

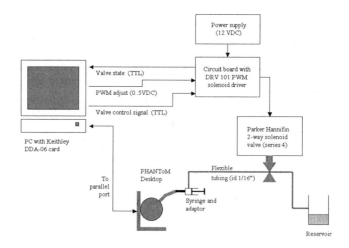

Figure 1. Schematic overview of simulator setup

Collisions between the needle tip and the tissue layers are detected with the "Neighborhood Watch" algorithm [8], an efficient method that makes use of oriented bounding boxes for initial contact recognition and a hierarchical representation of the geometry for collision detection once a preceding contact point is known. The haptic representation of the vertebrae is given by a spring-damper model. A piecewise linear series of Voigt elements has been proposed in [5] to govern the feedback forces in viscoelastic tissues. We have generalized this model for the three-dimensional case and added a set of logical rules to apply different forces when the needle is advanced or withdrawn from already ruptured layers. Internal Coulomb friction has been implemented and an additional force component based on a spring-damper model limits the lateral movement of the needle in the tissues.

In the current version of our simulator, the parameters of the tissue layers are determined following a perceptual approach. Experienced professionals adjust the model so that the feel of the simulated forces resemble the feel encountered in a real epidural injection. For this purpose, slider controls have been established to manipulate the coefficients of each tissue during run-time, such as the thickness of the tissues, spring and damping constants, widths of elements in the Voigt series and friction coefficients. The sliders may also be used for creating various virtual patients with different tissue characteristics. If empirically determined tissue properties are available, they can be easily incorporated into the model and simulation.

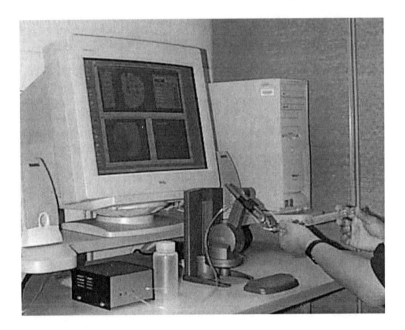

Figure 2. Epidural Injection Simulator with attached syringe

Loss of Resistance Simulation

In order to employ "loss of resistance" method, a syringe filled with either air or water can be attached to the Phantom at any time during the simulation. A two-way solenoid valve controls the flow through the syringe. The solenoid is driven by a pulse-width modulated input signal, thus allowing adjustment of different flow rates. In the current version of the simulator, the valve is only switching between two states, enabling flow when the needlepoint has entered the epidural space and closing the valve otherwise.

Visualization

During a training session, simulated front and lateral view x-ray images that show the current needle position can be displayed. The user can also select a 3D visualization of the vertebrae and tissue models that form the haptic scene.

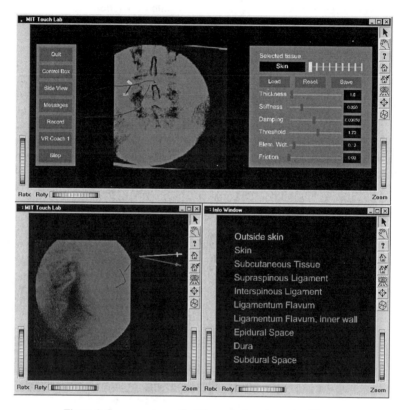

Figure 3. Screen capture with slider controls and tunnel guidance

Training Features

When starting the simulation, the trainee chooses the position of the virtual patient. In the current version of the simulator, seated or prone (lying with front of body facing downwards) positions are available for selection. In accordance to the experience of the user, different levels of additional visual and audio information can be provided during training. For example, a text window indicates the tissue in which the epidural needle is currently placed or the computer can announce important landmarks by playing corresponding audio files. These features should be gradually disabled as the trainee proceeds to more advanced training phases. The simulator also allows for recording of injection trials for further evaluation of the trainee's performance.

Related to recording of injection trials is "Haptic Guidance". The basic idea behind this feature is that a virtual instructor guides the hand of the novice through the injection procedure. We have experimented with several versions, two of which were found most promising. In the first approach, the simulator displays a second ("guiding") needle on the screen that moves along the same path and with the same speed as an expert in a previously recorded trial. If the user's needle position exactly matches the position of the guiding needle, the user will feel the same forces as the expert while the injection procedure was recorded. If there is a discrepancy between the actual and the guiding needle, the "virtual instructor" applies a force to pull the trainee back to the recorded trajectory. If the discrepancy exceeds a threshold value, the guiding needle changes its color and replay is paused until the user returns to the recorded position.

The second implemented version of haptic guidance discards the time-dependency of the recorded data, i.e. the user can perform the injection at his or her own speed. Here, the complete recorded path of the expert is displayed graphically and the movement of the needle is limited to the recorded trajectory, thus allowing the user to solely concentrate on the encountered tissue forces. "Tunnel Guidance" might be a suitable term to describe this feature.

3. Expert Evaluation and preliminary results

Experienced anesthetists and pain management specialists at UT Southwestern Medical Center at Dallas have evaluated the simulation in regard to its accuracy and utility as a training tool. Further evaluations are currently taking place at the MIT Laboratory of Human and Machine Haptics.

On a ten-point scale with ten indicating the best possible rating, the experts rated the likeliness of the simulated tissue forces at an average value of 6.4. The highest ratings (8.5) were achieved for the simulation of the "loss of resistance" effect. All interviewed experts indicated, that the "loss of resistance" was also the most reliable feedback in real-life procedures. Overall, the subjects rated the utility of the simulation as a training tool at 7.4.

4. Future Work and Conclusions

A shortcoming of using the Phantom Desktop model for our simulator is the inability to control the orientation of the needle. However, this limitation can be overcome by using haptic interfaces with full force and torque feedback, such as the Phantom 6DOF. Another promising method we have used to solve this problem in other contexts is the use of two Phantoms and ray-based haptic rendering techniques that have been developed at the MIT Touch Lab [9, 10].

Further work on the simulator will include improvement of the tissue models in regard to the feedback forces and the tissue geometries, and the attachment of a human low-back mannequin, as suggested by several interviewed experts. Overall, the expert feedback was encouraging and the preliminary evaluation results indicate that the simulator has considerable potential to become a useful aid in medical training.

Acknowledgments

The authors would like to thank the PM&R-ERF grant for funding part of this project and the MIT Germany Program and the DaimlerChrysler Scholarship Program Research & Technology for their support of Thao Dang.

References

[1] Gillespie, B. and L.B. Rosenberg, Design of High-Fidelity Haptic Display for One-Dimensional Force Reflection Applications, *Proceedings of SPIE - The International Society for Optical Engineering*, (1995).

[2] Popa, D.O. and S.K. Singh, Creating Realistic Force Sensations in a Virtual Environment: Experimental System, Fundamental Issues and Results, *Proceedings of IEEE International Conference on Robotics & Automation*, (1998).

[3] Singh, S.K., M. Bostrum, D. Popa, C. Wiley, Design of An Interactive Lumbar Puncture Simulator With Tactile Feedback, *Proceedings of IEEE Conference on Robotics and Automation* (1994) 1734-1752.

[4] Stredney, D., D. Sessanna, J.S. McDonald, L. Hiemenz, and L.B. Rosenberg, A Virtual Simulation Environment for Learning Epidural Anesthesia, *Proceedings of Medicine Meets Virtual Reality IV: Healthcare in the Information Age*, (1996).

[5] Brett, P.N., T.J. Parker, A.J. Harrison, T.A. Thomas and A. Carr, Simulation of resistance forces acting on surgical needles, *Proceedings of Institution of Mechanical Engineers*, **211** (1997) 335-347.

[6] Gorman, P., T. Krummel, R. Webster, M. Smith, D. Hutchens, A Prototype Haptic Lumbar Puncture Simulator, *Proceedings of Medicine Meets Virtual Reality*, (2000) 106-109.

[7] *Web-Based Surgical Simulators and Medical Education Tools*, <http://synaptic.mvc.mcc.ac.uk/simulators.html>. Manchester Visualization Centre, University of Manchester.

[8] Ho, C.-H., C. Basdogan, and M.A. Srinivasan, Efficient Point-Based Rendering Techniques for Haptic Display of Virtual Objects. Presence, **8**(5) (1999) 477-491.

[9] Basdogan, C., C-H. Ho, and M.A. Srinivasan, Ray-based Haptic Rendering Technique for Displaying Shape and Texture of 3D Objects in Virtual Environments, *Proceedings of the ASME Dynamic Systems and Control Division*, **61**, (1997) 77-84.

[10] Ho C-H., C. Basdogan, and M.A. Srinivasan, Ray-based Haptic Rendering: Force and Torque Interactions Between a Line Probe and 3D Objects in Virtual Environments, *International Journal of Robotics Research*, **19**(7), (2000) 668-683.

Medicine Meets Virtual Reality 2001
J.D. Westwood et al. (Eds.)
IOS Press, 2001

Statistical analysis of the morphology of three-dimensional objects and pathologic structures using spherical harmonics

*Sascha Däuber, *Jörg Raczkowsky,
**Jakob Brief , **Stefan Hassfeld and *Heinz Wörn
*University of Karlsruhe (TH), Institute for Process Control and Robotics,
Kaiserstraße 12, 76128 Karlsruhe, Germany
** University of Heidelberg, Clinic of Cranio-Maxillo-Facial Surgery*

Abstract. To support diagnosis and therapy, it is a fundamental aim of medical image processing to describe morphological characteristics of pathological structures or image objects in general. Different authors propose quantitative methods of description like bounding boxes[1], fourier descriptors[2] or contour moments[3]. Unfortunately, these methods either don't supply a complete, respectively precise description of the object or only operate on two-dimensional images.

Among the range of application are systems to classify lung nodules [4] or to help the diagnosis of brain tumors [5]. In this paper we present a method to analyze the morphology or shape of any three-dimensional object in order to describe it mathematically well-defined. We show how the description can be used to perform statistical operations on morphologies. The method presented in this paper was developed to assist the planning of craniofacial surgery. We analyze the shape of a given set of skull CT-data and use the mathematical description to statistically calculate the average shape of the skulls.

1. Introduction

While planning craniofacial surgical interventions the patient's ideal appearance is very important[6]. Appearance should be as close as possible to the aspect he/she would have without any defects. Thus it's necessary to obtain precise information about the look of a patient, just as if he/she was healthy. It is for this reason and for the fact that the skull dominates the look of the head that we build a 3D norm database[6], containing "ideal", averaged skulls, one for each age and sex. The surgeon is now able to form the pathological skull to an ideal shape given by the averaged skull. To calculate the norm data out of a set of CT-images, it is necessary to describe the morphology of the skull in a way which makes an averaging process possible.

This paper is splitted into two parts. In the first and more important part we describe, how we decompose the shape of a skull or any three-dimensional object using spherical harmonics. We calculate an one-dimensional set of scalar data, where each scalar represents the share of a particular spherical harmonic function of the object, thus forming its spectrum. We explain how we can achieve, limited only by computing time and memory, any desired degree of precision. We will reconstruct the object only using the spectrum and will afterwards compare it with original object, enabling us to verify the decompostion. The second part describes how we use the spectrum to average several CT-images.

2. Mathematical methods

To analyze the objects, we use the so-called spherical harmonics[7][8](the symbol j denotes the imaginary unit and P_l^m an associated Legendre polynomial):

$$Y_i(\vartheta,\varphi) = \sqrt{\frac{(2n+1)(l-m)!}{4\pi(l+m)!}} P_l^m(\cos\vartheta)e^{jm\varphi} \text{ , where} \tag{1}$$

$$l = 0,1,2,...$$

$$m = -l,-l+1,-l+2,...,l-1,l$$

$$i = 2l + m$$

They form a complete set of orthogonal functions. Analogous to the analysis of any function $f(x)$ with a set of functions $cos(ix)$ and $sin(ix)$ (the fourier series), any function $r(\theta,\varphi)$ defined on the unit sphere may be analyzed with the spherical harmonics as shown in equation (2).

$$r(\vartheta,\varphi) = \sum_i c_i Y_i(\vartheta,\varphi) \tag{2}$$

The coefficients are given as:

$$c_i = \iint Y_i(\vartheta,\varphi)^* r(\vartheta,\varphi)d\vartheta d\varphi \tag{3}$$

$Y_i(\vartheta,\varphi)^*$ denotes the complex conjugate of $Y_i(\vartheta,\varphi)$.

3. Analysis of the data

As shown in chapter 2, the object must be available in a functional form $r(\theta,\varphi)$. Unfortunately medical image data is normally available as voxel data $g(x,y,z)$ of CT/MRT-scans. To convert the voxel data $g(x,y,z)$, where g is a representation of physical parameters like attenuation and scatter coefficients, we first of all have to extract the desired objects in a segmentation process. Afterwards we calculate a point cloud with a contouring algorithm like "Marching Cubes". Finally the data is resampled where the distance r of the center of mass to the surface for each steradian (θ,φ) is calculated. This function of distance $r(\theta,\varphi)$ is the desired functional form of the shape of an object.

Now we can use equations (1) and (3) to calculate the various c_i. They form the shape-spectrum of the analyzed object, where the index parameter i varies from 0 to ∞. Only using the infinite number of c_i assures the precise and complete description of the object. Fortunately coarse structures of the object are described by low numbers of i, and only the low scale changes of the shape need to be described by high numbers of i. The higher the maximal value

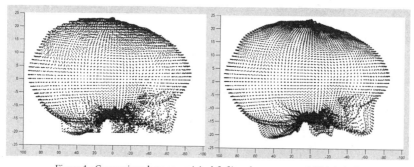

Figure 1.: Comparison between original (left) and reconstructed (right) skull

of i the more accurate the calculation. Thus the amount of coefficients c_i, i.e. the depth of the analysis, is adjustable to the needs of precision. In practice we use a few hundred coefficients to give a sufficient description of an object.

4. Verification method

To verify the precision of the above analysis we use equation (2) to reconstruct the original surface function $r(\theta,\varphi)$ with a sum over the calculated morphological parameters c_i.

By comparing the original function with the reconstructed one, the analysis process can be validated. The right part of figure 1 shows the reconstructed morphology of a skull using 1245 scalar parameters c_i. As you can see, the reconstruction is precise in smooth areas and shows deviations near fine structures e.g. the nose. Higher amounts of parameters c_i provide a more precise reconstruction.

5. Statistical method

The set of calculated parameters c_i can now be used to perform any statistical operation. In our application we analyzed several skulls, calculated the average set of parameters $c_{i,mean}$ which we used to reconstruct an average skull.

6. Results

The verifying process showed that complex structures like the skull are well represented by 1300 scalar parameters which we gained automatically. Simple shapes like tumors are described precisely with roughly three hundred parameters.

Our system is able to describe mathematically well defined the shape of three-dimensional objects with only a few scalar values. They can be used to depict the chronological development of objects, to classify them or to perform statistical operations like averaging on them. In our application it is used to calculate 3D norm data to assist craniofacial surgery planning.

The development of the algorithms is completed and now the method is applied to calculate the norm data. Work in the near future is to apply the method to a greater amount (so far 20) of images and to verify the averaging process.

References

[1] Sonka et. al., Image Processing, Analysis and Machine Vision, Chapman & Hall, London, 1993

[2] Reiss, T.H., Recognizing Planar Objects Using Invariant Image Features, Springer Verlag, Berlin, 1992

[3] Gupta, L. und Srinath, D., „Contour Sequence Moments for the Classification of Closed Planar Shapes", Pattern Recognition, 20(3), 1987

[4] Reeves AP, Kostis WJ; Computer-aided diagnosis of small pulmonary nodules; *Semin Ultrasound CT MR* 2000 Apr;21(2):116-28

[5] Handels, H. Roßmanith, C., Rinast, E., Weiss, H.-D. und Pöppl, S.J., „Objektbezogene Bildanalyse von Hirntumoren zur Unterstützung der neuroradiologischen Diagnostik", H.J. Trampisch und S. Lange (eds.), Medizinische Forschung – Ärztliches Handeln, MMV Medizin Verlag, München, 1995

[6] Brief, J., Hassfeld, S., Redlich, T., Mühling, J., Walz, M., Krempien, R., Münchenberg, J., Wörn, H., Rembold, U., Grabowski, H., Raczkowsky, J., Burgert, O., Salb, T. & Dillmann, R. (1999). *3D norm data- the first step towards semiautomatic virtual craniofacial surgery.* In Proceedings of the 13th International Congress and Exhibition on Computer Assisted Radiology and Surgery (CARS'99) (pp. 559-563). Paris: Elsevier Press

[7] Bronstejn, Il'ja N.: *Taschenbuch der Mathematik,* Stuttgart, Leipzig: B.G. Teubner

[8] http://mathworld.wolfram.com/SphericalHarmonic.html

Medicine Meets Virtual Reality 2001
J.D. Westwood et al. (Eds.)
IOS Press, 2001

Modeling and Simulation for Space Medicine Operations: Preliminary Requirements Considered

David L. Dawson MD*, Roger D. Billica MD*, P. Vernon McDonald PhD**
Space Medicine and Health Care Systems Office, NASA Johnson Space Center
**Medical Operations, Advanced Projects, Wyle Laboratories, Inc.*
Houston, Texas 77058 USA

1. Abstract

The NASA Space Medicine program is now developing plans for more extensive use of high-fidelity medical simulation systems. The use of simulation is seen as means to more effectively use the limited time available for astronaut medical training. Training systems should be adaptable for use in a variety of training environments, including classrooms or laboratories, space vehicle mockups, analog environments, and in microgravity.

Modeling and simulation can also provide the space medicine development program a mechanism for evaluation of other medical technologies under operationally realistic conditions. Systems and procedures need preflight verification with ground-based testing. Traditionally, component testing has been accomplished, but practical means for "human in the loop" verification of patient care systems have been lacking. Medical modeling and simulation technology offer potential means to accomplish such validation work.

Initial considerations in the development of functional requirements and design standards for simulation systems for space medicine are discussed.

2. Introduction

The Johnson Space Center (JSC) has operational responsibilities for implementing medical support for NASA's human space flight program. JSC space medicine specialists have the primary responsibility within NASA for the definition of operational medical requirements, medical procedures, specifications of medical hardware and systems, and their support. Within this context, the JSC Space Medicine program is now developing plans for more extensive use of high-fidelity medical simulation systems.

Astronaut Crew Medical Officers (CMOs), supported by ground-based flight surgeons, provide the routine and emergency medical care to astronaut crews during space flights. CMOs—who are generally not physicians—are trained to perform diagnostic and therapeutic procedures. At present, evacuation to a definitive care medical facility is planned if serious injury or illness occurs on orbit, but there may still be a delay of up to 24 hours between the evacuation decision and arrival at the definitive medical care facility (perhaps longer, in some circumstances). In the interim, CMOs will be responsible for the evaluation, initial resuscitation, stabilization, and monitoring of the patient until landing.

Medical plans for in-space resuscitation and emergency care have been developed and refined over the past two decades of the Space Shuttle program. The expanded capabilities planned for the International Space Station (ISS) have built on this foundation of experience, supplemented by operational experience from the Shuttle-Mir program.[1] The ISS will become a test-bed for the development and validation of medical systems that will support human exploration missions beyond Low Earth Orbit (LEO).

Modeling and simulation (M&S) are recognized as important technologies for Space Medicine. Current training systems are limited by amount of astronaut training time available and the limited medical background of non-physician CMOs. Use of simulation is seen as means to more effectively use the limited training time. Several approaches to medical M&S have been identified (Table 1), but no one is ideal for all applications.

Integration of high-level simulators in NASA's clinical space medicine development program can also provide a mechanism for evaluation of other NASA technologies under operational conditions. Portability of currently available simulator systems makes their use possible in operationally-relevant environments, including the Crew Return Vehicle for the ISS, the ISS mockup, and in microgravity (such as during KC-135 parabolic flight).

Table 1

Approaches to Medical Modeling and Simulation	Features	Current Shortcomings	Examples
PC-based interactive multimedia training systems	Inexpensive, readily available, portable	Inconsistent standards, less suitable for task training	Trauma Patient Simulator™ (Research Triangle Institute)
Digitally Enhanced Mannequins	Commercial-off-the-shelf technology, suitable for team training	Limited stand-alone capability, more complex and expensive than PC-based platform	Human Patient Simulator™ (METI)
Virtual Workbenches	Rapid technical development, facilitates practice of minimally invasive surgical procedures and team training	Limited stand-alone capability, haptic feedback limited by current technology, less portable than PC-based system	ImmersaDesk™ (Fakespace)
Total Immersion Virtual Reality (TIVR)	Evolving technology, provides realistic environmental simulation	High development costs, requires support systems and larger facility	University of Michigan Cave Automated Virtual Environment (CAVE)
Comprehensive Computational Models Combining Function and Structure	Integrated modeling of human systems, from molecular to system level; predicts problems, simulates responses to countermeasures or interventions	Integrated models proposed, but do not yet exist; high development costs anticipated	"Digital Human" National Biomedical Research Institute (NSBRI), Integrated Human Function Team

"Virtual Human" Oak Ridge National Laboratory, Life Sciences Division |

Adapted from Proceedings of February 2000 meeting of US Army Medical Research and Material Command (USAMRMC), Medical Modeling and Simulation (MM&S) Integrated Research Team.

3. Medical Risks in Space Flight

There are a number of physiologic responses and adaptations that occur during space flight. The principal known physiologic effects of space flight are due to microgravity. These include cardiovascular alterations, bone demineralization, muscle alterations and atrophy, neurovestibular adaptation, human performance factors, and effects on sleep and chronobiology.[2, 3,4] Based a review of space and analog environment operational experience, the risk of a significant medical events in LEO has been estimated to be 0.06 to 0.07 per person-year.

Some factors are of particular concern when considering future potential missions that would take crews beyond LEO. These missions are likely to be lengthy, with prolonged delays in evacuation to terrestrial medical care. Radiation in deep space—beyond the Earth's protective magnetosphere—is of greater concern. Not only is there electromagnetic radiation (x-rays), but there are also risks from Galactic Cosmic Radiation and Solar Particle Events.[4-6] Clearly, the CMO must be robustly trained, but there is no way to train for all possible scenarios. The pre-flight and in-flight training systems must consider expected illnesses and ambulatory medical problems, acute medical emergencies that could occur in space, and some types of chronic disease. (Table 2) Also, skills and knowledge degrade over time. Therefore, there will be a need for refresher or "just-in-time" training during a long duration exploration mission.

Table 2

Expected Illnesses and Ambulatory Medical Problems
Orthopedic and musculoskeletal problems
Infectious, hematological, and immune related diseases
Dermatological, ophthalmologic, and ear/nose/throat problems
Acute Medical Emergencies in Space
Wounds, lacerations, and burns
Toxic exposure and acute anaphylaxis
Acute radiation illness
Dental emergencies
Ophthalmologic emergencies
Psychiatric emergencies
Chronic Diseases
Radiation induced problems
Responses to environmental exposures, including lunar or planetary dusts
Presentation or acute manifestation of nascent illness

4. Space Medicine Operational Constraints

The practice of space medicine must contend with environmental and programmatic challenges.[5,6] The mass, volume, communication bandwidth requirements, and power consumption of medical systems must be optimized, as they compete with vehicle and payload systems. Communication capabilities will constrained, both now and in the future.

The orbital track and configuration of the ISS causes it to be out of direct communication with Mission Control Center 45-50% of the time.

Operational features of future exploration missions will require CMOs to function with even greater autonomy. Communication latency due to the great distances involved will prohibit real-time communication and remote operation of critical medical systems. For example, there is 7-40 minute round-trip communication to Mars. Relative positions of the Earth, Sun, and Mars may impose communication blackouts for up to 30 days. Medical systems must contend with bandwidth limitations, but these challenges may be mitigated by future technological advances, such as the establishment of interplanetary internet or broadband optical communication links.

There are many constraints imposed by distance. Without resupply capability, all consumables must be carried on board or generated *in situ*. Drugs and similar items need long shelf-lives. Device failure risks should be minimized by the use of highly-reliable systems, built-in fault management, functional redundancies, or by allowing astronaut servicing. Additionally, the long transit times of exploration missions impose physiological and psychological stresses due to the prolonged isolation and confinement. These factors may have effects on human performance and should be considered in the design of medical care systems.

Crew time, however, remains one of the space program's most precious and limited resources. This means that CMO training time is severely restricted. During the several years of preparation for an ISS mission, astronauts receive less than three weeks of dedicated medical training. Also notable, is that in NASA's current operational paradigm, there is no specialized training or proficiency maintenance program for the subset of astronauts who are physicians. While a graduate medical education program specific to in-flight space medicine practice has been envisioned [7], no such program exists. Thus, it is an imperative to optimize the limited medical training time available. The use of medical M&S technology is recognized as one means to achieve this goal.

Medical operations must be an integrated part of the overall mission. All systems for space flight must meet specific design, safety, and operational requirements. Not only must hardware items, software, and procedures be tested individually to be certified for flight, each component needs to be verified as a functional part of the overall system. The standard yardstick is to perform end-to-end testing in the "as flown" configuration.

Medical systems and procedures need preflight verification with ground-based testing. Traditionally, component testing has been accomplished, but practical means for "human in the loop" verification of patient care systems have been lacking. Medical M&S technologies offer potential means to accomplish such validation work.

5. Current "Real World" Applications of Modeling and Simulation: The ISS Era

Goals for ground-based simulation training include familiarization with medical systems and procedures, critical incident response, and team training. In the short term, high fidelity medical simulation systems should be incorporated into astronaut CMO and flight surgeon training. Currently available systems facilitate practice of individual psychomotor skills and have features that are adaptable to various levels of trainee knowledge and experience. Potential applications include part task training for basic CMO skills (orientation to medical kit use, patient assessment, airway management, procedures, etc.), Advanced Cardiac Life Support (ACLS) training, and to provide proficiency training for crewmembers who have completed the Emergency Medical Technician-Basic course. Simulation is not viewed as a replacement for clinical practice, rather, as a means to enrich limited clinical experiences. Unusual scenarios can be modeled, allowing emergency procedures to be drilled.[8,9]

Risk assessments suggest that in-flight medical events that would require immediate life-saving intervention will be extremely uncommon. Still, the medical kits and the associated CMO training are designed to provide for resuscitation and stabilization, should such an event occur. Considering the baseline health of the crews, age and gender factors, operational or environmental risks, past experiences from space flight or operations in analogous environments, and other relevant data, the most likely scenarios that might require such intervention can be anticipated. These include:

- acute airway obstruction
- severe decompression sickness
- hemorrhage
- major thermal or electrical injury
- myocardial infarction
- pneumothorax
- pulmonary embolism

- respiratory failure (aspiration or inhalational injury)
- sepsis
- severe anaphylaxis
- stroke or closed head injury
- unstable supraventricular tachycardia

Medical team training concepts have been developed as analogs to courses in aviation Crew (or Cockpit) Resource Management (CRM).[8,9] This type of training has been found to be especially useful for medical professionals as they transition to more complex roles and settings. The incorporation of CRM principles into CMO training naturally follows. As the ISS has multinational and multicultural crews, team training is of particular value to minimize miscommunication due to cultural nuances.[10]

6. Desired Features of Simulation System for Training Applications

While many training requirements of the space medicine program are conventional, there are some mission-specific requirements that should be considered.

The need to model microgravity effects is the most unique requirement for space medicine training applications.[5,11] Microgravity is known to alter cardiovascular physiology, autonomic function, fluid distribution, mineral metabolism, pharmacokinetics, pharmacodynamics, and other functions. Clinically significant effects on immune function and wound healing are suspected. Microgravity effects on fluid distribution also have effects on the presentation and course of certain conditions.

Training systems should be adaptable for use in a variety of training environments. These include classrooms or laboratories, space vehicle mockups, analog environments (such as field training settings, or in the BIO-Plex, a long-term closed habitat being constructed at JSC for research in advanced life support systems). Systems should also function in microgravity, to support medical training in the KC-135.

General characteristics desired include portability (manageable size, weight, and logistic support requirements); ability to function in various environments (tolerance of moisture, vibration, changes in temperature and barometric pressure); adaptability (usable for a variety of training objectives) and safe operation (no hazards to users and operators, and no interference with other critical systems).

7. Simulation for Evaluation of Medical Devices and Procedures for Space Flight

Other candidate uses for medical M&S tools include evolution and validation of new on-orbit medical procedures and for evaluation of on-orbit medical equipment human factors (design verification and validation). Scenario-based simulations provide a valuable tool for evaluating capabilities and identifying deficiencies in the medical infrastructure, as well as for the validation of clinical procedures and equipment. Clinical scenarios, developed from published literature or operational experience and model the presentation and time course of patient conditions, provide means for testing many aspects of the medical care delivery system, including training, equipment, communication, and other relevant factors. Better documentation of standards of care for each patient condition, along with the identification of new care procedures for each condition, result.

A new generation of intelligent devices could be incorporated into an advanced version of the ISS medical system. An envisioned networked device array could provide a simplified user interface to assist on-orbit care. A fully evolved system should provide (1) a single scaleable user interface for monitoring, controlling, documenting and guidance; (2) interactive context-sensitive diagnosis and management checklists; (3) integrated medical data storage and downlink capability; and (4) plug-and-play medical device modularity.

8. Long-Term Vision: Applications of Medical Modeling and Simulation

Exploration missions beyond LEO will require a level of autonomy far beyond that of the human space flight experience of the 20th century.[11] While it is difficult to project the state of technology in the future decades when humans may venture beyond Earth's neighborhood, a consensus of opinion of operational space medicine experts has identified desirable features of future on-board medical systems:

- non- or minimally invasive approaches for diagnosis and treatment
- built-in, distributed intelligence and automation (smart medical systems)
- consultative, diagnostic, and therapeutic telemedicine capabilities
- assistive technologies
- intuitive interfaces
- reconfigurable to various accommodate skill levels and levels of medical training
- comprehensive user support & feedback
- minimal mass, volume, power needs
- high degree of reliability, to ensure function throughout mission

Systems should be maintainable, upgradeable, reconfigurable, and multi-functional. Ideally, systems supporting medical care should be adaptable to non-medical applications.

9. Initial Plans for Modeling and Simulation Use in Space Medicine

The JSC space medicine programs is now taking the following steps:

- Identifying collaborators for development of simulator clinical training program.
- Developing initial recommendations for use of medical simulators in training of Space Shuttle CMOs, ISS CMOs, flight surgeons, and others.
- Identifying clinical training experiences that best complement simulator training.
- Identifying and prioritizing candidate technologies.
- Definition of human factors issues in the design and implementation of CMO medical simulator training programs.
- Establish protocols and procedures for optimal use of simulation facilities

Dialogue and collaboration are sought.

References

[1] National Aeronautics and Space Administration, Lyndon B. Johnson Space Center. International Space Station Crew Medical Officer Training Syllabus (JSC 28046). 1998.

[2] Barratt M. Medical support for the International Space Station. *Aviat Space Environ Med* 1999 Feb; 70(2):155-161.

[3] Sawin CF. Biomedical investigations conducted in support of the Extended Duration Orbiter Medical Project. *Aviat Space Environ Med* 1999 Feb; 70(2):169-180.

[4] Nicogossian AE, Huntoon CL, Pool SL. [Eds] *Space Medicine and Physiology*. vol 3, New York: Lea & Febiger, 1994.

[5] Davis JR. Medical issues for a mission to Mars. *Aviat Space Environ Med* 1999 Feb; 70(2):162-168.

[6] Jennings RT, Pool SL. Space medicine: what lies ahead? *Aviat Space Environ Med* 1999 Feb; 70(2):153-154.

[7] McGinnis PJ, Harris BA Jr. The re-emergence of space medicine as a distinct discipline. *Aviat Space Environ Med* 1998 Nov; 69(11):1107-1011.

[8] Holzman RS, Cooper JB, Gaba DM, Philip JH, Small SD, Feinstein D. Anesthesia crisis resource management: real-life simulation training in operating room crises. *J Clin Anesth* 1995; 8:675-687.

[9] Howard SK, Gaba DM, Fish, KJ, Yang G, Sarnquist FH. Anesthesia crisis resource management training: teaching anesthesiologists to handle critical incidents. *Aviat Space Environ Med* 1992; 63:763-770.

[10] Helmriech RL, Merritt AC. Culture at work in aviation and medicine. National, organization and professional influences. Aldershot, England: Ashgate Publishing Ltd., 1998.

[11] Campbell MR. Surgical care in space. Aviat Space Environ Med 1999 Feb; 70(2):181-184.

[12] Stuster J. Bold endeavors: lessons from polar and space exploration. Annapolis, MD: Naval Institute Press, 1996.

Medicine Meets Virtual Reality 2001
J.D. Westwood et al. (Eds.)
IOS Press, 2001

A Meshless Numerical Technique for Physically Based Real Time Medical Simulations

S. De, J. Kim and M. A. Srinivasan

Laboratory for Human and Machine Haptics, Department of Mechanical Engineering,
Massachusetts Institute of Technology, Cambridge, MA 02139, USA

Abstract. This work introduces, for the first time, a meshless modeling technique, the method of finite spheres, for physically based, real time rendering of soft tissues in medical simulations. The technique is conceptually similar to the traditional finite element techniques. However, while the finite element techniques requires a slow mesh generation process, this new technique has significant potential for multimodal medical simulations of the future since it does not use a mesh. Several examples are presented showing the effectiveness of the scheme.

1. Introduction

In this paper, we present a novel "meshless" numerical scheme for computations underlying virtual reality based medical simulations. This technique enables the user to interact with physically based tissue and organ models in real time, using both visual and haptic sensory modalities. Of special interest are surgical simulations involving contact interactions between long slender tools and deformable organs. Laparoscopic surgery is a particular example of such a procedure.

The success of a laparoscopic surgeon depends heavily on his or her training. An efficient laparoscopic surgery simulator will not only result in customized practice environments for medical students, but will also reduce the use of animals and cadavers that are currently used for such training.

An important issue in medical simulation is the modeling of soft tissues. From a purely mechanistic viewpoint, soft tissues exhibit complex material properties [1]. They are nonlinear, anisotropic, viscoelastic and nonhomogeneous (usually layered). Moreover, soft tissues deform considerably under the application of relatively small loads. In addition, it is quite difficult to obtain *in vivo* material properties of living tissues. Therefore a challenging task is to develop efficient models for living tissues so that realistic simulation of tool-tissue interaction can be performed in real time.

For real time visual display an update rate of 30 Hz is sufficient. For haptic display, we use the Phantom haptic interface device (SensAble Technologies, Inc). For stable simulation, the haptic loop requires an update rate of about 1kHz. This imposes severe restrictions on the complexity of the models that can be rendered haptically. Therefore simulation speed is the prime consideration.

Various techniques can be found in literature for the simulation and display of deformable objects. These techniques can be categorized into two main approaches: "geometrically based" approaches and "physically based" approaches [2]. The "geometrically based" modeling approaches, such as Bezier/B-spline based procedures and free form deformation techniques, do not account for the physics of deformation, but are simpler to implement.

In contrast, the "physically based" approaches, such as the lumped parameter spring-mass-damper models [3] attempt to model the underlying physics. These models are simple and computationally very efficient. However, the construction of an optimal network of springs in 3D is a complicated process. Moreover, under certain conditions, mass-spring systems may become oscillatory or even go unstable during simulation.

The finite element technique is widely used in engineering analysis for the simulation of deformable objects [4]. Several researchers have applied finite element techniques for real time surgical simulations [5, 6]. However, finite element techniques suffer from certain drawbacks in real time simulations. First, the contact between tool and tissues must occur at nodal points. Therefore, to prevent loss of resolution, the density of nodal points should be sufficiently high. This requires extensive memory resources and high computational overhead. Second, cutting or tearing requires an expensive remeshing process during simulation. This means precomputed data of the object becomes, at least locally, useless and all data must be computed in real time. The computation time increases approximately as the cube of the number of nodal unknowns. This poses significant obstacles in real time applications, given the high rate of force updates required.

A solution to the problems that are faced by the finite element techniques is to use a numerical technique that does not use a mesh. The method of finite spheres (MFS) is one such "meshless" computational technique [7]. In this paper we present a specialized version of the method of finite spheres for the purpose of real time medical simulations. Nodal points are sprinkled around the surgical tool tip (not the entire domain) and the interpolation is performed by functions that are nonzero only on spheres surrounding the nodes. A point collocation technique is used to generate the discrete equations that are solved in real time.

The localization provided by the finite influence zones of the nodes as well as the elimination of numerical integration results in a highly accelerated numerical scheme. The flexibility in the placement of nodes allows complex operations like cutting to take place relatively easily. In addition, since the differential equations governing the tool tissue interactions are being solved in the vicinity of the tool tip, the solution procedure is physically based.

In the next section we briefly introduce the numerical technique. In section 3 we discuss numerical implementation issues and finally present some examples in section 4.

2. The numerical scheme

In this section we briefly introduce the theory behind the method of finite spheres (refer to [7] for details). In this technique, we distribute nodal points around the surgical tool tip and define spherical "influence zones" around each node (see Figure 1). The approximation u_h of a variable u (e.g. displacement), using 'N' spheres, may be written as

$$u_h(\mathbf{x}) = \sum_{J=1}^{N} h_J(\mathbf{x})\alpha_J \tag{1}$$

where α_J is the nodal unknown at node J. The nodal shape function $h_J(\mathbf{x})$ at node J is generated using a moving least squares technique [8]

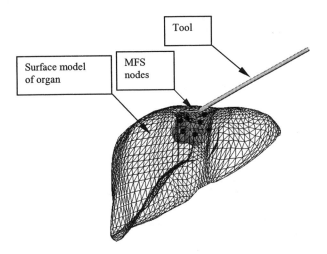

Figure 1. A laparoscopic surgical tool interacting with the surface model of a liver. MFS nodes are distributed in the vicinity of the tool tip to obtain a localized discretization.

$$h_J(\mathbf{x}) = W_J(\mathbf{x})\mathbf{P}(\mathbf{x})^T \mathbf{A}^{-1}(\mathbf{x})\mathbf{P}(\mathbf{x}_J) \qquad J=1,\ldots, N \tag{2}$$

where

$$\mathbf{A}(\mathbf{x}) = \sum_{I=1}^{N} W_I(\mathbf{x})\mathbf{P}(\mathbf{x}_I)\mathbf{P}(\mathbf{x}_I)^T . \tag{3}$$

The vector $\mathbf{P}(\mathbf{x})$ contains polynomials ensuring consistency up to a desired order (in our implementation we have chosen $\mathbf{P}(\mathbf{x}) = \{1,x,y,z\}^T$ to ensure a first order accurate scheme in 3D, similar to bilinear finite elements). W_J is a compactly supported radial weighting function at node J (which we have chosen as a quartic spline function).

We assume linear elastic tissue behavior. A point collocation technique is used to generate the discrete equations

$$\mathbf{KU} = \mathbf{f} \tag{4}$$

where $\mathbf{K}$ is the stiffness matrix and $\mathbf{f}$ is the vector containing nodal loads.

In surgical simulation, the tool tip may be modeled as having point interaction with the tissue (see Figure 2). A node is placed at the tool tip and all other nodes are placed such that their spheres do not intersect the node at the tool tip (or do so only minimally to ensure the invertibility of $\mathbf{A}(\mathbf{x})$ in Eq (3)). The nodal displacement at the tool tip is equal to the applied displacement, $\mathbf{U}_{\text{tooltip}}$.

The stiffness matrix in Eq (3) may be partitioned as

$$\mathbf{K} = \begin{bmatrix} \mathbf{K}_{aa} & \mathbf{K}_{ab} \\ \mathbf{K}_{ba} & \mathbf{K}_{bb} \end{bmatrix} \tag{5}$$

corresponding to a partitioning of the vector of nodal parameters as $\mathbf{U} = \begin{bmatrix} \mathbf{U}_{\text{tooltip}} & \mathbf{U}_b \end{bmatrix}^T$ where $\mathbf{U}_b$ is the vector of nodal unknowns which maybe obtained as $\mathbf{U}_b = -\mathbf{K}_{bb}^{-1}\mathbf{K}_{ba}\mathbf{U}_{\text{tooltip}}$. The reaction force to be delivered to the haptic interface device is obtained as $\mathbf{f}_{\text{tooltip}} = \mathbf{K}_{aa}\mathbf{U}_{\text{tooltip}} + \mathbf{K}_{ab}\mathbf{U}_b$.

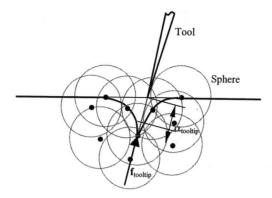

Figure 2. Placement of nodes at the tool tip. $\alpha_{tooltip}$ and $f_{tooltip}$ are the prescribed displacement and reaction force at the tool tip, respectively.

3. Real time issues

To simulate tissue palpation through a tool, collision detection, placement of the nodal points and computation of organ surface deformation and tool tip reaction force have to be performed in real time. The organ model is usually a polygon (triangular) based surface model. We use a fast collision detection algorithm developed by Ho et. al. [9] where we establish a hierarchical database of geometric primitives, with each primitive having pointers to neighboring primitives. The collision detection time is independent of the total number of polygons in the model and the process is, of course, real time (i.e. 1kHz and higher).

As soon as a collision point is detected, MFS nodes are sprinkled around the tool tip, both on the surface of the organ model as well as inside. This is a computationally intensive process. Therefore the location of the nodes relative to the tool tip is defined offline but the computation of tissue deformation is performed in real time. Another important issue is the choice of the radii of the spheres. While spheres with larger radii provide greater covering for fewer spheres, they increase the bandwidth of the stiffness matrix and also result in coarser approximation. Details regarding these issues may be found in [10].

4. Simulation demonstration

We have implemented the point collocation based method of finite spheres for real time simulation and display of deformation and tool tip reaction force for certain simple 3D geometries such as a hemisphere (see Figure 3) and a liver model (see Figure 4). In both cases, linear elastic tissue behavior has been assumed. These example problems illustrate the applicability of the new scheme proposed here to the simulation of tissue palpation.

In Figure 3 we compare the displacement solution results obtained for the hemisphere problem using the method of finite spheres (using 34 nodes) and the finite element technique (using the commercial finite element package ADINA and 27 noded volumetric brick elements). In the vicinity of the tool tip the displacement profile computed using the method of finite spheres is observed to match the much slower finite element solution and hence is quite accurate. However, increasing divergence is observed away from the tool tip. For the purpose of surgical simulation, this displacement profile based on MFS may be admissible.

The point collocation based method of finite spheres is however very fast. We were able to achieve a computational rate of about 100Hz for the example shown in Figure 2 when 34 spheres were used for discretization. Real time rendering rates of about 1 kHz was then obtained using a force extrapolation technique (refer to [10] for details).

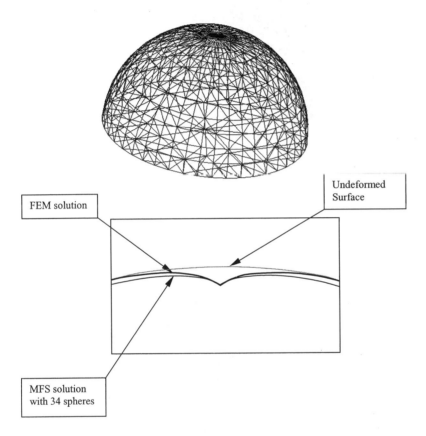

Figure 3. The deformation field obtained when MFS is used for the simulation of a surgical tool tip interacting with a hemispherical object is shown. The undeformed surface and the deformation field obtained using a finite element discretization are also shown.

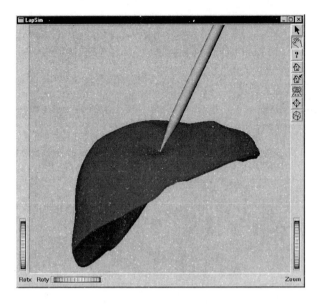

Figure 4. A snapshot of the laparoscopic surgical simulator LapSim showing a surgical tool interacting with a liver model.

References

[1] S. De and M. A. Srinivasan, Thin Walled Models for Haptic and Graphical Rendering of Soft Tissues in Surgical Simulation, *Proceeding of MMVR 7 Conference* (1999) 94-99.

[2] D. Terzopoulos, J. Platt, A. Barr and K. Fleischer, Elastically Deformable Models, *Computer Graphics* **21**(4) (1987) 205-214.

[3] D. Terzopoulos and K. Waters, Physically Based Facial Modeling, Analysis and Animation, *Journal of Visualization and Computer Animation* **1** (1990) 73-80.

[4] K. J. Bathe, Finite Element Procedures, Prentice Hall, 1996.

[5] M. Bro-Nielsen and S. Cotin, Real Time Volumetric Deformable Models for Surgery Simulation Using Finite Elements and Condensation, *Proceeding of Computer Graphics Forum, Eurographics 96* (1996) 57-66.

[6] S. Cotin, H. Delingette, J. M. Clement, V. Tassetti, J. Marescaux and N. Ayache, Geometric and Physical Representations for a Simulator of Hepatic Surgery, *Proceedings of MMVR 4 Conference* (1996)139-151.

[7] S. De and K. J. Bathe, The Method of Finite Spheres. Computational Mechanics, **25** (2000) 329-345.

[8] S.De and K. J.Bathe, Towards an Efficient Meshless Computational Technique: The Method of Finite Spheres, to appear in *Engineering Computations*.

[9] C. Ho, C. Basdogan and M. A. Srinivasan, Efficient Point-Based Rendering Techniques for Haptic Display of Virtual Objects, *Presence* **8** (1999) 477-491.

[10] S. De, J. Kim and M. A. Srinivasan, The Method of Finite Spheres in Real Time Multimodal Medical Simulations, to appear.

Medicine Meets Virtual Reality 2001
J.D. Westwood et al. (Eds.)
IOS Press, 2001

Manipulation of Volumetric Patient Data in a Distributed Virtual Reality Environment

Fred Dech, Zhuming Ai and Jonathan C. Silverstein
University of Illinois at Chicago
VRMedLab, HHSB M/C 530
Chicago, IL 60612-7249
fdech@uic.edu, zai@uic.edu, jsilver@uic.edu

Abstract. Due to increases in network speed and bandwidth, distributed exploration of medical data in immersive Virtual Reality (VR) environments is becoming increasingly feasible. The volumetric display of radiological data in such environments presents a unique set of challenges. The shear size and complexity of the datasets involved not only make them difficult to transmit to remote sites, but these datasets also require extensive user interaction in order to make them understandable to the investigator and manageable to the rendering hardware. A sophisticated VR user interface is required in order for the clinician to focus on the aspects of the data that will provide educational and/or diagnostic insight.

We will describe a software system of data acquisition, data display, Tele-Immersion, and data manipulation that supports interactive, collaborative investigation of large radiological datasets. The hardware required in this strategy is still at the high-end of the graphics workstation market. Future software ports to Linux and NT, along with the rapid development of PC graphics cards, open the possibility for later work with Linux or NT PCs and PC clusters.

1. Introduction

Real-time display of volumetric CT and MR data is challenging. There is the initial task of acquiring the data from the scanning workstation. We have chosen the DICOM de facto standard as our data format of choice. In addition, we have written numerous classes and dynamically shared object libraries to facilitate the input of this data into our visualization applications [1]. Managing a real-time frame-rate for larger and larger datasets requires the right high-end hardware and the appropriate volume-rendering approach. However, maintaining this frame-rate becomes increasingly difficult as the size of the volume exceeds the texture memory limits of the graphics platform. Add multi-site, networked Tele-collaboration in a VR environment to this equation and the difficulties of maintaining a coherent and productive environment for the clinician become daunting.

It is not enough to display radiological data (e.g., CT, MRI) in real-time. In order for this data visualization to be useful, there must be a high-level of interactivity between the user and the data being displayed. This interactivity and its results must also be available to the other networked participants in a Tele-collaborative exercise in order for the collaboration to be meaningful to these remote participants.

Research in the area of interactive, networked volume visualization is scarce. First, real-time volume rendering normally requires expensive hardware at all sites that are involved in the collaboration. Secondly, distributing volumetric information (even over high-speed networks) to multiple sites is problematic. And thirdly, high-level tools for manipulating complex volumes are needed in order for insights to be gained from the VR interaction. In this paper we will describe work-in-progress and propose solutions to these obstacles.

2. Methods and Tools

The applications and tools to be discussed are based on an object-oriented integration of C++ and C libraries. Current working models require both IRIS Performer (a high-level, high-performance C++ graphics library) and CAVElib™ (a VR Device Programmer's Interface (DPI)) [2].

2.1. Data Acquisition

A sniffer daemon based on Mallinckrodt CTN software toolkit's [3] simplestorage application automatically reads DICOM data files at a network port to which the files have been pushed from a remote CT or MR workstation. For our research purposes, all patient-specific information is currently stripped from the header during the transfer procedure in order to avoid the possibility of compromising medical record confidentiality.

As reported in earlier work [1], we have developed DICOM loaders for IRIS Performer. These loaders are written using CTN to interpret and parse the DICOM files. Currently we have several loaders, some of which are sub-classed from the IRIS Performer pfMemory class. This ensures that the data is available in shared memory and that it remains accessible to the IRIS Performer APP processes running across multiple processors in the visualization application.

2.2. Data Display

Current data types supported are 8-bit and 16 (12)-bit grayscale, along with 8-bit and 16-bit pseudo-color. Once the data has been loaded into shared memory, it is converted and segmented into *memory bricks* within an IRIS Performer geometry class. This class contains all of the OpenGL Volumizer (an OpenGL C++ volume rendering library) [4] construction routines. The construction process is forked off as part of the IRIS Performer APP process. The actual polygonization and rendering of the volume occurs in a separate IRIS Performer DRAW process.

Briefly, OGL Volumizer uses an approach whereby geometry and appearance are defined independently of one another. The three-dimensional geometric primitive is a tetrahedron. In the DRAW process, Volumizer uses a volume-slicing method which sequentially computes all points on a plane orthogonal to the line of sight. Consequently, Volumizer is much faster than other approaches (e.g., ray casting) because computations are performed by the dedicated texture mapping hardware rather than by the CPU. The volume is reduced to a series of texture-mapped, translucent polygons. Volumizer memory bricks are sections of the voxel data small enough to fit into available texture memory. It is possible to have multiple bricks representing a single volume. During the DRAW process, these bricks are swapped in and out of texture memory to complete the image rendering. Therefore, having enough texture memory to fit the entire volume into a single brick, or small number of bricks is the optimal scenario. Most of our volume-rendering research has been conducted on SGI Onyx2 IR2 platforms. A single IR2 graphics pipe can have up to 64 MB of available texture memory per raster manager. The texel primitive on these platforms is four bytes in length. However, by using a technique known as texture interleaving, two 2-byte bricks can be overlapped to make complete use of the 4-byte word texels. Therefore, on a fully configured IR2 a 2-byte 512x512x244 volume can remain resident in texture memory producing frame-rates upwards of 30 fps. A volume that requires less than 10 texture bricks may still produce frame-rates of 15-20 fps. This remains well within the range of interactive speed. Much larger volumes can be studied if the volume's geometry is made smaller than the actual voxel dimensions of the volume. Using this approach, one can interactively roam through small subsets of the volume. This method is known as *region-of-interest* (ROI) manipulation.

With CAVElib, the applications become integrated into the VR environment platforms in a straightforward fashion. CAVElib is a library for developing OpenGL and IRIS Performer VR applications. It supports the CAVE®, ImmersaDesk® [5]. The hardware-specific tasks (e.g., tracking, multi-screen display) needed for these devices are handled by the CAVE library and remain transparent to the application. Current research is being conducted primarily on ImmersaDesk and ImmersaDesk2® platforms.

2.3. Tele-Immersion

Tele-Immersion, or the real-time collaboration of remotely connected sites in a VR environment, is an essential ingredient to the remote teaching of, and remote, collaborative investigation of radiological patient data. The difficulties and variables involved in developing a successful Tele-Immersive application are many. Shared or synchronized databases, application hand-shaking, streaming audio and video, and network management are just a few of the issues that require detailed attention.

In previous work, we have developed applications incorporating CAVERNsoft G1 (a toolkit for developing Tele-Immersive applications) [6]. We have successfully linked multiple VR sites together into one shared, interactive environment. Within the last twelve months, CAVERNsoft G2 has been released. Unlike G1, which is a large monolithic system, G2 has been completely re-designed as a modular and flexible object-oriented library. G2 supports various forms of UDP, TCP and multicast communication, and its higher-level classes incorporate CAVElib and IRIS Performer. We will be porting our VR applications to G2 in the near future.

When conducting a Tele-Immersive examination of radiological data, all sites normally should be viewing the same data in exactly the same way, while not necessarily from the same perspective. Each remote participant must be aware of what the other participants are saying and doing; thus the need for audio transmission and a representation of the other participants within the shared virtual environment. This representation, or avatar, can often be sufficiently expressed by the location of the participants' hands and an indication of where they are pointing. All participating sites should also remain informed as new participants join and others leave. If a user has control of the data and is manipulating it in some way, these changes need to be broadcast to all remote users involved. CAVERNsoft G2 has flexible high-level methods for constructing communication channels that enable such complex, multi-site interaction to occur.

2.4. Data Manipulation

Volumetric data is incredibly rich in information. For example, density ranges and variations in water content in CT and MR data respectively can reveal dramatically different details when the opacity and contrast along their dynamic range is varied. Because of the number and complexity of attributes in volumetric radiological datasets, some sort of VR Graphical User Interface (GUI) is required in order to manipulate these attributes successfully. We have developed a library of widget classes, *vwLib* [7], to facilitate the construction of complex GUIs in a CAVElib, IRIS Performer environment. This widget library uses an *Observer Pattern* with a *Mediator Pattern*, an object-oriented approach to event generation and propagation [8]. A Mediator handles the event mapping between event generating widgets (Subjects) and the recipients of these events (Observers). The result is an extremely straightforward and efficient event model. Currently, we have Button classes, Slider classes, various Frame classes and an Incrementor class. Menus are described by a well-defined configuration file making many modifications possible without the need for re-compilation.

3. Results

Using a main-menu structure, where various selections spawn off sub-menus or special interactive states, we have had promising results in the task of manipulating volumes in a collaborative, VR environment. To date, we have used the WAND™ and WANDA™ 3D pointing devices to select and manipulate the 3D widgets in these interfaces. Other, 3D-interaction devices are also supported. In the following paragraphs, we offer a brief account of the functionality supported in our current research applications.

Windowing of volume data can be manipulated in real-time using a group of specialized sliders and incrementors (Figure 1). Simultaneously, the volume can be picked and rotated about its centroid, translated arbitrarily, clipped arbitrarily and the data windowed in standard fashion for radiological data by selection of center and width of the data window. All of this manipulation is done by changing the user's hand (WAND) orientation and position including menu (state) selection. To date, only one data window is supported. This will be enhanced shortly to allow simultaneous windowing of two discrete regions of the volume data.

The size and location of the volume's geometric region can be modified with various sliders (Figure 2). Along with the use of multiple, arbitrarily oriented clipping planes, this allows users to focus in on details and maintain a favorable frame-rate. The location sliders will soon be replaced with a *roaming* interface whereby a user will be able to pick the ROI with the WAND and move it through the volume in arbitrary directions, or in fixed axial directions.

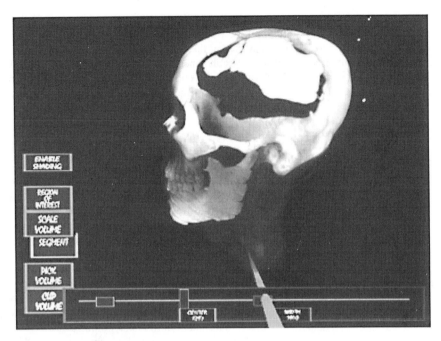

Figure 1: CT data with data-windowing sub-menu. Specialized sliders and incrementors control the width and location of the data window.

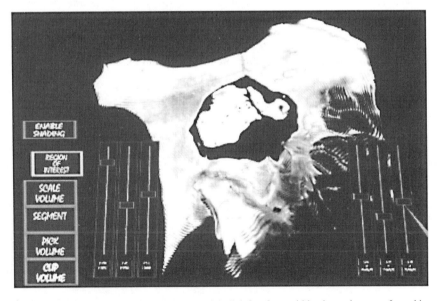

Figure 2: CT data with ROI sub-menu. Close-up of skull defect from within also makes use of an arbitrary clipping plane.

We have also implemented a gradient-shading method option that can be toggled at any time and used with all of the other features. This provides the user with shadowing of the three-dimensional contours displayed as though there was a natural light source. Gradient shading can be useful when examining certain types of details but does carry with it a heavy performance penalty when activated, as the entire volume must be rendering three or more times per frame in order to generate the shaded image. Finally, the volume can be scaled up or down from the original real size.

4. Conclusions

We have largely succeeded in overcoming the significant challenges of real-time stereoscopic display and manipulation of volumetric CT and MR data. Our software system of data acquisition, data display, Tele-Immersion, and data manipulation is built on modular architecture and supports interactive, collaborative investigation of large radiological datasets. Specifically, we have succeeded in developing a robust distributed virtual reality environment in which remotely collaborating participants can load, extensively manipulate in real-time, and share visualizations of standard three-dimensional radiological data.

Future work will include the expansion of our collaborative capabilities with CAVERNsoft G2, further development of our multi-volume display capabilities, enhanced and expanded data manipulation tools and performance optimizations.

The hardware required in our strategy is still at the high-end of the graphics workstation market. Future software ports to Linux and NT, along with the rapid development of PC graphics cards, open the possibility for later work with Linux or NT PCs and PC clusters.

Applications such as this coupled with the advanced network features of the Next Generation Internet will soon bring sophisticated visualization techniques directly into the hands of clinicians. Such intuitive environments will finally permit custom visualizations to be rapidly generated directly by clinicians for a variety of purposes including education, research, diagnostics, pre-surgical planning, and even intra-operative decision support.

5. Acknowledgments

This project has been funded in whole or in part with Federal funds from the National Library of Medicine, National Institutes of Health, under Contract No. N01-LM-9-3543.

References

1. Z. Ai, F. Dech, M. Rasmussen, and J. C. Silverstein. Radiological Tele-Immersion for Next Generation Networks, *Stud Health Technol Inform 2000*;70, 2000, pp 4-9.

2. C. Cruz-Neira, D. J. Sandin, and T. A. DeFanti. Surround-screen Projection-Based Virtual Reality: The Design and Implementation of the CAVE. *ACM SIGGRAPH '93 Proceedings*, Anaheim CA, August 1993.

3. Developed as part of the 1993 – 1995 DICOM Central Test Node project for the Radiological Society of North America by Washington University's Mallinckrodt Institute of Radiology, St. Louis MO.

4. R. Grzeszczuk, C. Henn, and R. Yagel. Advanced Geometric Techniques for Ray Casting Volumes, *ACM SIGGRAPH '98 Course Notes,* Volume 4, Orlando FL, April 1998.

5. M. Czernuszenko, D. Pape, D. Sandin, T. DeFanti, G. L. Dawe, and M. D. Brown. The ImmersaDesk and Infinity Wall Projection-Based Virtual Reality Displays, *Computer Graphics*, Vol. 31 Number 2, May 1997 pp 46-49.

6. K. Park, Y. J. Cho, N. K. Krishnaprasad, C. Scharver, M. J. Lewis, J. Leigh, and A. E. Johnson. CAVERsoft G2: A Toolkit for High Performance Tele-Immersive Collaboration, *ACM 7th Annual Symposium on Virtual Reality Software & Technology (VRST),* Seoul, Korea, 2000, to appear.

7. http://www.evl.uic.edu/fred/vwLib/docs

8. E. Gamma, R. Helm, R. Johnson, and J. Vlissides. Design Patterns – Elements of Reusable Object-Oriented Software, pp. 273-282 and 293-303, Reading MA. Addison-Wesley, 1995.

Medicine Meets Virtual Reality 2001
J.D. Westwood et al. (Eds.)
IOS Press, 2001

Bimanual Haptic Workstation
for Laparoscopic Surgery Simulation

Venkat Devarajan[1], Daniel Scott[2], Daniel Jones[2], Robert Rege[2], Robert Eberhart[2]

Charlie Lindahl[1], Peter Tanguy[3], Raul Fernandez

[1]Dept of Electrical engineering, 410 Yates Street

M/S 19077 Arlington, TX 76019

The University of Texas at Arlington

[2] The University of Texas Southwestern Medical Center at Dallas and

Southwestern Center for Minimally Invasive Surgery

[3]Automation and Robotic research institute

The University of Texas at Arlington

ABSTRACT: *Realistic laparoscopic surgical simulators will require real-time graphic imaging and tactile feedback. Our research objective is to develop a cost-effective haptic workstation for the simulation of laparoscopic procedures for training and treatment planning. The physical station consists of a custom-built frame into which laparoscopic trocars and surgical tools may be attached/inserted and which are continuously adjustable to various positions and orientations to simulate multiple laparoscopic surgical approaches. Instruments inserted through the trocars are attached to end effectors of two haptic devices and interfaced to a high speed PC with fast graphics capability. The haptic device transduces 3D motion of the two manually operated surgical instruments into slave maneuvers in virtual space. The slave instrument tips probe the simulated organ. Simulations currently in progress include: 1) Surface-only renderings, deformation, and haptic interactions with elements in the gall gladder surgical field; 2) Voxel-based simulations of the bulk manipulation of tissue; 3) laparoscopic herniorrhaphy. This system provides force feed-forward from the grasped tools to the contact tissue in virtual space, with deformation of the tissue by the virtual probe, and force feedback from the deformed tissue to the operator's hands.*

1.Introduction

The objective of this project is to develop a realistic and cost effective virtual surgery trainer with tactile feedback. This will be useful tool for training, treatment planning and surgical performance measurement. Realistic surgery simulations need real time graphics and fast haptic update. To achieve this we have a high-end graphics workstation with dual processors and a force-feed device called PHANToM from SensAble technologies. One of the interesting aspects of our work is the development of a mechanical frame for placing surgical tools. This ergonomically designed frame gives the flexibility of using various surgical tools for simulating various laparoscopic procedures. Currently we are working on laparoscopic herniorrhaphy which is a difficult procedure needing a lot of training and skill. We believe our work will have a significant impact in this area.

2 System Description

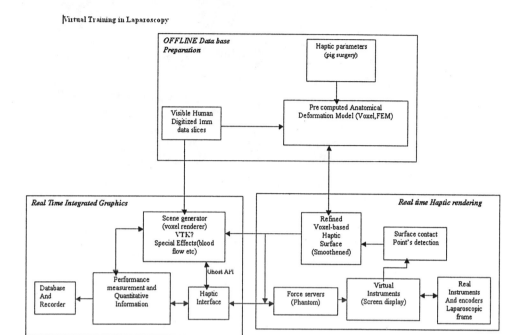

Figure 1 Block Diagram of the Laparoscopic Trainer

The basic block diagram shown in Fig.1 consists of Offline Data base, Real time Haptic Rendering and Real time Integrated Graphics.

The offline Database has data sets of CT, MRI and digitized images from the National library of medicine. The pre computed anatomical deformation model is still in development. The visible human data set is rendered with VTK (Visualization Tool Kit, Kitware Inc.). We have polygonal bone and skin models that can be rendered. We also have a voxel model of the anatomy. We will be conducting a porcine surgery to obtain the in vivo tissue forced feedback parameters to properly calibrate our haptics.

In Real Time Haptic rendering we are working on a refined voxel based haptic surface that will provide realistic volumetric smoothened surface. We are also working on a smoothing algorithm to reduce the blockiness of voxel-based haptic rendering

In Real time Integrated Graphics we have a VTK based renderor with pre-computed deformation model. We will be performing the actual measurements and gather performance measurements and quantitative information that should provide valuable feedback to laparoscopic surgeons. We also have a database that will record all the information and can be accessed for future analysis.

3. Haptic workstation

Our haptic workstation consists of an ergonomically designed frame with mounted trocars (See Fig 2). This interfaces the generic force feedback device called Phantom (the black device) to the surgical instrument. The instrument inserted through a trocar is connected to the Phantom wand through which tactile feedback is passed.

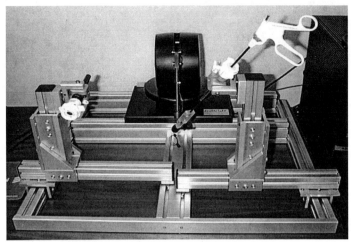

Figure 2 The Frameset for Trocars and the Surgical Instruments

Some of the unique features of our haptic workstation are (1) it can accommodate one or two Phantom devices, (2) it provides for surgical tools held in either/both the left and/or right hand(s),(3) trocars can be interchanged, (4) these trocars can accommodate a variety of surgical tools, (5) to use other trocars with this fixture, custom-fit, low-cost adapters can be designed and fabricated, (5) surgical tools can be interchanged and (6) the spatial relationship between the pivot point of the trocar (representing the entry point at the abdominal wall) and the interface between the tool tip and the Phantom (representing the tool's point of contact inside the abdominal cavity) is adjustable. By simple adjustment of its slides and clamps, the fixture can accommodate many different configurations.

For surgical simulation, we have developed deformable surface and volumetric models from the Visible Human data (from the National Institute of Health) and using the Visualization Tool Kit (VTK from Kitware Inc.).We have added haptics in our surface model of the gall bladder, which consists of a texture-mapped mesh with deformation and a mass spring model.

Our present work also includes a preliminary volumetric deformation model for the inguinal region, and a deformation model to give both visual and haptic clues. Also, we are working on special graphic effects such as blood vessel puncture or transection, to simulate hemorrhage, thereby adding realism to the simulation.

4. Results
Our preliminary results with surface models show no observable latency in image manipulation. Our surgery consultants deem the fast graphic displays and haptics to be realistic. They have had no problem operating, over a wide range of motion, laparoscopic tools inserted in the frame and attached to the PHANToM.

The wire frame model of the gall bladder field consists of 100,000 nodes and interconnects, and includes gall bladder and connecting ducts, liver, omentum and intestine. The haptics overlay currently consists of a 16 node rectangular array, with scalable spring and damping elements. Extension to a compromise density of the very realistic wire frame model is currently underway.

Our next goal is to achieve realistic results with volumetric model simulating difficult procedures like laparoscopic herniorrhaphy. The workstation is also designed to measure the operator's performance during the virtual surgery thereby giving a large scope for improvement and honing operative skills.

Medicine Meets Virtual Reality 2001
J.D. Westwood et al. (Eds.)
IOS Press, 2001

Cubby: A Unified Interaction Space for Precision Manipulation

J.P. Djajadiningrat   **P.J. Stappers**   **C.J. Overbeeke**
ID-StudioLab, Department of Industrial Design, Delft University of Technology
Jaffalaan 9, 2628 BX Delft, The Netherlands

Abstract. Precision manipulation in surgical simulation poses special requirements on a VR system. One such requirement is unification, i.e. that the user manipulates a virtual object where it appears. We have designed Cubby, a system of which the visualization part was presented at MMVR97 [3], for precision manipulation and unification. In an experiment Cubby was compared with a single screen head-tracked display, both in a unified and a non-unified version. The results show that subjects could manipulate virtual objects in Cubby with significantly higher accuracy and preferred it to the single screen head-tracked display. Though no significant difference in accuracy between the unified and non-unified conditions could be shown, subjects did prefer the unified over the non-unified condition within both setups.

1. Introduction

Surgical simulations are prime examples of precision manipulation tasks. It is hard to support such tasks with currently available VR systems. Systems based on helmet mounted displays (HMDs) typically lack the resolution and tracking accuracy required for precision manipulation. And with the current devices for head and hand tracking, it is not possible to realize high accuracy within a large space, such as a CAVE [2]. Given the currently available technology, head-tracked displays offer a smaller, but more stable workspace [1] [9].

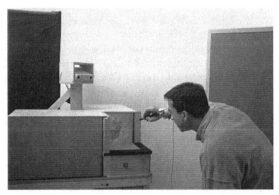

Figure 1   Cubby is a unified VR system: the user manipulates virtual objects at the place where they appear.

To create a VR system optimized for precision manipulation, we have taken natural skills in precision tasks as our starting point. In the natural environment, people pick up and manipulate objects where they appear, unlike the typical computer setup where we see virtual objects on a screen but act on these objects through a pointing device held at another position. We call a VR system in which we can manipulate virtual objects where they appear a unified system, since it unifies the display and manipulation spaces. Unification is worth pursuing since experimental literature shows that disruptions of hand-eye coordination have a negative impact on manipulation performance. For example, in an endoscopy task, performance decreased considerably when the angle between the display and manipulation space exceeded 45° [8]. Everyday tasks are also impeded when visual feedback is transformed (See, e.g., [6] for a discussion and overview). As we will explain, a unified system poses its own problems and challenges though. For instance, your hands block your view.

In this paper the emphasis is on accurate, unified manipulation. We start with the requirements for unified systems and the perceptual conflicts which these requirements lead to. We then present a VR system named Cubby (Figure 1) which was designed to solve these problems. We discuss the decisions made in the design of Cubby and argue why Cubby is well-suited to precision manipulation. Finally, Cubby is tested in an experiment on accuracy and unification.

2. Unification

In a unified system, the surgeon wields his instruments within the scene. He must be able to reach as many parts of the scene as possible, both visually and physically. In designing unified systems, we are confronted with the following related problems: Accessibility, head-tracking support, occlusion conflicts, and clipping.

Accessibility—This means that the surgeon's physical tools must be able to enter the virtual scene, and not be blocked, e.g., by the display as in most stereo- or Fishtank-VR systems, where half the scene cannot be reached because it lies within the computer monitor.

Head-tracking support—Head movements are needed when instruments or parts of the scene hide other parts from view. The user can move his head to get another view on the scene, but this movement needs to be matched by a corresponding change in the perspective image on the display: the display must be head-tracked.

Occlusion conflicts—These occur when the user inserts a physical object, such as a hand or an instrument, between virtual objects positioned in front of the display surface and the display surface itself (Figure 2) [10]. While the virtual objects should occlude the physical instrument since they are frontmost, this does not happen as the physical instrument prevents the user from seeing the representation of the virtual objects on the display surface. As a result, the depth impression can collapse, and spatial performance drops with it.

Clipping—Virtual displays can make objects float in front of the display, but only within the visual pyramid whose base is the display and whose apex is the eye of the user. As the user moves, parts of the scene that lie outside of the pyramid get 'cut off' optically by the edges of the display behind them. This effect is not prominent when visual angles are large (as in a CAVE), but becomes a noticeable and disturbing problem with regular display angles, as in Figure 2.

3. Cubby: A design solution for unification

The VR system Cubby [1][4][5] was developed to solve the aforementioned problems (http://www.io.tudelft.nl/id-studiolab/cubby/index.html). Cubby uses three orthogonal head-

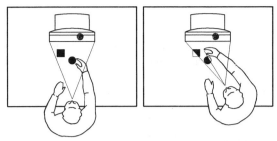

Figure 2 Problems with unified systems. The grey virtual sphere behind the screen is inaccessible to the user. When the user moves his hand behind the black virtual sphere, this object cannot occlude the hand. When the user moves sideways from the neutral position, the cube is clipped by the left edge of the display.

tracked displays which form a cubic space. Through the use of head-coupled perspective on all three screens, the illusion is created that virtual objects stand inside the cubic space. Manipulation in Cuby is done by means of an instrument which behaves as a pair of tweezers. Figure 1 shows a user manipulating virtual objects in Cuby. In Cuby the problems associated with unified systems have been eliminated or at least alleviated.

Accessibility—In Cuby the virtual objects are directly accessible to an instrument, since they appear inside the cubic space and in front of the screens.

Head-tracking support—All three screens feature head-tracking. As the user moves his head, his view of the virtual scene changes in the same way as his view onto his hands.

Occlusion conflicts—To reduce the occlusion problem, Cuby uses a hybrid instrument with a physical barrel and a virtual tip. This approach is similar to that of [7], with the difference that with Cuby the instrument is not mounted on a mechanical, force-feedback arm. The tip is rendered as an extension of the physical barrel (Figure 4). The virtual pointer is rendered with the scene and can be moved behind a virtual object without occlusion anomalies occurring. Moreover, the user can choose a viewpoint from where objects in the virtual scene are not in conflict with the physical part of the pointer.

Clipping—Cuby's display layout greatly reduces the clipping problem. When a virtual object is clipped by the inner edge of one screen, the clipped part appears on the adjacent screen. As a result, the user can view the scene from many sides, and virtual objects can be placed in a larger workspace (see illustrations in [3]).

In addition to these unification related properties we also addressed the following issues which influence precision manipulation.

Non-encumbering—If the user is to perform with accuracy, a VR system should influence his movements as little as possible. In Cuby, the head-sensor is wireless. While the instrument is not wireless, it minimally hinders the user and is easy to pick up and put down. These choices for head and instrument tracking make it easy for the user to detach from the system.

Accurate depth perception from a wide range of angles—For the current Cuby prototype we decided to use head-tracking, but no stereo. Head-tracking by itself offers a convincing depth impression [9], as one can experience by manipulating in the real world with one eye closed. Not using stereo has two advantages. From a user-friendliness point of view, this setup requires very little headware. From a technical point of view, using only head-tracking requires half the calibration and rendering power. That being said, accuracy of depth perception could be further improved by adding stereoscopy in a trade off with headware.

Accurate manipulation within the workspace—Because the electro-magnetic instrument tracker is not used to track head-position, it can be dedicated to cover only the much smaller workspace. This is advantageous, since electro-magnetic tracking systems are more accurate at a small range.

4. Experiment

In an experiment, we compared Cubby to a standard single-screen VR display configuration which we name 'Solo'. Aim of the experiment was to establish quantitative evidence for the design decisions underlying Cubby. Earlier experience and user reports strongly suggested in favour of these choices, but produced only anecdotal evidence. In this experiment we tried to construct a task that could be carried out in each of the systems and be compared between them. This task can therefore only use part of Cubby's functionality; e.g., tasks that require large freedom of head movements simply cannot be done in Solo, so larger head movements should not be necessary for subjects to complete the task. The experiment therefore could not be a fair total evaluation between Cubby and Solo, but only tests some aspects of the design in a highly controlled setting.

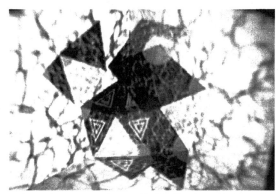

Figure 3 One of several puzzle arrangements with the fixed puzzle base (marked with concentric triangles) and three puzzle pieces which the subject could move.

Subjects performed a spatial composition task: put together pieces of a puzzle into a solid icosahedron (Figure 3). This task involves precise 3D vision and spatial manipulation, resembling the needs of surgical tasks. Each of the pieces could fit only in a single position and orientation, so success of the placement was measured as the distance and angular errors of the pieces. The interaction between instrument and puzzle is shown inFigure 4.

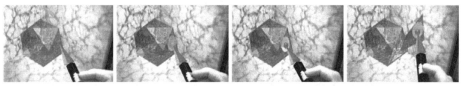

Figure 4 Visual feedback (from left to right): The instrument approaches (1). As the virtual tip enters the sensitive zone of a polygon the inscribed circle lights up, a green sphere appears at the point of contact and a collision sound is heard (2). The closer the tip gets to the polygon, the brighter the inscribed circle. After the user presses the button on the instrument, the sphere turns from green to red (3), and the puzzle piece follows the instrument in both orientation and position (4).

Subjects performed the task in four conditions, ordered by two variables: unification (unified versus non-unified) and display configuration (Cubby versus Solo) (Figure 5). In the unified conditions, the coupling between instrument and virtual tip is absolute by necessity. In the non-unified conditions, we made it absolute to allow a fair comparison. In the non-unified conditions, the manipulation space was translated by 200mm in the direction shown .

Twelve subjects, all of them students of Industrial Design Engineering or Architecture, took part in the experiment. Each subject completed two sessions lasting two hours each, in which the puzzle task was performed in the four conditions (order of conditions was counterbalanced). In each condition, the subject performed two practice trial, followed by five measurement trials. Trials lasted a maximum of three minutes, with a warning sound ten seconds before the end. A trial was terminated if the subject indicated he was satisfied with the composed shape. At the end of each session, the subjects were asked to rank the conditions in order of preference.

Dependent variables were the error in position and orientation of the three pieces of the puzzle. The expectation of the experimenters was that errors in the Cubby condition would be lower than with Solo, and errors in the unified condition lower than in the non-unified condition. Similarly, we expected users to prefer the former conditions over the latter ones.

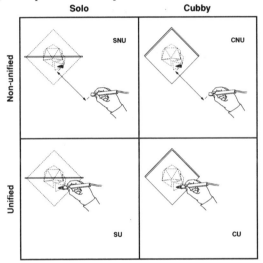

Figure 5 The four conditions of the manipulation experiment

5. RESULTS

Analysis of the data showed that in many trials subjects had not got round to adjusting all of the puzzle pieces within the three minutes. Puzzle pieces which had not been adjusted showed high positional and rotational errors. These were deemed to not be representative of performance in a certain condition, yet they had a considerable impact on the mean error. Such non-representative data were reduced in a two step process. The first step was to exclude from the analysis those puzzle pieces which had a rotational error of 30 degrees or more. As the typical rotational error was in the order of five degrees such a large rotational error meant that the subject had not got round to adjusting the piece or had run out of time whilst adjusting it. In this way, 6.7% of the data in session 1, and 2.1% of the data in session 2 was eliminated from analysis (see Table 1 for the exact remaining number of puzzle piece placements). The second step was to use the median instead of the mean as a measure of central tendency, because the mean is sensitive to extreme values of positional or rotational error.

Session 1—Because of the large variability, conditions were compared through the extension of the median test . This was done both for rotational and positional error (Table 1). The null-hypothesis of equal medians was rejected both for the rotational and positional errors: the four conditions did not share the same median. We therefore proceeded by comparing the pairs of

Table 1   Extension of the median tests (% of pieces with an error <= common median)

session	type of error	CU	CNU	SU	SNU	χ^2	p
1	rotational	58.4	57.9	44.4	39.9	18.06	<0.001**
	positional	53.3	57.9	49.1	40.5	10.95	<0.05*
2	rotational	55.4	60.8	38.3	45.8	21.17	<0.001**
	postional	54.8	53.8	43.3	48.0	6.45	0.1<p<0.2

conditions which differ along one dimension: CU-CNU, SU-SNU, CU-SU and CNU-SNU (Table 2). CU and SU differ significantly in terms of rotational error. CNU and SNU differ significantly both in rotational and positional error. All other pairwise comparisons show no significant differences.

Session 2—Again we started with the extension of the median test to investigate whether the four conditions shared the same median, for rotational error and for positional error (Table 1). Since the null-hypothesis could not be rejected for the positional error, the pairwise testing only needed to be carried out on the rotational error (Table 2). CU-SU and CNU-SNU differed significantly in terms of rotational error. All other pairwise comparisons showed no significant differences. Cubby thus allows subjects to manipulate virtual objects with higher accuracy than is possible with Solo.

The ranks for both sessions are shown in Figure 6. Not only do subjects prefer Cubby over the single screen Solo setup, within these setups they also prefer the unified conditions over the non-unified conditions.

6. Discussion

The results show that subjects can manipulate virtual objects with significantly higher accuracy in Cubby than in Solo. The higher performance in Cubby may be the result of reduced distortion, as compared to the single screen setup. No differences in accuracy could be found between the unified and non-unified conditions for either Cubby or Solo. However, rating the conditions according to preference, shows not only that Cubby is preferred over the single screen head-tracked setup, but also that within each setup the unified condition is preferred over the non-unified condition.

It should be emphasized that Cubby's main advantages were not exploited in this experiment: a larger accessible work space and a wide range of viewing angles without clipping. With Solo the space behind the screen is for the larger part inaccessible to the user's instrument in the unified condition. With regards to the viewing angles, with Cubby it is possible to look down on the display space without clipping occurring. In many precision manipulation tasks it is an advantage to be able to look down onto the scene.

Table 2   Significant pairwise median tests, p<0.05 (% of pieces with an error <= common median)

session	type of error		%		%	χ^2	p
1	rotational	CU	57.3	SU	42.6	6.92	0.0005<p<0.005*
	rotational	CNU	59.9	SNU	41.0	10.73	0.0005<p<0.005*
	positional	CNU	58.6	SNU	42.2	8.36	0.0005<p<0.005*
2	rotational	CU	57.8	SU	41.8	10.42	0.0005<p<0.005*
	rotational	CNU	56.7	SNU	45.0	5.56	0.005<p<0.01*

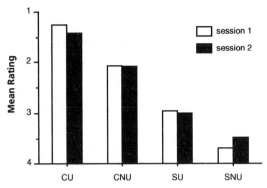

Figure 6 The mean rating for session 1 and 2.

7. Conclusions

Unlike most VR systems, Cubby was designed with precision manipulation in mind. Unification of display and manipulation spaces formed an important part of our approach. Cubby shows that it is possible to offer unification, whilst avoiding occlusion and clipping problems. An experiment showed that subjects could manipulate virtual objects in Cubby with significantly higher accuracy and preferred it to a single screen head-tracked display. Though no significant difference in performance between the unified and non-unified conditions could be found, subjects did prefer the unified over non-unified condition within both setups. Moreover, Cubby offers two advantages that were not tested in the experiment. Cubby's first advantage is that the accessible workspace is larger than that of a single screen head-tracked display. Cubby's second advantage is that the user can look down onto the scene. In general, we think that the design of Cubby reflects that the design of task specific VR devices with a human-centric approach is a worthwhile pursuit.

8. References

[1]   Buxton, W. & Fitzmaurice, G.W. (1998). HMDs, Caves & Chameleon: A human centric analysis of interaction in virtual space. Computer Graphics, The SIGGRAPH Quarterly, 32(4), 64-68.
[2]   Cruz-Neira, C., Sandin, D.J., & DeFanti, T.A. (1993). Surround-screen projection based virtual reality: The design and implementation of the CAVE. *Proceedings of SIGGRAPH'93*, 135-142.
[3]   Djajadiningrat, J.P., Overbeeke, C.J., & Smets, G.J.F. (1997). Cubby: A medical virtual environment based on multiscreen movement parallax. In: K.S. Morgan et al. (Eds), *Medicine Meets Virtual Reality*, Amsterdam: IOS Press, 387-394.
[4]   Djajadiningrat, J.P., Smets, G.J.F., & Overbeeke, C.J. (1997). Cubby: a multiscreen movement parallax display for direct manual manipulation. *Displays*, 17, 191-197.
[5]   Djajadiningrat, J.P. (1998). *Cubby: What you see is where you act. Interlacing the display and manipulation spaces*. Doctoral dissertation. Delft University of Technology, Delft, The Netherlands.
[6]   Dolezal, H. (1982). *Living in a world transformed. Perceptual and performatory adaptation to visual distortion*. NY: Academic Press.
[7]   Ishii, I., Karasawa, T., & Makino, H. (1994). A method of handling virtual objects that incorporates the sense of touch. *Systems and Computers in Japan*, 25 (10), 72-81.
[8]   Tendick, F., Jennings, R.W., Tharp, G., & Stark, L. (1993). Sensing and manipulation problems in endoscopic surgery: experiment, analysis, and observation. *Presence*, 2 (1), 66-81.
[9]   Ware, C., Arthur, K., & Booth, K.S. (1993). Fish tank virtual reality. *Proceedings of the INTERCHI'93*, 37-42.
[10] Ware, C. (1990). Using hand position for virtual object placement. *The Visual Computer*, 6, 245-253.

Medicine Meets Virtual Reality 2001
J.D. Westwood et al. (Eds.)
IOS Press, 2001

A methodological tool for computer-assisted surgery interface design: its application to computer-assisted pericardial puncture

Emmanuel Dubois ([1, 2]), Laurence Nigay ([2]), Jocelyne Troccaz ([1]),
Lionel Carrat ([1]), Olivier Chavanon ([3])

([1]) TIMC-IMAG / GMCAO	*([2]) CLIPS-IMAG / IIHM*	*([3]) Cardiac Surgery*
School of Medicine, IAB	*Rue de la bibliothèque*	*Department,*
Domaine de la Merci	*BP 53*	*Grenoble University Hospital,*
F - 38706 La Tronche Cedex.	*F - 38041 Grenoble Cedex9.*	*F - 38700 La Tronche.*

[Emmanuel.Dubois, Laurence.Nigay, Jocelyne.Troccaz]@imag.fr

Abstract

Computer Assisted Surgery systems are becoming more and more prevalent. Design processes currently used, pay only a small attention to the surgeon's interaction. To address this lack in design, we propose the OP-a-S notation: OP-a-S modeling of a system adopts an interaction-centered point of view and highlights the links between the real world and the virtual world. Based on an OP-a-S modeling, predictive usability analysis can be performed by considering the ergonomic property. We illustrate our method on the retro-design of a computer assisted surgical application, CASPER.

1. Introduction

Very few attention has been paid to interface design in CAS although we think it is a very important key to success and clinical acceptation. This work is based on our 15 years experience of Computer-assisted surgery (CAS) system development and evaluation. We launched, four years ago, a cooperative work based on the following partnership: a Computer Aided Medical Intervention group, a group specialized in man-machine interface design and the university hospital. This cooperation resulted in the development of methodological tools for CAS interface design and evaluation. These principles were used to evaluate a particular clinical application from the interaction point of view and to propose new developments which are in progress.

This work describes a new concept for man-machine interface design in CAS and makes uses of a clinical application for which a first release of computer-assistance exists and is entering clinical validation.

2. Our CAS Application: CASPER

A pericardial puncture consists in the manual insertion of a needle near the heart to remove a build up of a pathological fluid in the pericardium. In order to face some dangers of this surgery, mainly organs effraction, we have developed a computer assisted system that provides helpful guidance information to the surgeon performing the puncture. The first version consisted in the combined use of both an infrared based localizer tracking the patient, the needle and the imaging sensor (ultrasound probe) and a computer screen used to display the guidance information (planned and current trajectories). This system called CASPER, Computer Assisted PERicardial puncture is being validated at the Grenoble University Hospital [1].

From previous animal experiments, several drawbacks concerning the user interaction were identified. For example, the surgeon has to look at the patient but also at the screen to get the guidance information; he has to push the needle to cross several layers of tissues whilst controlling the insertion depth which is the critical parameter. An additional analysis based on our OP-a-S notation [2] has helped us to identify and explain other problems linked to the interaction. The next paragraph highlights two of them and briefly present the solutions we developed to overcome them.

3. Results

Our OP-a-S notation is a methodological tool that decomposes an interactive system into four kinds of components: user(s) (P), computer system (S), real objects (Ot and Oo) and adapters (IA and OA) that aim at transferring information from the real to the virtual (or electronic) world. Additionally, OP-a-S relations, i.e. exchange of information between OP-a-S components, enable the identification of the several parts of the interaction supported by the system. A diagrammatic representation of the system results from an OP-a-S analysis. Examples may be found in [2] and [3]. On the basis of a diagrammatic modeling, designers are then able to evaluate ergonomic properties to characterize the interaction. Next paragraphs illustrate the process on CASPER.

3.1. Cognitive consistency

With the OP-a-S modeling of CASPER shown in Figure 1, we were able to methodologically explain why the surgeon had some difficulties to interpret the guidance information displayed by the system. During the intervention, the surgeon manipulates a surgical needle in a 3D environment. But, the guidance information provided is represented with a 2D model. This consideration is an instance of the *cognitive consistency* ergonomic property that OP-a-S helps to identify: information caught by the user must be preferably expressed in a common "language". Our solution to this has been to develop a 3D representation of the planned and executed trajectories, in order to reduce the cognitive process of data interpretation during the intervention. An ultrasound image on which is superimposed a 3D cone, that represents the planned trajectory, constitutes the scene displayed to the surgeon. A representation of the needle is also perceivable. Experiments are in progress with psychologists to select the best reference system to display fully understandable information.

3.2. Perceptual consistency

OP-a-S has also highlighted the difficulty for the surgeon to catch alternatively information on the screen and in the surgical field. This difficulty is linked to the more generic property of *perceptual consistency*. Perceptual consistency is expressed in OP-a-S modeling by a set of relations linked to the surgeon, carrying information of importance but perceivable at different locations. In CASPER, this is clearly the case with the trajectory information: the real one is perceived on top of the patient, while the "virtual" one is displayed on the monitor. Our solution to this second outcome has consisted in using a see-through Head-Mounted Display (HMD) in which guidance information are displayed and through which the surgeon can directly look at the position and orientation of the real puncture needle. In this case, the point of view of the information is the surgeon's point of view. Surgeon's head tracking is realized thanks a rigid-body mounted on top of the HMD. To be able to display the virtual information merged with the real one, a calibration of the HMD is required.

The calibration process we have implemented is composed of two steps. The first step consists in determining the position of each corner of both screens of the HMD. For each screen, averaging the coordinates of the four points provides a position that approximately correspond to the position of the eye of the surgeon. These positions are then used to generate the left and right images needed to display stereoscopic 3D information in the HMD. The second step permits the definition of the gaze direction. The surgeon is asked to look straight forward and to align the tip of a pointer with an OpenGL sphere displayed in the middle of the screen. Later, during the execution, this gaze direction is used to set the orientation of the OpenGL cameras. The Figure 1 is a picture taken through the HMD screens on which you can see that real and virtual data are aligned.

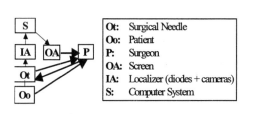
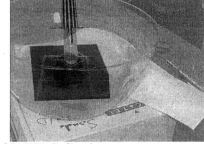

Figure 1: OP-a-S modeling of CASPER (Left) and
view of the trajectory and the reality through the Head-Mounted Display (Right).

3.3.Limitations

Currently the matching error between real and virtual data is far too big (up to 2 cm). This is clearly unacceptable in regard to traditional CAS applications. Most of this imprecision is due to a low accuracy of the HMD-calibration phase. However, work is in course to increase the precision of the calibration. Other methods will be implemented and tested.

Another limitation is directly linked to the actual state of see-through technologies. None of the devices we tried, permitted to modify the focus distance of the HMD. This means that the surgeon have to focus at 4 meters in front of him to get a real 3D stereoscopic information; the patient on which the surgeon is working, is never so far away from him. Nevertheless, we are quite sure that such devices will soon be usable.

4. Conclusion

Our methodological approach for the analysis of an existing system has revealed a set of deficiencies in the induced interaction. Future works will explore other ergonomic properties. Moreover, our approach has already proved to be valuable for the design of new interaction techniques, better suited to the surgeon's activity. Additionally, it has led us to the investigation of the optical see-through device domain which allows the surgeon to stay in direct contact with the real operating theatre. In regard to traditional VR or Video-See-Through techniques, the accuracy is not yet satisfying enough. Further work is still necessary to make it clinically usable.

5. References

[1] Chavanon, O., Barbe, C., Troccaz, J., Carrat, L., Ribuot, C., Blin, D., Accurate guidance for percutaneous access to a specific target in soft tissues, Journal of Laparoendoscopic and Advanced Surgical techniques, Vol. 9, No 3, (1999), p. 259-266.
[2] Dubois, E., Nigay, L., Troccaz, J., Chavanon, O., Carrat, L., Classification space for augmented surgery, an augmented reality case study, Conference Proceedings of Interact'99, Edinburgh - UK, (1999), p. 353-359.
[3] Dubois, E., Nigay, L., Augmented Reality: Which Augmentation for Which Reality ?, Conference Proceedings of DARE'2000, ACM, Elsinore - Danemark, (2000), p.165-167.

Medicine Meets Virtual Reality 2001
J.D. Westwood et al. (Eds.)
IOS Press, 2001

Measurement and Display of Regional Myocardial Motion During Post Infarct Treatment

Christian D. Eusemann, Erik L. Ritman, Thomas R. Behrenbeck and Richard A. Robb

Mayo Foundation/Clinic, Rochester, MN 55905 USA

Abstract.   Quantitative assessment of 3-D regional heart motion has significant potential to provide more specific diagnosis of cardiac malfunction than currently possible. Using functional parametric mapping, regional myocardial motion during a cardiac cycle can be color-mapped onto a deformable heart model to provide better understanding of the structure-to-function relationships in the myocardium, including regional patterns of akinesis or dyskinesis associated with ischemia or infarction. In this study, 3-D reconstructions of human hearts were obtained from Electron-Beam Computed Tomography [1] (EB-CT), comparing stages of treatment after myocardial infarction.

1. Introduction

Cardiovascular disease (CVD) is the most common cause of death in the United States. In 1996, CVD claimed 959,227 lives in the United States[2]. For effective treatment of heart disease, accurate diagnosis is needed. For disease affecting the myocardium, information about the structure and regional mechanical behavior of the heartwall is important. Previous studies have used 3-D data sets acquired from MRI, especially MRI tagging[3,4], 3-D X-ray CT (DSR)[5,6] and Ultrasound[7] for the quantitative assessment of dynamic heart motion. The DSR is a unique high-resolution three-dimensional imaging scanner, which operates on the principles of computerized tomography (CT). It allows very high temporal and spatial image sequences without gating, which results in high accuracy.

This paper describes a method to measure and visualize myocardial structure and function using a fast, modality independent algorithm applied to heart images acquired in three sequential stages of treatment during a controlled study. This method is based on a technique introduced previously using DSR data[8]. The method can be applied to any 4-D data set provided by a fast 3-D scanning system. The technique is based on deformable surface reconstruction, involving creation of a polygonal surface mesh to represent the myocardial walls. From these polygonal models, regional excursions and velocities of each vertex representing a unit of myocardium can be calculated for successive time intervals. The calculated results may be visualized by specially formatted static images.

The algorithm was tested, to determine if it could convey pathophysically meaningful changes in cardiac mechanics during treatment.

2. Methods

2.1 Image Acquisition

Myocardial reconstructions were obtained using electron beam CT (EBCT). The data was acquired during the course of treatment for myocardial infarction. Following 3D data sets were acquired over the course of treatment: (1) immediately following hospital admission for myocardial infarct, (2) 6 weeks after infarction, and (3) 6 months after infarction. The EBCT data sets are the basis for 5D visualizations - 3 spatial dimensions, 1 time dimension, and 1 functional dimension. Each data set consists of 13 time points throughout a cardiac cycle with a heart rates between 58 and 82 beats/min respectively. The individual time point volumes include two scans with 6 adjacent slices with a 20 – 30sec relaxation time in-between scans. The in-plane pixel size is 0.969 mm^2 and the imaged slice thickness is 8mm. Circulatory contrast agents to enhance the visibility of chambers and vessels was injected intravenously during the scans

2.2 Image Segmentation

Segmentation of anatomic structures, which isolates specific objects in an image, is often the initial step in image analysis. The segmentation of cardiac images was performed using the AnalyzeAVW[9,10] software package developed in the Biomedical Imaging Resource at Mayo Clinic. The first processing step was the registration of the volumes. The data sets collected immediately and 6 weeks after infarct required adjustment in the lateral direction, whereas the third data set required adjustments in the lateral and anterior directions. The actual segmentation was done using fast and convinient tracing of the region of interest. After segmentation, the data were transformed from greyscale to binary, which is the data type required for the interpolation program. The interpolation algorithm used in the program is based upon shape-based interpolation[11].

2.2 Surface reconstruction

Surface reconstruction is the transformation from a binary image volume to a geometric description of an object surface[12]. An adaptive deformable surface reconstruction program was used to model the physical structure of the LV volumes, The physical structure is represented as a set of nodes (polygon vertices) interconnected by adjustable "springs" (polygon edges). The physical structure of the end diastolic volume was used as an initial triangular mesh. This initial triangular mesh gradually deforms from time point volume to time point volume to preserve the same number of vertices and triangles for each volume throughout the cardiac cycle. Each vertex is assigned to the closest voxel of the subsequent time-point surface.

2.3 Motion tracking, analysis and visualization

The goal of this research was to measure, compute and visualize the instantaneous regional myocardial motion throughout the cardiac cycle. The software used to perform these computations was written in C/C++ and Open Inventor.

2.3.1 Tracking and Analysis

The myocardium shifts globally within the chest throughout the cardiac cycle, which has a confounding influence on quantifying the intrinsic cardiac motion. To minimize this problem, the epicardial apex of the left ventricle was chosen as a fixed reference point to describe cardiac shift[13]. Using this anatomic fiducial marker, the heart shift could be determined and used to compensate for myocardial motion.

To calculate the specific motion of the LV, the deformation constraint was based on the surface reconstruction algorithm used. Since each vertex describes the pathway of a single surface point, computation of the dynamic properties of myocardial function is straightforward. Excursion is the vector length between any selected vertex in space and the initial vertex. Velocity is the vector length between two successive time point vertices.

2.3.2 Visualization

To visualize instantaneous regional myocardial motion, reference displays with value equivalent colors had to be designed. Conversely, for this publication grayscale values were assigned. Each dynamic property was divided into fifteen reference colors (grayscale values) which were assigned to each time point in the cardiac cycle. The excursion value colors were assigned in 1.25 voxel (1.25 mm) increments, and the velocity value colors in 0.6 voxel (0.6mm) increments. To display the dynamic properties, the assigned color values were mapped onto the myocardial polygon surface representing the endocardial surface of the myocardial wall at end diastole. The color of each surface triangle was determined by interpolating the colors of the three connecting triangular vertices. The images of these functional structure maps can be displayed. To simplify these illustrations a reference grayscale with reference values is always included.

3. Results

Figure 1 illustrates regional excursion values of the left ventricle, displayed on the end diastolic volume. The top row displays the excursion map on data acquired immediately after the infarction. The second row illustrates the excursion values of the ventricle after 6 weeks of treatment, and the third row illustrates the excursion values of the ventricle after 6 months of treatment. These parametric mappings use light shading to visualize small excursions and dark saturation to illustrate high excursion. Figure 2 illustrates the velocity values of the left ventricle during the cardiac cycle, displayed on the end diastolic volume. The top row shows the parametric velocity maps of data acquired immediately after the infarction. The second row illustrates the velocity maps for the ventricle after 6 weeks of treatment and the third row illustrates the velocity values for the ventricle after 6 months of treatment. The shown parametric mappings also use light shading to illustrate small excursion and dark saturation to illustrate high excursion. The validity of these representations are dependent on the preprocessing of the data and the poor 3-D spatial resolution of the EBCT image data. Although, the methodology has been shown valid (12) for high-spatial resolution data.

4. Discussion and Future work

The main problem contributing to the sub optimal results in this analysis is the poor out of plain resolution of the EB-CT scans, which results in thick slices. Because of slice thickness, anatomical structures are incompletely imaged due to partial volume "blurring". For example the left papillary muscle is in the data set acquired 6 weeks after infarction and visible in only one slice due to orientation of slice relative to papillary. The actual problem occurs during the shape-based interpolation of such thick sections. The algorithm interpolates around the anatomical structure of the papillary muscle, which produces an anatomical distortion of the ventricle. A similar error can be seen in Figure1. The ventricle image on the left in the third row shows a groove. These are only two very obvious examples, but the error caused by the slice thickness can be observed throughout all volumes. Since the parametric mapping algorithm uses the deformation constraint, which is based on the surface reconstruction algorithm, it is not surprising that the mapping algorithm is prone to changes of the anatomical structure created during interpolation.

The next step, therefore, will include attempt at improvement of the interpolation algorithm and/or the use of data with smaller slice thickness. Recent availability of fast multi thin slice helical CT should improve application of the algorithm

Acknowledgements

The author expresses thanks to Wei-te Lin for development of the deformable surface reconstruction program and David R. Holmes III for technical advice.

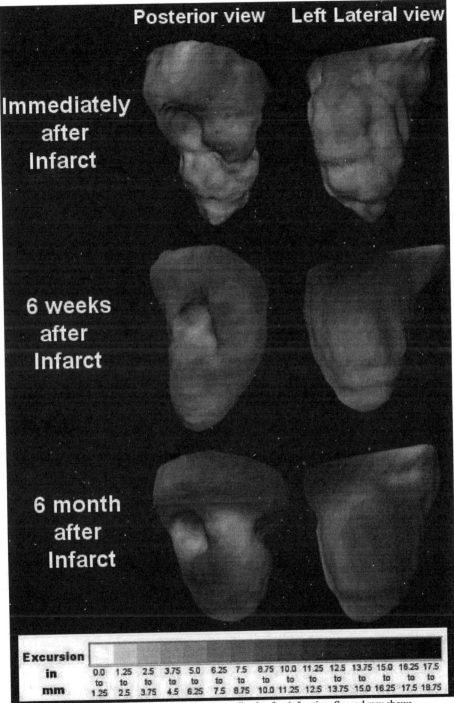

Figure 1: Excursion - Top shows Left Ventricle immediately after infarction. Second row shows Left Ventricle after six weeks and the third row after 6 month of treatment.

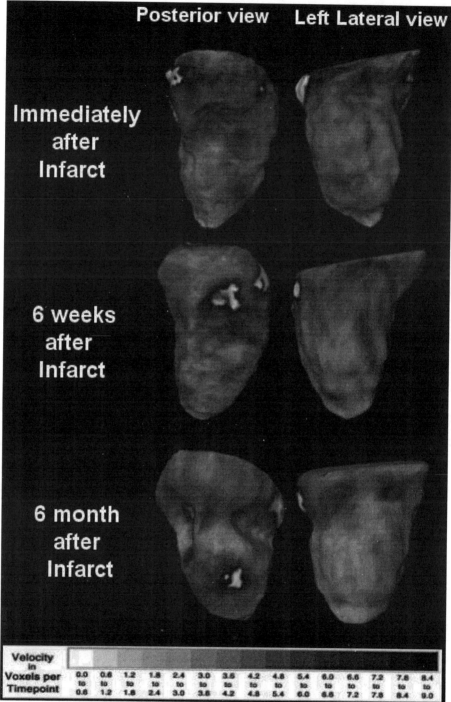

Figure 2: Velocity - Top shows Left Ventricle immediately after infarction. Second row shows Left Ventricle after six weeks and the third row after 6 month of treatment.

References

[1] J.A. Rumberger, P.F. Sheedy, J.F. Breen, L.A. Fitzpatrick, R.S. Schwartz, "Electron Beam Computed Tomography and Coronary Artery Disease: Scanning for Coronary Artery Calcification", Mayo Clinic Proceedings, 1996, Vol71(4), pp 369-377

[2] American Heart Association, 1999 Heart and Stroke – Statistical Update, 1999

[3] P. Croissile, C.C. Moore, R.M. Judd, J.A.C. Lima, M. Arai, E.R. McVeigh, L.C. Becker, E.A. Zerhouni, Differentiation of viable and nonviable myocardium by the use of three-dimensional tagged MRI in 2-day-old reperfused infarcts", Circulation, 99:284-291,1999

[4] P. Shi, A. Amini, G. Robinson, A. Sinusas, C.T. Constable, J.S. Duncan, "ShapeBased 4D Left Ventricular Myocardial Function Analysis", http://ipag.med.yale.edu/alums/xship/work/work.html

[5] D. Friboulet, I. E. Magnin, C. Mathieu, A. Pommert, K.H. Hoehne, "Assessment and Visualization of the Curvature of the Left Ventricle from 3D Medical Images", Computerized Medical Imaging and Graphics 1993, Vol. 4/5:257-262

[6] J.M. Gorce, D. Friboulet, P. Clarysse, I.E. Magnin, "Three-dimensional Velocity Field Estimation of Moving Cardiac Walls", Computers in Cardiology 1994, Vol. 0276-6547/94:489-492

[7] X. Papademetris, A.J. Sinusas, D.P. Dione, J.S. Duncan, "3D Cardiac Deformation from Ultrasound Images", Proceedings of Medical Image Computing and Computer-Assisted Intervention", 1679:420-429,1999

[8] C.E. Eusemann, M.E. Bellemann, R.A.Robb, "Quantitative Analysis and Parametric Display of Regional Myocardial Mechanics", Proceedings of Medical Image …

[9] R.A. Robb, D.P. Hanson, "The ANALYZE software system for visualization and analysis in surgery simulation", chap. In Computer Integrated Surgery (Cambridge, MA: MIT Press, 1995)

[10] R.A. Robb, "Three-Dimensional Biomedical Imaging - Principles and Practice", VCH Publishers, New York, NY 1995

[11] S.P. Raya, J.K. Udepa, " Shape-Based Interpolation of Multidimensional Objects", IEEE Transactions on Medical Imaging, Vol.9, No.1: 32-42, 1990

[12] W.T. Lin, R.A. Robb," Realistic Visualization for Surgery Simulation Using Dynamic Volume Texture Mapping and Model Deformation", Proceedings of SPIE, Medical Imaging 1999, Vol. 3658:308-314

[13] E.A. Hoffman, E.L. Ritman, "Invariant total heart volume in the intact thorax", Am. J. Physiol. 249 (Heart Circ. Physiol. 18): H883-H890, 1985

Medicine Meets Virtual Reality 2001
J.D. Westwood et al. (Eds.)
IOS Press, 2001

Spatial Ability and Learning the Use of an Angled Laparoscope in a Virtual Environment

Roy Eyal and Frank Tendick
Department of Surgery, University of California, San Francisco, CA 94143-0475
frankt@itsa.ucsf.edu

Abstract. Little is known about the cognitive demands that underlie surgical performance. Several studies have suggested that spatial ability plays a substantial role in surgical skill. An example of a skill in which spatial cognition appears to be of importance is the use of the angled laparoscope. This paper describes a virtual environment designed to assess and train the use of the angled laparoscope. The learning rates of novices learning the skill for the first time in the virtual environment were measured. The rates were found to be highly variable and strongly correlated with spatial ability.

1. Introduction

Despite the importance to society of ensuring the competence of surgeons, there has been surprisingly little research on surgical skill and training. Although the perceptual motor consequences of degraded visual information, reduced dexterity, and limited haptic sensation in laparoscopic surgery have been identified [1,2] and detailed time and motion studies have also been performed [3,4], these studies have done little to elucidate the underlying cognitive demands in surgery.

Several studies have shown strong correlations between standardized tests of spatial ability and performance ratings on a variety of tasks in open surgery [5-8]. Spatial cognition is the study of how humans acquire, store, retrieve, and process knowledge of the spatial properties of objects, events, and places in the world. Spatial properties include location, movement, extent, shape and connectivity. Although skilled surgeons are often said to have "good hands," in fact, performance in surgery is strongly dependent on spatial skills. The surgeon must develop a mental image of three-dimensional anatomy based on a surface view or cross sections from X-ray, CT, MRI, or ultrasound images. From this model and a goal state based on experience and anatomical knowledge, he or she must plan a strategy to gain exposure of the important anatomy and obtain the desired result. This plan requires complex coordination between a team of assistants using an array of instruments. With the advent of minimally invasive techniques such as laparoscopic surgery, the surgeon must rely on a video image of the internal anatomy and use instruments constrained by a fulcrum at their passage through the skin. This requires additional mental transformations of the image and careful planning to handle the constraints.

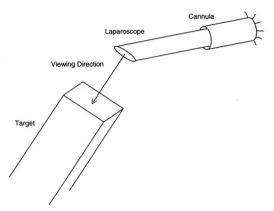

Figure 1. Angled laparoscope concept. The laparoscope passes through a cannula, which is constrained by the fulcrum at the abdominal wall. The objective lens is angled with respect to the laparoscope axis.

An example of a skill that requires the use of spatial cognition is guiding an angled laparoscope. In laparoscopic surgery, the fulcrum at the abdominal wall limits the range of motion of the laparoscope. Consequently, the viewing perspective within the abdomen is also limited. If the objective lens is aligned with the laparoscope axis, it is only possible to view from directions centered at the fulcrum. Some regions may be obscured by neighboring organs, or it may be impossible to view important structures *en face*. Laparoscopes with the objective lens at an angle with respect to the laparoscope axis are preferred and are often essential for many procedures, as they expand the range of viewing orientations (Figure 1).

Although the concept of the angled laparoscope is simple, in practice its use can be difficult. For example, to look into a narrow cavity (shown as a box in Figure 1), the laparoscope objective must point along a line into the cavity. Because of the constrained motion of the laparoscope, there is only one position and orientation of the laparoscope that will place the lens view along this line. (Or, more strictly, there is a narrow range of position and orientation that will suffice, depending on the width of the cavity and the field of view of the laparoscope.) The viewer can only see the location of the cavity relative to the current video image, and consequently must use spatial reasoning to estimate how to achieve the necessary laparoscope location.

Exacerbating the difficulty of using a laparoscope is the fact that often the least experienced person in the operating room handles the scope. The nurse, resident, or medical student serving as camera operator usually has no specific training in its use. Unskilled use of the laparoscope makes it difficult to obtain adequate exposure, potentially resulting in errors.

A major reason for the poor state of surgical training has been the lack of suitable media for training and assessing skills. Books, videos, and CD-ROMs are poor media for training skills; they are 2-D and the user cannot physically interact with them. Cadavers, animals, and in vitro training models made of synthetic materials can be useful, but they are scarce and expensive. Virtual environments are a promising new medium for assessing and understanding the nature of surgical skill as well as for training [9]. In this paper, we use a virtual environment developed to study and teach the use of an angled laparoscope. In the simulation, described in section 2, the user must steer the scope to view the inside of five target boxes suspended in different positions and orientations in space.

In earlier studies, the simulation was tested informally at UCSF in a one-day course for first year surgical residents and in advanced three-day courses for practicing surgeons.

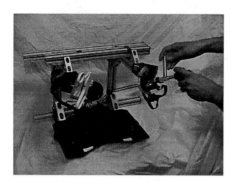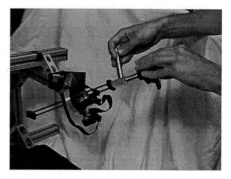

Figure 2. The interface to the simulation (left). Close-up of handle, in which the user's right hand controls the "light cable" and the left stabilizes the "camera" (right).

The former group had little prior experience in handling the laparoscope in the operating room (mean of 6.5 cases, range 0 to 30, n = 13). Each had experience operating an angled laparoscope in one procedure performed in a pig during the day. The median time to complete the test was 94 seconds, with a range of 35 seconds (for the subject with 30 procedures experience) to 305 seconds (for a subject with no prior experience). We have seen an even wider range of performance among the experienced surgeons than in the basic course. One participant needed over 26 minutes to complete the task, even with substantial coaching from the experimenter, and despite having used angled laparoscopes in his practice. It is clear that some surgeons do not achieve competence in this skill even with experience in the operating room.

We suspected that spatial ability might play a role in the use of the angled scope and the ease with which people learn the skill. To test this hypothesis, we measured learning rates in novices using the virtual environment and compared them with performance on standard tests of spatial ability.

2. Methods

2.1 Simulation

The simulation runs in C and OpenGL on Silicon Graphics Octane or O2 workstations. Input to the simulation is through a custom interface with optical encoders to measure motion of a handle in four degrees of freedom (plus one additional DOF to simulate camera rotation relative to the laparoscope), with kinematics identical to a laparoscope passing through a fulcrum (Figure 2). The handle is similar in shape to a laparoscope with a camera and light cable. By turning the handle about its axis, the orientation of the simulated laparoscope is changed. The simulation models the effect of a 45 degree laparoscope. All the encoders are tracked with an external interface board, which communicates with the computer through the serial port 30 times per second.

The environment comprises five targets, each a tall box suspended in space at a different position and orientation (Figure 3). The test begins with the laparoscope view centered. One of the targets changes color, and the subject must position and orient the laparoscope to see into the target box. The simulation detects when this view is demonstrated for one second, and the process is repeated for the next target in sequence. A two-minute time limit is enforced for each target, after which the next box in sequence becomes the target. The simulation records the movement trajectories as well as the time to locate each target.

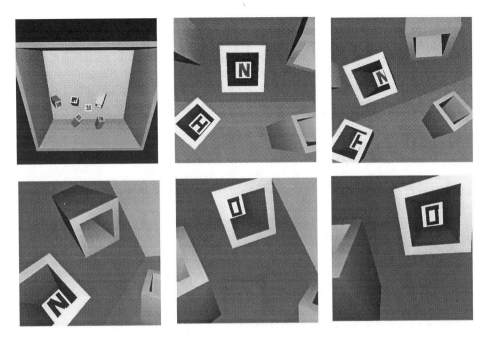

Figure 3. Angled laparoscope simulation. Upper left shows distant view of targets suspended at different positions and orientations. Remaining images show a sequence as the user smoothly changes the laparoscope position and orientation from view of target "N" to target "O".

Six target sets were used. The first three sets increased in difficulty from very easy to moderate; the last three target sets were difficult. Subjects completed the first three sets, then cycled through the last three until the time limit was reached. The score for each subject was the number of targets successfully achieved in two ten-minute sessions using the simulation.

2.2 Experiments

Subjects were novices, Berkeley undergraduates (14 males, 13 females, ages 18-25) who were not previously familiar with laparoscopic instruments. They were recruited through posters placed around campus and paid for their participation. Subjects were given a brief description of laparoscopic surgery and the role of the laparoscope. Then the researcher pointed out each part of a real scope, and described its function. This included the camera, light cable, scope shaft, and angled lens. Subjects were told that the most common way to hold the scope is with one hand on the light cable, to control the view direction, and one hand on the camera, to ensure an upright view. After some time to manipulate the real scope, the subjects were introduced to the simulation. Alternating between an external view of the scope in the virtual environment and the view through the scope, each of the four possible movements were demonstrated: left-right, up-down, in-out, and axial rotation. Then the subjects were given hints. The first was to pull the scope out at the begining of the search for the next target. In this position most of the virtual environment can be seen. Next, the subjects were advised to start their movement toward the target by orienting the view direction using the light cable, and then advance toward the target. After this explanation, the subject were asked to complete one target set as a practice, and were encouraged to ask questions about the procedure.

Subjects were tested in the simulation on target sets of increasing difficulty in three periods of 10 minutes. The measure of performance in the simulation was the total number of targets completed in the first two periods. Although the third period of the test was not included in the subjects' scores, data was collected for future analysis of movement trajectories to model the strategies the subjects developed.

After each period, the subject was given a test of spatial ability. The first, Card Rotations from the French kit [10] requires subjects to determine whether or not one shape is the rotated image of another. In the second, Paper Folding from the French kit [10], subjects imagine the folding of pieces of paper, imagine having a hole punched through the thickness of the paper in its folded position, and visualize where the holes would be when the paper is unfolded. The third test, Perspective Taking developed by Hegarty and Kozhevnikov, requires subjects to imagine the angular relationship between two objects in a plane as if viewed from a third object's location [11].

3. Results

There was a very wide range of performance in the simulation, ranging from 13 to 92 targets completed. Significant correlations were found with each of the tests of spatial ability: Pearson's $r = 0.39$ ($p < 0.05$) with Card Rotations, $r = 0.58$ ($p < 0.001$) with Paper Folding, $r = 0.40$ ($p < 0.05$) with Perspective Taking (Figure 4). A combined Z score was formed for each subject by summing their normal deviate from the mean of each of the three tests. The correlation between the combined score and performance on the simulation was $r = 0.52$ ($p < 0.005$). Furthermore, in each test the subjects scoring lowest were also among the poorest performers in the simulation.

4. Discussion

The wide range of performance in the simulation demonstrates the large variation in learning rates for this skill. The strong correlations with standard tests demonstrate the role of spatial ability in learning this skill. In particular, the fact that the lowest scorers on each test were also the poorest performers in the simulation implies that some degree of spatial ability is a prerequisite for adequate learning, at least with the minimal instruction provided in this experiment (and typically provided to those who must use an angled scope in the operating room). We are now developing training methods within the simulation that we hope will improve learning among those with lower spatial ability, for example by teaching strategies that do not depend strongly on mental visualization. These methods will be evaluated by measuring transfer to performance in vivo.

It might be argued that the population of surgeons could differ from the sample of undergraduates used in this experiment, for example if primarily those medical students with high spatial ability choose to become surgeons. However, in studies now going on at UCSF, we have so far found that experienced laparoscopic surgeons attending our courses are comparable to college students in their performance on the Paper Folding test [M. Hegarty, unpublished data]. There are, of course, many abilities and factors that contribute to success in a complex domain like surgery. However, the fact that the lowest scorers on the spatial tests consistently had difficulty learning to use the angled scope in the simulation implies that people with low spatial ability may require focused instruction in this skill and possibly other laparoscopic skills. Although similar tests could eventually be used in a battery to assess aptitude for success in laparoscopic surgery, such prediction has proven to be difficult in other domains.

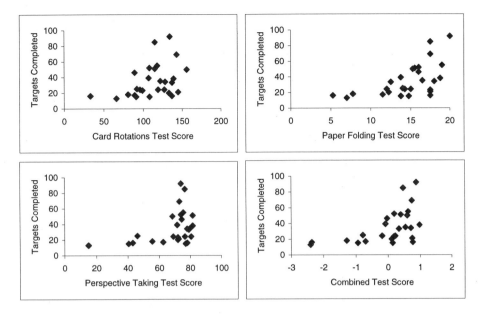

Figure 4. Subjects' performance in the simulation (number of targets completed) compared to their scores on the spatial ability tests.

Although the angled laparoscope virtual environment obviously is not intended to simulate surgical anatomy, our research group is developing simulations to simulate realistic skills [9]. The emphasis is on exposure skills and teaching correct performance of the procedural steps that can lead to major complications if performed incorrectly. As the skills are developed and validated, a major goal will be to develop models of task performance and relate these models to the underlying cognitive demands.

Acknowledgments

This research was supported in part by the National Science Foundation through grants CDA-9726362 and BCS-9980122 and the Office of Naval Research under grant N14-96-1-1200. We thank Sue-Lynn Wu for her work in designing the interface to the simulation and Mary Hegarty for providing the Perspective Taking test.

References

[1] F. Tendick, R. Jennings, G. Tharp, and L. Stark, "Sensing and manipulation problems in endoscopic surgery: experiment, analysis and observation," *Presence* 2, 66–81, 1993.
[2] P. Breedveld, P. *Observation, manipulation, and eye-hand coordination in minimally invasive surgery.* Technical Report Report N-510, Delft University of Technology, Man-Machine Systems and Control Group, 1998.
[3.] C. Cao, C. MacKenzie, and S. Payandeh, "Task and motion analyses in endoscopic surgery." In K. Danai, ed., *Proc. ASME Dynamic Systems and Control Division*, 1996.
[4] W. Sjoerdsma. *Surgeons at Work: Time and Actions Analysis of the Laparoscopic Surgical Process.* PhD thesis, Delft University of Technology, 1998.
[5] R. Gibbons, C. Gudas, and S. Gibbons, "A study of the relationship between flexibility of closure and surgical skill," *J. Am. Podiatr. Assoc.*, 73(1):12–6, 1983.

[6] R. Gibbons, R. Baker, and D. Skinner, D, "Field articulation testing: a predictor of technical skills in surgical residents," *J Surg. Res.* 41:53–7, 1986.

[7] A. Schueneman, J. Pickleman, R. Hesslein, and R. Freeark, "Neuropsychologic predictors of operative skill among general surgery residents," *Surgery* 96(2):288–295, 1984.

[8] R. Steele, C. Walder, and M. Herbert, M. (1992), "Psychomotor testing and the ability to perform an anastomosis in junior surgical trainees," *Br. J. Surg.* 79:1065–7, 1992.

[9] F. Tendick, M. Downes, T. Goktekin, M.C. Cavusoglu, D. Feygin, X. Wu, R. Eyal, M. Hegarty, and L.W. Way, "A virtual environment testbed for training laparoscopic surgical skills," *Presence* 9(3), 236–255, June 2000.

[10] R.B. Ekstrom, J.W. French, and H.H. Harman, *Manual for Kit of Factor Referenced Cognitive Tests.* Educational Testing Service, Princeton, NJ, 1976.

[11] M. Kozhevnikov and M. Hegarty, "Perspective-taking ability is distinct from mental rotation ability," paper presented at the Annual Meeting of the Psychonomics Society, Los Angeles, CA, November, 1999.

Medicine Meets Virtual Reality 2001
J.D. Westwood et al. (Eds.)
IOS Press, 2001

Wireless Vital Sign Telemetry to Hand Held Computers

Alex Gandsas, MD[1]; Kevin Montgomery, PhD[3], Katie McIntire [3]and Rodolfo Altrudi, MD[4]

1-Department of Surgery, University of Kentucky, 800 Rose Street Rd. Room #349 Lexington, KY 40536
2-NASA Ames Research Ct. – National Biocomputation Center, Stanford University, Palo Alto, CA
3-Duke University Medical Center. School of Medicine, Durham, North Carolina
4. Department of Surgery, Hospital Santojanni, Buenos Aires, Argentina

Abstract: Most physicians and other health care providers share/access patient information via hard copy chart records, telephone conversations, or through hospital computer networks. These modalities are cumbersome when physicians are away from the hospital and ground wiring infrastructure is not readily available. In a prior study, we used wireless in-flight telephony and the Internet to transmit vital signs from an airborne Boeing 757 to three remote locations on the ground. However, because all recipient stations relied on an institutional network to receive the information, it was not possible to transfer data to a given location beyond the hospital campus. We now propose an innovative system capable of transmitting telemetry information from any location in the globe to a single portable computer using Wireless Application Protocol (WAP) technology for the Internet. Medical data including blood pressure, pulse, respiratory rate, end tidal CO_2, oxygen saturation and EKG tracings were transferred from a G2 (digital cellular) phone linked to a hand held computer to a remote hand held device and were viewed in real time using customized software. Cellular Digital Packet Protocols (CDPD) enabled data transfer speeds up to 19,200 bps. Advances including the Internet and wireless computer technology may revolutionize the way medical information is shared, making it possible for physicians and health allies to directly access patient data from anywhere at any time.

1. Introduction

Telemedicine refers to health care services delivered across distances using information and communication technology. Telemedicine applications have been a growing research interest since the late 1980's with a burst of popularity in the 1990's as computer hardware and software have become more powerful, easier to use and more affordable [1]. Using telemedicine applications, off-site specialists may be consulted by transferring medical data stored in different formats such as audio, video, still images, and/or text. Telemedicine is becoming an integral component of comprehensive health care delivery systems, and, in recent years, the federal government and some insurance companies have begun to reimburse telemedicine services [2]. However, despite the growing role of telemedicine in health care delivery, many rural institutions that may stand to benefit most from this technology are not yet connected to a telemedicine network [2-3]. Therefore, we propose an innovative system that uses wireless technology to transfer data to distant sites making the exchange of medical information possible in regions where a ground wired infrastructure is not readily available [2].

A major barrier to the widespread use of telemedicine services is that the consultant must be present at a telemedicine center or must possess a personal computer with telemedicine capabilities in order to receive medical data.   A wired infrastructure connecting the two locations (transmitter and recipient) is required and serves as the platform on which data may be sent and delivered. The required connection speed or bandwidth varies depending on the type of data being shared. A 12-lead electrocardiogram can be easily transmitted over copper telephone lines with a bandwidth up to 56 kilobits per second (Kbps) while more complex data such as a 30-frame-per-second video or audio require a larger bandwidth up to 1.5 Megabits per second (Mbps). Although bandwidth availability using fiber optic networks working with satellites can reach a speed as high as one gigabyte per second (1 billion bits), the system is too costly for practical or clinical purposes. Cellular phone technology and the Internet represent a potential, cost-effective solution.

In 1997, we successfully piloted a system capable of transmitting vital signs from commercial aircraft to the ground using G1 analog phones and the Internet [4]. A computer equipped with customized client software was connected to the Internet and received medical data that was then displayed in real-time through a graphic interface. In that study, data transfer was limited to locations within the hospital campus as all recipient stations relied on an institutional network to receive the information. To address this limitation, we now propose an innovative system capable of transmitting telemetry information from any location in the globe to a single portable computer using Wireless Application Protocol (WAP) technology for the Internet. Medical data including blood pressure, pulse, respiratory rate, end tidal CO_2, oxygen saturation and EKG tracings were transmitted from a G2 (digital cellular) phone linked to a hand held computer to a recipient hand held device and were viewed in real time using customized software. Data transfer speeds up to 19,200 bps were accomplished using Cellular Digital Packet Data (CDPD) protocols.   This system demonstrates the feasibility of using wireless technology to facilitate the practice of telemedicine.

Our system has the potential to make specialized medical expertise available to remote locations for stat consultation. Furthermore, the real time nature of data transmission promotes the concept of the "virtual physician" and may facilitate prompt adequate treatment when physicians are off-site.

2. Materials and Methods

The hardware platform consisted of a portable medical monitoring system (Propaq 106 , Protocol Systems-Beaverton, Oregon) a handheld PC (Cassiopeia E115), a compact card for wireless communication (Xircom GSM card) and a digital cellular phone (Ericsson CF 688) for Internet connectivity. The handheld PC was loaded with a Microsoft Pocket/Windows CE 3.0 operating system and was optimized to run on a 131 MHz MIPS VR4121 processor with 32 MB of RAM and 16 MB of ROM. Additional features of the device included a 240x320 TFT liquid crystal with 65535-color display, an IrDA 1.0 (115Kbps infrared port), a serial RS232C port (115Kbps) and a Type I/II CompactFlash slot. Internet connectivity with a data transfer rate of 9600 bps (full duplex) was achieved by plugging the Xircom GSM card into the handheld Type II CompactFlash slot and the cellular phone. The software used for our previous in-flight telemetry study was recoded for the Microsoft Windows CE environment such that four "live" waveforms could be transmitted in a single session [4]. The four transmitted waveforms included any combination of the following data types: EKG1, EKG2, blood pressure, end-tidal carbon dioxide, arterial oxygen saturation and respiratory rate.

Upon starting the system, the handheld PC automatically created a connection with the portable monitor then communicated with the Xircom card/cellular phone to establish a link to the Sprint PCS (Personal Communication Services) network using WAP over SMS (Short Messaging Service). This routine generated a socket connection to a known server running Solaris 2.6. A client version of our customized software that displays streaming data in real time was launched in Solaris 2.6 by clicking on a web page with the appropriate link.

An identical setup was tested to view vital signs through a handheld PC device that acted as a recipient station. The client (recipient) machine achieved connectivity to the Internet using similar hardware. Once the connection was established, the web page on the server was reached using WAP, and the browser spawned our helper application enabling a socket connection to the server. After the socket was active, streaming data (vital signs) were displayed in real time on the recipient handheld PC.

3. Results

Multiple connections were successfully established between the transmitting handheld PC and the server over a wireless cellular connection. The Internet link-up was achieved in less that one minute. All data was transmitted in real time with a maximum delay of one second using any combination of seven physiologic parameters with a maximum of four live waveforms per session. Vital signs were successfully received by a recipient handheld PC that was connected to the Internet in a similar fashion. The wireless connection was stable during data transmission but dropped when the digital signal was out of range from the cell tower. The system needed to be restarted if the combination of data types was changed.

4. Discussion

Analog devices were the first cellular phones to appear on the market. They use radio waves that are modulated to recreate the voice signal of the transmitting station. Analog phones are not capable of data transmission unless a modem is used to convert the analog signal to digital (bits/bytes) and vice-versa. The bandwidth achieved with this scheme ranges from 4 to 10 Kbps. Second generation (G2) digital phones were introduced in the early 1990s. The analog signal is converted to digital format within the phone and delivered through modulated microwaves. Unlike analog counterparts, digital phones do not require a modem to translate the signal when connected to a computer. Despite this technological advancement, the bandwidth is still limited to a maximum of 19 Kbps, which is only adequate for voice and text messages [5]. This narrow pipeline is not sufficient to transmit the type of content Hypertext Markup Language (HTML) could offer as seen in regular browsers (text, pictures, sound and movies). Therefore, a new "low bandwidth" language was designed, Wireless Application Protocol (WAP) [6].

The user with a WAP-enabled cellular phone sends a request in digital format over modulated microwaves to a cellular phone transmission tower. The signal is relayed through the ground to a server that is linked to the Internet. The server then picks up the requested web page from the Internet and transforms the web page HTML into a text-solo version known as Wireless Markup Language (WML) using special coding software that filters all graphics and multimedia, keeping the text format. This process may result in errors of format interpretation and may also constitute a bridge in security when encrypted data transmitted to the server needs to be unlocked for WML formatting [5].

Although wireless technology opens new opportunities for health care delivery, WAP technology presents a potential confidentiality problem when patient information is shared over such a large network. In this study, our application uses WAP to establish a link to the server and launch proprietary software that enables real time vital signs monitoring. Security was not of concern as the recipient wireless station must be equipped with specialized software to decode the data. In our previous study, vital signs were transmitted as a single dataset to a single recipient station. We have now implemented a server connected to the Internet, acting as a switchboard, with the ability to handle up to 65,000 datasets. Therefore, several telemetry units may send signals simultaneously. However, due to WAP's low bandwidth, it is not unreasonable to think that this technology may not be the platform on which wireless medical data will be exchanged. New technologies and networks that may provide a faster wireless platform for medical data are currently being assessed.

The Ericsson CF 688 cellular phone used in this study, was built to operate on a 900 MHz frequency on a Global System for Mobile (GSM) network. This technology, primarily found in Europe, allows many signals (users) to simultaneously share a given frequency channel. Although they are popular, the data transmission speed of GSM phones is insufficient to deliver content in a multimedia format. A new generation (G3) is currently being designed with the objective of increasing the data transfer speed to between 2 and 2.4 Mbps. This increase would allow physicians to download or upload content rich in multimedia such as video or sound. Unfortunately, G3 cell phone networks will be designed so that individual devices will share the bandwidth offered from a single cell tower, creating a situation similar to that encountered by those who access the Internet using cable-modems (the signal from a main pipeline is usually shared by many households). Therefore, the final bandwidth, after compensating for splitting among many users, will achieve an estimated data transfer speed of only 64Kbps. According to current compression protocols, 64Kbps is insufficient to view multimedia [7]. Wideband Code Division Multiple Access (W-CDMA) is a growing technology for wireless networks that divides a signal into "chips" of data that are then spread over a large bandwidth of frequencies. W-CDMA increases the transmission speed to a maximum of 2 Megabits per second (5). Many believe that current GSM networks will be replaced by W-CDMA in the years to come. [7]. In the meantime, emerging technologies such as Wireless Local Loop (WLL) networking may provide high bandwidth solutions for rural areas with inadequate wired infrastructures [8].

In conclusion, this study demonstrates the feasibility of using G2 cellular telephony combined with handheld computers to effectively transmit vital signs in real-time over the Internet in a wireless fashion. Advances including the Internet and wireless computer technology may revolutionize the way medical information is shared, making it possible for physicians and health allies to directly access patient data from anywhere at any time.

5. References

1. Kvedar JC, Menn E, Loughlin KR. Telemedicine. Present Applications and Future Prospects. Urologic Clinics of North America. Urol Clin North Am. 1998; 25(1):137-49.

2. Grigsby J; Sanders JH. Telemedicine: where it is and where it's going. *Ann Intern Med* - 1998; 129(2): 123-7

3. Williams ME, Remmes WD and Thompson BG. Nine reasons why healthcare delivery using advanced communications technology should be reimbursed. J Am Geriatr Soc 1996; 44(12):1477-8

4. Gandsas A, Montgomery K, Mc Kenas D et al. In-flight continuous vital signs telemetry via the Internet. Aviat Space Environ Med. 2000; 71(1): 68-71.

5. Harvey F. The Internet in your Hands. Scientific American. 2000; 283 (4):40-45.

6. Bannan K. The Promise and Perils of WAP. Scientific American. 2000; 283 (4):46-48.

7. Kahney L. The Third-Generation Gap. Scientific American. 2000; 283 (4):54-57.

8. Derfler F. Your Digital Future. Infrastructure. PC Magazine, 2000; :149-151.

Medicine Meets Virtual Reality 2001
J.D. Westwood et al. (Eds.)
IOS Press, 2001

Measurable Models of Abdominal Aortic Aneurysm on the Web

Andrea Giachetti, Massimiliano Tuveri, Gianluigi Zanetti
CRS4, VI Strada Ovest, Z.I. Macchiareddu, UTA (CA), Italy

Abstract In this paper we describe a method for 3D reconstruction and web distribution of vessel structures specifically designed to allow the remote measurement of parameters of surgical interest. Deformable models are used for segmentation, while VRML and ECMA scripting are used to obtain 3D models that are not only viewable from any VRML97 enabled browser, but that also allow users to interact with the model, navigate along the vessel lumen and perform guided measurements of distances and angles.

1. Introduction

Since the introduction of VRML97 it has been possible to generate three dimensional models of organs from CT or MR data using standard image processing software, and convert them to a format that could be visualized on any web browser. The application of this technique has been mostly limited to proof of concepts, see, for instance, the nice demos of surgical simulation proposed in [1], but not to tasks immediately useful to clinical applications.

Here, we show an example of a 3D web based application directly motivated by a specific clinical need: the measurement of the geometrical characteristics of Abdominal Aortic Aneurysms. Recent advances in the endovascular treatment of this kind of pathology require, in fact, a precise knowledge of the 3D structure of the specific patient abdominal aortic aneurysm in order to evaluate risk factors, decide if the intervention is necessary, select the prostheses to be used, plan the surgical procedure [2].

The system proposed in this paper builds enhanced patient specific VRML97 models of AAA, which contain also specialized guided measurement tools. These models enable surgeons to perform 3D measurements needed in endovascular AAA intervention planning directly from their web browsers. The structure of the system is naturally suited for the operation of an Internet based image processing service that receives in input DICOM data obtained from hospitals acquisition modalities and returns WWW browsable models.

2. Segmentation techniques

In order to support the relevant measurements on vascular geometries, we needed a segmentation algorithm able to extract both the complete surface mesh with no holes for the vessels internal surface and a series of 1D lines representing the vessels centerline. We organized these data in a dedicated data structure called *arterial tree*. We adopted two different metods to build arterial trees: a 2d contour based method and a 3D segmentation based on Simplex Meshes. The first consists of generating single tubes from series of contours located in the 3D space and then joining them with basic operations. Contours are extracted from 2D slices (with arbitrary orientation) using customized region growing or balloon snakes [3] algorithms, and can be modified and controlled through a specialized user interface. Tubes segments are then generated from contour series and their centerlines are also built from contours centers of mass. The operations introduced to join the contours are three: simple joint, anastomosis and bifurcation. The first connects two tubes at their extrema, the second joins two intersecting tubes, the third joins three different tubes in a bifurcation structure.

The same procedure of the balloon evolution, can be performed directly in 3D starting from a small sphere first put inside the data set and then grown driven by an internal pressure, regularizing forces and voxel based forces. We found a good 3D geometrical structure to be used as a basis to implement the balloon in the Simplex Meshes introduced by Delingette el al. [4]. Simplex Meshes are very simple surface meshes where each node is connected exactly to three neighbours. This makes very easy to write the code for the dynamics and the algorithms obtained are simple and fast. The only problem of this method is that the geometry obtained is composed by non-planar polygons. We overcame the latter by saving for rendering a dual triangulation of the surface, obtained from nodes placed at the center of each simplex face connected with the other nodes corresponding to the neighbouring faces of the simplex mesh. We control the size of the faces by splitting them if they overshoot either an area or an elongation threshold and by merging them if under another threshold. The Simplex balloon method we implemented do not provide an Arterial Tree as output, but only the external surface of the vessel. We reconstruct in this case the centerline directly from the dataset, after binarization. This step can be done by voxel coding technique by Zhou [5]. The simplex reconstruction is more regular than the 2d contour based method near the bifurcations and it is usually better with irregular vessels. However, in case of plaques or local structures it is convenient to correct locally the reconstruction with 2d contour information.

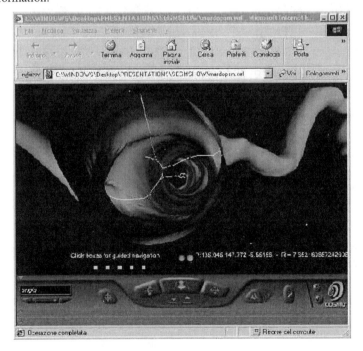

Fig.1 Virtual endoscopy with measurement of radii on the browser

3. VRML97 generation

VRML97 files are generated, including surfaces, centerline and also an user interface that can be used to start guided navigation inside the vessel's branches, and to select the measurement mode preferred. Different "nodes" of VRML97 have been used to represent the geometry of the vessel surface and the vessel centerline; to make easier the measurement of angles and distances the centerline is also duplicated in another part of the scene. The Viewpoint node is used to define a set of privileged points of view (at the end of each vessel branch and an external global view). The simple VRML user interface allows the control of pre-defined animations. Our conversion script automatically creates a guided navigation along each branch of the tree along the vessel centerline. The VRML97 language specification includes a particular node called Script that allows the introduction of code inside the file using ECMAScript or Java. The output of the node can be used to change the value of variables in the other VRML nodes instantiated. Using ECMA scripting we implemented a method to measure parameters, with three main options. The first consists of printing the 3D coordinates and the distance from the centerline for an arbitrary point on the surface, selected with the mouse (Fig.1). The second consists of measuring the distance traveled by a point moving along the centerline between two user selected reference points (Fig. 2 A). This is an extremely useful measure, since usual measurements of vessel length done with 2D imaging or endoscopy are often wrong due to the effect of vessel curvature [2]. The last one is the measurements of angles defined selecting three points on the centerline (Fig. 2 B). With these tools the end user can perform many useful computations on realistic models that can be distributed worldwide a few hours after the image acquisition and just by using standard web browser.

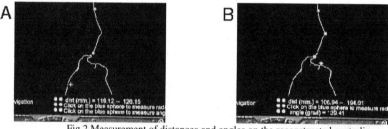

Fig.2 Measurement of distances and angles on the reconstructed centerline

4. Results

With our software tools, 3D models can be created and distributed within a few hours from the image acquisition. The scripting code allows quick measurements of the parameters used by the surgeon; the accuracy of these measurements is currently under test on controlled data sets

5. Conclusions

In this paper we have shown how it is possible to harness VRML technology to provide surgeons with a new tool directly applicable to clinical practice.

References
[1] John, N.W., Phillips, N., Vawda, R., Perrin, J., "A VRML Simulator for Ventricular Catheterisation" In Proceedings of the Eurographics UK conference, Cambridge, UK. April (1999)
[2] K.M. Baskin et al., "Volumetric Analysis of Abdominal Aortic Aneurysm" in Medical Imaging 1996: Physiology and Function from Multidimensional Images, Eric A. Hoffman, Editor, Proc. SPIE 2709, p. 323-337 (1996).
[3] L.D. Cohen and Isaac Cohen, "A finite element method applied to new active contour models and 3D reconstructions from cross-sections" Proc. of 3rd Int. Conf. on Comp. Vision, pp. 587--591 (1990).
[4] H. Delingette, "Simplex meshes: a general representation for 3d shape reconstruction", in CVPR94, pp. 856-859, 1994.
[5] Y. Zhou and A.W. Toga, "Efficient skeletonization of volumetric objects", TVCG, vol. 5, 1999.

Medicine Meets Virtual Reality 2001
J.D. Westwood et al. (Eds.)
IOS Press, 2001

Interactive Stereoscopic Full-Color Direct Volume Visualization for Virtual Reality Applications in Medicine

Vicente Pimentel de Sampaio Góes
Liliane dos Santos Machado
Márcio Calixto Cabral
Ricardo Bittencourt Vidigal Leitão
Roseli de Deus Lopes
Marcelo Knörich Zuffo

Laboratório de Sistemas Integráveis – Universidade de São Paulo
Av. Prof. Luciano Gualberto N. 158 Travessa 3 Cidade Universitária
São Paulo – SP, 05508-900
{vigoes, liliane, mcabral, ricardo, roseli, mkzuffo}@lsi.usp.br

Abstract: Only recently, advanced direct volume visualization techniques have been widely used due to the availability of low cost hardware accelerators; such techniques have a great potential of use for many applications of the virtual reality in medicine. We proposed and implemented a low cost system for interactive and stereoscopic 3D visualization of the full color visible human dataset. Potential use of the proposed system includes anatomical atlases and surgical simulators. A prototype of the proposed system is rendering full color volumes with 256x152x470 in real time (15-20Hz) with stereoscopy.

1. Introduction

The majority of the currently available virtual reality applications are based on traditional polygon oriented graphics systems. Recently advanced direct volume rendering techniques such as the ray-casting based on the shear-warp factorization have been implemented in low cost hardware making possible real time and accurate visualization of volumetric data. We believe that these advances will open a broad range of applications in the medical field when we consider the availability of non-invasive high-resolution volumetric data such as the helicoidal computer topography, functional magnetic resonance and SPECT imaging.

Potential applications could consider also non-conventional data sources such as the volumetric full color slices made available by the Visible Human Project [13], where two corpses (a male one and a female one) were cut in sub-millimeter slices and color photographed in high resolution. Intense research has been done related with the 3D interactive visualization of such datasets, however many approaches consider the use of very expensive supercomputers and high performance parallel computing systems that make impossible the disseminated use of these costly visualization systems.

We proposed and implemented a system for the interactive and stereoscopic direct volume visualization of the visible human color dataset. Our approach is based on the use of low cost hardware platform to make available desktop virtual reality medical applications.

2. The Visible Human Project

In 1989, the National Library of Medicine (NLM) began The Visible Human Project to create a digital atlas of the human anatomy [10]. The digital atlas is based in two datasets: The Visible Man and The Visible Woman. Multimodal 3D medical imaging that includes X-ray Computed Tomography and Magnetic Resonance Imaging (MRI) and axial physical cross-sections composes each dataset.

Full color images (RGB) based on photographs of physical sections of both cadavers are also available. To obtain these images the cadavers were embedded in gelatin, frozen and sliced from head to the toe. As each layer was exposed, a color RGB (24Bits) photograph was taken with a resolution of 2048 by 1216 pixels.

The axial anatomical cross-sections images of the Visible Man are at 1mm intervals and coincide with the X-ray CT images, resulting in 1871 full color and CT images. The axial anatomical cross-sections images of the Visible Woman are at 0.33mm intervals, resulting in 5.000 anatomical images. Since the availability of such datasets to the international scientific community [Tiede et al [15], Lorensen [7, 8] and Reinig et al. [12]), to build applications has been a challenge for many research groups.

3. Volume Visualization and Virtual Reality

Stereoscopic Volume Visualization

The term volume visualization often refers to the images created from volumetric datasets and then displayed as a parallel projection onto a flat CRT screen. Perspective projection is not so often used since it considers the depth in the overall computation of the projections that significant increases the computational cost of the resampling in the volume rendering. Stereoscopic volume visualization adds the additional depth cue of stereopsis that potentially could have many applications on the virtual reality field. When an observer looks at a 3D scene, the horizontal separations of the eye means that the images projected in the back of each eye for any particular point in the scene differ in their horizontal position, this effect is referred to as binocular disparity or binocular parallax [4].

Time-multiplexed stereoscopic systems present the stereoscopic image pair by alternating right and left eye of an object on a CRT. Current implementations use an alternation rate of around 120Hz (60Hz image rate for the left eye and 60Hz image rate for the right eye).

Particularly, Direct Volume Rendering [1, 3, 5, 6] is a term to designate that set of rendering algorithms that do a direct mapping among voxels and pixels offering accurate image renderings from the volumetric data set. Volume Visualization deals with potentially huge amounts of data, considering for example the full color visible Woman dataset with 2048x1216x5000 voxels we have around 12Gigabytes.

The VolumePro Real-Time Ray-Casting Accelerator Board

The Volume-Pro system is the first low-cost real-time direct volume rendering accelerator board for consumer PCs [11] made available in august 1999. The introduction of this system made a major impact in the developing of real time applications with this visualization technique that could be available before only in very expensive supercomputers or graphics superworkstations such as the SGI Onyx II machines.

The VolumePro implements the ray-casting direct volume rendering method based on the shear-warp factorization of the viewing matrix, which allows parallel slice-by-slice processing. The system incorporates hardware for gradient estimation, classification and Phong illumination. The system renders 500 Million interpolated Phong illuminated, composited samples per second enabling real-time volume rendering up to 16 million voxels (256^3) at 30 frames per-second.

Color&Opacity Classification and Bilinear Interpolation

The rendering pipeline implemented in VolumePro assigns RGBA values to interpolated samples as opposed to many volume-rendering methods, which usually classify voxels values first and then interpolate RGBA. The system supports 8 and 12 bit scalar voxels and classification is based on full color 24bit RGB tables and 12bit Alpha (opacity) tables. We call these tables RGBA classification tables.

This RGBA classification scheme results in great accuracy for non-linear mappings from data to color and opacity, however direct rendering of volumes that have been pre-classified in RGBA materials such as the full color Visible Human is not possible.

One major advantage of the ray-casting factorization when compared with related ray-casting methods is that a volume is processed in slice-by-slice order and then bi-linear interpolations instead of tri-linear interpolations delivering a significant reduce of the computing complexity. However, when we consider the interpolation index of color tables, color artifacts are introduced resulting on a poor quality image. Some existing quantization algorithms can be used to minimize this problem, but in this case color tables need to be computed for every new image rendering decreasing dramatically the frame rate. In section 4 we propose a volume rendering pipeline to solve these drawbacks.

4. The Proposed System

The proposed system is based on the "Fish-Tank" model, where a large desktop screen will establish a "portal" to the virtual world. The time-multiplexed stereoscopic and additional haptic devices specific for each application deliver the sense of immersion to the users with minimal body movements restrictions. Groups up to 5 physicians can easily share the same virtual world with a good sense of immersion. The main problem of such approach is that the sense of immersion is completely lost when users move their view out of the computer screen.

Hardware and Software Platforms

The hardware platform is a Pentium III 600MHz with 128Mytes RAM with PCI and AGP buses. The graphics adapter is a 3Dlabs Oxygen GVX1-AGP board with support to stereoscopy. One PCI bus is used to connect the VolumePro500 board with 128Mbytes RAM. To support stereoscopy we used the StereoGraphics CrystalEyes shutter glasses [14] with wireless infrared connection, with three shutter glasses. Finally to support time-multiplexed stereoscopy a Sony-UltraScan 1600HS 21" monitor is attached to the system.

The software was implemented in C++, using the VLI VolumePro API [9] on NT, the warping and display was implemented in NT OpenGL, the resampling, segmentation and filtering were implemented in C.

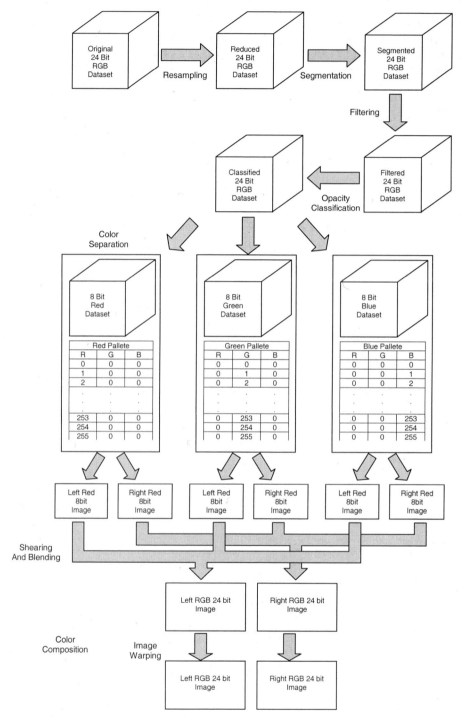

Figure 1. The Volume Rendering Pipeline

The Visualization Pipeline

The proposed visualization pipeline is showed in Figure 1.

The first step of the visualization pipeline is the resampling of the visible human dataset in order to fit it on the VolumePro memory. We choose 377 slices from the original Visible Man color dataset resulting in a volume with 2048x1216x377 color voxels. The volume was reduced by an 8x8x2 factor resulting in a 256x152x470 voxels.

The resampled volume was segmented to remove the blue gelatine; the segmentation was based on the region growing with tolerance of 20% related to the original RGB seed. A mean 3x3x3 filter was applied to remove additional noise not removed by the segmentation. To classify the voxel opacity we used two methods: gradient modulation and direct opacity mapping.

Since the VolumePro does not have capabilities to render full color pre-classified datasets, our approach was based on the splitting of the original RGB 24 bit volume in three monochromatic 8 bit volumes, respectively the Red, Green and Blue volumes. The VolumePro independently rendered each of these three volumes resulting in monochromatic three stereo pairs. The stereo pairs were generated with parallel projection (since VolumePro do not implement yet perspective projection) with the binocular parallax of 7.0.

The three monochromatic stereo pairs were composed on a RGB stereo pair, which is transferred to the GL board for the final image warping and then it is displayed to the user.

5. Results

Figure 2 shows some images rendered by our system. Figure 2 (a) and (b) shows two different views of the 256x15x470 dataset without segmentation and filtering, in this case opacity was assigned to maximize the transparency of the gelatin. Figure 2 (c) and (d) shows different views of the 256x152x470 dataset segmented and filtered, Figure 2-(d) shows the dataset with two cutting planes to show the body interior. Figure 2-(e) shows the whole body. These images were generated in full screen (1280x1024) with stereoscopy at a frame rate ranging from 15 to 25 Hz.

We tested the system with different users and all of them accepted well the stereoscopy. We consider that this high level of acceptance is based on the fact that the renderings are from semi-transparent objects with a large color dynamic range that can facilitate the binocular disparity even considering that the objects are not projected with perspective projection.

Additional interactive Virtual Reality features have also been added such as haptic touching. Our implementation is based on the marching cubes algorithm to generate an invisible surface used as reference to a Phantom Desktop haptic system.

6. Conclusions and Future Work

In this paper we proposed and implemented a low cost 3D stereoscopic full color direct volume visualization system for virtual reality medical applications. Currently the system is rendering full color volumes of 256x152x470 in real time with stereoscopy. The availability of a system like that will open a great potential of applications on medicine that includes anatomical atlases, surgical simulators and related clinical invasive procedures.

Currently we are expanding the proposed system in order to offer a full immersive low cost Volumetric Virtual Reality system. Basically we are building a cluster based 5-side CAVE with the architecture proposed in Figure 3. This implementation considers 5 high-end PCs with Graphics Accelerators and Volume Pro boards attached to them and high-speed synchronization provided by a Gigabit-Ethernet switch.

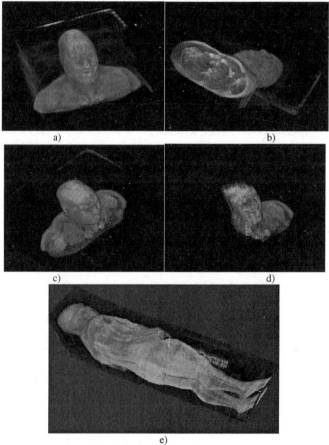

Figure 2. Rendered Images From the Visible Man Dataset

7. Acknowledgments

This work was supported by RECOPE-FINEP project Visualization in Engineering and FAPESP project #. 99/01583-0. The authors would like to thanks Marco Antonio Simon Dal Poz and Fábio José Ayres for their support managing the Visible Human files.

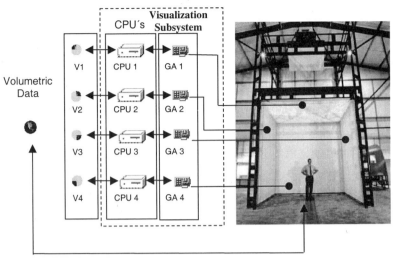

Figure 3 - The CAVE Volumetric System Architecture

References

[1]   B. Cabral, N. Cam, and J. Foran. "Accelerated volume rendering and tomographic reconstruction using texture mapping hardware", In 1994 Workshop on Volume Visualization, pp. 91-98, Washington, DC, October 1994.

[2]   R. A. Drebin, L. Carpenter, P. Hanrahan, "Volume Rendering", SIGGRAPH'88, August 1988,

[3]   Foley et al, Computer Graphics Principles and Practice, 2d ed., Addison Wesley, 1990

[4]   L. Hodges, "Tutorial: Time-Multiplexed Stereoscopic Computer Graphics", IEEE Computer Graphics & Applications, March 1992, pp. 20-30.

[5]   P. Lacroute and M. Levoy. "Fast volume rendering using a shear-warp factorization of the viewing transform", in Computer Graphics, Proceedings of SIGGRAPH94, p. 451-457, July 1994.

[6]   M. Levoy, "Display of Surfaces from Volume Data", IEEE Computer Graphics and Applications, Volume 8, Number 5, May 1988, pp. 29-37.

[7]   W.E. Lorensen, H.E. Cline, "Marching Cubes: A high-resolution 3D Surface Construction Algorithm", Computer Graphics, vol. 21, # 4, July 1987, pp. 163-169.

[8]   Lorensen, W. E. "Marching Through the Visible Human", Proceeding of Visualization 95, IEEE Press, October 1995, pp. 368-373.

[9]   Mitsubishi, Volume Library Interface User's Guide, V1.0, Mitsubishi Electric Information Technology Center America, Inc., 1999.

[10]   National Library of Medicine NLM, "Fact Sheet The Visible Human Project", http://www.nlm.nih.gov/pubs/factssheets/visible_human.html

[11]   H. Pfister et al., "The Volume Pro Real-Time Ray-Casting System", SIGGRAPH'99, 1999, pp. 251-260.

[12]   K. D. Reinig, C. G. Rush, Helen L. Pelster, Victor M. Spitzer, J. A. Heath., "Real Time Visually and Haptically Accurate Surgical Simulation", available at: http://w1.uchsc.edu/sm/chs/research/MMVR4.html.

[13]   V. Spitzer et al. "The Visible Human Male: A Technical Report", Journal of the American Medical Informatics Association, 1995.

[14]   Stereographics, Developer Handbook, StereoGraphics Corp., 1997.

[15]   U. Tiede; T. Schiemann and K. H. Höhne, "Visualizing the Visible Human", IEEE Computer Graphics and Applications, January 1996, pp. 7-9.

Medicine Meets Virtual Reality 2001
J.D. Westwood et al. (Eds.)
IOS Press, 2001

Virtual simulation system for collision avoidance for medical robot

L. Gonchar, D. Engel, J. Raczkowsky, H. Wörn
University of Karlsruhe, Institute for Process Control and Robotics

For the collision avoidance with a medical robot with 6 DOF a virtual simulation system is presented. Manipulator and obstacles are modelled by geometric primitives. Collisions are detected in the Cartesian workspace by hierarchical distance computation based on the given CAD model. The application initially being addressed is maxillofacial surgery, where the safety of the patient is the main requirement, because of the closeness to vital parts. The simulation system allows the surgeon to check up the trajectory of the robot before the current operation begins.

1. Introduction

Virtual simulation has proved to be a cost-effective tool in path planning avoiding costly errors in judgement. Computerised systems for path planning have been developed for redundant manipulators [1] and for 6-DOF industrial robots [2], but are not used in medical applications where high precision of moving control is required.

This work focuses on the use of 3D simulation for collision detection and avoidance. The 3D simulation has been developed using ROBCAD.

2. Requirements of a Surgical Application

The goal of our medical application is to support the surgeon in maxillofacial surgery doing sawing, drilling, and milling jobs placed on the human skull.

The simulation system accepts the data file from the trajectory planning application and according to these data initial position of the robot is defined. The optimal relative position and the start configuration of the robot are determined by using the simulation system preoperatively.

Before the current operation begins, the physicians or assistants move the robot to the initial calculated position. For more convenience, the personal is guided using the navigation system. Nevertheless, the position will differ from the preoperative planned, so that the current position is handed over to simulation and collision check once more.

Figure 1 illustrates the operation sequence. The following steps will be the patient registration and the operation itself.

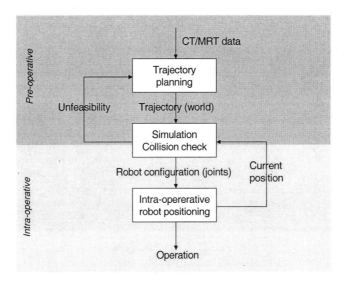

Figure 1: Simulation in the operation time sequence

3. The Collisions Detection

Collisions are detected by a fast, hierarchical distance computation in 3D workspace, based on the polyhedral model of the environment and the robot provided by special ROBCAD system. [3]. The Cartesian distances are then transformed into joint angles in order to define the state ("free" or "prohibited") of the regarded configuration. For obtaining similar joint intervals, thus implicating an efficient distance exploitation, the optimal joint discretization is automatically computed based on the method presented in [4]. Collision are detected in the explicit workspace by computing the minimum distance between robot R and obstacles W_i (Figure 2).

4. The Collisions Avoidance

A frequent approach to collision avoidance is the calculation of a penalty function, which value is increased in case of the robot removal from the goal [1]. Other approaches work in the explicit representation of the free C-space [2].

Here a method "the hypothesis–test" is presented. The first step is definition of possible collisions as non-zero geometrical crossing between models of the manipulator and obstacles. The second step is modification of the trajectory. Updating occurs at first on axis z, which keeps upward orientation of the trajectory. If it is a necessary, then the path is modified on the other axes.

5. The Simulation System Realization

The system was implemented on a SGI IRIX in the programming language C.

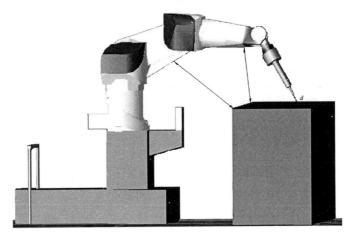

Figure 2: Collision detection

The 3D simulation model provides a robust visualisation tool helping reveal and prevent a potential collision.

The application of results, obtained by the present work, was carried out at the Institute for Process Control and Robotics (University of Karlsruhe, Germany) in the form of a software package for control of the 6-DOF manipulator.

6. Conclusion and Future Goals

The virtual simulation system for collision avoidance of medical robot has been presented. The paper shows the use of 3D graphics for support of the visualisation of the planned robot motion along the trajectory. The collision detection is done in the Cartesian workspace by distance computation. This avoid the time and memory consuming obstacle transformation and C-space calculation. The collision avoidance is based on the "the hypothesis–test" method and provide the supervising surgeon a good overview over all robot activities. Based on these results, we focus next on developing means of communication between the robot control system and the developed simulation system.

References

[1] Yussupova, N.I., Gonchar, L.E., Nikiforov, D.V., Rembold, U., Iterative Recursive Algorithm For Path Planning For Redundant Manipulators. In Highly Constrained Environment IAF-97, Turin, Italy, p.1-9.

[2] Wurll, C., Multi-goal path planning for industrial robots. PhD thesis, University Karlsruhe, 1999.

[3] Heinrich D., Fast motion planning by parallel processing – A review. In: Journal of Intelligent and Robotic Systems, vol 20, no 1, pp. 45-69, sept 1997.

[4] Qin C., Heinrich D., Path planning for industrial robot arms – A parallel randomized approach. In Proc. Of the International Symposium on Intelligent Robotic Systems (SIRS'96), Lissabon, Portugal, pp. 65-72, July 22-26, 1996.

Medicine Meets Virtual Reality 2001
J.D. Westwood et al. (Eds.)
IOS Press, 2001

A Virtual Reality Surgical Trainer for Navigation in Laparoscopic Surgery

Randy S. Haluck MD[1], Roger W. Webster PhD[2], Alan J. Snyder PhD[1],
Michael G. Melkonian MD[1], Betty J. Mohler[2], Mike L. Dise[2], Andrew Lefever[2]

[1]*Department of Surgery, Penn State College of Medicine, MC H070, PO Box 850, Hershey, PA 17033*
[2]*Department of Computer Science, School of Science and Mathematics, Millersville University of Pennsylvania, Millersville, PA 17551*

Abstract. A virtual reality trainer was designed to familiarize students and surgeons with surgical navigation using an angled laparoscopic lens and camera system. Previous laparoscopic trainers have been devoted to task or procedure training. Our system is exclusively devoted to laparoscope manipulation and navigation. Laparoscopic experts scored better than novices in this system suggesting construct validity. The trainer received favorable subjective ratings. This simulator may provide for improved navigation in the operating room and become a useful tool for residents and practicing surgeons.

1. Background/Problem

All surgical procedures require some degree of visual navigation within an operative field. Different visuospatial skills however, are required for navigation with a laparoscopic lens within the complex three-dimensional environment of a body cavity [1]. In traditional open surgery, unaided eyes track and focus without higher cognitive input. In video-endoscopic or laparoscopic surgery, the "vision" of the operation must be directed manually, requiring a different set of skills and possibly higher cognitive function.

Most commercially available angled laparoscopic lens systems consist of a long slender lens that allows change in direction of view through rotation of the lens itself. The angled view allows for another degree of freedom for inspection, i.e. the ability to look around corners. This is coupled to an independently rotating video camera. The camera and lens system must be rotated independently in order to achieve the desired angle of view while maintaining correct right-side-up orientation. The function, orientation, and manipulation of an angled laparoscopic lens in combination with an independently rotating camera system may not be intuitive.

Several simulators have been developed for training laparoendoscopic surgery, but most focus on task or part-task trainers, designed to provide instruction in the motor component required for laparoscopic surgery [2-7]. One such computer-based trainer is the MIST VR, which was designed to train in the special "hand-eye" coordinated movements that are basic to laparoscopic surgery [8]. Aside from motor skill learning, the acquisition of visuospatial skills may be important to operating surgeons [9-13]. Our simulator is concerned with the visuospatial issues of manipulating an angled laparoscope. To date, no simulator has been developed for instruction in laparoscopic navigation.

Often, the duty of "driving the camera" is delegated to an assistant or a junior member of the team while the operating surgeon performs the procedure. In this arrangement, the camera / lens operator must serve as the eyes for the entire surgical team. A facile understanding of the function, operation, and manipulation of the laparoscope is essential. While stationary and robotic camera-positioning devices are available, the surgeon must still have a fluid understanding of the manipulation of the laparoscope. A computer-based simulator designed to replicate the maneuvers necessary and provide instruction in angled laparoscopic lens "driving" in a controlled setting would theoretically provide for a better understanding of the camera lens system and more efficient navigation in the operating room.

The purpose of this project was to develop a computer-based training system that would provide instruction to relative novices at laparoscopic navigation using an angled lens. The software was designed to challenge the participants so that a wide variety of angular and rotational maneuvers would be required to identify visual targets while maintaining right-side-up orientation. Additionally, a timer and error scoring system was developed and included.

2. Methods and Tools

2a. Hardware Platform

The Virtual Laparoscopic Interface (VLI) (Immersion Corporation, San Jose, CA), was utilized as the input device as it provides a fast, effective means of tracking simulated laparoscopic motion. The VLI is a human-computer interface tool designed for virtual reality (VR) simulations of laparoscopic and endoscopic surgical procedures. The frame unit acts as a sensored trocar that is connected via a serial port on a Windows™ NT workstation with dual pentium processors and Wildcat OpenGL™ graphics. Different surgical tool handles can be attached to the sensory unit. The VLI tracks the motion of a pair of laparoscopic surgical instruments, each moving in 5 degrees of freedom. The trocar sensors provide an angular resolution of 0.088 degrees, a linear position resolution of 0.0005 inches, and can move up to 8 inches along the insertion axis. The latency is less than 1 ms. The VLI system provides a fast, effective means of tracking laparoscopic and endoscopic surgical procedures.

2b. Modeling and Software

The task for the laparoscopic surgical training session entails identifying randomly placed arrows in an "endotower". The endotower is a three dimensional (3D) block tower with holes drilled out within its various arms (Figure 1). The endotower provides a relatively complex three-dimensional structure for exploration with the angled lens. In the simulator, 3D arrows of varying colors and directional orientation are randomly placed inside the cylindrical cut-outs. Arrows were chosen as the targets so that participants would be required to maintain right-side-up orientation in order to be able to properly identify them. Arrows could have one of four colors and six directional orientations giving 24 possible combinations. Six arrows were randomly placed on and within the virtual endotower (Figure 2).

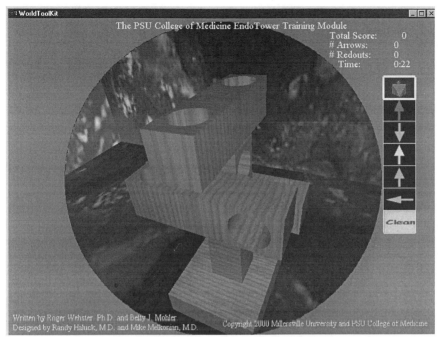

Figure 1: The three dimensional endotower

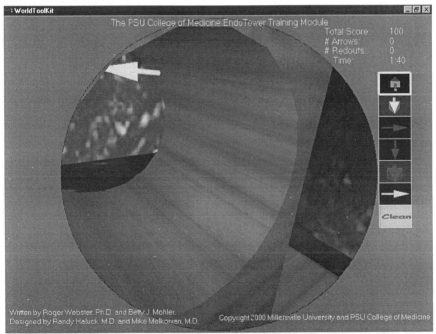

Figure 2: A randomly paced arrow within the virtual endotower

To operate the simulator, the practicing surgeon holds one of the VLI laparoscopic tools, which simulates the angled lens laparoscope. Rotation of this tool rotates the angle of view from the longitudinal axis of the virtual laparoscope. The other laparoscopic tool is used to simulate the laparoscopic camera and rotations of this instrument change the up and down orientation of the surgeons' view. These separations of functions, in contrast to the coaxial controls of a standard laparoscopic camera, are due to the limitations of the present VLI hardware. In the virtual world, the user's viewpoint is placed at the tip of the laparoscopic tool. Due to the 3D nature of the endotower and the cylindrical cutouts, identifying all the arrows entails manipulating the laparoscope to many different and challenging orientations and positions.

Once a target arrow is identified, the student selects the matching arrow from a list. The user's score goes up for each arrow correctly identified. Any collision with the endotower causes the view to become fuzzy and blurry with 'red out', simulating touching the laparoscope to an organ and smudging the lens with blood (Figure 3). The learner must withdraw the virtual laparoscope and await a cleaning mode, thus penalizing the user's score in terms of time efficiency and errors. The scoring mechanism keeps track of the amount of time to correctly identify the color and orientation of each arrow, the number of times the users dirties the camera lens (collides with the endotower), and the rotational efficiency. It also records the amount of time to complete the entire training procedure.

The three dimensional models of the virtual laparoscopic tool and endotower model were built in 3D Studio Max and are stored as 3ds files. These models are loaded into the graphics simulation. The graphics software modules make calls to EAI/Sense8's WorldToolkit API of OpenGL calls.

Another software module records the motions of the user by continuously recording the positions and orientation of the endoscope and the lens rotations. Thus, 3D graphics can be used to replay the movements, showing the user what they did during the training session. The replay can be done either from the laparoscopic viewpoint or from a bystander viewpoint.

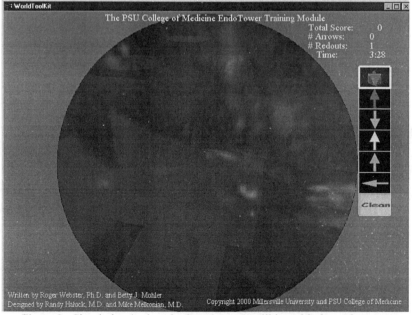

Figure 3: Simulating 'red-out' when the user collides with the endotower

3. Results

Two small groups of surgeons, novices and experts, were enlisted to test the fidelity of the simulator and test the validity of the scoring mechanism. Novices included medical students who had never performed a laparoscopic procedure. Experts included the surgical chief residents and minimally invasive surgical staff. All of the users found that the graphics of the simulator were adequate, however, 86% of the users found the hardware tools/handles interface to be inadequate for this type of simulation. Seventy-one percent of the users believed that the laparoscopic surgical endotower training simulator would be useful as a training tool for laparoscopic surgery and that it has the capability of teaching a novice the 30 degree angle scope.

All of the users went through a training program with an expert instructor, which included practice sessions. The two groups of surgeons performed three scoring sessions with the endotower simulator in a maximum time frame for each session of 240 seconds. Table 1 summarizes the mean and standard deviation of the data. Comparisons between the two groups was done with the Student T test. All six randomly placed colored arrows were identified within the allotted time frame 88.9% by the experts and 58.3% of the time by the novices. With the novices, only one run was error free (i.e. no red-outs), while a third of the expert runs were error free.

Table 1: Mean and Standard Deviation of the number of arrows correctly identified and number of errors

	Novices	Experts	P value
Correctly identified Arrows	5.3 ± 1.1	5.9 ± 0.3	0.045
Errors ('Red-outs')	3.1 ± 3.1	1.0 ± 0.9	0.023

4. Discussion / Conclusions

Our endotower laparoscopic navigation simulator has successfully reproduced the optics and movements of a 30 degree angled lens. We are able to portray a realistic view of a three dimensional object as it is navigated with a virtual laparoscope. All of our test users found the graphical user interface to be adequate. The dual pentium personal computer with an OPENGL graphic accelerator provides a system with fast frame rates and the VLI system provides an economical laparoscopic simulator interface with no perceived lag.

More work is needed on the tool handle interface. The Immersion device was designed to portray two laparoscopic instruments and not a lens/camera laparoscope. Our current system has the user using the right instrument as the navigating camera and the left instrument purely for rotation of the scope. Most of our users found this to be somewhat cumbersome. Whereas true angled laparoscope have the camera and lens held in the same hand, we developed our system using the VLI and a two handed technique as an economical alternative. We are currently developing plans to provide a more accurate hardware tools/handles user interface for the simulator.

Initial tests using experienced surgeons and novices to compare scores on the simulator suggest that manipulating a 30 degree laparoscope is a skill that is not intuitive but rather acquired. More errors were made by the novice than the experts. These findings suggest construct validity for the simulator in the scoring system.

Times varied widely in our novice group and may represent the underlying differences in understanding visuospatial relationships. This could suggest that there are subgroups novices that may be more adept at tasks involving visuospatial skills than others.

Ongoing development is focused upon providing users more feedback and adding functions to output and analyze motion metrics [14]. The intent is to provide a method to learn how to efficiently manipulate a laparoscope by measuring surgical skills in a simulator. Future plans include improving the hardware tools/handles interface, adapting the environment to clinical situations, and validating that acquisition of skills using the simulator that will affect performance in live situations.

5. Acknowledgments

This project was funded, in part, by the National Science Foundation under grant numbers DUE-9950742 and DUE-9651237, a Penn State College of Medicine Department of Surgery Feasibility Grant, the Eberly Medical Research Innovation Fund, the Millersville University Neimeyer-Hodgson Grants Program, and by the Faculty Grants Committee of Millersville University. Thanks to Cindy Miller for her editorial expertise.

6. References/Literature

[1] Medina M. Image rotation and reversal – major obstacles in learning intracorporeal suturing and knot-tying. J Soc Laparoendosc Surg 1997;1:331-6.

[2] Bro-Nielsen M, Tasto JL, Cunningham R, Merril GL. PREOP endoscopic simulator: a PC-based immersive training system for bronchoscopy. Stud Health Technol Inform 1999;62:76-82.

[3] Kukuk M, Geiger B. Registration of real and virtual endoscopy - a model and image based approach. Stud Health Technol Inform 2000;70:168-74.

[4] Auer LM, Auer DP. Virtual endoscopy for planning and simulation of minimally invasive neurosurgery. Neurosurgery 1998;43:529-48.

[5] Tasto JL, Verstreken K, Brown JM, Bauer JJ. PreOp endoscopy simulator: from bronchoscopy to ureteroscopy. Stud Health Technol Inform 2000;70:344-9.

[6] Jang DP, Han MH, Kim SI. Virtual endoscopy using surface rendering and perspective volume rendering. Stud Health Technol Inform 1999;62:161-6.

[7] Baur C, Guzzoni D, Georg O. VIRGY: a virtual reality and force feedback based endoscopic surgery simulator. Stud Health Technol Inform 1998;50:110-6.

[8] Sutton C, McCloy R, Middlebrook A, Chater P, Wilson M, Stone R. MIST VR. A laparoscopic surgery procedures trainer and evaluator. Stud Health Technol Inform 1997;39:598-607.

[9] Harris CJ, Herbert M, Steele RJ. Psychomotor skills of surgical trainees compared with those of different medical specialists. Br J Surg 1994;81:382-3.

[10] Squire D, Giachino AA, Proffit AW, Heaney C. Objective comparison of manual dexterity in physicians and surgeons. Can J Surg 1989;32:467-70.

[11] Schueneman AL, Pickleman J, Hesslein R, Freeark RJ. Neuropsychological predictors of operative skill among general surgery residents. Surgery 1984;96:288-95.

[12] Gibbons RD, Baker RJ, Skinner DB. Field articulation testing: A predictor of technical skills in surgical residents. J Surg Res 1986;41:53-7.

[13] Risucci D, Tortolani A, Horowitz M. Neuropsychological assessment of general surgery interns. Focus Surg Edu 1991;10:14-5.

[14] Millersville University and Penn State College of Medicine. Joint Research Project in Surgical Simulation. Available at http://cs.millersville.edu/haptics/index.html. Accessed October 10, 2000.

Medicine Meets Virtual Reality 2001
J.D. Westwood et al. (Eds.)
IOS Press, 2001

Quantification of the Gravity-Dependent Change in the C-arm Image Center for Image Compensation in Fluoroscopic Spinal Neuronavigation

Sanaz Hariri, Hamid Reza Abbasi, Shao Chin, Gary Steinberg, Ramin Shahidi
Image Guidance Laboratory, Department of Neurosurgery, Stanford School of Medicine

Abstract. In the quest to develop a viable, frameless spinal navigation system, many researchers are utilizing the C-arm fluoroscope. However, there is a significant problem with the C-arm that must be quantified: the gravity-dependent sag effect resulting from the geometry of the C-arm and aggravated by the inequity of weight at each end of the C-arm. This study quantified the C-arm sag effect, giving researchers the protocol and data needed to develop a program that accounts for this distortion. The development of spinal navigation algorithms that account for the C-arm sag effect should produce a more accurate spinal navigation system.

1. Introduction

Mobile fluoroscopic devices (C-arms) are already part of the standard equipment of many operating rooms. For example, in orthopedic surgeries, setting the C-arm in a constant or pulsed mode, the surgeon can obtain real-time feedback of bone and surgical tool positions. C-arms are becoming increasingly important in neurosurgery due to their potential use in spinal neuronavigation. In such a system, a CT of the patient can be used to create a reconstructed 3D "virtual patient." A virtual fluoroscopic image of that virtual patient can be obtained and matched to a real fluoroscopic image of the patient, telling the neuronavigation system where the patient is in space intraoperatively. This technology will allow the surgeon to visualize the spinal anatomy in 3D and see where his instruments are with respect to the anatomy.

Such a spinal navigation system is dependent on an algorithm involving three steps: calibration, tracking, and registration. In the process of calibration, the image distortion must be corrected and two parameters (the length between the scanner and the source and the location of the image center on the scanner) must be determined. Ideally, the source intersects the plate at the plate's center and the distance between the source and the scanner is constant. However, the geometry of the C-arm produces a gravity-dependent "sag effect" that is least when the source-to-scanner line is perpendicular to the ground and is greatest when the source-to-scanner line is parallel to the ground. Further aggravating the sag effect is the weight inequity due to the scanner end of the C-arm being heavier than the source end. The aim of this study is to precisely quantify the sag effect by tracking the movement of the image center as the C-arm is rotated.

2.   Materials and Methods

This study quantified the sag effect for the two degrees of freedom that affect the geometry of the mobile fluoroscopic device (C-Arm, GE, Milwaukee, WI, USA): movement in planes perpendicular to and parallel to the length of the patient (Figure 1). Sliding the C-arm so that the scanner-to-source line is perpendicular to the plane of the ground (defined as 0° "angle"), the experimenter adjusted a mechanical arm holding a laser pointer so that the pointer is mounted at the exact center of one end of the fluoroscope and the red dot is exactly at the center of the other end (Figure 1). This is the ideal image center and served as the baseline calibration point throughout the experiment.

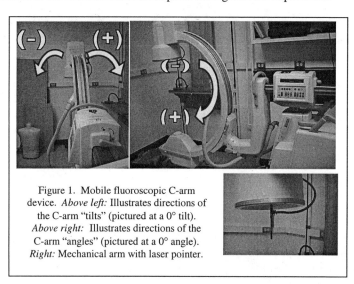

Figure 1. Mobile fluoroscopic C-arm device. *Above left:* Illustrates directions of the C-arm "tilts" (pictured at a 0° tilt). *Above right:* Illustrates directions of the C-arm "angles" (pictured at a 0° angle). *Right:* Mechanical arm with laser pointer.

Beginning with the C-arm plane exactly parallel to the length of the patient (0° tilt), a series of measurements were taken at every 15° angles for the whole range of the C-arm (-24° to 90°). A measurement was defined as the x- and y-values for distance from the calibration baseline. This series of measurements was repeated three times at three different C-arm "tilts" (0° tilt = plane of C-arm parallel to wall, 45° tilt = plane of C-arm tilted 45° towards the nearest wall, -45° tilt = plane of C-arm tilted away from the nearest wall). Between each discrete measurement, the C-arm was returned to its baseline to ensure that the laser pointer remained calibrated correctly. In all, 81 measurements (each measurement consisting of an x- and y-value) were obtained.

3.   Results

It was found that at all tilts of the C-arm, the laser pointer dot moved further away from the baseline center the more the C-arm was rotated away from its original position (baseline was when the scanner-to-source line is perpendicular to the plane of the ground, defined as 0° angle). For each C-arm tilt, maximum sag was found to be 11.8 mm at a 90° angle in the 0° tilt, 9.28 mm at a 90° angle in the 45° tilt, and 9.33 mm at a 90° angle in the -45° tilt.

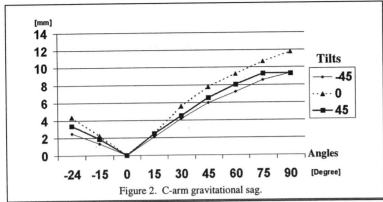

Figure 2. C-arm gravitational sag.

Angle	-45° tilt			0° tilt			45° tilt		
	xAve	yAve	VectorAve	xAve	yAve	VectorAve	xAve	yAve	VectorAve
-24	-2.32	0.83	2.49	-4.38	0.00	4.38	-3.13	-1.20	3.38
-15	-1.10	0.73	1.35	-2.27	0.00	2.27	-1.73	-0.57	1.87
0	0.00	0.00	0.00	0.00	0.00	0.00	0.00	0.00	0.00
15	2.08	0.00	2.08	2.50	0.00	2.50	2.43	0.35	2.47
30	4.18	0.00	4.18	5.57	0.00	5.57	4.40	0.90	4.49
45	5.93	-0.15	5.94	7.78	0.00	7.78	6.35	1.62	6.55
60	7.17	-0.77	7.21	9.27	0.00	9.27	7.83	1.85	8.05
75	8.33	-1.90	8.55	10.65	0.00	10.65	9.00	2.22	9.28
90	8.82	-2.97	9.33	11.80	0.00	11.80	9.00	2.22	9.28

Table 1. C-arm gravitational sag (values are average of three measurements).

4. Discussion

Quantification of the gravity-dependent change in the C-arm image center is critical data for researchers creating fluoroscopic spinal neuronavigation systems. Image compensation in these system algorithms are necessary for the development of a maximally accurate system needed to perform delicate spinal surgeries in sensitive areas such as the cervical and upper thoracic regions. For example, the Image Guidance Laboratory spinal navigation algorithm has an overall error of 1.41 mm. At every 15° increment, this algorithm only makes an approximately 0.5mm adjustment for C-arm sag, whereas this study shows that more than 0.5mm of sag occurs in every 15° increment.

We are aware that the sag effect of a C-arm is probably specific to the mechanical properties of that particular type of C-arm, and so the sag effect will be different for different systems. However, the protocol used to determine C-arm sag in this study can be applied to any C-arm.

5. References

1. Nolte LP, Slomczykowski MA, Berlemann U, Strauss MJ, Hofstetter R, Schlenzka D, Laine T, Lund T. "A new approach to computer-aided spine surgery: fluoroscopy-based surgical navigation." *Eur Spine J.* 2000 Feb;9 Suppl 1:S78-88.
2. Hofstetter R, Slomczykowski M, Sati M, Nolte LP. "Fluoroscopy as an imaging means for computer-assisted surgical navigation." *Comput Aided Surg.* 1999;4(2):65-76.
3. Samset E, Hirschberg H. "Neuronavigation in intraoperative MRI." *Comput Aided Surg.* 1999;4(4):200-7.
4. de Mey J, Op de Beeck B, Meysman M, Noppen M, De Maeseneer M, Vanhoey M, Vincken W, Osteaux M. "Real time CT-fluoroscopy: diagnostic and therapeutic applications." *Eur J Radiol.* 2000 Apr;34(1):32-40.

Medicine Meets Virtual Reality 2001
J.D. Westwood et al. (Eds.)
IOS Press, 2001

Force Models for Needle Insertion Created from Measured Needle Puncture Data

Leslie L. Hiemenz Holton, Ph.D.

Center for Human Simulation
University of Colorado
leslie@chs.uchsc.edu

Abstract. The focus of this paper is to present a force-feedback model that has been developed for the epidural needle insertion procedure. The model is based on data collected from biomaterials testing studies, and consists of separate force models for each of the tissue types relevant to the epidural needle insertion procedure. These tissue force models were generalized to create force-feedback models to drive haptic devices for needle insertion simulation.

1. Introduction

Needle insertion training is a natural application for haptic-based VR simulation because needle insertion techniques rely heavily on perception of force to localize the tip of the needle. As evidenced in prior year's proceedings from MMVR, many research groups are developing needle insertion simulators for a wide range of techniques. Most of these simulators are created using force-feedback models derived from expert opinion, as little data is available on the amount of force required to puncture human tissues.

More realistic and flexible force models can be created through biomaterials testing, by measuring actual needle penetration forces and then creating force models from those measurements. These models offer several advantages over models derived from expert opinion. Since they are derived from measured data they are more accurate. These models are verifiable since the output of the force-feedback device can be compared against the measured data. Because the models are based on penetration depth into the tissue, patient variance can be incorporated into the simulation by developing multiple virtual patients with differing tissue widths.

The focus of this paper is to present a force-feedback model that has been developed for the epidural needle insertion procedure. This model was developed as part of the author's dissertation research at The Ohio State University. [1] The model is based on data collected from biomaterials testing studies, following the modeling methodology presented by the author at MMVR, 1998. [2] The force-feedback model includes separate force models for each of the tissue types relevant to the epidural needle insertion procedure: skin, fat, muscle, interspinous ligament, ligamentum flavum, epidural space, and bone. These tissue force models were generalized to create force-feedback models to drive haptic devices for epidural needle insertion simulation.

2. Methods

The tissue force models were developed from needle force puncture data collected during three studies using human skin and fat tissue samples, and four newly sacrificed porcine cadavers. The first step for each specimen was to obtain high-resolution MRI images in order to be able to identify the internal structure at each location where a needle was to be subsequently inserted. Insertion locations were registered using a grid of oil soaked yarn placed on the surface of the specimen.

Next, a materials testing system [Bionix 858, MTS Corporation, Eden Prairie, MN] was used to measure load vs. displacement curves for the tip of an 18-gauge Tuohy needle as it was inserted into the test objects under displacement control. Figure 1 shows a swine cadaver under test on the MTS machine.

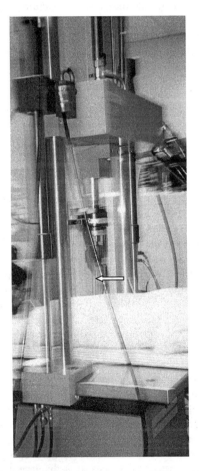

Figure 1: Photograph of swine cadaver under test on the MTS machine. Note: the needle is attached to the end of the insertion rod (indicated by the white arrow).

The measured load versus displacement curves were filtered using a 7-point moving average filter to remove machine noise from the signal. Through correlation of the penetration depth and the MRI images, the curves were broken down into smaller curves representing the different tissue layers. The individual tissue layer curves were then averaged across trials to create a general force profile for the given tissue type. Finally, curve fitting was performed to create tissue force models.

The derived equations were programmed into a needle insertion simulator. The force output displayed by the simulator's force-feedback device at any point was calculated from type of tissue at the tip of the virtual needle, the depth of needle penetration into that tissue type, and the derived equation for that tissue type.

Several assumptions regarding the mechanics of needle puncture were made in developing the needle insertion force models. These assumptions are:

1. *Puncture force is independent of insertion speed.* The forces felt at the tip of the needle were independent of the insertion speed across the range of speeds typical for epidural needle insertion (0.4 to 10 mm/sec).

2. *Skin puncture force is independent of the initial insertion angle.* The difference in forces obtained during initial skin puncture due to angle of insertion is immeasurably small.

3. *Muscle puncture force is independent of the initial angle of insertion.* The difference in forces obtained due to angle of insertion with respect to the muscle fiber is immeasurably small.

4. *Puncture forces are axial.* The puncture force is purely axial along the trajectory of the needle.

5. *The trajectory of the needle can be identified prior to needle insertion.* There is no deflection in the needle trajectory as the needle is inserted.

Assumptions 1, 2, and 3 were tested during pilot studies for this research and found to be valid. Details of the assumptions and testing of the assumptions can be found in [2].

Three force measurement studies were performed. The goal of the first study was to collect needle puncture force data for human skin and fat. The samples were excised pieces from the posterior surface of the arm and were comprised of a layer of skin over a thick layer of fat. These samples were mounted in round acrylic containers over a piece of Styrofoam. Fourteen force curves were obtained using the MTS machine at a needle insertion speed of 0.2 mm/sec as the needle was inserted under displacement control.

The goal of the second study was to collect needle puncture force data for a close analogue to the human back. Three freshly sacrificed young swine cadavers were mounted on wooden boards and secured with tie wraps. The backs were palpated and the lumbar spinal region was approximately identified. A centerline was drawn through this region, and marks made each centimeter along this line. A grid of oil soaked yarn was placed over the marks for registration of the subsequent needle insertion locations on the MRI images. MRI images were obtained of each cadaver. Force curves were obtained at each marked location using the MTS machine with an insertion speed of 0.1 mm/sec. Testing was completed within 26 hours of sacrifice.

One limitation with the second study was that none of the trials resulted in placing the needle into the epidural space because the needle insertions locations were preset, and each missed the small opening between the vertebrae. The goal of the third study was to dissect a single swine cadaver to expose the spinal column, and thus collect needle puncture data for the ligamentum flavum and the epidural space. In this study the needle was inserted into 5 exposed vertebral spaces at a displacement rate of 0.1mm/s. The testing was completed within 4 hours of sacrifice.

3. Results

The force models for skin and fat were created from the data collected in the human tissue sample study. The data curves were broken into three pieces: pre-puncture (increase in force to the point of skin puncture), post-puncture (decrease in force until the steady-state is reached), and fat (the steady-state). The skin and fat puncture models were calculated to be:

Skin pre-puncture: $F(X) = 0.0235 + 0.0116(X - X_s) - 0.0046(X - X_s)^2$
$+ 0.0025(X - X_s)^3$; for $F(X) <=$ Skin puncture force, $X < X_p$
Skin puncture force: $F(X) = 6.0372$ N; $X_p = X$
Skin post-puncture: $F(X) = 6.0372 + 0.4516(X - X_p) - 0.5287(X - X_p)^2$
    for $X > X_p$ and $F(X) >=$ Fat puncture force.
Fat puncture force: $F(X) = 1.974$
    X = Needle penetration depth (mm)
    X_s = Skin surface depth (location of the surface of the skin relative to the start of the needle movement) (mm)
    X_p = Skin puncture depth (mm)

The force-feedback model for muscle was created from data collected in the first swine study. The muscle curve was a distinct curve found in most of the data sets from the MTS trials, and appears as a second puncture curve after the fat is reached.

The models were created using data from swine, but are intended to approximate needle puncture of human tissue. The force model for puncturing human fat was 1.974 N; however, for the swine fat the average puncture force was 6.027 N. This discrepancy was caused by the increased frictional force from the tougher and thicker swine skin. Therefore, a correction factor of 4.053 N will be used to adapt from the calculated swine muscle puncture models to models for human muscle. The muscle puncture models were calculated to be:

Muscle pre-puncture: $F(X) = (6.0266 + 0.8287(X - X_m) + 0.1078(X - X_m)^2) - 4.053$
    for $F(X) <=$ Muscle puncture force, $X < X_p$
Muscle puncture force: $F(X) = 4.354$; $X_p = X$
Muscle post-puncture: $F(X) = (8.407 - 2.2543(X - X_p) + 0.2902(X - X_p)^2) - 4.053$
    for $X > X_p$ and $F(X) >= 3.675$
Muscle steady-state: $F(X) = 3.675$
    X = Needle penetration depth (mm)
    X_m = Muscle surface depth (mm)
    X_p = Muscle puncture depth (mm)

The force-feedback model for the interspinous ligament (ISL) was created from data collected in the first swine study. The interspinous ligament was not punctured in every data trial, but with the MRI data set as a reference, several trials were found in which interspinous ligament was punctured. There was not a distinct drop in force after puncture because of the thickness and density of the tissue. The interspinous ligament puncture models were calculated to be:

ISL pre-puncture: $F(X) = (8.4592 + 0.9598 * (X - X_{ISL})) - 4.053$
    for $F(X) <=$ ISL puncture force, $X < X_p$
ISL puncture force: $F(X) = 7.467$; $X_p = X$
ISL steady-state: $F(X) = 4.053$
    X = Needle penetration depth (mm)
    X_{isl} = ISL surface depth (mm)
    X_p = ISL puncture depth (mm)

The force-feedback model for the ligamentum flavum was created from data collected from the second swine study. In this study the cadaver was dissected down to the ligamentum flavum. Five trials were collected, but only three of these trials were used to calculate the force models. Trial 1 was discarded because the needle went through cartilage, not ligamentum flavum. Trial 3 was discarded because the forces were significantly lower than for the other 3 trials, indicating that again ligamentum flavum was not punctured.

The collected force curves represent puncture directly into the ligamentum flavum, and do not contain the shear force caused by friction on the needle from previous layers. A correction factor of 6.0 N was added to correct for this lack of shear force. This constant was based on the qualitative knowledge that the ligamentum flavum is significantly tougher than the skin, and the measured puncture force for the two was roughly equivalent (skin = 6.0372, ligamentum flavum = 6.1330). Further biomaterials testing, such as in-vivo needle puncture measurements during the procedure, will be necessary to create accurate ligamentum flavum force models. These ligamentum flavum (LF) models were calculated to be:

> *LF pre-puncture:* $F(X) = (-0.0085 + 1.5029 (X - X_{LF}) - 0.0583 (X - X_{LF})^2) + 6.0$
> for $F(X) <= LF$ puncture force, $X < X_p$
> *LF puncture force:* $F(X) = 12.1330; X_p = X$
> *LF post-puncture:* $F(X) = (6.1330 - 3.4693 (X - X_p) - 0.7177 (X - X_p)^2) + 6.0$
> for $X > X_p$
> X = Needle penetration depth (mm)
> X_{LF} LF surface location (mm)
> X_p = LF puncture depth (mm)

The force-feedback model for the epidural space and subdural tissue was created from data collected from the second swine study. These curves were broken into three pieces. The epidural space ad subdural tissue layers correspond to the steady-state level reached before the trial ended or bone was encountered. These two tissues were grouped together because there was no apparent change in the force curve when the dura was punctured. This indicated the dural puncture was too small of a force change to be picked up by the machine. From discussions with anesthesiologists, this correlates with what is actually felt during epidural needle insertion as they usually cannot feel a distinct dural puncture. The epidural space and subdural tissue constant was calculated to be:

> *Epidural Space and Subdural Tissue puncture force:* $F(X) = 2.437$ N

The force-feedback model for the bone was created from data collected in the first swine study. The bone curve was a distinct curve found in most of the data sets from the MTS trials, and appears as a large increase in force followed by halting the data collection trial since the MTS machine was set to stop if the puncture force exceeded 20 N. The bone models were calculated to be:

> *Bone strike force:* $F(X) = (8.0265 + 2.210(X - X_b) + 1.4814(X - X_b)^2) - 4.053$
> for, $X < X_{max}$
> X = Needle penetration Depth (mm)
> X_b = Bone surface depth (mm)

An MRI scan was performed on an average-sized female and the width of each type of tissue encountered if a needle was inserted on the midline at the second lumbar vertebrae was measured. Figure 2 shows the calculated needle puncture force curve for this needle insertion. The graph illustrates the skin curve (13.5mm to 27mm), followed by a small amount of fat (27mm to 27.1mm). Note that this does not indicate the fat layer is only 0.1 mm thick because the needle is puncturing fat on the down slope of the skin curve. A slight muscle puncture curve is shown (27.1 mm to 29 mm) but the interspinous ligament is hit before the muscle reaches its steady state value (29 mm to 47mm). Next is the LF puncture (47 mm to 54.4 mm) and a drop to the epidural space and dura puncture before hitting bone at 63mm.

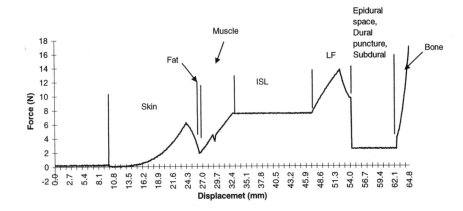

Figure 2: Force curve developed from the force models and an MRI image from
an average female. Each layer of the force curve is identified.

4. Model Limitations

The force model developed is a result of curve fitting to measured data. As such, it
is inherently dependent on a specific layering of tissues, and to a specific needle gauge and
tip-type. The layering of tissues affects the pre-puncture curves, as they are in part due to
the compression of the underlying tissues. The needle gauge and tip-type affect the
puncture force. More data must be collected in order to evaluate which properties of these
curves are intrinsic to the tissues and which are dependent on other factors. The developed
model is for the epidural procedure, using an 18-gauge Tuohy needle. Future research
goals are to develop force models that can be generalized to other needle insertion
procedures and other needles.

A limitation inherent to using the MTS system for measuring the forces was that
there was no interactive control of the needle during the data collection process. The
specimen was placed below the needle to allow for needle insertion into a pre-specified
location, and then the needle was inserted to a pre-specified depth. This limited the choice
of specimens to cadavers.

It is common practice to use swine models in biomaterials research as analogues to
humans; however, dead pigs are not equivalent to live humans so there are limitations to
the resultant force models. One such limitation is that swine skin is tougher than human
skin. The average puncture force for human skin was found to be 6.0 ± 0.7 N, whereas for
the swine skin this force was 12.9 ± 2.6 N.

Although all biomechanical testing was performed within 26 hours of sacrifice on
unembalmed animal cadavers, there are physical changes that occur with death such as
rigor mortis, and the pooling of liquids at the base of the cadaver due to gravity. No
attempt was made to quantify what effects these changes may have on the puncture force.

5. Conclusion

The force-feedback model developed through this series of biomaterials testing
studies is a first approximation of the forces involved in the epidural needle insertion
procedure. The limitation of the force-feedback models is that they have been pieced
together from data collected from tissue samples and porcine cadavers. However, these
models do provide a foundation for force models for the epidural procedure.

The current focus of my research is to develop an instrumented sterile needle that could be used to measure forces during needle insertion procedure on live patients. Data collected *in vivo* from live human trials will provide the most accurate force curves possible, and allow for more exact modeling of the needle insertion procedure. This data will be used to refine the models, and to generalize the models across a larger range of procedures and for a range of needle types.

Future research also includes incorporating these models into a thoracic epidural simulator, and doing user testing to evaluate the realism of the models and the effects of the simulation on user training.

Bibliography

[1]   L. Hiemenz Holton, Development of a Haptic Feedback Model for Computer Simulation of the Epidural Anesthesia Needle Insertion Procedure, Doctoral Dissertation, The Ohio State University, 2000.

[2]   L. Hiemenz, D. Stredney, P. Schmalbrock, Development of the Force Feedback Model for an Epidural Needle Insertion Simulator, In: JD Westwood, et al, eds, Medicine Meets Virtual Reality, IOS Press and Ohmsha, Amsterdam, 1998, 272-277.

Medicine Meets Virtual Reality 2001
J.D. Westwood et al. (Eds.)
IOS Press, 2001

Development of an Experimental Paradigm In Which to Examine Human Learning Using Two Computer-Based Formats

Helene M. Hoffman[1] Ph.D., Henri G. Colt[2] M.D., and Ariel Haas[1]

<hhoffman@ucsd.edu>, <hcolt@ucsd.edu>

University of California at San Diego (UCSD), School of Medicine
[1]*Learning Resources Center, 9500 Gilman Drive, La Jolla CA 92093-0661*
[2]*Interventional Pulmonary Services, 9300 Campus Point Drive, La Jolla CA 92037-7372*

Abstract: Computer-based self-instructional programs are frequently promoted as means to augment or replace the traditional anatomy curricula taught in medical schools. These programs may range from static slide shows to fully immersive virtual environments. However, the impact of these learning technologies on knowledge acquisition, and their comparative cost/benefit to education remain unclear. As a consequence, we are embarking on a series of experiments to compare knowledge acquisition and the meaningful use of information among students who are learning anatomy using one of two different computer-based self-instructional formats. These studies will be based on a specially developed learning module on basic lung anatomy; they will utilize a variety of assessment tools to measure factual knowledge, conceptual understanding of spatial-anatomic relationships, and the ability to apply newly acquired knowledge of anatomy to clinical problem-solving scenarios. The primary object of this paper is to describe the design and development of the underlying test module and to outline the two computer-based formats that will be evaluated. The virtual reality (VR) environment, UCSD's Anatomic VisualizeR, provides dynamic access to 3-dimensional polygonal models of the lesson content and supports student-centered exploration and learning. The multimedia environment, Microsoft PowerPoint, provides a structured presentation of the lesson content and illustrates important anatomic structures through the use of 2-dimensional images derived by screen captures of models available in the VR learning module. This paper also provides an overview of the first experiment in the series, a pilot study using first-year medical students without previous participation in a medical school anatomy curriculum. For this study, students will be prospectively randomized into two groups, each group learning the lung anatomy lesson using one of the computer-based formats described. Immediate knowledge retention will be measured by asking students to complete the assessment instrument immediately after completing their learning module. The results of the pilot study will be used to refine and improve the design of the remainder of studies planned in this experimental series.

1. Introduction

Human anatomy is found at the very core of all medical knowledge, yet it is extremely challenging to teach and learn. Traditionally, anatomy is taught through a combination of textbooks, lectures, and laboratory dissections. While still considered the "gold standard" against which alternatives are judged, the above practices in anatomy education do not fully support students' need to develop the necessary conceptual understanding of spatial-anatomic relationships and to apply anatomic knowledge to clinical problem-solving scenarios [1]. These pedagogical challenges are further complicated by reduced hours available to anatomy education [2-3] and a growing need to find alternatives for cadaver and animal specimens resulting from scarcity, costs, and environmental concerns [1,4].

Computer-based self-instructional programs are frequently promoted as means to augment or replace the traditional anatomy curriculum. The most commonly used are multimedia programs which range from static slide shows to interactive dissection manuals [5-6]. Virtual reality (VR)-based environments, increasingly advocated as a means to practice surgical and procedural skills, have not yet gained widespread acceptance with anatomy educators. This reluctance to embrace the newer simulation-based applications may be due to: (1) reservations about embracing new technology without scientific proof that it improves learning and retention; (2) fear that students will avoid traditional classroom and didactic teaching methods in favor of computer-based learning; and (3) costs. Each of these valid concerns must be addressed before technology-based resources are considered for implementation in today's educational context.

As a consequence, we are embarking on a series of studies to compare the efficacy and efficiency of new and conventional computer-based learning formats. The initial study, which will commence shortly at UCSD, will compare knowledge acquisition and the meaningful use of information among medical students who are learning an anatomy lesson using one of two different computer-based self-instructional modalities: multimedia (Microsoft PowerPoint [7]) or VR (UCSD's Anatomic VisualizeR [8-11]). The multimedia application, a 2-dimensional (2D) learning module with pre-selected idealized views of anatomic structures; and the VR application, a 3-dimensional (3D) learning module with student-selected visualization options; will provide equivalent lesson content, but will differ in their level of interactivity. In this manuscript we will describe the content and process of lesson building and the overall experimental strategy that will be employed in this pilot study.

2. Methods

2.1 Building a basic lung anatomy learning module

The topic selected for this experimental series was basic lung anatomy. One challenge has been to plan a test lesson that maintains a level of complexity consistent with an introductory medical school anatomy curriculum, yet can be completed by students in less than one hour. Moreover, the planned lesson also had to be fully self-instructional and deliverable via both the multimedia and VR formats.

The learning module that has been designed provides focused information pertaining to the thoracic cage, lungs, pleura and fissures, tracheobronchial tree, mediastinum, and pulmonary vessels. The anatomic models that form the core of the lesson materials have been derived from the National Library of Medicine's Visible Human database [12] or developed at UCSD [11]. Digital still and video images (labeled chest radiographs, computed tomography scans, photographs of gross anatomy, gough sections from the UCSD Department of Pathology's Liebow collection, drawings, and images obtained during endoscopic procedures such as flexible or rigid bronchoscopy and thoracoscopy) have also been included in the lesson plan. These resources are intended to provide a clinical context for the lesson as well as to enhance the learning process by introducing anatomic structures from a variety of clinically relevant viewpoints. The limited use of text in the lesson design (e.g., action phrases and directed questions with short-answer feedback) is intended to stimulate student exploration and to promote learning through self-discovery.

2.2 Implementing the learning module in Anatomic VisualizeR

The lung anatomy lesson plan is currently being realized in VR using Anatomic VisualizeR's Lesson Editor [11]. The virtual Study Guide is being used to organize the lesson into the primary topics, displayed to the user as tabbed sections. Depending on the learning objectives, one or more pages are being created under each tab with varying lesson content loaded, placed, or removed. The Study Guide is also being used to deliver the short action phrases and questions as well as to provide selectable links for feedback and additional information. All 3D polygonal models and 2D adjunctive materials have been prepared by methods described previously [11] and incorporated into the VisualizeR database. An example of the VR implementation is shown in Figure 1.

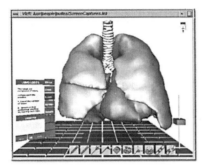 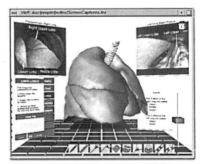

Figure 1: The learning module as implemented in Anatomic VisualizeR. These images represent one scene from the lung module, captured at different times in the exercise. The image on the left is the initial scene presented to the student upon entering into the Lung section of the lesson. Students are able to directly interact with the 3D models, use tools to link/unlink structures, dynamically create cross-sectional views, change opacity and view interior structures. The image on the right demonstrates the additional resources (an explanatory text file and clinical images) requested by the student during the exploratory exercise.

2.3 Implementing the learning module in PowerPoint

The lung anatomy lesson plan is also now being realized using Microsoft PowerPoint, with display and navigation options designed to provide intuitive access to the instructional elements. An index page is being used to organize the lesson topics and to provide a cognitive framework for students using this computer-based format. The anatomic images found in the multimedia lesson have been created by screen captures of 3D models in the virtual environment. Because of the static nature of the PowerPoint format, active manipulation of these images is not possible. Consequently, significant effort has been made to capture the perspective that best illustrates a learning objective or to provide multiple views. The supporting 2D imagery (diagrams, clinical photographs, etc.) and the descriptive text (with only slight modification of the short action phrases) are identical in both lessons. The implementation of the multimedia-based lesson is shown in Figure 2.

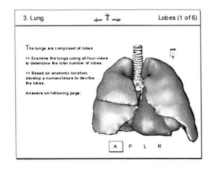 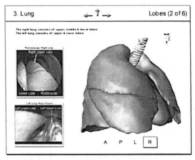

Figure 2: The learning module as implemented in Microsoft PowerPoint. These images are sequential screens from the multimedia version of the lung anatomy learning module. The image on the left is the first screen of the Lung section and the image on the right shows the additional resources (explanatory text and clinical images) in the following screen of this lesson.

2.4 Experimental Protocol Overview

This pilot study will use first-year medical students, who because of UCSD curriculum [13] will not take the Human Anatomy course until the beginning of their second year. All volunteers will be accepted into the study, but a minimum of twenty students will be required before the protocol is initiated.

The study will begin with a one-hour orientation session during which the students will be introduced to the two computer-based formats, have an opportunity for hands-on training on an unrelated learning module, and complete a demographic questionnaire. At the conclusion of the orientation, the students will be prospectively randomized into two groups: one assigned to use the multimedia environment (PowerPoint), the other to the VR environment (Anatomic VisualizeR). Each group will then be given 60 minutes to complete their lesson. Immediately thereafter, students will take an identical written examination and complete a short follow-up questionnaire.

2.5 Developing the Assessment Tool

The assessments to be used in the educational studies will be comprehensive and keyed to several levels of cognitive performance and standardized sets of learning goals. The written examination has been designed to test factual knowledge, conceptual understanding of spatial-anatomic relationships, and the ability to apply newly acquired knowledge of lung anatomy to clinical problem-solving scenarios. The questionnaires will be used to measure the perceived quality of the educational experience as well as various demographic and attitudinal dimensions. As a consequence, the impact of learning environment (multimedia vs. VR) and learner demographics on student achievement and attitude will be evaluated.

3 Discussion

Establishing the experimental paradigm for these studies has been challenging. The obstacles encountered in the development of the learning module and its implementation in two computer-based formats cannot be trivialized. Considerable effort has been expended in obtaining the underlying 3D and 2D materials. Creation of high-quality polygonal models of the thoracic region has been a major undertaking, but has produced outstanding results. Equally daunting has been the efforts to acquire, retouch, annotate, label, and catalog large quantities of multimedia resources. Authoring the learning module, the largest self-instruction anatomy module ever developed by this group, has also been a challenge. Much consideration has been given to text presentation because the words used are intended to be an important catalyst in the learning process, yet cannot be a dominant feature of either presentation format. Developing the syntax for short action phrases and questions, and establishing uniform criteria for their placement within the lesson framework, have been among the most arduous of these activities. The VR implementation has required the design of virtual scenes that compel students to actively explore the 3D models, to ask and answer their own questions, yet contain sufficient structure to ensure that the underlying learning objectives are realized. The multimedia implementation has been equally difficult since it required the use of PowerPoint and other multimedia tools to create a completely new program with high-quality interface and interaction options and access to the requisite instructional elements. While the VR and multimedia implementations of the test lesson have not yet been fully realized, this has already been an important learning experience for the development team and has produced lesson authoring guidelines and multimedia standards that will serve as the foundation for subsequent efforts.

The educational experiences afforded by VR are frequently touted as being superior to those of other computer-based learning modalities. Virtual environments, such as Anatomic VisualizeR are predicated on the notion of student exploration, discovery, and active self-learning. Using Anatomic VisualizeR, students are able to disassemble and reconstruct spatial anatomic relationships while participating actively in the virtual learning environment. These design features are certainly consistent with currently accepted best practices in education [14-16]. Moreover, it can be argued that the cognitive processes evoked in a virtual learning environment are similar to those employed when people acquire knowledge from authentic real-life experiences, and are therefore potentially superior. One might further argue that the direct physical links between the learner's actions and effects within the simulation (e.g., interacting with 3D models, using tools to link/unlink structures, dynamically creating cross-sectional views, changing opacity to view interior structures, etc.) enable a greater understanding of complex spatial relationships [17]. However, this positive view of virtual learning and 3D visualization is not universally accepted and one recent account has suggested that students remember objects as limited 2D views, making 3D representation extraneous and burdensome [18]. Clearly, further investigation into the efficiency and effectiveness of learning anatomy with multimedia and VR formats is required. Only by systematically comparing the efficacy of VR and multimedia formats, will we hope to elucidate the appropriate roles for virtual and conventional representations in anatomy education.

References

[1] **Rosse** C., *The Potential of Computerized Representations of Anatomy in the Training of Health Care Providers.* Academic Medicine 70 (6): 499-505, **1995**.

[2] **Yeager** V., *Learning Gross Anatomy: Dissection and Prosection.* Clinical Anatomy 9(1): 57-9, **1996**.

[3] **Hubbell** D., Byers P., McKeown P., *Clinical Anatomy Instruction in the Operating Room.* Clinical Anatomy 9 (6): 405-7, **1996**.

[4] **Jones** D., *Reassessing the Importance of Dissection: A Critique and Elaboration.* Clinical Anatomy 10:123-127, **1997**.

[5] **Carmichael** S.W., Pawlina W., *Animated PowerPoint as a Tool to Teach Anatomy.* Anatomical Record 261(2): 83-8, **2000**.

[6] **Chen** M.Y., Boehme J.M., Schwarz D.L., Liebkemann W.D., Bartholmai B.J., Wolfman N.T., *Radiographic anatomy. Multimedia Interactive Instructional Software on CD-ROM.* American Journal of Roentgenology 173(5): 1181-4, **1999**.

[7] **Microsoft PowerPoint** (http://www.microsoft.com/office/powerpoint/default.htm).

[8] **Hoffman** H., Murray M., Irwin A.E., McCracken T., *Developing a Virtual Reality Multimedia System for Anatomy Training.* Studies in Health Technology Informatics 29:204-10, **1996**.

[9] **Hoffman** H.M., Irwin A.E., Prayaga R., Danks M., Murray, M., *Virtual Anatomy from the Visible Man: Creating Tools for Medical Education.* In: Visible Human Project Conference Proceedings, NLM, Office of High Performance Computing and Communications, **1996**.

[10] **Hoffman** H.M., Murray M., Danks M., Prayaga R., Irwin A.E., Vu, D., *A Flexible and Extensible Object-Oriented 3D Architecture: an Application in the Development of Virtual Anatomy Lessons.* Studies in Health Technology Informatics. (39): 461-466, **1997**.

[11] **Hoffman** H., Murray M., *Anatomic VisualizeR: Realizing the Vision of a VR-based learning Environment.* Studies in Health Technology and Informatics, 62:134-40, **1999**.

[12] **Ackerman** M.J., *The Visible Human Project.* Proceedings of the IEEE, 86(3): 504-11, **1998**.

[13] **UCSD SOM Catalog** (http://medschool.ucsd.edu/Catalog/78.html).

[14] **Montgomery** J. R., *Global Trend In Education: Shifting From A Teaching Focus To A Learning Focus.* International Experiential Learning Conference, Nov. 9-12, Washington, DC, **1994**.

[15] **Lake** D. A., *Active Learning: Student Performance And Perceptions Compared With Lecture.* Selected papers from the 11th International Conference on College Teaching and Learning, Jacksonville, FL., 119-124, **2000**.

[16] **Hetzroni** O.E., *Effects of Active versus Passive Computer Instruction on the Learning of Element and Compound Blissymbols.* Augmentative & Alternative Communication. June 16 (2): 95-106, **2000**.

[17] **Salzman** M.C., Dede C., Bowen Loftin R., Chen J., *A Model for Understanding how Virtual Reality Aids Complex Conceptual Learning.* Presence 8(3): 293-316, **1999**.

[18] **Garg** A., Norman G.R., Spero L., Maheshwari P., *Do Virtual Computer Models Hinder Anatomy Learning?* Academic Medicine 74:S87-S89, **1999**.

Acknowledgments

This work was sponsored in part by a grant from the Defense Advanced Research Projects Agency (DAMD 17-94-J-4487) and a contract from the Henry M. Jackson Foundation for the Advancement of Military Medicine (#13225). The authors would also like to acknowledge Alicia Fritchle (3D modeling) and Christina Tsang (technical support) for their important contributions to this endeavor.

Medicine Meets Virtual Reality 2001
J.D. Westwood et al. (Eds.)
IOS Press, 2001

Retraining Movement in Patients with Acquired Brain Injury using a Virtual Environment

Maureen K. Holden, Ph.D., P.T.[1]; Annegret Dettwiler, Ed.D., P.T.[2]; Thomas Dyar, B.S.[1]; George Niemann, Ph.D.[2] and Emilio Bizzi, M.D.[1]

[1]Department of Brain and Cognitive Sciences, MIT, Bldg. E-25-526b, 45 Carleton Street, Cambridge, MA 02139
[2]Bancroft NeuroHealth, Hopkins Lane, P.O. Box 20, Haddonfield, N.J.

Abstract. We report preliminary results of an ongoing study in which a virtual environment (VE) system is used to facilitate motor relearning of a pouring task in patients with Acquired Brain Injury (ABI). Four subjects were evaluated pre-and post-VE training using virtual-world and real-world tests in which subjects performed a pouring motion while holding a cup. Standard clinical tests of motor and functional ability were also used. Three of four subjects demonstrated improvement in end-point trajectories (cup path) performed during the virtual and real world tests. Clinical test scores also improved. Results indicate that subjects with ABI were able to learn a movement in VE, and generalize this ability to real-world performance of similar and unrelated tasks. VE training appears to be a feasible and promising approach to the rehabilitation of subjects with ABI.

1. Introduction

Acquired brain injury (ABI) is one of the leading causes of death and disability in the United States. Every 15 seconds, someone suffers a head injury and every five minutes a person becomes permanently disabled by ABI. Survivors with severe ABI typically face 5-10 years of intensive health related services with an estimated lifetime cost of $4 million dollars[1-3]. Individuals who survive severe ABI face long-term problems with impaired motor control and cognitive function. The gravity of this problem calls for new ideas and methods in the rehabilitation of these individuals, particularly in the area of motor control.

Recent findings in the field of neuroscience, from animal studies of motor control, suggest that both the normal adult brain and the damaged brain are capable of much greater plastic change than was previously thought possible. In addition, the nature of physical rehabilitation following injury has been found to be an important variable in the type and extent of plastic changes that occur during the recovery process [4-8].

One new method that may allow us to develop this untapped potential for motor recovery in patients with brain damage is the use of computer generated virtual environments (VE) for training. By VE we mean an interactive computer technology that is capable of creating the illusion of being in an artificial world in which one can move around, and examine or manipulate objects. In VE, the visual aspects of the computer-generated environment can be presented via a head-mounted display or on a conventional desktop monitor. In the latter case, the user feels as if he is looking through a window at the virtual environment [9-10].

Several reports describing the potential usefulness of VE in ABI rehabilitation [9-12]. However, to our knowledge, no studies which examine the effects of VR training on motor rehabilitation in actual individuals with ABI have been published. Several reports of

VE use in the rehabilitation of individuals with other types (i.e., not ABI) of disabilities have appeared. For example, Wilson et al. reported successful learning of a spatial task (directional pointing to object location in a 3-level building) in physically disabled children as compared to untrained normal controls, following VE training [13]. Holden et al. reported improved reaching ability in stroke patients following a course of training using VE [14]. Burdea and colleagues have reported on the use of VE for orthopaedic rehabilitation [15]. In normal subjects, several reports of motor learning following virtual practice have been reported [16-18], but transfer of motor learning in VE to real world performance has not always been found [19].

In this paper, we report preliminary results from an ongoing clinical study in which we use a novel motor-training system based upon augmented feedback in a virtual environment (VE) to facilitate motor relearning in patients with acquired brain injury (ABI). The purpose of our study is to assess the feasibility of VE training with the ABI population, to test whether motor learning can be achieved in VE, and to assess whether motor skills acquired in VE can generalize to similar real world tasks, or to untrained tasks.

2. Method

2.1 Design

A single-subject AABABAA design was used. Subjects received an evaluation battery 2x, 1-2 wk. apart prior to treatment (AA), followed by 16 one-hr. treatment sessions, (frequency 3x/week) (B), a mid-way evaluation (A), then a second block of 16 treatments (B), followed by 2 post treatment evaluations (AA).

2.2 Subjects

Four male subjects w/ chronic ABI have been tested and trained thus far. Duration post-injury ranged from 3 yr. to 18 yr.; ages from 16 yr. to 37yr. Three subjects had much greater impairment on the right (R); one on the left (L).

2.3 Apparatus

The VE training system consists of a computer, specially developed software [20], and an electromagnetic motion-tracking device. A central feature of the system is the simultaneous display on the computer screen of the prerecorded arm movements of a "teacher" and the arm movements of the patient using the motion tracking device. During training, the patient is asked to imitate the teacher's trajectory, as it is displayed ("learning by imitation"). The difference between the teacher's trajectory and that of the patient's provides the augmented feedback. This feedback can be enhanced in a variety of ways by optional features. For example, distance and orientation error can be highlighted, the teacher speed can vary, sound cues can be added to enhance timing, a static trace of the teacher trajectory can be used to enhance spatial learning.

2.4 Treatment

Subjects were trained in VE on the functional task of pouring from a cup through practice in virtual scenes. A desktop display was used. In each scene, a 'teacher' was displayed performing the pouring movement. During practice, subjects' held a real cup in their hand, and tried to imitate the teacher by watching their 'virtual' cup as it moved on the computer screen in concert with their movement. For subjects 1 and 2, only two pour' scenes were used for training; for subjects 3 and 4, some additional scenes were added. These scenes worked on the control of wrist motion and repeated reciprocal movements of the elbow. Only the near center workspace location was trained in VE.

2.5 Measures

Four tests were used to evaluate motor performance: 1) a "Virtual" motor test; here the subject performed the trained movement in VE (pouring from one virtual cup to another), but without teacher feedback; 2) a "Real World" test, in which the subject performed the same task as that trained in VE, but in the real world. In our case, the subject poured real oatmeal from one cup to another. This was performed at the trained location (center-near), and at five other workspace locations. During both virtual and real world tests, 3D kinematics of the arm were recorded using a motion tracker. Finally, two standard Clinical Tests were used: 3) the Fugl-Meyer Test of Motor Recovery (FM) [21]; and 4) the Emory test of Upper Extremity (UE) Function (timed tasks)[22].

The 'Virtual' motor test was administered at regular intervals during VE training sessions; the 'Real World' (RW) and Clinical Tests were administered before and after each 16 session treatment block.

3. Results

Subject 1 (S1) had 32 sessions with no midway testing. Subject 2 (S2) dropped out following the first 16-session treatment block. Subjects 3 (S3) and 4 (S4) completed the two 16 session blocks for a total of 32 sessions. We now present the results of our VE training in three sections: Virtual performance, Real World performance, and the Clinical Tests (FM and Emory).

3.1 Virtual Pouring Performance

Qualitative analysis of the end point trajectories (cup path) during virtual 'pouring' indicated an improvement following training. Trajectories performed in VE become straighter, especially during the first 3/4 of the movement. An example is shown in Figure 1 below.

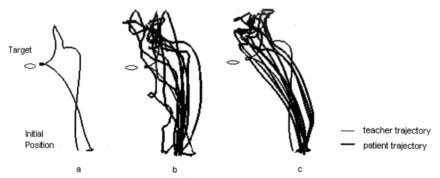

Figure 1. Raw data graphs of endpoint trajectories for S4 during 5 repeated level 1 pouring motions of 1st block of 16 training sessions. Circles represent the location of the container towards which subject was performing the pouring motion. a) teacher trajectory; b) teacher trajectory with five superimposed end-point trajectories of pre-training session, involved upper extremity; c) teacher trajectory with five superimposed end-point trajectories of post-training session, involved upper extremity.

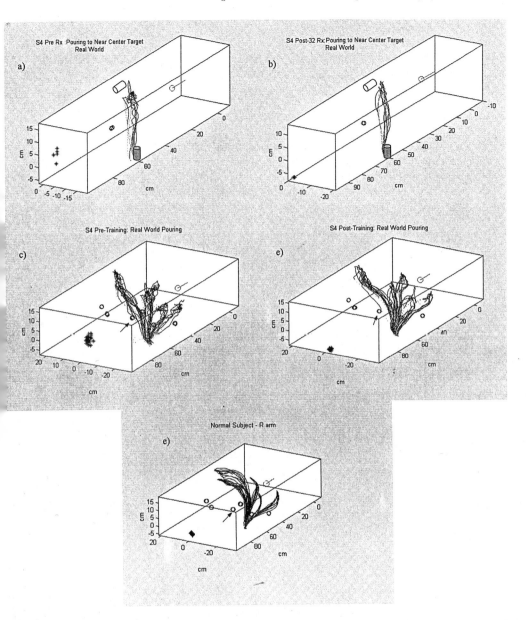

Figure 2. Trajectories (cup path) for S4 while performing the pouring task in the real world. Perspective is as if one were looking downward over the subject's right shoulder. For top 2 panels, dark gray cup shows starting position of held cup (hand by the side); white cup shows its end position for the trained location (near-center). The red circles indicate the target cup positions; arrow indicates trained location. Crosses near front indicate trunk position; red sphere in back shows transmitter location; a) pouring to midline center with right arm Pre-Training and b) Post-Training; c) pouring to 6 workspace locations (5 were untrained) Pre-Training and d) Post-Training; e) normal subject performing same task for comparison.

3.2 Real World Pouring Performance

Three of the 4 subjects (S2, S3 and S4) showed qualitative improvement in their trajectories when performing the pouring movement in the real world near the same location trained in the VE (i.e. to midline center, 8 cm. from table edge). The trajectories were smoother, straighter and more accurate. Of the three subjects who improved, S4 showed the most change. While improvement was greatest near the trained location, improvement was also noted for pouring performed in the five workspace locations that were not trained in VE (i.e., 20 cm to right and left of near center targets; 30 cm to either side of the far target; far target was 20 cm. from table edge). For S3 and S4, these changes were fairly large. For S2, they were slight; S1 showed no change. Figure 2 illustrates the changes in real world pouring performance for S4. Data from a normal subject, performing the same tasks, is shown for comparison. Quantitative analysis of these data are currently underway.

In addition to the trajectory changes, we noted that all subjects displayed fewer spills during real world pouring following VE training. (Oatmeal was substituted for liquid during pouring because of the proximity to electronic equipment.)

3.3 Clinical Tests

Results for the upper extremity portion of the FM test of motor recovery are shown below in Figure 3. Total FM includes the pain, range of motion, sensory and motor subscores; Motor FM is motor subscore only. The test assesses active movement control, quality of movement, intralimb joint coordination and reflex function.

S1 and S2 showed less than 5 % improvement (essentially no change) on the FM. S3 showed little change after the first treatment block, but improved by 21% on his Motor score and by 11% on his Total FM score following the second block. S4 improved the most, by 40% Motor, 17% Total in block 1, and by an additional 14% Motor, 5% Total after treatment block 2.

Results for the Emory UE Functional test are shown in Figure 4. The test measures the time required by subjects to perform fifteen different functional tasks. S1 had slightly slower median times following treatment. S2 improved the most, by 48%. S3 worsened slightly in block 1, but improved by 36% in the 2nd half of training. S4 had little change in the first block of treatments, but improved by 34% following the second block. S4 also improved his total time Emory score by 50% across the two blocks.

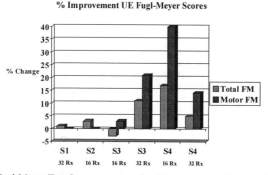

Figure 3. Fugl-Meyer Test Scores, expressed as % improvement from pre to post VE training. Note that S1 had the 32 Rx as one block, S2 had only block 1 of 16 sessions. S3 and S4 had both treatment blocks and results are shown seperately for each block.

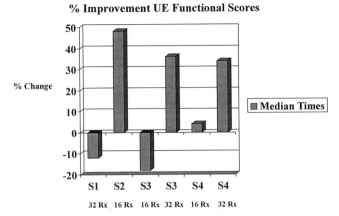

Figure 4. Emory Test Scores, expressed as % improvement from pre to post VE training. Note that S1 had the 32 treatments as one block, S2 had only block 1 of 16 sessions. S3 and S4 had both treatment blocks and results are shown separately for each block.

4. Discussion

We found improvement for 3 of the 4 subjects trained in VE for all of our measures: motor performance of the trained task in the virtual world, motor performance in the real world for similar and related tasks, and for standard clinical tests of UE motor recovery and function. Since all our subjects sustained their brain injuries between 3-18 yr. prior to the study, it seems reasonable to attribute the improvements we found to the VE treatment, as the expected time for spontaneous recovery had passed.

The changes in performance in VE (Fig. 1) indicate that subjects with ABI, despite significant impairments and time post injury, *can* learn motor tasks in VE. Even more encouraging is the transfer of this improved performance to the same task in the real world. All three of our subjects who 'learned' in the virtual world achieved this transfer. Two subjects also improved their trajectories for real world pouring performance in parts of the workspace which were not trained in VE, i.e., forward and to the right and left of the trained location (Fig.2). If these findings are confirmed in additional subjects, and by quantitative analysis, it would imply that therapists could achieve improvements in many related functional movements by training just one type of movement. Our most intriguing finding is the improvement on the standard clinical tests. These results indicate a greater degree of motor generalization, as tasks tested on these clinical measures were very different from our training task, in terms of limb configuration, workspace location, and muscle activation patterns required. Given that we trained only the pouring movement and its components, this degree of generalization is very surprising.

The greatest changes were seen in S3 and S4. Several factors may have influenced this result. For these subjects, we added some additional scenes to the training. These scenes were designed to address the specific deficits of each subject in performing the pour movement. For S3, this was reciprocal movement at the elbow; for S4 it was control of wrist extension while maintaining a grip. These elements were practiced however, in the same general workspace as the pour movement, and in combination with similar movements at the other UE joints. Differences in other clinical factors may have accounted for the greater success of these subjects, e.g. initial Emory scores were lowest (better) for S3 and S4. However, S1 and S3 had the highest pre-training FM scores. We are currently investigating whether cognitive and perceptual impairments account for the differences in effectivness of the VE treatment in our subjects.

5. Conclusions

VE motor training appears to be feasible for use with ABI subjects. We believe this new method holds promise for improved neurorehabilitation outcomes in patients with ABI.

References

[1]   JF. Kraus, Epidemiology of Head Injury. In: RR. Cooper (ed.), Head Injury. William and Wilkins Co, Baltimore, 1987, pp.1-19.
[2]   BR. Selecki et al., Trauma to the Central and Peripheral Nervous Systems: An Overview of Mortality, Morbidity, and Costs, NSW 1977, Aust NZ J Surg 52 (1982) 93-102.
[3]   ZL. Fulop et al., Pharmacology of Traumatic Brain Injury: Experimental models and clinical implications, Neurology Report 22 (3) (1998) 100-109.
[4]   RJ. Nudo et al., Use dependent Alterations of Movement Representation in Primary Motor Cortex of Adult Squirrel Monkeys, J Neuroscience 16 (2) (1996) 785-807.
[5]   RJ. Nudo et al., Neural Substrates for the Effects of Rehabilitative Training on Motor Recovery after Ischemic Infarct, Science 272 (1996) 1791-1794.
[6]   RJ. Nudo et al., Reorganization of Movement Representation in Primary Motor Cortex following Focal Ischemic Infarcts in Adult Squirrel Monkeys, J Neurophysiol 75 (1996) 2144-2149.
[7]   RJ. Nudo, Role of Cortical Plasticity in Motor Recovery after Stroke, Neurology Report 22 (2) (1998) 61-67.
[8]   JM. Held, Environmental Enrichment Enhances Sparing and Recovery of Function Following Brain Damage, Neurology Report 22(2) (1998) 74-78.
[9]   PN. Wilson et al., Virtual Reality, Disability and Rehabilitation, Disability and Rehabilitation 19(6) (1997) 213-220.
[10] FD. Rose et al., Virtual Reality, an Assistive Technology in Neurological Rehabilitation, Curr Opin in Neurol 9 (1996) 461-467.
[11] FD. Rose, Virtual Reality in Brain Damage Rehabilitation, Med Sci Res 22 (2) (1994) 82.
[12] T. Kuhlen, Virtual Reality for Physically Disabled People, Comp in Biol and Med 25(2) (1995) 205-211.
[13] PN. Wilson et al., Transfer of Spatial Information from a Virutal to a Real Environment in Physically Disabled Children, Disabil and Rehabil 18 (12) (1996) 633-637.
[14] M. Holden et al., Virtual Environment Training Improves Motor Performance in two Patients with Stroke, Neurology Report 23(2) (1999) 57-67.
[15] G. Burdea et al., Virtual Reality-Based Orthopedic Telerehabilitation. IEEE Trans Rehabil Eng, 8(3) (2000) 430-432.
[16] E. Todorov et al., Augmented Feedback Presented in a Virtual Environment Accelerates Learning of a Difficult Motor Task, J Motor Behav 29 (1997) 147-158.
[17] DR. Lampton et al., The Virutal Environment Performance Assessment Battery (VEPAB): Development and Evaluation., Presence 3 (1994) 145-157.
[18] JW Regian et al., Virtual Reality: An Instructional Medium for Visual Spatial Tasks, J Communication 42 (1992) 136-149.
[19] JJ Kozak JJ et al., Transfer of Training from Virtual Reality, Ergonomics 36 (1993) 777-784.
[20] E. Bizzi et al., System for Human Trajectory Learning in Virtual Environments, MIT Patent No. 5,554,033. (Spet.1996).
[21] AR. Fugl-Meyer et al., the Post-Stroke Hemiplegic Patient: A method for evaluation of physical performance, Scandinavian Journal of Rehabilitation Medicine 7 (1975) 13-31.
[22] SL.Wolf et al., Comparison of Motor Copy and Targeted Biofeedback Training Techniques for Restitution of Upper Extremity Function among Patients with Neurologic Disorders, Physical Therapy 69 (1989a) 719-735.

Medicine Meets Virtual Reality 2001
J.D. Westwood et al. (Eds.)
IOS Press, 2001

3D Localization of Implanted Radioactive Sources in the Prostate Using Trans-Urethral Ultrasound

David R. Holmes III(a), Brian J. Davis(b), Richard A. Robb(a)

(a) *Biomedical Imaging Resource, Mayo Clinic and Foundation, Rochester, MN*
(b) *Division of Radiation Oncology, Mayo Clinic and Foundation, Rochester, MN*

Abstract: Prostate cancer is the most common cancer diagnosed in men in the United States. Many techniques have been developed to diagnose and treat prostate cancer. 3D Trans-Urethral Ultrasound (TUUS) is a new technique for the diagnosis and treatment of prostate disease. This research focuses on the potential of TUUS for therapy-guidance during and after transperineal interstitial permanent prostate brachytherapy (TIPPB). Computed tomography (CT) is currently used to determine the source locations and the effective radiation dose distribution throughout the tissue after the completion of the procedure. TUUS may be a viable alternative to CT for determining source locations within the prostate. Placement of the TUUS catheter into the urethra provides excellent 2D images of the prostate. In addition, the catheter can be used to acquire 3D volumetric data for 3D analysis of the prostate, associated tissue, and radioactive sources.

Initial work on source localization was conducted on an ultrasound-equivalent prostate phantom. Cylindrical dummy radiation sources with diameter of .8 mm and length of 4.5 mm were placed into the prostate phantom for assessment with TUUS. The TUUS imaging device is a 10fr catheter with a linear array of ultrasonic crystals at one end. The ultrasound catheter operates at 10MHz and is controlled by the Acuson Sequoia ultrasound workstation. The catheter was placed in the phantom urethra and 3D scans were acquired. A corresponding CT was acquired for comparative purposes. Segmentation of the prostate capsule was done semi-automatically. Dummy radiation seed segmentation was conducted manually. Additional processing was necessary to account for image artifact and correctly reconstruct the seeds.

The prostate shell and radioactive source reconstructions provide an excellent 3D representation. Comparison to the CT data suggests that the TUUS data provided: 1) greater resolution and 2) better soft tissue differentiation. The reconstructed sources were measured and corresponded to the physical dimensions of those placed in the phantoms. The method is now being evaluated on cadavers and patients.

1. Introduction

Study of methods for diagnosis and treatment of prostate cancer is motivated by the near 200,000 new cases and 40,000 deaths resulting from this disease. Currently, trans-rectal ultrasound (TRUS) is often used to confirm diagnosis of the disease. In particular, TRUS is used during prostate biopsies to determine cancer foci[1]. TRUS is also used as a therapy-planning tool. Prior to surgery and/or radiation treatment, TRUS images are collected to build a model of the prostate. Recent work with trans-urethral ultrasound (TUUS) devices has suggested that this new technology may be a viable alternative to TRUS for diagnosis and treatment guidance[8,9]. Previous reports of this technology focused on TUUS as a potential diagnostic tool[7,8]. This work addresses TUUS as a therapy guidance tool during and after transperineal interstitial permanent prostate brachytherapy(TIPPB).

TIPPB therapy has become an increasingly popular alternative to prostatectomy[11] due to the less invasive nature of the procedure. During a typical TIPPB procedure, 100 or more radioactive sources (referred to as seeds) are placed into and around the prostate using needles inserted through the perineum. The goal of this procedure is to provide adequate radiation dose to the prostate to slow or stop the growth of cancerous tissue. In order to provide uniform dose coverage and minimize radiation exposure to the surrounding tissues, the procedure is planned pre-operatively with acquired TRUS data. During the procedure, the seeds are placed into the prostate tissue according to the prescription. Both TRUS and x-ray fluoroscopy are used to guide the placement of the seeds. X-ray fluoroscopy can effectively image the seeds, but poorly distinguishes the prostate tissue[4,5]. TRUS, on the other hand, adequately images the prostate tissue, but cannot effectively image the individual seeds. For these reasons, post-operative CT scans are used to determine the seed locations and calculate the actual dose delivery. This work explores TUUS as an intra-operative tool for assessing seed locations and dose distributions.

TUUS provides real-time, high resolution images of the prostate. Because of the central location of the urethra, the TUUS devices can use higher frequency than TRUS, since there is less tissue to traverse to the prostate borders. The higher frequency device produces higher resolution and better quality images. These devices provide other useful imaging tools such as PW Doppler imaging for looking at the blood flow into and out of the prostate. The potential benefits to using TUUS in TIPPB procedures are two fold: 1) higher resolution provides excellent tissue differentiation, and 2) image radiation seeds may be imaged better by avoiding image shadowing. As a result, TUUS may overcome some of the problems with TRUS and x-ray fluoroscopy imaging. In addition, due to the compact size of the device and real-time operation, the device can be rolled into the procedure room for actual intra-operative assessment of seed location and dose distribution.

Potential use of this device in the procedure room requires adequate study under controlled conditions. In particular, prostate phantoms can provide a robust experimental environment for the assessment of the TUUS imaging device. Our hypothesis is that TUUS will provide excellent tissue differentiation in phantoms, including differentiation of dummy radiation seeds both in two and three dimensions which can be used for the calculation of dose distribution.

2. Methods

The study consisted of the examination of a prostate phantom with a specially designed US catheter imaging device[2,10]. The imaging device is a 10 French catheter with a 3.5-10.0 MHz vector phased array transducer located at the tip of the catheter. This device is controlled with the Acuson Sequoia workstation and can provide many different acquisition modes, including Doppler imaging. The device scans along a longitudinal plane and can be rotated to acquire 3D datasets.

The prostate phantom, designed by Computerized Imaging Reference Systems, is commonly used as a practice tool for placing seeds using TRUS and provides tissue-equivalent ultrasound images. Dummy radiation seeds measuring 4.5 mm in length and 800 microns in diameter were placed in the phantom by a clinician in the Dept. of Radiation Oncology prior to the TUUS exam. The dummy seeds were also designed to mimic the actual seeds in CT and US.

A CT scan was acquired as the gold standard for comparison to the TUUS data. The resolution of the scan was .35mm x .35mm x 3mm which is consistent with clinical acquisitions. The dummy seeds were segmented using simple thresholding with some post-processing to refine the data. Because of the large slice thickness, many of the seeds appeared to run together in the data and required further processing. In addition, the boundaries of the prostate were segmented manually for volumetric calculations. Visualizations of the CT data can be seen in Figure 1.

The TUUS exam consisted of 2D exploration of the prostate as well as several 3D acquisitions. The in-plane resolution of the TUUS images is .1mm x .1mm. This permitted accurate segmentation of the prostate tissue and the seminal vesicles. 2D images of the phantom can be seen in Figure 2. Also, due to the high resolution of the images, measurements of the dummy seeds were precise and accurate.

3D datasets consisted of rotating the imaging catheter 360 degrees while acquiring equi-spaced images. The resulting datasets prior to reconstruction contained 576x456x300 voxels. Torodial reconstruction reformats the original data(Xo, Yo, Yo) into Cartesian coordinates(X, Y, Z). An illustration of torodial reconstruction can be seen in Figure 3. The resulting volume of data has a slice thickness is .1mm. The in-plane resolution is radially dependent according to the following equation $l = 2 \cdot r \cdot \tan(\theta/2)$. For this particular data $\theta = 1.2°$, which suggests that the lowest in-plane resolution is $l = 0.02 \cdot r$. The focal distance of the transducer was set to 25mm with a maximum depth of 45mm which suggests a lower bound resolution of $l = 0.5mm$ and $l = 2.25mm$, respectively. In actuality, most of the data has an in-plane resolution of .1mm x .1mm which is therefore used as the grid spacing.

Segmentation of the prostate tissue and seeds was conducted on the original data before reconstruction. Segmentation of the prostate was a three-step process. The first step required manual delineation the prostate border in 6-8 representative slices. These manual segmentations were used as control points for a directed graph search algorithm[6] to segment the entire dataset. The final step was also manual editing for regions where the graph search failed to segment the prostate border. Automatic segmentation of the seeds proved difficult due to image speckle and other artifacts. However, manual segmentation of the seeds was successful.

Reconstruction of the segmented prostate was straightforward (See Figure 4), however, reconstruction of the seeds in 3D was a challenge due to the poor out-of-plane resolution of the imaging catheter. As expected, the out-of-plane resolution deteriorates with distance from the imaging device. The result of this artifact is that each seed is reconstructed as a "patch" in Cartesian space. The "patch," although correct in length and thickness, is incorrect in width. For this reason, each segmented seed requires segmentation with an auto-correction feature. As each seed is reconstructed, the seed is assessed for artifact based on the distance away from the transducer and the dimensions of the incorrectly reconstructed seed. The error in measurement is symmetrically removed from the seed during reconstruction to provide an accurate image of the seed. An example of the incorrect and correct reconstructed seed can be seen in Figure 5.

Dose distribution calculations were conducted on both the 2D data and 3D data. The actual dose is dependent on the radioisotope chosen, however, the distribution is effectively $1/r^2$. This can be calculated based on the seed locations. A chamfer distance algorithm[3] was applied to rapidly compute the distance from each seed. The resulting distance image was scaled, squared and inverted to provide the dose information. For presentation purposes, dose rings were labeled at magnitudes of 10 and superimposed onto the data. Examples in 2D are illustrated in Figure 6. 3D dose maps are illustrated in Figure 7.

3. Results

The CT images proved to be useful only as a qualitative tool. Because of the thick sections of the data, the seeds were not easily segmented for comparison. In addition, the poor tissue differentiation made it difficult to segment the prostate tissue from the rest of the phantom. Due to inconsistent segmentation of the prostate tissue, the volume measurements from the CT were not acceptable to use.

The 2D TUUS examination of the prostate phantom clearly showed the different regions of the phantom including the prostate, seminal vesicles, and phantom floor. In addition, the 2D images clearly differentiated the dummy radiation seeds. The measurements taken on the seeds give an average size of .5mm in diameter and 4.3mm in length. This is close to the actual size of the seeds which are .8mm in diameter and 4.5mm in diameter. Discrepancies could be attributed to partial volume effects, different imaging parameters at the ends of the seeds, and/or off-axis seeds. The process of calculating dose distribution in 2D is rapid, however, the chamfer distance measure appears to provide a "blocky" result.

The segmentation of the data before 3D reconstruction was particularly effective due to the high resolution of the data and excellent tissue differentiation. The three-step process for segmenting the prostate shell was rapid (<5 minutes per volume), but still requires additional study. The segmentation of the seeds was relatively slow due to the image artifacts resulting from the seeds themselves and other energy scatterers.

Reconstruction was rapid and automated with minimal loss in resolution. Additional processing was necessary on the seeds because of the poor out-of-plane resolution. The auto-correction of the seeds during reconstruction was effective and provided accurate representations of the seeds and phantom. Calculation of 3D dose distribution was similar to 2D dose calculations. The 3D algorithm suffers somewhat from the "blocky" nature of the distance algorithm. Visualizations of the 3D images confirmed that TUUS could be used for dose calculations and presentation of the dose maps.

4. Discussion

Preliminary results using TUUS demonstrate several benefits over CT for post-operative procedure assessment. These benefits include higher resolution and better tissue differentiation. It has yet to be determined if TUUS can distinguish and segment all of the seeds placed in a patient's prostate. In addition to the imaging benefits, TUUS also has the advantage over CT in that it is inexpensive and mobile. Thus, one institution may purchase one machine and move it from procedure to procedure. The compact size of the device allows acquisition in the TIIBP procedure room.

TUUS is a high resolution "practical" imaging technology that can be applied to many different medical scenarios. Previous work has suggested that TUUS can be useful in diagnosis. This work suggests that TUUS may be useful in therapy-guidance. The disadvantages of TUUS are limitations of the device, rather than the imaging techniques. New catheters under development may overcome some of these limitations therefore making TUUS an even more powerful tool in the hands of the clinician.

Future work will include refinement of the imaging parameters to provide better images. Improvements in the image processing will provide more rapid and accurate results. Segmentation algorithms are still manual/semi-manual, and advances need to be made in the automated segmentation of the data. In-depth examination of the dose calculation technique may prove useful. Finally, this imaging techniquewill be implemented and evaluated on in a true clinical setting.

5. Acknowledgements

The author would like to acknowledge Dr. Charles Bruce of the Department of Cardiology, Mayo Clinic, for being an important collaborator on this work. His expertise with the ultrasound catheter and system is invaluable. The author would also like to acknowledge the help of the BIR staff and students for providing support and software tools used in this. In addition, the authors would like to thank Wayne LaJoie for providing the data to be processed.

6. References

1) Aarnink RG et al., Trans-rectal ultrasound of the prostate: innovations and future applications. J Urol, 159(5):1568-79, 1998.

2) Bruce CJ et al. Feasibility study: transesophageal echocardiography with a 10F, multifrequency (5.5- to 10-MHz) ultrasound catheter in a small rabbit model. Journal of the American Society of Echocardiography, 12(7):596-600, 1999.

3) Borgefors, G. "Distance Transformations in Arbitrary Dimensions." Comput. Vision, Graphics, Image Processing, 27:321 - 345, 1984.

4) Grado GL, Larson TR, Balch CS, Grado MM, Collins JM, Kriegshauser JS, Swanson GP, et al. Actuarial disease-free survival after prostate cancer brachytherapy using interactive techniques with biplane ultrasound and fluoroscopic guidance. Int J Rad Onco Bio Phys, 42:289-98, 1998.

5) Holm HH. The history of interstitial brachytherapy of prostate cancer, 13(6):431-437, 1997.

6) Holmes DR and Robb RA. Processing, segmentation, and visualization of pre- and post-stent coronary arteries using IVUS. Proc. SPIE, 3335: 72-82, 1998.

7) Holmes DR and Robb RA. Trans-Urethral Ultrasound (TUUS) Imaging for Visualization and Analysis of the Prostate and Associated Tissues, Proc. Medicine Meets Virtual Reality, 70: 126-132,2000.

8) Holmes DR and Robb RA. Novel Imaging Methods for Visualization and Analysis of the Prostate and Associated Tissues, Proc. SPIE, 3976: 22-27, 2000.

9) Holmes DR and Robb RA. 3-D Trans-ureathral Ultrasound: A New View of the Prostate Gland. Computer Aided Radiology and Surgery 2000.

10) Seward JB et al., Ultrasound cardioscopy: embarking on a new journey. Mayo Clinic Proceedings, 71(7):629-35, 1996.

11) Prestidge BR. Radioisotopic implantation for carcinoma of the prostate: does it work better than it used to? Sem Rand Onc, 8:124-131, 1998.

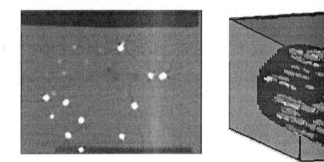

Figure 1 – The picture on the left shows a 2D slice of the CT data. Although the seeds are apparent, the prostate tissue is difficult to differentiate. The picture on the right is a 3D volume rendering of the data. It is evident that the thick slices degrade the image quality.

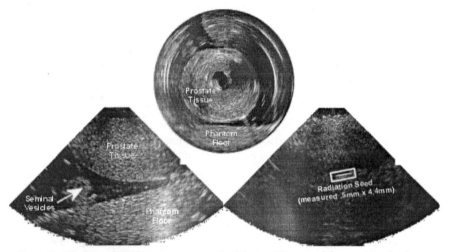

Figure 2 – The above TUUS images were acquired during 2D scans of the prostate phantom. The picture on the right shows excellent differentiation between tissues. The middle picture also shows differentiation in the fully reconstructed data. The picture on the right highlights the ability to image radiation seeds. The measurements taken on this image show that the seed measures .5mm in diameter and 4.4mm in length. The actual dimensions are .8mm in diameter and 4.5mm in length.

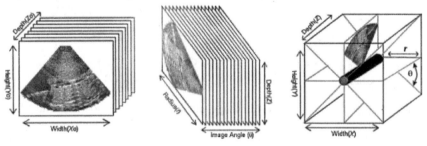

Figure 3 – Torodial reconstruction begins with a stacked set of images in acquisition coordinates (Xo,Yo,Zo) [Left picture]. After reformatting the data[Middle picture], the data is in radial coordinates with the actual slices (θ,r,Z). By applying a radial transformation to each slice, the data is reformatted into standard Cartesian coordinates (X,Y,Z)[Right picture].

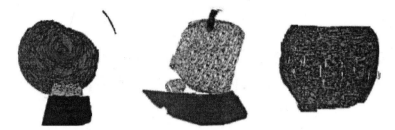

Figure 4 – Visualizations of the reconstructed prostate from TUUS data. The image on the left show excellent detail of the prostate, seminal vesicles, phantom floor, and includes one incorrectly reconstructed seed. The middle image provides similar information. The image on the right shows the prostate with correctly reconstructed seeds located within the boundaries of the prostate.

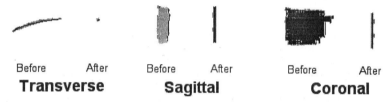

Before   After   Before   After   Before   After
Transverse   **Sagittal**   **Coronal**

Figure 5 – Above are orthogonal volume renderings of seeds before and after auto-correction resulting from out-of-plane resolution of the imaging device. Before correction, the seeds appear as patches. After correction, they have the appearance of the actual seeds. It is also noted that the measured size of the seeds corresponds well with the corrected seeds.

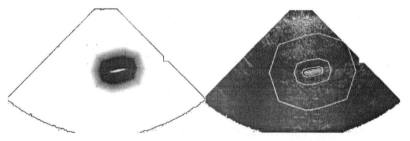

Figure 6 – Reconstructed seeds are used in the calculation of dose distribution. The effective fall off of radiation is $1/r^2$ and is calculated efficiently with a chamfer distance algorithm. The image on the left shows one of the seeds and the dose distribution. The image on the right illustrates superimposed dose rings onto the original data.

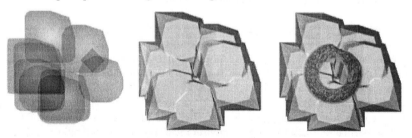

Figure 7 – 3D dose maps can be calculated with the reconstructed seeds. On the left, a slice through the dose map. In the middle, a 3D rendering of the dose map. On the right, the dose map and prostate boundary superimposed.

206

Medicine Meets Virtual Reality 2001
J.D. Westwood et al. (Eds.)
IOS Press, 2001

Intraoperative Visualization of Surgical Planning Data Using Video Projectors

*Harald Hoppe, *Sascha Däuber, *Jörg Raczkowsky,
*Heinz Wörn, and **José Luis Moctezuma
*University of Karlsruhe (TH), Institute for Process Control and Robotics,
Kaiserstraße 12, 76128 Karlsruhe, Germany
**Stryker Leibinger GmbH & Co KG, Freiburg, Germany

Abstract. The Institute for Process Control and Robotics has developed a new system using projector based augmented reality for the intraoperative visualization of preoperatively defined surgical planning data. Projector based augmented reality in medical applications represents a new field of research and gives an alternative solution to the commonly used Head Mounted Display technology. Moreover, the projector is not only used for visualization, but also for registration of the patient without the usage of invasive fiducial techniques as e.g. screw markers or frames. Recent results showed an achieved accuracy of ±1.5 mm which roughly meets clinical demands.

1. Introduction

In recent years, different methods for the intraoperative visualization of preoperatively defined surgical planning data have become a field of considerable interest [1]. Normally, preprocessed diagnostic image data from CT or MRI serve as basis for the planning task. The intraoperative usage of surgical planning data mostly traces back to one of the following methods:

- The surgeon manually transfers the planning data to the area of interest by surveying the monitor screen and memorizing unequivocal anatomical landmarks.
- The surgeon is guided and supported by a navigation system overlaying the current pointer position with corresponding data on the computer screen.
- A robot performs parts of the surgical intervention.

The latter two methods often require the use of artificial markers which are fixed to the patient's bones before acquiring the diagnostic image data and remain there for intra-operative registration of the patient's position. Furthermore, the surgeon is constrained to persistently reorient his view from the patient to the monitor and vice versa, which influences the surgeon's general practice.

Great efforts are being made to directly visualize the surgical planning data in the operation area. Most commonly used devices are Head Mounted Displays (HMDs) which superimpose virtual objects to the real environment. But in consideration of precision,

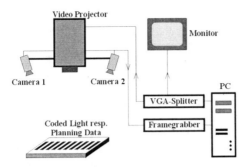

Fig. 1 Schematic system configuration

resolution, display refresh rate, and sterility, HMDs still show great disadvantages and often lead to queasiness of the wearer. However, directly visualizing the results of a preparatory surgical planning in the area of interest entails significant advantages.

The Institute for Process Control and Robotics (IPR) has developed a new system which allows to directly visualize the surgical planning data on the patient's surfaces (skin, bone, tissue) by using an off the shelf video projector [2]. The latter is both used for visualization and registration of the patient which will be explained in the subsequent section.

2. System description

The presented system (see Fig. 1) consists of an off-the-shelf video projector, two CCD-cameras and a state-of-the-art PC (800 MHz CPU, 256 MByte RAM) and assumes the availability of an appropriate operation planning system to define trajectories, boreholes, osteotomy lines or other relevant features. It is assumed that regions of interest are preoperatively generated by analyzing and segmenting appropriate images from CT or MRI. In addition to defining the actual surgical plan it is necessary to generate a so-called distance tomogram, which stores the shortest distances of all voxels to the surface (skin) of the area of interest by assigning the corresponding value to the voxels (appropriate tools were developed at the IPR). The distance tomogram intraoperatively serves to register the patient which will be explained further below.

The essential part of the developed system is formed by a 3D surface scanner which is used to intraoperatively generate a 3D point cloud of the patient's surface. This is accomplished by projecting a sequence of stripe patterns (coded light) on top of the region of interest with the aid of the integrated video projector. The corresponding images are acquired by the cameras, analyzed in consideration of emerging Moiré-patterns and yield a 3D point cloud of the scanned area [3]. After removing inevitable outliers, the resulting point cloud can be matched to the preoperatively segmented surface of the diagnostic image data (CT, MRI) on which the surgical plan was defined.

At this stage, most known matching algorithms require user interaction in order to find an adequate starting position for the matching process. Since matching algorithms commonly work by optimizing an appropriate failure function, this step ensures that the global (and not only the nearest local) optimum is found. In order to realize a system that needs no helping hands from outside, we developed a new matching algorithm which imitates the human strategy for the matching process of two corresponding surfaces. The global optimum of the failure function which is computed with the aid of the described distance tomogram is found by reducing the dimensionality of the search space from commonly six parameters (rotation and translation) to three. Only those transformations are considered which move around the point cloud on top of the CT or MRI surface. After an adequate starting position is found, the fine tuning is realized by using an arbitrary matching algorithm (e. g. [4], [5]).

The matching process provides an initial transformation T_{ini} from the coordinate system of the diagnostic image data to the initial position of the patient. Since intraoperative conditions impede continuous scanning and in order to avoid attaching rigid fixations to the patient, succeeding registrations are performed by tracking markers stuck to the area of interest. These are tracked and registered by analyzing corresponding images from the integrated cameras using Hough-transformations [6]. This step yields a second transformation $T_{cur}(t)$ mapping the patient's initial to his current position.

The global transformation $T_{global}(t) = T_{cur}(t)T_{ini}$ now allows to continuously transfer the surgical planning data to the patient's coordinate system thus taking into account the actual position. The corresponding two-dimensional projector-bitmap which is projected onto the three-dimensional patient's surface is edited in order to avoid or minimize distortion in areas of steep and bended surfaces. Maintaining lengths and angles, however, requires a triangulated surface (e.g. Delaunay-Triangulation) in order to predict and correct deformations by using normal vectors and other features.

3. Results and discussion

The described method enables the surgeon to visualize planning data on top of any preoperatively segmented and triangulated surface (skin, bone, etc.) with direct line of sight during the operation. Furthermore, the tracking system allows dynamic adjustment of the data to the patient's current position and therefore eliminates the need for rigid fixation with stereotactic frames or similar devices. The system is particularly attractive due to the fact that both the video projector and the cameras are multiply used (registration/ visualization and registration/tracking respectively). While systems using HMDs generally require expensive navigation systems, the cost of the presented system is much lower than that of a corresponding system based on HMDs. Furthermore, it is currently superior to any HMD with regard to accuracy and resolution. Assuming the area of interest to be 200 x 250 mm, the planning data can be visualized using a resolution of 0.33 mm or less (SVGA or higher). Thereby, the currently achieved accuracy of the projected surgical planning data is about 1.5 mm (which nearly meets clinical demands) and will be further improved.

Moreover, neither the surgeon is obliged to wear encumbering devices on his head, nor the patient is affected by unpleasant, additionally burdening screw markers or similar devices.

References

[1]　S. Tang, C. Kwoh, M. Teo, N. W. Sing, and K. Ling, "Augmented Reality Systems for Medical Applications", IEEE Engineering in Medicine and Biology (May/June 1998), pp. 49-58, 1998.
[2]　C. Loullingen, "Lagebestimmung mit Hilfe eines 3D-Oberflächenscanners", Master Thesis IPR, University of Karlsruhe, 1998.
[3]　H. Gärtner, "Quantitative 3D-Vermessung mit codierter Beleuchtung", Institut für Technische Optik, Universität Stuttgart, 1998.
[4]　K. S. Arun, T. S. Huang, and S. D. Blostein, "Least-Squares Fitting of Two 3-D Point Sets", IEEE Transactions on PAMI, vol. 9, no. 5, pp. 698-700, 1987.
[5]　J. M. Fitzpatrick, J. B. West, and C. R. Maurer, "Predicting Error in Rigid-Body Point.-Based Registration", IEEE Transactions On MI, vol. 17, no. 5, pp. 694-702, 1998.
[6]　C. F. Olson, "Constrained Hough Transforms for Curve Detection", Computer Vision and Image Understanding, vol. 73, no. 3, pp. 329-345, 1999.

Medicine Meets Virtual Reality 2001
J.D. Westwood et al. (Eds.)
IOS Press, 2001

The development of the virtual reality system for the treatment of the fears of public speaking

Hang Joon Jo, J. H. Ku, D. P. Jang, M. B. Shin, H. B. Ahn, J. M. Lee, B. H. Cho, Sun I. Kim

Department of Biomedical Engineering, College of Medicine, Hanyang University, Seoul, Korea

Abstract. The fear of public speaking is a kind of social phobias. The patients having the fear of public speaking show some symptoms like shame and timidity in the daily personal relationship. They are afraid that the other person would be puzzled, feel insulted, and they also fear that they should be underestimated for their mistakes. For the treatment of the fear of public speaking, the cognitive-behavioral therapy has been generally used. The cognitive-behavioral therapy is the method that makes the patients gradually experience some situations inducing the fears and overcome those at last. Recently, the virtual reality technology has been introduced as an alternative method for providing phobic situations. In this study, we developed the public speaking simulator and the virtual environments for the treatment of the fear of public speaking. The head-mounted display, the head-tracker and the 3 dimensional sound system were used for the immersive virtual environment. The imagery of the virtual environment consists of a seminar room and 8 virtual audiences. The patient will speak in front of these virtual audiences and the therapist can control motions, facial expressions, sounds, and voices of each virtual audience.

1. Introduction

The fear of public speaking is a kind of social phobias. The patients having the fear of public speaking show some symptoms like shame and timidity in the daily personal relationship. They are afraid that the other person would be puzzled, feel insulted, and they also fear that they should be underestimated for their mistakes[1]. For the treatment of the fear of public speaking, the cognitive-behavioral therapy has been generally used. The cognitive-behavioral therapy is the method that makes the patients gradually experience some situations inducing the fears and overcome those at last. Recently, the virtual reality technology has been introduced as an alternative method for providing phobic situations[2][3][4]. In this study, we developed the public speaking simulator and the virtual environments for the treatment of the fear of public speaking.

2. Method

System

This public speaking simulator was based on a *Pentium III* class PC. A head-mounted display (*Proview XL50*) was used for covering user's visual fields in, and a head-tracker (*Polhemus Fastrak*) was attached to the HMD for more immersive experience. Moreover, this system is equipped with a 3-dimemsional sound system for generating realistic voices and sounds.

Virtual Environment

The main program of this simulator was developed in *Visual C++ 6.0* and *DirectX 7.0a SDK*. 3-dimensional modeling tools (*3D Studio MAX* and *Rhinoceros*) is used for making virtual objects and audiences. In the virtual environment, the eight virtual audiences are sitting down on the chairs in the seminar room.

Virtual Audience

The virtual audience has some motions, facial expressions, and voices. The virtual audiences perform a certain action continuously for themselves. Moreover, the therapist can control the motions, facial expressions, sounds, and voices of each virtual audience. The connection between two motions is naturally continuous, because each virtual audience starts motions from the specific position and ends to the same. The detail motions and facial expressions of virtual audiences are presented in Table 1.

Detail Motion	Facial Expression
Chatting	Speaking
Hands clapping	Smile
Folding arms	Making a wry face
Yawning	Laugh
Looking around	Grumbling
Getting out of the room	Blinking

Table 1. Animations of virtual audiences

3. Results

Figure 1 shows the virtual environment that the eight virtual audiences are sitting down on the chairs. Figure 2 shows examples of the virtual audience's motions. (a), (b), (c) and (d) of Figure 2 successively shows the motions and facial expressions in the meaning of protesting, chatting, clapping and getting out of the room.

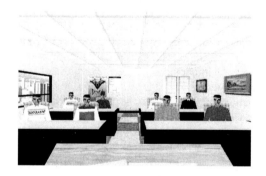

Figure 1. The virtual environment

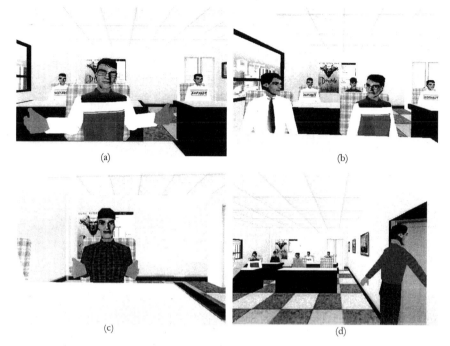

(a)

(b)

(c)

(d)

Figure 2. Variable motions of the virtual audiences

(a) Protesting (b) Chatting (c) Clapping (d) Getting out of the room

Acknowledgments

The National Research Laboratory (NRL) Program at Korea Institute of Science & Technology Evaluation and Planning funded this study.

4. References

[1] M. M Antony, "*Assessment and Treatment of Social Phobia*", Can J Psychiatry, Vol.42, pp.826-834, October 1997

[2] M. North, S. M. North, and J. R. Coble, "*Virtual Reality Therapy: An Effective Treatment for Psychological Disorders*", Virtual Reality in Neuro-Psycho-Physiology IOS Press, 1997

[3] D. Strickland, L. Hodges, M. North, S. Weghorst, "*Overcoming Phobias by Virtual Exposure*", Comm.ACM, Vol.40, No.8, pp.34-39, 1997

[4] R. W Bloom, "*Psychiatric Therapeutic Applications of Virtual Reality Technology (VRT): Research Prospectus and Phenomenological Critique*", Medicine Meets Virtual Reality IOS Press, 1997

Medicine Meets Virtual Reality 2001
J.D. Westwood et al. (Eds.)
IOS Press, 2001

Web-based Surgical Educational Tools

Nigel W. John[1], Mark Riding[1], Nicholas I. Phillips[2], Sean Mackay[3], Leif Steineke[4], Bernard Fontaine[4], Gerhard Reitmayr[5], Vojko Valenčič[6], Nikolaj Zimic[6], Ad Emmen[7], Elena Manolakaki[8], Diamantis Theodoros[9]

[1]*Manchester Visualization Centre, University of Manchester, UK*
[2]*Department of Neurosurgery, Leeds General Infirmary, UK*
[3]*Imperial College School of Medicine at St Mary's, UK*
[4]*SAS, Belgium*
[5]*uma Holding GmbH, Austria*
[6]*Faculty of Electrical Engineering, University of Ljubljana, Slovenia*
[7]*Genias Benelux b.v., The Netherlands*
[8]*IDEC, Greece*
[9]*University Hospital, Athens, Greece*

Abstract. This paper describes work being undertaken as part of the WebSET (Web-based Standard Educational Tools) project. The project is producing a standardised suite of interactive three-dimensional educational tools, delivered across the WWW. The major focus will be the use of open technology and standards, and the production of learning components that can be used as building blocks for further development in a wide range of application areas. Two learning disciplines have been selected for the development of the WebSET tools: surgical training, and physiological education. A high quality consortium from across Europe has been assembled with complementary skills in the technologies needed by the project. The project is partly funded by the European Commission.

1. Background

The rapid decline in the cost of computer-based and communications technologies during the last decade have enabled attractive alternatives to the conventional lecture method of providing instruction. Cost savings can be demonstrated if the teacher-pupil ratio is increased. By moving the training environment to the World Wide Web (WWW) this criterion can be easily met, and over the last decade, many academic institutions and other organisations have embraced the Internet as a way to enhance face-to-face instruction and to deliver distance learning.

Today surgical training has little changed from the apprenticeship model. This is a situation that can certainly be improved and surgical training too can benefit from the Internet revolution, particularly as multimedia and 3D tools become more common. The authors have already presented web-based simulators for procedures such as Ventricular Catheterisation [1][2]. WebSET (Web-based Standard Education Tools) is a project that has subsequently been part funded by the European Commission to build and extend on this work and deliver an integrated suite of surgical training tools based on open Web standards.

WebSET aims to provide quality training on surgical procedures. The fidelity is not as high as the real operation or as complete as totally immersive virtual reality, however, the fidelity is more than adequate to learn and practice procedures and, most importantly, will not be costly to implement and use. Lessons learned by surgeons during training and in performing the procedure will be provided to the learner and others.

An equally important goal is to disseminate the WebSET ideas to more general educational fields such as physiology teaching in schools.

2. Methods & Tools

2.1 User Requirements Analysis

The WebSET consortium includes key surgical end user groups from several European countries. During the first phase of the project, a detailed User Requirements Analysis was carried out using their input. They identified appropriate applications for the simulators, determined target groups, and outlined the validation process to be applied to the simulators. The major requirements identified were:

- Develop web-deliverable virtual environment training tools. Existing prototype tools for Ventricular Catheterisation and Lumbar Puncture procedures are being used as a starting point. The modular design of these applications makes re-use simplistic, and allows additional features to be included with minimal extra effort.
- Include both single and multi-user features to allow collaborative and single end user training. The ability to allow a trainee to be given online tuition and demonstrations of correct procedure is a very important requirement of web-based educational software. The software must facilitate this interaction, and also allow a trainee to practice a procedure alone, when the tutor is not available.
- Include an on-line tutorial for single user training. A trainee should be able to use the software without the tuition of another; therefore there should be adequate instructions and demonstration both of how to use the simulation, and of how to perform a correct procedure.
- Assess and record user progress, to determine when competence is achieved. The software should be able to monitor user progress, and to record results in a database for evaluation at a later date.
- Make the content web-deliverable. All content should be deliverable over the Internet, making best use of existing web technologies. Consideration needs to be given to the time required to download the simulation, for those users without direct connections to the web.
- Use realistic anatomical 3D models. Any 3D models used in the simulations should be anatomically correct.

A series of desirable features was also identified, such as the need to maintain a simple and intuitive user interface, and include support for optional cost effective haptic feedback [3]. Other appropriate training modules were highlighted, for example a training module to simulate skin suturing, and a module to simulate the insufflation procedure prior to laparoscopy.

2.2 Current Implementation

Use of Multimedia on the Web to supplement the traditional media of text and graphics is growing fast. Multimedia content includes video, audio, animation, and 3D technologies. When multimedia is used, client-side response time must be taken into account [4]. For example, users demand a one tenth of a second response time when directly manipulating objects on the screen e.g. to rotate a 3D object. Large multimedia files can also take a very long time to download to the client. The equipment used by the target audience and their likely network bandwidths are therefore very important factors when using multimedia. In the WebSET project, the target audience will be at hospitals and schools. Here a mid range PC with 64 – 128 MB RAM and an average graphics card is the best configuration that can be expected.

Figure 1 illustrates the functional architecture of the WebSET application. Each learner can make use of WebSET alone without interacting with others and without others observing what he is doing. However any other learner or teacher can join and interact in a number of ways, by passively observing or by actively taking part in the learning session. Similarly each learner can leave a learning session and continue learning alone.

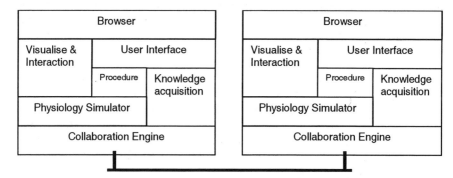

Figure 1: Functional Architecture

The WebSET applications are being implemented using the Extensible Markup Language (XML) [5], which provides a framework for defining document structures independent of the layout. Apart from describing information, XML is also widely used to glue different applications together. How this is being done within WebSET is described in detail in [6]. The resulting document objects are suitable for producing reusable information material. The aim is to provide a procedure-authoring tool that will define and integrate the components shown in Fig.1.

The Virtual Reality Modeling Language (VRML) ISO standard is being utilised to provide visualisation and interaction, and integrated with other learning materials to deliver a comprehensive training package. It is also intended to utilise X3D, the new standard for 3D graphics on the web. X3D has a subset of VRML functionality and features an XML based file format.

A physiology simulator module is being developed using Java software called JaCoB (Java Constructive Objects) [7]. JaCoB is designed to facilitate conceptual learning of natural sciences and can be used to provide physiology within virtual experiments by means of particle constructive objects simulations. This technology is applicable to a wide range of learning disciplines.

From the outset, WebSET is being developed in a multi-user environment so that collaborative training across the WWW is possible. Following an evaluation of the available solutions for multi-user VRML, an open technology based virtual environment system called Deep Matrix [8] has been selected, and is being developed further for this task (see Fig. 2). We are currently using the Deep Matrix Shout3D client. Shout3D is a Java based rendering engine for Shout Interactive's X3D proposal. Shout's proposal defines a subset of VRML97 nodes and a new definition of node fields.

2.3 Knowledge Acquisition

One important requirement from the project is to identify a standard taxonomy for surgical learning and associated meta-data for surgical learning objects. Meta-data covers categories such as the educational and pedagogic features of the resource, and the features that deal with the conditions of use for the resource.

The "Dublin Core Metadata" [9] should therefore being adhered to. This standard is specifically intended to support resource discovery. The IEEE P1484.12 Learning Object Metadata Working Group (LOM) [10] provides a basis for specifying the syntax and semantics of learning objects and we are starting to use this within WebSET. As far as the implementation is concerned, we are following the general trend for XML-based solutions.

2.4 Evaluation

The evaluation of the tools is a key part of WebSET and will be completed in the next phase of the project. Trainee surgeons will have seen but not performed the procedure and before they start performing the procedure they will use the surgical simulation. The aim of the simulation will be to:

- Give an overview of the procedure.
- Teach three-dimensional anatomy.
- Teach the concepts that many seemingly complex surgical procedures are a series of simpler steps, thus allowing trainees to have a fall-back position in surgery should the procedure not go to plan.

The test simulation scenario then proceeds as follows:

(1) The trainee will log onto the web server from his local PC running a web browser with appropriate plug-ins installed.
(2) If a trainer is involved he also logs onto the same server and can view the trainee's progress. He will also be able to contribute by annotation on the trainees' screen. The trainer and the trainee and the web server can be at geographically distant sites.
(3) Having downloaded this small file from the web server into the VRML capable browser, the trainees can begin the simulation, either on their own or with input and assessment from the trainer. Conversely the trainee can use this simulation on his own in what is effectively a tutorial mode.
(4) The trainee will carry out the simulation several times as his action and speed in the simulation is logged.
(5) When the trainee has reached the desired standard he will be assessed as capable by the trainer, progressing to actually performing the operation.

We also need to evaluate, as well as the trainee, the simulation itself and there are trainer aspects and web aspect to this. If the simulation is a good simulation the trainee should get better with practice and the trained surgeon should be for the same exposure to the trainer, better than the trainee at performing the task. Thus the simulation is being designed to differentiate between trainer and trainee. We will assess trainees for their feeling of how this has helped them when they go on to perform the actual operation and compare this to trainees who have not used the simulation.

The web aspects of the simulation largely revolve around the ease of download of the files and accessibility and the speed of inter-active software feedback. WebSET provides test scenarios where medical students, trainees and trained surgeons will carry out the simulations repeatedly and be accurately assessed for speed of response, number of mouse moves, accuracy, decision-making and learning.

3. Results

Several of the WebSET components described above have now been implemented and are providing a useful surgical training tool. Figure 2, for example, shows a snapshot of the Lumbar Puncture simulator being used in a collaborative environment. The instructor and a student are accessing the simulator over the WWW, they can communicate with each other using the "chat" area, and they can monitor each others use of the simulator.

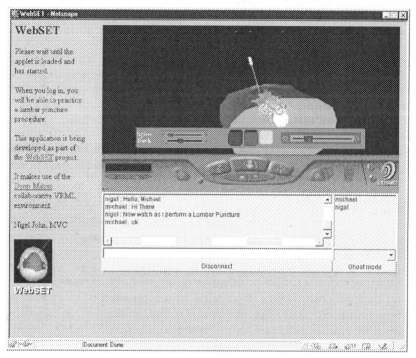

Figure 2: WebSET Collaborative Environment

The progress being made by WebSET is being demonstrated by the results of the evaluation of the initial applications in hospitals. In particular, over the next year the surgical tools will be introduced into the training curriculum of the courses already taught at the WebSET user group sites. These groups have vast experience in the training process and the evaluation of a student's performance. We are using the models of ventricular catheterisation and lumbar puncture as a test bed on which we can decide on what makes a good surgical trainer. With these generic characteristics we can define some principles for the production of future surgical simulators.

4. Conclusions

WebSET is providing quality training on surgical procedures and is intended to complement the apprenticeship model of learning. The fidelity is not as high as the real operation or as complete as totally immersive virtual reality, however, the fidelity is more than adequate to learn and practice procedures and, most importantly, is not costly to implement and use. Furthermore WebSET is allowing training 'anywhere' and 'at anytime' as well as at the convenience of the learner. All that is required is a PC to access the lessons. The training can be performed alone, with no one checking what mistakes the trainee makes or in a group or with a teacher. This freedom to access the training is already a great improvement upon current practice

Although still in its first year of development, the potential of the WebSET approach is clear. Low fidelity training simulators can make a contribution to the education of a trainee surgeon/clinician. By delivering the solutions over the World Wide Web, the accessibility of these tools is excellent. Further these low cost solutions are ideal for most hospitals where only PCs of average capacity will be available for use. We are confident that the final versions of the WebSET tools will prove their worth and be readily accepted by the surgical profession.

References

[1] N.I. Phillips and N.W. John, Web-based Surgical Simulation for Ventricular Catheterisation, Neurosurgery: Official Journal of the Congress of Neurosurgical Surgeons, Vol. 46, No. 4, pp933-937, April 2000.

[2] N.W. John and N.I. Phillips, Surgical Simulators Using the WWW, Medicine Meets Virtual Reality 2000, Newport Beach, California, January 2000.

[3] M. Riding and N. W. John, Force-feedback in Web-based Surgical Simulators, Medicine Meets Virtual Reality 2001, Newport Beach, California, January 2001.

[4] J. Nielsen, Designing Web Usability, New Riders Publishing, ISBN 1-56205-810-X

[5] http://www.w3.org/TR/REC-xml

[6] A. Emmen, N.W. John, and L. Versweyveld, WebSET: Integrated XML and VR components for collaborative medical training, MEDNET 2000, Brussels, November 2000

[7] V. Valencic, Electricity and Magnetism by Virtual Experiment, Zalozba FER and FRI, Ljubljana, 1999

[8] http://www.geometrek.com; http://www.deepmatrix.com

[9] Dublin Core Metadata Initiative, http://purl.org/DC/

[10] IEEE P1484.2 Learner Model Working Group http://ltsc.ieee.org/wg2/

Acknowledgements

The work described in this paper was performed as part of the WebSET project (Web-based Standard Educational Tools), which is part funded under contract IST-1999-10632 of the European Community. The project is a collaboration between University of Manchester, SAS NV, uma Holdings GmbH, University of Ljubljana, Leeds General Infirmary, Imperial College School of Medicine at St. Mary's, Slovenian Ministry of Education and Sport, Industrial Development Education Centre, and Medical School of University of Athens.

Medicine Meets Virtual Reality 2001
J.D. Westwood et al. (Eds.)
IOS Press, 2001

An Integrated Simulator for Surgery of the Petrous Bone

Nigel W. John[1], Neil Thacker[1], Maja Pokric[1], Alan Jackson[1], Gianluigi Zanetti[2], Enrico Gobbetti[2], Andrea Giachetti[2], Robert J.Stone[3], Joao Campos[4], Ad Emmen[5], Armin Schwerdtner[6], Emanuele Neri[7], Stefano Sellari Franceschini[7], Frederic Rubio[8]

[1]University of Manchester, UK
[2]CRS4, Italy
[3]MUSE Virtual Presence Ltd, UK
[4]UCL Institute of Laryngology and Otology, UK
[5]Genias Benelux b.v., The Netherlands
[6]University of Dresden, Germany
[7]University of Pisa, Italy
[8]CS-SI, France

Abstract. This paper describes work being undertaken as part of the IERAPSI (Integrated Environment for the Rehearsal and Panning of Surgical Intervention) project. The project is focussing on surgery for the petrous bone, and brings together a consortium of European clinicians and technology providers working in this field. The paper presents the results of a comprehensive user task analysis that has been carried out in the first phase of the IERAPSI project, and details the current status of development of a pre operative planning environment and a physically-based surgical simulator.

1. Background

Today, planning of surgical procedures makes poor use of imaging data. In most cases surgeons simply study medical images from MRI, CT, etc. prior to surgery and construct a mental 3D model of anatomy in each individual case. Previous knowledge of normal anatomy is essential. Furthermore the ability to rehearse the surgical procedure using patient specific data is extremely rare. The IERAPSI (Integrated Environment for the Rehearsal And Planning of Surgical Intervention) project is addressing these shortcomings for surgery of the petrous bone - a common surgical site with complex anatomy. A range of surgical procedures with escalating levels of complexity is being covered: Mastoidectomy; Cochlea electrode implantation; Acoustic Neuroma resection. Solutions for both surgical planning and surgical simulation are being implemented.

IERAPSI brings together a consortium of European clinicians and technology providers to create this integrated simulator for surgery of the petrous bone. The project is being partly funded by the European Commission.

2. Methods & Tools

2.1 User Task Analysis

The project began with a detailed user task analysis of surgeons carrying out the procedures being targeted. The task analysis [1] followed the ISO 13407 standard [2], and focused on activities that ensure involvement of users, and a clear understanding of user and task requirements (including context of use and how users might work with any future system evolving from the project). This initial exercise has provided an input into early system design processes. We are also repeating the analysis periodically to ensure that the recommendations do not produce any unforeseen human performance artefacts or safety-critical consequences.

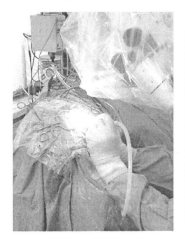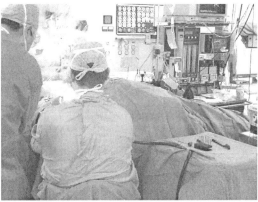

Figure 1: Translabyrinthine Acoustic Neuroma Resection in Progress. Note the use of additional "greens" to support the surgeon's left wrist and the need to clip the drill pneumatic supply pipe to avoid drag

With the support of the staff of the ENT unit, the Department of Otolaryngology, Head & Neck Surgery and the theatre personnel at Manchester's Royal Infirmary and the Institute of Laryngology and Otology, University College London, we were permitted to observe and, where possible, video record surgeon performance and close-in drilling activities (backed by additional important video contributions from the University of Pisa) – see Fig. 1, for example. Initially, five theatre sessions were analysed in detail, each lasting an average of six hours:

- Infantile Cochlea Implant.
- Middle Fossa Acoustic Neuroma.
- Translabyrinthine Acoustic Neuroma.
- Stapedectomy "Follow-Up" and Ossicle Prosthesis *(combined approach)*.

With regard to planning, whilst IERAPSI concentrates on the development of software modules to support the processing of radiological data, the way in which surgeons actually use the data must be considered early and refined by consultation with users as the concepts emerge. Initial human interface proposals resulting from the task analysis describe an off-line (pre-operative) system based around a multi-user real-time 3D display and appropriate interactive controls. Amongst the key anatomical features to be highlighted are the facial nerve (and any other key neuronal features), the jugular bulb and sigmoid sinus, blood vessels of secondary importance, the semi-circular canals and close proximity of brain tissue.

The training environment is designed to simulate those aspects of the surgeon's task that are characterised by special procedures and operative skills. The task analysis highlighted key human interface features, including stereoscopic vs. conventional display, haptic feedback, fidelity and coding techniques for initial bone exposure, drilling/burring effects, use of other virtual instruments and materials, and error/performance recording. Careful consideration must be given to the display-control stereotypes expected by temporal bone surgeons and those delivered by the final training interface. Otherwise, a fixed display (or display frame) moveable image solution might foster negative transfer of training from the virtual to the real.

2.2 System Requirements and Functional Specification

Using the task analysis as input, a detailed system requirements and functional specification has been prepared for the main components of IERAPSI.

The functionality of IERAPSI is being provided by three independent subsystems: pre-operation planning, surgical simulation, and educational and usage demonstrator. These components will be integrated as a single data handling pipe-line through data exchange based on common file formats, introducing and supporting a novel and innovative training strategy based on patient-specific pre operative and simulation environments. Relevant technological state-of-the-art, including hardware/software issues have been considered. IERAPSI is making extensive use of 3D visualization, physics based simulation, and virtual reality technologies, including autostereoscopic visual and bi-manual haptic feedback.

An implementation specification has been produced, which describes the software architecture, the link between the system components, as well as the required hardware configurations. The reference hardware for the pre-operative system will be a single-processor PC Linux/NT platform with the Dresden autosteroscopic display [3] for visual feedback. The surgical simulation system will be designed for being run on a multiprocessing PC Linux platform, using two PHANToMs for haptic feedback and a microscope-like display for visual feedback.

2.3 Pre-Operative Planning

A pre-operative planning module is currently under development containing a suite of image segmentation and visualization tools, and allowing rapid and accurate identification of individual structures based on their imaging characteristics. Techniques to allow the segmentation of the facial nerve are being investigated as part of this task. Different stages addressed involve: an automatic co-registration system to align the specified data sets based on mutual information, data non-uniformity correction [4], multi-spectral classification for data segmentation and optimal boundary representation for visualisation purposes.

The most principled approach to MRI, CT and MRA image segmentation is based on techniques that utilise statistical models. Devised multi-spectral classification system will make probability maps available for bone, blood vessels and soft tissues, which then can be used to segment regions or locate the boundaries between tissues. Availability of multiple images provides more information for separation of ambiguous regions present due to overlapping tissues and requires multivariate distribution model for each pure tissue and partial volume distribution.

The methodology of probabilistic data segmentation involves constructing a likelihood model for each tissue component present in data. A common approach involves modelling only pure tissue distributions, but in order to account for the fact that in a single voxel a mixture of tissues can be present, a partial distribution must also be modelled [5]. Pure tissues have been modelled using Gaussian distributions, P_t, while partial volume distributions for paired tissue combinations take the form of a triangular distribution convolved with a Gaussian, P_{ts}, which is intended to model the response function of the measurement system.

A multi-variate distribution for each pure tissue t is defined as:

$$P_t(g) = \alpha_t e^{-(g-G_t)^T C_t(g-G_t)}$$

where G_t is the mean tissue vector and C_t its covariance and α chosen to give unit normalisation.

Partial volume distributions are modelled along the line between two pure tissue means $G_t G_s$.

$$P_{ts}(g) = \beta_{ts} P_{ts}(h) e^{-(g-h.g/|h|)^T C_h(g-h.g/|h|)}$$

with $h = (g - G_s)C_h(G_t - G_s)/|(G_t - G_s)C_h(G_t - G_s)|$, $C_h = C_t h + C_s(1-h)$.

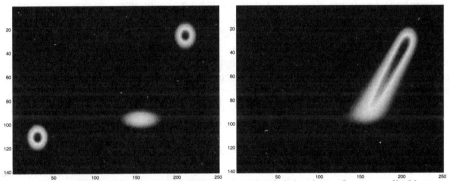

Figure 2: 2D probability density model for 3 pure tissues and their mixture for two medical images

The parameters for the density model must be determined using an optimisation algorithm to minimise the difference between the model and the data. Parameters can be iteratively estimated by taking weighted averages over the selected volume V using a maximum likelihood process generally referred to as Expectation Maximisation [6]. This approach is expected to deal successfully with multiple tissue segmentation from multiple images for boundary representation and data visualisation. Extension of this technique to deal with pathological (unmodelled) tissues can be incorporated by allowing an additional category for infrequently occurring outlier data [7].

2.4 Surgical Simulation

Physical modelling is a computationally expensive approach to virtual reality, but is essential in this specific field of application since it provides the only practical way to accommodate arbitrary positioning in the area affected by the operation of the surgical tools, e.g. drilling, and the use of realistic anatomical models derived from patients CT data. The computational costs due to physical modelling are partially mitigated by the fact that the surgical procedures mentioned above are constrained by a restrictive field of view and limited haptic interaction between the surgeon and the patient, and thus the overall computational cost is compatible with available computer technology.

Research and development for the real-time physically based simulator is at this stage focusing on physically motivated solutions for drilling into the petrous bone. The task analysis has indicated that the most common actions to be simulated are performed by three different manipulators: a burr reducing trabecular bone in fine dust, an irrigator introducing water that is mixed with the bone dust, and a sucker removing bone dust and water. In order to provide a useful training platform, the simulator should not model only the primary effect (bone removal), but should also be capable of replicating the secondary effects caused by the different physical processes (in particular, bone paste creation and obscuring effects). Wiet and colleagues [8] have done some preliminary work toward the simulation of temporal bone dissection, but their approach is purely geometric and limited to the modelling of the bone removal process.

In our simulator, different specific solvers cooperate in determining the time evolution of the model in response to external actions and in computing the feedback to be returned to the user. Our approach, as well as preliminary simulation results, is described in the following sections.

2.4.1 Bone drilling

Bone is hard and has a stress-strain relationship similar to many engineering materials. Hence, as discussed by Fung [9], stress analysis in bone can be made in a way similar to the usual engineering structural analysis. The simulation of the drilling of the petrous bone involves first the detection of collisions of the drill burr with the bone surface, then, depending on the type and location of the contact, a prediction on the amount of bone to be removed and of the forces that should be returned to the hand of the user via the haptic feed-back device. Given the particular nature of the process simulated, the natural way to model the petrous bone anatomy is by using a volumetric approach, with the initial configuration of the model directly derived from patient CT data.

Currently, we model the scene with a set of voxels, and we define each voxel of the scene as "empty", "bone" or "bone dust or water". The bone removal process is modelled with a set of rules that define what happens when the burr intersects the bone. This is simply obtained by cleaning voxels where the distance from the burr centre is less than the burr radius, and filling the first empty voxel with dust following some basic rules: if under the burr the space is empty, the material falls, if it is full, the material is put at the borders of the hole created. The force to be returned to the hand of the user via the haptic feedback device is computed using an inverse dynamics approach.

2.4.2 Bone dust and paste

The behaviour of bone dust and of the dust paste created by the mixing of blood, water, and dust, is modelled using a technique derived by sand-pile simulation [10, 11]. The problem in our application is that the material cannot be modelled as a single height field, so the evolution algorithm is more complex. At each simulation step, we consider each voxel in a region around the burr and check if it contains dust. In this case, we look at the surrounding columns of dust and measure the local height difference. A redistribution algorithm is then applied to move the system to a more stable state. The algorithm is defined by a set of evolution rules that are derived from the equations that describe the physical behaviour of dust. As in [11], we use the Mohr-Coulomb theory to determine shear stress and shear strength and then calculate the critical slope angle and the forces, which push material along a failure plane.

2.4.3 Irrigation and suction

The irrigator is modelled as a source generating a flow of water particles. These particles have a velocity and are affected by gravity. When they are close to a dust or bone voxel they interact with the material. In our first implementation, we consider only an extremely simplified model, where particles that collide with a "dust" voxel are merged with it, creating a new dust voxel with a "wet" attribute. The sand pile falling threshold of wet voxels is set to zero, thus the created "mud" will behave like a liquid.

The sucker, removing bone dust and water, is the simplest element in the simulation. A process that empties all the "mud" voxels in contact with the sucker tip models it. Force feedback for the irrigator and sucker is computed using a simple collision model that considers only the bone voxels.

3. Results

The modules produced for the pre-operative planning tool are providing high image quality 3D visualization, and segmentation precision to increase available information for operation planning. Algorithms based on probabilistic labelling and deformable templates are performing well. The new techniques being developed for multiple tissue segmentation from multiple images for boundary representation and data visualisation augurs particularly well.

Research and development for the physically based simulator is at this stage focussing on real-time physically motivated solutions for drilling into the petrous bone. We are currently in the phase of testing our system off-line, without connection to the I/O devices, by modelling the effect of pre-determined instrument actions on test datasets. Figure 3 shows a sequence of frames in a bone drilling simulation. The combined effects of the different simulation components are clearly visible.

 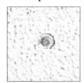 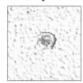 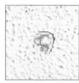

Figure 3: Sequence of frames in a bone drilling simulation. The drill is excavating a flat bone structure. The bone dust accumulates around the hole following a sand pile dynamics. The irrigator drops of water are visible.

It is planned to use two 6 DOF/3 DOF PHANToM haptic devices for the user interface, although a lower specification device could be used for the non-dominant hand.

Anatomical models are provided from the pre-operative tool and a process to augment the segmented voxel data with information on the organ's physical properties is being developed.

4. Conclusions

Other groups are developing simulators for surgical procedures of the petrous, or temporal, bone [8, 12-15]. This project, however, introduces several novel factors: a detailed user task analysis (based on ISO 13407); the use of patient specific data with tight integration between the medical image analysis and simulator components; the use of new autostereoscopic technology.

The use of patient specific data with tight integration between the medical image analysis and simulator components is proving to be an effective approach. At the end of the project we expect a high-fidelity solution for surgical planning and training in the field of otology, providing:

- A high quality user interface designed through ergonomic task analysis.

- A state-of-the-art system for pre-operative planning using advanced image analysis and visualization techniques.
- A leading system for physics-based surgical simulation.
- Innovative use of 3D display technology for a clinical application.

In addition, the project partners will have established a framework on which further surgical applications can be developed.

References

[1] R.J. Stone, A Human-Centred Definition of Surgical Procedures, IERAPSI (IST-1999-12175), Work Package 2, Deliverable D2 (Part 1), July 2000

[2] International Standard ISO 13407, Human-Centered Design Processes for Interactive Systems (ISO, 1999).

[3] A. Schwerdtner and H. Heidrich, Dresden 3D Display: A Flat Autostereoscopic Display, Electronic Imaging / Photonics West 1998, San Jose, California, 1998.

[4] E.Vokurka, N.Thacker, and A.Jackson, A Fast Model Independant Method for Automatic Correction of Correction of Intensity Non-Uniformity in MRI Data, JMRI, 10, 4, 550-562, 1999.

[5] D.H. Laidlaw, K.W. Fleischer, and A.H Barr, Partial-volume bayesian classification of material mixtures in MR volume data using voxel histograms, IEEE Trans. Med. Imag., vol. 17, no. 1, 74-86, Feb. 1998.

[6] W.M.Wells, E.L.Grimson, R.Kikinis et al. Adaptive segmentation of MRI data, IEEE Trans. on Medical Imaging, 15(4), 429-442, 1996.

[7] K.Fukenaga, Introduction to Statistical Pattern Recognition, 2ed, Academic Press, San Diego (1990).

[8] G. Wiet, J. Bryan, D. Sessanna, D. Streadney, P. Schmalbrock, and B. Welling. Virtual Temporal Bone Dissection Simulation, in Proc. Medicine Meets Virtual Reality 2000, Newport Beach, CA.

[9] Y.C. Fung, Biomechanics: Properties of Living Tissues, Springer-Verlag Inc., New York, NY, USA, 1993.

[10] R.W. Sumner, J.F. O'Brien, J.K. Hodgins, Animating Sand, Mud and Snow, Computer Graphics Forum, 18(1), 1999.

[11] X. Li and J.M. Moshell, Modelling Soil: Realtime Dynamic Models for Soil Slippage and Manipulation, Computer Graphics Proceedings, Annual Conference Series, 1993.

[12] C.V. Edmond, et al., Simulation for ENT Endoscopic Surgical Training, in Proc. Medicine Meets Virtual Reality 5, San Diego, CA, January 1997.

[13] S. Weghorst, et al., Validation of the Madigan ESS Simulator, in Proc. Medicine Meets Virtual Reality 6, San Diego, CA, January 1998.

[14] T. Harada, S Ishii, N Tayama, Three-dimensional Reconstruction of the Temporal Bone From Histological Sections, Arch Otolaryngol Head Neck Surg, 1998 114

[15] T.P. Mason, et al., The Virtual Temporal Bone, in Proc. Medicine Meets Virtual Reality 6, San Diego, CA, January 1998.

Acknowledgements

The IERAPSI Project is part funded by the European Community under the IST Project IST-1999-12175.

We wish to acknowledge the clinical contributions made by Prof. Richard Ramsden, Prof. Anthony Taylor, Mr Ghassan Alusi, Dr Hugh Wheatley, Dr Nigel Biggs, Dr Simon Hargreaves, and theatre staff, nurses and secretaries.

Medicine Meets Virtual Reality 2001
J.D. Westwood et al. (Eds.)
IOS Press, 2001

VIRTUAL FLUOROSCOPY: A TOOL FOR DECREASING RADIATION EXPOSURE DURING FEMORAL INTRAMEDULLARY NAILING

David M. KAHLER, M.D.

Department of Orthopaedic Surgery, Division of Trauma
University of Virginia Health System
Charlottesville, VA, 22908-0159
Dmk7y@virginia.edu

INTRODUCTION

Orthopaedic trauma has long been identified as a potential impact area for the relatively new field of computer assisted orthopaedic surgery. 3D-based computer assisted surgical guidance has been shown to significantly decrease radiation exposure and operative time when compared to standard fluoroscopic technique for the fixation of posterior pelvic ring disruptions [1,2]. Unfortunately, the 3D-based technology requires a dedicated CT scan preoperatively, rendering it unsuitable for fracture cases in which a reduction will be performed after obtaining the CT [3]. This dilemma has led to the development of *virtual fluoroscopy* for placement of fixation devices in fracture surgery. Virtual fluoroscopy gives the surgeon the ability to update images in the operating room after fracture reduction, and allows use of the updated images for surgical navigation. This development greatly expands the potential applications for computer assisted surgical guidance.

In virtual fluoroscopic navigation, a 3D model need not be obtained preoperatively. Instead, the surgeon harvests and stores standard two-dimensional C-arm fluoroscopic images in the operating room. The position of the patient and the fluoroscopy unit are tracked using optoelectronic markers. The stored images are then used to provide surgical guidance by displaying the position of optically tracked instruments relative to the images. A formal registration step is not required, as there is no need to relate a three-dimensional virtual model to an actual object in the operating room. The images used for navigation may be readily updated following fracture reduction maneuvers. This development has expanded the scope of computer assisted orthopaedic surgery to more routine cases, such as hip fracture fixation and intramedullary nailing of long bone fractures. These two applications account for the majority of the fluoroscopy time used in most hospital operating rooms.

CLINICAL RELEVANCE

Closed antegrade intramedullary nailing of diaphyseal femoral fractures (OTA 32-A,B,C) allows minimally invasive stabilization of these injuries at the expense of significant ionizing radiation exposure to both patient and operative team. The procedure typically requires several minutes of fluoroscopy time. Multiple C-arm images are usually obtained during the three critical portions of the procedure: identification of the starting point for reaming; fracture reduction; and insertion of distal locking screws. The total radiation exposure has historically been approximately four minutes during these steps, and over one hundred individual images are often obtained. Many of these images must be obtained with the surgeon's hands in the radiation field, particularly during fracture reduction and distal freehand interlocking.

Virtual fluoroscopy allows the performance of the critical portions of the femoral nailing procedure with as few as six individual images and only a few seconds of fluoroscopy time. The surgeon may be well away from the fluoroscope during imaging, and no additional imaging is required during virtual guidance. A virtual fluoroscopic technique for femoral nailing, including fracture reduction, is described.

METHODS

A standard analog C-arm unit is retrofitted with a calibration target and an array of light emitting diodes (LED's) to allow tracking of the unit by an optical digital camera. The calibration target and a software package are used to warp each fluoroscopic image to render them optically correct. A reference array of LED's is then attached to the patient to allow tracking of the femur during the procedure. The fluoroscopy unit and camera are interfaced with a CAOS workstation and computer monitor (Ion/FluoroNav, Medtronic/Sofamor Danek, Memphis, TN). Standard fluoroscopic images are stored on the workstation, and up to four images in different planes may be displayed simultaneously. The real time position of surgical instruments, such as a drill guide or reduction rod, may be overlaid onto the stored images. The virtual images are updated several times per second, allowing real-time feedback as the instruments are moved. This has allowed performance of each of the three critical portions of the femoral nailing procedure to be performed using only two stored images of the relevant anatomy, without the need for constantly reacquiring fluoroscopic images during the surgical procedure.

The antegrade femoral nailing procedure is performed with the patient supine on a fracture table. The patient's legs are scissored, with the injured leg placed in traction with slight flexion and adduction at the hip. The reference arc is attached to the greater trochanter with a single Schanz pin and toothy cannula. Antero-posterior (AP) and lateral C-arm images of the piriformis fossa are obtained and stored (Figure 1). The starting point for nail insertion is identified using virtual fluoroscopic guidance. A trajectory "look ahead" feature is used to align the drill guide with the femoral canal in both views, and a 3.2 mm guide wire is inserted through the piriformis fossa into the center of the intramedullary canal. The wire is then overdrilled with a rigid compound reamer to open a working channel in the proximal femur.

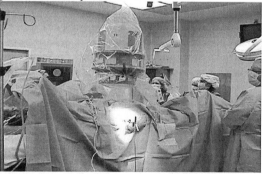

Figure 1. Operating room setup with calibration target and reference frame.

The next step is fracture reduction. Recent developments allow this step to be performed under virtual guidance. The fracture is slightly overdistracted by applying traction through the fracture table, and standard AP and lateral C-arm views of the fracture site are obtained. The reference arc is moved to the distal fracture fragment and attached to the anterolateral metaphysis of the femur. A special reduction rod instrumented with LED's (TriGen, Smith and Nephew, Memphis, TN) is inserted into the proximal fragment and advanced to the fracture site under virtual guidance. The position of the reduction rod within the femur is represented as a red line on the stored images. This process defines the axis and intramedullary canal of the proximal fragment. The fracture is manipulated manually until the virtual axis of the proximal fragment is aligned with the distal fragment. This step is somewhat disconcerting for the untrained observer, as the stored images show no change in the displaced position of the fracture fragments. The goal of this task is to align the proximal fragment, as defined by the position of the reduction rod, with the distal fragment being tracked by the reference arc. Fracture reduction is confirmed when the virtual image of the guide rod can be advanced into the distal fracture segment. A guide wire is then passed through the cannula in the reduction rod, and the rod is removed to allow reaming over the guide wire. If desired, additional images may be obtained to confirm reduction and restoration of normal length and alignment of the femur.

Following insertion of the femoral nail, the distal locking screws are inserted to provide rotational stability. A perfect lateral view of the locking screw holes in the nail must be obtained for adequate guidance. An AP image is also helpful to confirm that the drill guide is perpendicular to the femoral nail. The universal drill guide is then used to drill the holes for the locking screws under virtual fluoroscopic guidance (Figure 2 below). Alternatively, a captured self-drilling, self-tapping screw may be inserted in a single step without predrilling. The trajectory length feature of the system acts as a virtual depth gauge for selection of the proper screw length. An illustrative case will be presented.

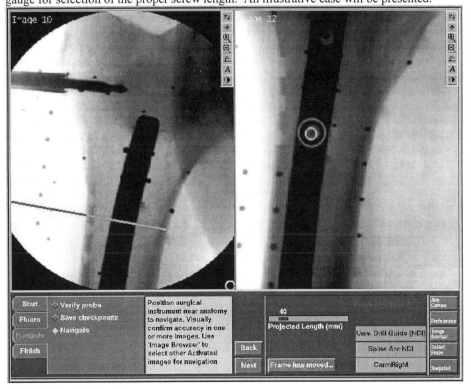

Figure 2.

RESULTS

All three critical portions of the femoral nailing procedure have been performed using virtual fluoroscopic guidance. Hand radiation exposure and additional imaging during reduction have been eliminated using this technique. In actual practice, several trial fluoroscopic images must be obtained for each step; the optimal images are then activated and displayed for virtual fluoroscopic guidance. Early clinical experience suggests that intraoperative radiation exposure during femoral nailing may be decreased by an order of magnitude when compared to standard fluoroscopic technique. The setup time for the computer is offset by the operative time savings during implant placement.

DISCUSSION/CONCLUSION

Ionizing radiation exposure is an underappreciated risk for both trauma surgeons and trauma patients. One minute of intraoperative fluoroscopy is equivalent to 40 mSv (4 Rads, 4,000 mrem) of radiation, or approximately equivalent to 250 chest x-rays. The fluoroscopy time required for femoral nailing is routinely reported to be over 4 minutes, and this is consistent with our internal data. The careful surgeon absorbs very little direct radiation, but is still subject to scatter from the patients anatomy; the patient absorbs most of the radiation dose. In actual practice, surgeons frequently place their hands in the radiation beam, especially during fracture reduction and freehand locking. The Occupational Safety and Health Administration's guidelines recommend no more than 50 rem per year of hand exposure, and this corresponds to only 12 minutes per year. It is very easy for an Orthopaedic Surgeon to exceed this threshold.

Measurable health effects occur at much lower doses of radiation. Career high-altitude airline pilots receive only about 3-6 mSv of radiation over environmental background per year. Nonetheless, they have a fivefold increase in myeloid malignancies and a threefold increase in skin cancers when compared to the population at large [4].

Virtual fluoroscopy, a new development in the field of CAOS, has numerous potential applications in the field of orthopaedic trauma. Using this technique, the femoral nailing procedure has been routinely be performed using less than one minute of fluoroscopy time. Despite the need for specialized equipment and instruments, this technology has the potential to greatly decrease the orthopaedic surgeon's reliance on intraoperative ionizing radiation during the performance of minimally invasive surgery. A prospective randomized trial is underway comparing virtual fluoroscopy to standard technique, with regard to operative time and radiation exposure.

The author gratefully acknowledges the assistance of Tony Melkent and Tommy Carls, Medtronic/Sofamor Danek, and David Simon, Medtronic/Surgical Navigation Technologies.

REFERENCES

1. Kahler DM, Mallik K. Computer assisted iliosacral screw placement compared to standard fluoroscopic technique. Computer Aided Surgery 4(6): 348, 1999.
2. Kahler DM. Computer-assisted percutaneous fixation of acetabular fractures and pelvic ring disruptions. Operative Techniques in Orthopaedics 10(1): 20-24, 2000.
3. Zura R, Kahler DM. A transverse acetabular nonunion treated with computer assisted percutaneous internal fixation. Journal of Bone and Joint Surgery 82A: 219-224, 2000.
4. Lancet 354:2029-2031, 1999.

Medicine Meets Virtual Reality 2001
J.D. Westwood et al. (Eds.)
IOS Press, 2001

229

Ghost Imaging in MRI

Leon Kaufman, David M Goldhaber, David M Kramer and Christine Hawryszko
Toshiba America MRI, Inc., Radiologic Imaging Laboratory
South San Francisco, CA
and
Dianne Georgian-Smith and David Haynor
Department of Radiology, University of Washington Medical Center
Seattle, WA

Abstract. Needle biopsies and other interventions done under MR Fluoroscopy sometimes do not show the target well, either because the rapid sequence does not have adequate contrast or because a contrast agent may have washed out of the target. In these cases, an image that shows the target can be saved and scaled to match the spatial parameters of the fluoroscopic sequence, and used as a virtual or ghost field upon which the fluoroscopic images are superimposed, thus providing a view of the target, useful for needle pre-localization and for monitoring its progress as it is inserted.

1. Introduction

In MRI interventional work it is sometimes the case that the target of the intervention is identified through a relatively long imaging procedure or by the injection of a contrast agent which clears in times that are rapid compared to the intervention time itself.

Contrast agents currently used in magnetic resonance imaging (MRI) and computerized tomography (CT) first diffuse into the extracellular fluid space and are then cleared by the kidneys. Thus, the contrast changes they produce are transient. Contrast media concentrations are highest during the bolus phase and decrease as dilution occurs. Thus, tumors that are visualized best early following injection may become indistinguishable from adjacent normal tissue relatively quickly. An example of this is breast biopsy. Performing a needle biopsy on a breast cancer patient before the contrast agent has cleared can be challenging, even with a second injection (Kuhl et al [1]).

A technique that can be used to aid in these cases is ghost imaging. In ghost imaging, images are stored for future reference to be subsequently superimposed upon an on-going real-time imaging procedure. This capability allows a mass to be imaged during peak enhancement and the image to be stored. When that image is used as the ghost image, it may be used to guide a biopsy needle in near real-time even after the lesion is no longer visible [2]. In this manner a diagnostic procedure and the biopsy can be performed following a single injection of contrast media.

2. Methodology

A single procedure involves three closely interlocked processes: Acquisition, processing and biopsy.

a. Acquisition. The acquisition of data is performed in "stream" mode, a continuous acquisition and storing of time domain or k-space data, in our case from +k to -k immediately followed by another acquisition from +k to -k, and so on. We typically acquire 25 frames, each of 11 slices, in approximately 15 seconds each, for a total time of just over 6 minutes. Injection is performed soon after the second frame is completed, but the time of injection is not critical nor does it need to be recorded. A total of 275 images are generated in this way.

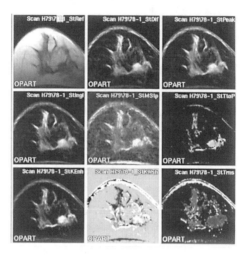

Figure 1. Automated image output from a contrast enhanced breast study. From left to right and top to bottom; average of pre contrast arrival images; subtraction image at the time point at which contrast enhancement is maximum; image of the peak enhancement reached by each pixel; integral of the enhancement over the study time; the maximum enhancement step between any two consecutive time frames; the time at which enhancement reached peak in each pixel, early times being more intense; the enhancement slope, high slope showing with higher intensity; the washout slope, gray being flat, bright for decreasing enhancement after peak is reached and dark for continuing enhancement after the initial fast component occurs; and the transit time, which in this kind of study is not relevant. Note that although the spicule (vertical structure near the center of the image) enhances as much as the tumor (rounded structure right of center), their time-course characteristics are quite distinct, with the tumor enhancing earlier and clearing faster.

b. Processing. There are various methods to detect the presence of contrast media in breast imaging. What appears to be robust and effective is to subtract the pre-contrast image from the post-contrast one. Commonly, serial pictures of the breast are obtained for a few minutes after injection. Images pre-injection are subtracted from the post injection ones and the resultant images analyzed (see, for instance, [3] and references therein). The criteria on which to diagnose accurately are not well established. Diagnostic specificity has been variously ascribed to the degree of enhancement (how much the signal increases due to contrast media intake), the rapidity of the intake, and/or to the washout characteristics [4]. Typically, time curves are obtained from suspicious areas so that these parameters can evaluated. The decisions as to where to obtain the time information have to be made from the examination of a very large number of images, as there are many time points per slice. This work is tedious, can have built in biases and is not easily adapted to routine clinical practice. In addition, such a process presupposes a selection of what regions of the image may be of interest, which in itself biases the diagnosis.

For 30 years, in nuclear medicine, people have generated parametric images where time analysis is done on a pixel by pixel basis, with varying degrees of operator input. We have put together a package that computes, without operator intervention, a number of desired parameters and displays them as an image. The package automatically selects the pre-injection images, calculates the arrival time of the contrast agent, performs the subtraction so as to maximize signal-to-noise, and computes various images. Not only does this make the process operator-independent and convenient for generalized use, but it also avoids the pitfall that a region has to be recognized as abnormal before a region can be defined, whereas the generation of parametric images presents the physician with all pixels at once.

The frames are examined by the computer to find the maximum enhancement and then earlier frames are examined to find the first in time when enhancement reached 10% of peak. One frame before it is eliminated (unless that is the first frame) and the other early ones are averaged to maximize S/N in the subtracted images. A set of subtracted images (frames as of time of enhancement minus the reference image) are generated. From these parametric images are calculated. Some examples of the output are:

1. The reference magnitude image, its components automatically selected and averaged for maximum S/N

2. The magnitude image where enhancement reached a peak

3. The subtraction of these two, i.e., the enhancement at peak value.

4. An image of the peak enhancement for every pixel irrespective of the time when it occurred.

5. The integral of the enhancement curve

6. The maximum step between two time points at any time during the enhancement process.

7. The time at which the peak value was reached

8. The slope of the enhancement portion of the curve

9. The slope of the washout portion

10. The transit time

The process does not involve operator intervention and takes 2-3 min. for a full data set. Figure 1 shows an example.

c. Biopsy

MRI provides a fluoroscopic operating mode (MRF) where data are acquired continuously and the reconstruction proceeds asynchronously using the latest full data set. A needle can be guided to target in this manner. Nevertheless, it is useful to be able to initiate the puncture with as much certainty as possible as to where the needle is aimed. For this purpose, we have developed the ghost imaging technique, basically a virtual reality process: An appropriate image is selected and superimposed on MRF images as they are acquired. The ghost image is automatically rescaled so as to match the MRF images spatially even if they are of different matrix size and/or resolution. The images can be added with variable weight or similarly subtracted.

The procedure consists of placing the sample or subject in the breast coil and positioning within the magnet using MRF. Once the desired position is achieved the diagnostic technique is run and processed. The table is then rolled out of the magnet and a mock needle with a tip phantom consisting of a 5 mm-diameter oil-filled torus with its own receiver coil is introduced and moved under real time feedback from MRF until the tip of the needle overlaps the target tumor in the ghost image. The needle holder settings are noted and locked and the needle is withdrawn. The table is returned to its previous position and the location of the target is confirmed by running MRF so as to subtract from the ghost image, this yielding edge artifacts if the breast or sample are improperly positioned. Location is also confirmed by matching oil-filled fiducials built into the receiver coil and sample holder. Once location is confirmed the MRF procedure runs so as to show both the real-time images and the superposition of one of them on the ghost. Thus, the biopsy

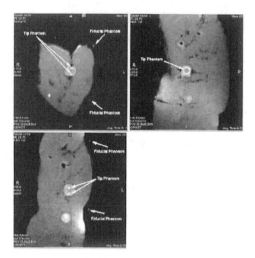

Figure 2. Three orthogonal ghost images of the bovine muscle/grape phantom with the live images of the needle phantom superimposed.

needle is aimed at a predetermined position while at the same time monitoring its progress on a real-time basis.

Initial tests of this procedure were done on tissue phantoms., constructed using bovine muscle at room temperature and grapes. Three phantoms were made each with 5-10 grapes stuffed into holes made with a knife in the muscle. Each phantom was approximately 10 cm x 10 cm x 20 cm. Five grapes were 25 mm in greatest diameter, and 15 grapes were approximately 15 mm in greatest diameter. The tissue phantom was placed into a prototype interventional breast coil. This coil immobilizes the contained tissue with light compression. There is an open rectangular window in the compression plate so that the tissue is accessible to the needle. Imaging was done in a Toshiba OPART open MRI operating at 0.35 Tesla.

The technique used initially to locate the grape-target was a multislice fast-spin echo (FSE) (TR=800-1500 ms, TE=100-120 ms) which simulated a brightly enhancing lesion. This image was saved as the ghost image and used for phantom needle placement (Figure 2). The other imaging parameters were: slice thickness, 5-6 mm; matrix, 128 x 256; field of view, 26 mm x 26 mm; imaging time, 13-17 s. A 14-gauge, 15 cm MR-compatible core biopsy needle (E-Z-EM Inc., Westbury, NY) was used for the biopsy. Its location was monitored by a multislice field echo (FE)(TR=120ms, TE= 20ms, flip angle= 10 degrees) imaging sequence. The grapes were not used for targeting the needle. The other imaging parameters were: matrix, 128 x 256; field of view, 20-26 mm square; imaging time 9-32 s. The shortest scans (9-10 s) were sufficient for tracking the needle progress. The longer scans (>10 s) were taken for higher signal-to-noise ratio and improved resolution.

The biopsy was then performed. A second pass was infrequently made when it was observed under MR fluoroscopy that the needle tip was deflected from a straight line. The needle was withdrawn prior to attempting a biopsy and reinserted using the same coordinates for the second pass. Immediately after the biopsy needle was fired, the needle was withdrawn and immediately inspected for grape pulp within the biopsy notch. Each

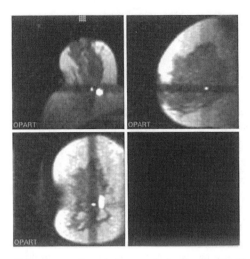

Figure 3. Three orthogonal ghost images through the target lesion in a breast with the live images of the phantom needle. (The phantom needle shown in these images is of a different design than the toroidal one used in the grape studies. Here the position of the biopsy needle's sampling area is marked with a single dot of oil and a larger volume oil phantom appears nearby to aid finding that small phantom while adjusting the coarse position of the device.)

grape was re-scanned to look for the course of the needle track. The grapes were all removed at the completion of all of the passes to inspect them for needle tracks and to note the course of the tracks in relationship to the center of the grape.

3. Results

All twenty grapes were hit by the biopsy needle. Grapes #1-#5 were 25 mm in diameter and #6-#20 were 15 mm in diameter. In four out of twenty passes, a second pass was made when the needle tip was observed not to be at the center of the "cross-hairs". The needle was reinserted prior to firing using the original coordinates. By observing pulp within the needle as evidence for successful biopsy, all five of the large grapes and 13 out of 15 of the smaller grapes were biopsied. However, inspection of the grapes for needle tracks revealed that all had been hit, although grapes #8 and #10 were grazed peripherally. Although all were centrally targeted, three grapes, including grapes #8 and #10, were hit eccentrically by as much as 5 to 6 mm. These grapes were included in the attempts that required a second pass. Each biopsy took approximately 1 hour.

Following work with phantoms we have performed 6 biopsies in patients with known breast tumors (Figure 3). With improvements in software and user interface, the patient procedure was completed in an hour as well. All tissue samples were examined by a pathologist. In 3 of these cases this examination revealed malignancy and confirmed the placement of the needle within the mass. In the remaining 3 cases, possible causes for the failure to obtain histopathologic confirmation are poor targeting accuracy in the procedure or insufficient sample size due to the design of the MRI-compatible biopsy needle. We observed in the breast cases, as we did in the grape experiments, that accuracy was limited

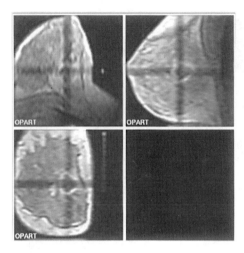

Figure 4. MR Fluoro images showing centering of the orthogonal planes on the contrast-enhanced lesion.

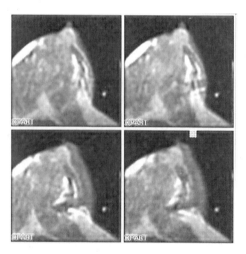

Figure 5. Progress of the needle monitored by MR Fluoro. Last frame, bottom right, shows the needle in the lesion, which at this time is no longer enhanced.

because of movement of tissue with needle insertion. This was more of a problem in the breast because of the dense and fibrous quality of the target masses. The unavoidable (but limited) motion of the patient with respect to the fiducial marks on the coil was probably also a factor. Figure 4 shows a fluoroscopic MRI scan where the point of intersection of the three orthogonal imaging planes is centered on the contrast-enhanced target lesion. Figure 5 shows a series of axial images taken as the biopsy needle was inserted. Each image is a composite live and superposed ghost image. The deflection of the lesion and much of the breast from the force of the needle is apparent.

4. Discussion

The advantages of ghost imaging and a phantom needle to find the correct initial trajectory are that a minimal number of realignment passes in the patient are needed to reach the target, thereby reducing patient trauma, and by using a non-magnetic needle phantom, geometric distortions due to magnetic susceptibility effects at the needle tip are eliminated, solving the imprecision of needle localization caused by blooming artifacts that affects all interventional MRI procedures.

References

[1]   Kuhl CK, Elevelt A, Leutner CC, Gieseke J, Pakos E, and Schild HH. Interventional Breast MR Imaging: Clinical use of a Stereotactic Localization and Biopsy Device. Radiology 204 (1997) 667-675.

[2]   Kaufman L, Kramer DM and Hawryszko C. Method and Apparatus for Performing Interventional Medical Procedures Using MR Imaging of Interventional Device Superimposed with Ghost Patient Image. U.S. Patent 5,155,435. Issued October 13, 1992.

[3]   Orel SG. Differentiating Benign From malignant Enhancing Lesions Identified at MR Imaging of the Breast: Are Time-Signal Intensity Curves an Accurate Predictor?, Radiology 211 (1999) 5-7.

[4]   Kuhl CK, Mielcareck P, Klaschik S, Leutner C, Wardelmann E, Gieseke J and Schild HH. Dynamic Breast MR Imaging: Are Signal Intensity Time Course Data Useful for Differential Diagnosis of Enhancing Lesions? Radiology 211 (1999) 101-110.

236

Medicine Meets Virtual Reality 2001
J.D. Westwood et al. (Eds.)
IOS Press, 2001

Trauma Training: Virtual Reality Applications

Christoph Kaufmann, MD
Alan Liu, Ph.D.

National Capital Area Medical Simulation Center
Uniformed Services University of the Health Sciences
Bethesda, MD 20814
ckaufmann/aliu@simcen.usuhs.mil
http://www.simcen.usuhs.mil

Abstract. Training medics, medical students, nurses, and residents to perform trauma care skills presents many obstacles. These include: emergent nature of the procedures, instructor time, availability of clinical material, and anatomic knowledge. Virtual Reality simulators address each of these obstacles. The National Capital Area Medical Simulation Center is a unique national asset that not only uses state-of-the-art simulators to teach trauma care skills to medical students and others, but adapts existing technology and develops new simulations to teach these skills. Most standard trauma training is performed on either mannequins or anesthetized animals and requires the constant presence of an instructor. VR applications can be stand-alone devices that have built-in scenarios and multiple patients to increase variation and/or level of technical expertise required to successfully complete the required steps of the trauma procedure. Commercial VR simulators to teach trauma skills include: CathSim Intravenous Simulator (HT Medical), UltraSim Ultrasound Simulator (MedSim), Limb Trauma Simulator (Musculographics/BDI), and the Human Patient Simulator (MedSim). Additionally, we have developed two additional simulators based on the HT CathSim; these are the pericardiocentesis simulator and the diagnostic peritoneal lavage simulator. Future applications include virtual environment triage simulation and surgical airway simulators.

1. Background

For over one thousand years, advances in trauma care have resulted from experience gained through care of wounds suffered on the battlefield. As the frequency of large-scale wars has decreased in the past several decades, advances in trauma care have resulted from the "battlefields" of large U.S. cities. This lack of exposure to military trauma patients has made it more and more difficult to train and maintain trauma skills for military medical care providers. Military medics, nurses, and doctors must be prepared with the necessary skills to be able to provide excellent care to the wounded soldier, sailor, airman, or marine from the very start of a war or conflict. A long learning curve to gain or refresh skills is not acceptable. The difficulty is to learn and maintain skills with little or no exposure to trauma patients. Medical simulation is one of the answers to this training dilemma.

2. Tools and Methods

The Surgical Simulation Laboratory of the National Capital Area Medical Simulation Center (NCAMSC) provides the ideal combination of teaching and research environments [1]. As a result of the DARPA program headed by Col. Richard Satava and the financial commitment of the medical school administration, the facility had a state-of-the-art suite of surgical simulators when the center opened in April, 2000 [2]. These included many with application to care of the injured patient, including CathSim Intravenous Simulator (HT Medical), UltraSim Ultrasound Simulator (MedSim), Limb Trauma Simulator (Musculographics), and the Human Patient Simulator (MedSim). The focus of the Surgical Simulation Laboratory is training resuscitation principles and techniques to Uniformed Services University medical students as well as engaging in research to improve this training. Initial trauma patient resuscitation should follow the A, B, C's of the American College of Surgeons Advanced Trauma Life Support (ATLS®) course: airway, breathing, circulation [3]. The first step is to establish an airway for the patient (and breathe for him/her as necessary) if the patient is obtunded, comatose, or has an obstructed airway. There are several methods available to secure the patient's airway, but the main challenge is time. If the patient is not getting enough oxygen he/she will rapidly die. If less invasive methods fail or are not appropriate, a surgical airway is the best approach. One way to achieve this is to insert a needle or tube through the cricothyroid membrane just cephalad to the trachea. As no VR simulators currently exist to teach this important procedure, this is currently being addressed at the NCAMSC.

Circulation, "C", consists of both stopping the bleeding and replenishing the intravascular volume with crystalloid solution and/or blood as required. Although many steps can and do occur simultaneously, control of bleeding is the most important factor after airway and breathing are addressed. The Limb Trauma Simulator (Musculographics/BDI) is an SGI Octane-based 3D simulator with two 1.5 Phantoms (Sensable) for haptics that depicts a high velocity gunshot wound to the leg (Fig. 1 left). The student must not only stop the bleeding by putting on virtual hemostats, but can also debride the wound (removing bone fragments in this case). Using the same workstation, the student can train to either start a peripheral intravenous line in the hand or a central venous catheter in the groin (femoral line). Another simulator that is designed to teach starting an intravenous line is the CathSim (HT Medical). The CathSim uses a two dimensional view of an arm or hand to teach starting an intravenous line and includes a haptic device to simulate the force feedback provided by the needle.

Following the A, B, C's of trauma patient care, further physical examination is required to explore for disability ("D"). The MedSim Human Patient mannequin can respond to questions (via the human operator) or has an electromechanical pain response if obtunded - similar to a real patient. He can also be exposed ("E") for complete examination to ensure there are no unexpected signs of injury.

After the initial assessment, the trauma patient may require specific diagnostic procedures to examine for life-threatening or potentially life-threatening injuries. One of these diagnostic procedures is the FAST exam or focused abdominal sonography for trauma. The UltraSim ultrasound simulator (MedSim) permits simulation of this diagnostic study with instructor-defined findings of positive or negative intra-abdominal bleeding depending on what the student is intended to find. Two other trauma diagnostic procedures have not been available as virtual reality training devices until now. Those are pericardiocentesis and diagnostic peritoneal lavage. These two simulations have been developed at the NCAMSC.

Pericardiocentesis is a needle-based procedure that can be both diagnostic and therapeutic. When performed in the trauma patient setting, clinical suspicion indicates that the patient has blood around the heart within the pericardial sac preventing proper filling and function of the heart. This emergency procedure does not allow for radiographic evaluation or other preliminary study as the patient will rapidly die if a cardiac tamponade is present and pericardiocentesis is not performed. Using animal models to learn this procedure is suboptimal as the anatomy is not correct and anatomical landmarks are the key to performing this procedure correctly. Cadavers may be used, but will uniformly give a negative result. Using a "hand-immersive" 3D VR tabletop workstation (Fig. 1 right), a prototype pericardiocentesis simulator was developed [4]. This simulator was immediately deemed too expensive for general use, so a 2D version was then

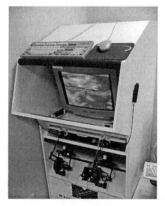 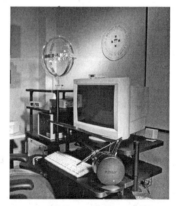

Fig. 1: Hand-immersive virtual environment generators. Left: Console version for limb trauma/ vascular anastomosis simulation. Right: Desktop version for simulator prototype development (e.g., pericardiocentesis).

created using the haptic feedback device of the HT CathSim as this is a commercially available piece of hardware. Fig. 2 (left) depicts the user interface from this simulator. The resulting simulator would be expected to cost approximately 10% as much as the 3D version with little loss in realism or utility.

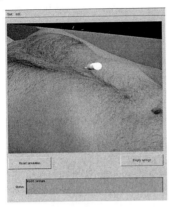 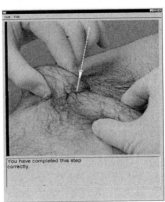

Fig. 2: (left) Pericardiocentesis simulator. (right) Diagnostic peritoneal lavage simulator.

Diagnostic peritoneal lavage (DPL) is also a needle-based procedure performed when there is suspicion of intra-abdominal bleeding in an injured patient. This is particularly true when the patient is unstable and there is not time to take the patient to the CT scanner for an abdomen and pelvis scan. There are more steps to this procedure than with pericardiocentesis as a wire must first be inserted into the abdomen before a catheter is inserted over the wire. Additionally, if immediate gross blood does not return from the catheter, crystalloid must be instilled and than drained to look for further evidence of intra-abdominal injury [5]. Fig. 2 (right) illustrates the catheter insertion step of our DPL simulator.

With both the pericardiocentesis simulator and the DPL simulators there exists the ability for the instructor to specify whether the result will be positive or negative. This is helpful when combining various simulators into a patient care scenario that may begin with triage in the field to the emergency department to the operating room and finally to the intensive care unit and beyond.

3. Results

These two new simulators, pericardiocentesis and diagnostic peritoneal lavage, have been used in several instructional opportunities at the NCAMSC. These include a day-long orientation to surgery for the third-year medical students and an ATLS® course.

The existing resources and new simulators have been integrated into a curriculum that provides the third year students with experience in abdominal examination, suturing and knot tying skills, resuscitation of a hypovolemic patient, and trauma care-related skills and procedures using the various computer-based simulators.

One ATLS® course has been taught at the NCAMSC to investigate these tools as a potential option for the surgical skills practicum. The students included surgery residents and staff surgeons. The majority felt the surgical skills were well-taught using the simulators.

4. Discussion

Trauma procedure training is important for both the military and civilian medical communities. Many medical care procedures can be taught in a comfortable and safe environment as they are not emergency procedures. This is not true of trauma care procedures. As the patient may die without rapid and effective diagnosis and treatment, there is little opportunity to practice these procedures when they are most needed. This necessarily results in the most skilled individual performing the procedure rather than the individual that most needs to learn the skill. Thus, the need for simulators in addressing these needs.

Trauma procedural skill simulators are primarily of three distinct types: "wet" models such as cadavers or anesthetized animals, plastic models or mannequins, and finally computer-based or virtual reality simulators. Each of these has its strengths and weaknesses.

Over centuries, cadavers and animals have served to educate medical professionals. The drawbacks of each are obvious. Today is the day of plastic models and mannequins which are achieving more and more realism and are used widely. They have some limitations in realism and there are costs to replaceable parts. Tomorrow is the age of computer-based virtual reality simulators [6]. Their realism continues to improve and they do not readily wear out or require any replaceable parts. A single VR simulator can be programmed to simulate many different patients with many different findings. There are never any "tracks" of the previous student to follow (as is true with the other models).

Another very important aspect of the computer-based trainers is that they can be stand alone. The student can learn in the absence of an instructor as the computer serves as the instructor. This leaves more time for the instructor to help those students most in need of his/her attention. The instructor may also elect to focus on testing the students' acquisition of knowledge and skills from the simulators. This will be particularly important until we have more objective information regarding the validity of various training simulators.

5. Conclusion

Trauma care skills are integral to the successful resuscitation of the injured patient, military or civilian. There are obstacles to mastering these skills using conventional training methods. Current lack of trauma care opportunities make it particularly difficult for military care providers to maintain these important skills. Virtual reality surgical procedural simulators are one answer to this problem. It is extremely likely that they will become integral to the training of all trauma care providers.

6. References

[1]   Kaufmann C., "Role of Surgical Simulators in Surgical Education", Asian J Surg; oct 1999, 22(4): p 398-401.

[2]   Satava R., "Medicine 2001 the king is dead". In: Satava R, Morgan K, Sieburg H, Mattheus R, Christensen J, eds. Interactive Technology and the New Paradigm for Healthcare. Amsterdam: IOS Press, 1995:334-339.

[3]   American College of Surgeons Committee on Trauma, "Advanced Trauma Life Support® for Doctors", 6th edition, Chicago, IL (1997).

[4]   Kaufmann C, Zakaluzny S., Liu A., "First Steps in Eliminating the Need for Animals and Cadavers in Advanced Trauma Life Support®". MICCAI 2000.

[5]   Liu A., Kaufmann C., Ritchie T., "A Computer-based Simulator for Diagnostic Peritoneal Lavage", Medicine Meets Virtual Reality 2001.

[6]   O'Toole R., Playter R., Krummel T., et al, "Measuring and developing suture technique with a virtual reality surgical simulator", J Am Coll Surg, Jul 1999, 189(1): p114-27.

Medicine Meets Virtual Reality 2001
J.D. Westwood et al. (Eds.)
IOS Press, 2001

Computer Assisted Treatment Of Pelvis Fractures

O. Krivonos[1 2 3], F. Gebhard[1], P. Keppler[1], L. Kinzl[1], J. Hesser[2 3], R. Männer[2 3]
[1]Trauma Department, University of Ulm, Germany
[2]Lehrstuhl für Informatik V, University of Mannheim, Germany
[3]Institute for Computational Medicine, Universities Mannheim and Heidelberg, Germany

Abstract. The presented approach is the realization of a minimal invasive treatment of pelvis fractures using the computer aided surgery (CAS). Main problem of tracking of major bone fragments after reposition is solved by implementing of 3D ultrasound to obtain intraoperative bone surfaces. Preoperative and intraoperative data sets are matched. Major fragments are tracked. The real time navigation is possible.

1. Objective

Orthopedic surgeons use widely methods like fluoroscopy, computer tomography and magnetic resonance imaging for diagnosis and computer aided surgery (CAS). However in reality their usage is frequently limited. CT and MRI do not provide the information about position of bones in real time when reposition of bones is possible. Implementation of fluoroscopy does not guarantee a good navigation after reposition. Main problem is the tracking of major bone fragments as well as matching using a non-touch technique, because data are taken from preoperative CT scans [1][2]. Using of fiducial markers for preoperative data does not also guarantee successful tracking during operation and moreover in majority is not possible. The problem is that each fragment being tracked must be marked by at least three points. In this case the total number of fiducial markers becomes too high for existing optical tracking devices (OTD) [3] and the density of these markers can be large, which reduces the probability of their recognition by OTD. Thereafter following reposition of bone fragments the navigation is not more possible. A minimal invasive treatment is almost not possible without real time navigation. During operation screws should be placed with very high accuracy, because thickness of pelvis bone is sometime close to diameter of screws and structures like hip joint and nervetrunks are very close. To solve this problem it is necessary to develop a real time navigation system based on the registration of pelvis bone surfaces taken from preoperative CT data and intraoperative data without additional damage of patient.

2. Materials and methods

A proposed new technique is the realisation of a minimal invasive treatment of pelvis fractures using a navigated 3D ultrasound device. We suppose that the surgery has three standard stages: planning, registration and plan execution. First, a CT scan of the patient's pelvis is taken for planning the operation process. Next, bones are segmented and the new data set is reconstructed, reflecting the actual position of each fragment. It allows to evaluate the extent personality of the fracture and create the operation plan. In accordance

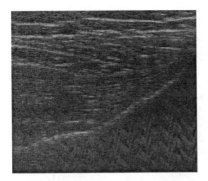 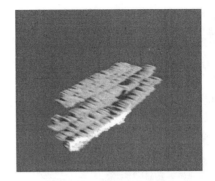

Figure 1 Example of US slice of pelvis   Figure 2 Reconstructed pelvic surface (20 slices)

with developed planes guiding or positioning instruments are fixed to bone fragments in order to move them. Now, the bone fragments can be rearranged using the instrument as a joy - stick. After that the surgical instrumentation can be done using navigated tools. Since for this operation the physician has no direct view onto the bone, the following technique is implemented.

The navigated ultrasound scanning device is moved over the operation area, ultrasound images are taken slice by slice. A sequence of morphological filters is used to remove speckle noise in the ultrasound data and to extract the bone surface, which reflects the actual position of each fragment. Because the interpretation of ultrasound images is difficult even for experienced physicians, this surface is matched with the preoperatively taken CT, and the movement of the bone parts during repositioning is determined. The actual position of the bone fragments is displayed using real time volume rendering. Thus, the physician can look at the operation area and sees the virtual bone fragments at their correct position and orientation relative to the patient.

3. Implementation of ultrasound

Recently the popularity of ultrasound imaging is growing [4][5]. Ultrasound provides flexible tools for diagnosis. These investigations are inexpensive and riskless. Despite of the fact that there are successful implementations of three-dimensional ultrasound images for visualization of fetus surfaces [5], ultrasound images have very big disadvantage. Existence of high level noise makes the segmentation and interpretation of ultrasound images particularly difficult (B-mode images). The reason of those artifacts is that skin and mussels have high reflection of ultrasound waves along their borders (Figure 1). Also there are shadow regions behind strong reflecting tissues, which can have bright spots inside. We use filter operations to improve quality of extracted surfaces and reduce artifacts. The Gaussian 5x5 filter improves initial images [6]. The closing $L_7(\pi/2)$ operator connects parts of bone surface [7] separated by small zones with low reflection in horizontal direction. Then the South Shadow filter with a 3x3 mask [[1,2,1],[0,1,0],[-1,-2,-1]] enhances the lower border of spikes. The image gray values are then scaled to a range between 0-2000 and image enhancement is implemented. Next, since there is a nearly complete reflection of ultrasound near the bone the impedance difference between bone and the surrounding soft tissue is very high. Thus, a forced rainfall algorithm is implemented in direction opposite to the direction of the ultrasound wave propagation.

This kind of segmentation algorithm is based on so-called directed thresholding. The threshold value is chosen to 1850. This directed thresholding is performed pixel by pixel in

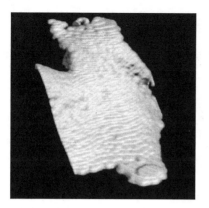

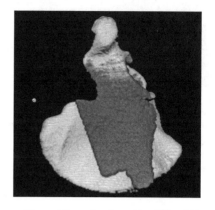

Figure 3 Reconstruction of the pelvis sawbone
surface from US

Figure 4 Example of matching US and CT
surfaces

given direction. It exploits the fact that ultrasound is completely reflected on the bone surface so that behind this surface there is no usable information (before, if we scan in opposite direction). In other words real bone surfaces are followed by shadow area behind. Thus, if an object with of high intensity is found, the length, area and altitude deviation of the "shadow" along the ultrasound ray direction are measured. In order to remove remaining artifacts additional a posteriori knowledge about the properties of the bone to be extracted is used. For example, only bright spots in the slices, which have a length of 7 pixels perpendicular to the propagation direction, an area of 20 pixels, a ratio of length to area more then 0.3 and "shadow" altitude standard deviation less then 0.3, belong to the bone and are thus filtered.

Since the interference patterns are horizontal, the filtered surface elements are often dissected in the vertical direction orthogonal to waves propagation. Thus closing with an $L_7(0)$ structured element on the 2-D slice is applied. From this step the filtering is performed on a volume generated by stacking the presegmented slices by the rainfall algorithm. The rest artifacts are removed by using the connected component labelling algorithm. The bone surface extracted by this way is not smooth. Its roughness is still a consequence of the interference patterns. For better visible inspection and comparison the surface is smoothed by an opening filter with a structured element 5x5, followed by a 3x3x3 closing filter. Finally a 5x5x5 Gaussian leads to smooth transitions of gray values and improves the visual quality. Figure 2 shows the segmentation result.

4. Surface registration

The interpretation of US surfaces is a complex task, especially when they describe complex anatomical structures or fractures. Thus, the registration process is very important for orthopedic surgery. It helps to establish a correspondence between two data sets representing two images. Multimodal registration in such case can significantly help the surgeon to understand the created virtual model. More over, the registration with surfaces extracted from the preoperative data (CT) solves the problem of tracking major bone fragments after reposition.

Lets consider that $N_p=|P|$ and $N_x=|X|$ are potencies of point sets representing bone surfaces respectively from intraoperative and preoperative data sets. We are implementing the Interactive Closest Point (ICP) algorithm for the registration of dense maps P and X respectively. When numbers N_p and N_x are relatively big the implementation of ICP algorithm is difficult for the real time registration of two data sets. The cause is a seek

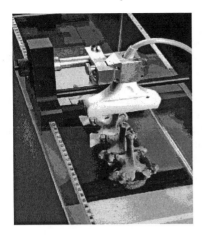
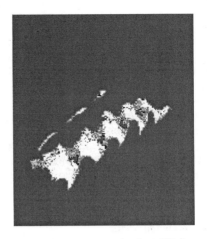

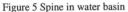

Figure 5 Spine in water basin   Figure 6 Spine reconstruction from US slices

strategy of closest point used in this algorithm. Its complexity is equal to $O(N_p*N_x)$[8], when the complexity of other parts of the algorithm remain $O(N_p)$. We propose a modification of ICP algorithm or more exactly an implementation of other seek strategy for closest points. As the X dense map is calculated from the preoperative data set, we have enough time for calculation a look-up-table for all possible distances to points from X. The idea is to implement the three dimensional internal Euclidean Distance Map (IEDM) [9] for the volume concerned surfaces extracted from CT data. The computational complexity of IEDM is equal $O(N)$, where N is size of the preoperative data set. This fact gives a possibility to implement IEDM calculation in real time with using hardware acceleration. Thus, the change of the seek strategy in our case results in final complexity of ICP algorithm $O(N_p)$. The proposed modification of registration algorithm belongs to group of local matching algorithms. Since the CT data is large then US data it is necessary to implement either a global registration algorithm or an initial transformation, which places surfaces closely to optimal position. Because the position and direction of US scans is known relatively to CT data, the position of matched data, i.e. the initial transformation is calculated in advance. Figures 3-4 show an example of multimodal registration.

5. Results

To evaluate the segmentation of bone surfaces from different modalities a feasibility study was done. Two bones (cadaveric spine and pelvis saw-bone) were selected, on the assumption that they have steep and flat surfaces respectively. Also the spine represents the worst case for segmentation, because its density is less then density of bone of a patient. Surfaces of bones where segmented from CT scans (Picker Mx8000). Then, each bone was placed in a water basin and conventional guided ultrasound slices (Siemens Sonoline 5 MHz, linear transducer) were taken (Figure 5). Pictures are accepted with 1 mm of distance between slices. The quality of segmented surfaces was estimated. A comparison with CT images shows a good agreement of the bone surfaces both from CT and ultrasound.

6. Conclusions

The main advantage of the presented technique is that no surgeon interaction is required for surface segmentation and registration processes. In addition no physical features about investigated anatomical structures are used during segmentation. It gives an opportunity to implement this approach for other part of the skeleton, where it is possible to receive an intraoperative data set that follows the reposition of fragments and shows their final position relatively to preoperative data set. For example the same technique could be used for correction of osteotomies of long bones.

Main difficulties from image processing view are to reach frame rate required for the real time tracking. Acceleration of segmentation algorithms is possible to reach at least 10 fps. Also implementation of the internal distance precalculation for volumes, which contain surfaces segmented from CT images, considerable reduces the complexity of the registration process. Implementation a multi-processor PC or FPGA-based PCI-boards can give acceleration of factor 10. Final speed could be reached within 100 ms for large data sets.

7. Acknowledgements

The project was granted by the AO/ASIF research funding 99-K43.

References

[1] F. Gebhard, O. Krivonos, U.C. Liener, P. Keppler, L. Kinzl, J. Hesser, Bone Extraction from Ultrasound Images and Surface Matching with CT. Proc. CAOS: Computer Assisted Orthopedic Surgery, Symposium, Davos, Switzerland, 2000.
[2] O. Krivonos, J. Hesser, R. Männer, F. Gebhard, U. Liener, P. Keppler, L. Kinzl, Minimal Invasive Surgery of the Pelvis using Ultrasound. In: 4th CAOSUSA Conference in Pittsburgh, Pennsylvania, 2000, pp 203-205.
[3] www.ndigital.com
[4] G. Sakas, L. Schreyer, M. Grimm, Case Study: Visualization of 3D Ultrasonic Data. In: Visualization'94 conference, 17-21 October 1994, Washington/DC, Proceedings, pp. 369-373.
[5] G. Sakas, S. Walter, Extracting Surfaces from Fuzzy 3D Ultrasonic Data. In: ACM Computer Graphics SIGGRAPH-95, Los Angeles/USA, 1995.
[6] R.C. Gonzalez, R.E. Wood, Digital Image Processing. Addison-Wesley Publishing Company; 1992.
[7] R.M. Haralick, S.R. Sternberg, X. Zhuang, Image Analysis Using Mathematical Morphology. IEEE Trans. on PAMI 9 4 (1987) 532-550.
[8] P. Besl, N. McKay, A Method for Registration of 3-D Shapes. In: IEEE Trans. On PAMI 14 2 (1992) 239-256.
[9] S. Sheynin, A. Tuzikov, O. Krivonos, Computation of the Opening Transform. In: Mathematical Morphology and its Applications to Image and Signal Processing, CWI, 1998, pp. 339-346.

Medicine Meets Virtual Reality 2001
J.D. Westwood et al. (Eds.)
IOS Press, 2001

Computer Simulation Of Osteotomy Correction

O. Krivonos[1 2 3], D. Moskalenko[1 2], P. Keppler[1], L. Kinzl[1],
J. Hesser[2 3], R. Männer[2 3]

[1]*Trauma Department, University of Ulm, Germany*
[2]*Lehrstuhl für Informatik V, University of Mannheim, Germany*
[3]*Institute for Computational Medicine, Universities Mannheim and Heidelberg, Germany*

Abstract. This paper describes a novel approach to correct osteotomy deformities
of long bones using virtual reality and image processing techniques on personal
computers. The discussed method allows to simulate osteotomy corrections by
implementing a single cut and a rearrangement of the dissected bone parts. It
allows the surgeon to directly control the pre-operative situation and the postoperative result of the simulation by comparing bone-length, angles, and torsion of
the bone. In addition, he or she obtains the coordinates and angles of the planned
cut relative to anatomical landmarks.

1. Background

As investigated in medical praxis, fracture treatment occasionally results in a mal-
alignment of bones. This post-traumatic deformities of bones causes pain and loss of limb
functionality. Also, adjacent joints are applied non-physiologic strain, which leads to early
arthrosis in these joints. Therefore, corrective osteotomies are required [1].

The goal of the osteotomy planning is to find an ideal plane, which allows correction
using one cut. In practice, the correction is made by a set of rotations in different planes
and translations of dissected bones. The procedure of a preoperative planning is as follows:
Several projections of the bone are exposed on x-ray films. A physician investigates
deformities by calculation of distances between anatomic landmarks, projection angles, and
torsion angle. After this step he or she use a simulation of osteotomy on a set of transparent
films to find optimal length, angles and torsion for the patient. Thus the position of a cut
plane and type of correction can be defined. However, this method leads to two problems:
The procedure of osteotomy planning becomes extremely difficult in case of 3D torsion
and of course it is very time consuming. Moreover even small deviations of the ideal
position of the cut plane can result in a failure of the whole operation.

2. Methods & Tools

A software prototype for planning osteotomies has been developed. The kernel of this
software was created on the base of VGL2.1®, powerful and flexible library from
VolumeGraphics GmbH. This library provides interactive visualization of volume data
with different render methods, shadowing effects, and manipulation of lightning sources
and effective memory management. The image processing part of prototype allows to
segment bone from low dose CT (using Marconi's MxTwin CT-system) in order to remove
possible artifacts interactively or in automatic mode. After the segmentation step a

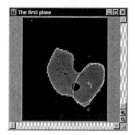

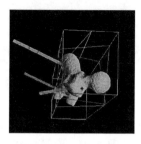

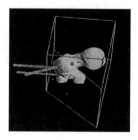

Figure 1 Placement of the marker **Figure 2** Excessive torsion angle measured by instruments **Figure 3** Corrected torsion angle

physician has to introduce anatomical markers, which can be determined in three perpendicular planes. These markers define an orientation and help to measure different features of investigated part of skeleton such as distances, angles and torsion based on marker points. For example, for the femur we define four 3D markers x_i, i=1..4 exactly in centre of the hip head, condyle medial, condyle lateral, and trochanter major respectively (Figure 1). First three markers define standard views on the bone and a reference plane. The program calculates distances $d_{i,j}(x_i,x_j)$ and angles between segments $[x_i,x_j]$ and $[x_j,x_k]$ automatically, where i,j,k=1..4, i≠j, i≠k, j≠k. Torsion angle is calculated between planes $P(x_1,x_2,x_3)$ and $P(x_1,x_4,x_5)$, where x_5 is a middle point of segment $[x_2,x_3]$, projection torsion angle is angle $(\text{proj}_{P(x1,x2,x3)}([x_1,x_4]), [x_1,x_4])$.

The program includes an interface for instrument simulation. The instrument position is defined by a given marker, and its orientation is specified moving the endpoints of the instrument in three perpendicular planes. Two instruments with non-zero common angle define a cut plane if their markers have the same position in 3D space. Length, diameter, and color of each instrument can be changed in special parameter section.

The surgeon can perform a virtual cut in the data volume. Dissected bone parts can be moved. The restriction is that the motion is confined to be along the cut plane. The rotation is limited to rotations about an axis that is parallel to a cut plane normal. In order to measure the success of a rearrangement, markers are grouped with the corresponding bone parts. Distances, angles, torsion, and projection torsion angles are updated automatically for the selected markers during the bone manipulations. This allows the surgeon to observe directly improvements of the bone position and to approach the optimal arrangement of it. There is a possibility to calculate angles between vectors parallel to orientation vectors of marked instruments (Figure 2-3). Additional correction of the bone position can be done with implementation of the open wedge transformation. The angle between equal wedge facets and its top are specified by the surgeon. Results of correction operations can be stored in a file and loaded on demand. Also an undo mechanism is applied when it is necessary to return to the step of cut plane definition.

To simplify the work with the program its interface includes a workflow panel. All main actions are divided on groups as sequence of steps and every step is represented by a button. Only one button is active at the moment. User actions are guided on each step by using on-line help from the same panel.

3. Results

When the planning of osteotomy is completed a physician can export data related to operation and also store different views of bones after virtual correction to be able to compare real view of the bone with its corrected model (Figure 2-3). Also based on the obtained data a wedge can be fabricated for the real operation. The computer aided

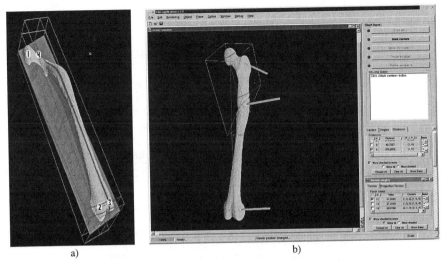

a) b)

Figure 4 Anatomical markers and reference plane a), and result of osteotomy simulation b)

planning gives the possibility to increase accuracy and precision of the operation and provides for surgeon complementary digital and visual information.

4. Conclusions

The presented software prototype simplifies significantly the process of osteotomy planning and allows to train a surgeon without or with lesser implementation of saw-bones. Excellent quality of realtime interactive visualization simplifies the understanding of anatomy and the user interface has been optimized for the task in cooperation with the surgeons (Figure 4 b). The program accelerates total time of the operation planning. In comparison with the hand drawings approach, if the planning of one dimensional osteotomy takes about three hours, our software needs less then twenty minutes for an experienced user. The next version will extend wedge types including close and dome wedges. Some new features as a real-time tracking based on 3D ultrasound navigated system [2] will be coupled with an optical instrument tracking system to use this program not only for simulation but also for computer-assisted surgery.

5. Acknowledgements

The authors would like to thank Volume Graphics GmbH (www.volumegraphics.com) for their cooperation in combining their software with our application.

References

[1] P. Keppler, D. Moskalenko, O. Krivonos, F. Gebhard, L. Kinzl, J. Hesser, R. Männer, Computer Aided Correction of Bone Deformations. In: Proc. CAOS: Computer Assisted Orthopedic Surgery, Symposium, Davos, Switzerland, 2000.
[2] F. Gebhard, O. Krivonos, UC. Liener, P. Keppler, L. Kinzl, J. Hesser. Bone Extraction from Ultrasound Images and Surface Matching with CT. In: Proc. CAOS: Computer Assisted Orthopedic Surgery, Symposium, Davos, Switzerland, 2000.

Medicine Meets Virtual Reality 2001
J.D. Westwood et al. (Eds.)
IOS Press, 2001

Development of Virtual Environment
for Treating Acrophobia

Jeonghun Ku, Dongpyo Jang, Minbo Shin, Hangjoon jo, Heebum Ahn, Jaemin Lee, Baekhwan Cho,
Sun I. Kim
Department of Biomedical Engineering, College of Medicine, Hanyang University, Seoul, Korea

Abstract. Virtual Reality (VR) is a new technology that makes humans
communicate with computer. It allows the user to see, hear, feel and interact in a
three-dimensional virtual world created graphically. Virtual Reality Therapy (VRT),
based on this sophisticated technology, has been recently used in the treatment of
subjects diagnosed with acrophobia, a disorder that is characterized by marked
anxiety upon exposure to heights, avoidance of heights, and a resulting interference
in functioning. Conventional virtual reality system for the treatment of acrophobia
has a limitation in scope that it is based on over-costly devices or somewhat
unrealistic graphic scene. The goal of this study was to develop a inexpensive and
more realistic virtual environment for the exposure therapy of acrophobia. We
constructed two types virtual environment. One is constituted a bungee-jump tower
in the middle of a city. It includes the open lift surrounded by props beside tower
that allowed the patient to feel sense of heights. Another is composed of diving
boards which have various heights. It provides a view of a lower diving board and
people swimming in the pool to serve the patient stimuli upon exposure to heights.

1. Introduction

Acrophobia is classified as a specific phobia in the Diagnostic and Statistical Manual of
Mental Disorders[1]. People who have this disorder are characterized by marked anxiety
upon exposure to heights, avoidance of heights, and a resulting interference in functioning.
Behavior dysfunction involves interference with normal routine or interpersonal
relationships.

Currently, the advancement of computer and display technology allows the creation of
virtual reality environment which can evoke stimuli as same phobia as in real phobic.
Virtual reality therapy, based on this sophisticated technology, has recently been suggested
by a few studies for the treatment of specific phobia including acrophobia. VRT is based on
systematic desensitization, one of behavioral therapy. VRT provides stimuli for the patient
who cannot imagine well. VRT adds advantage of greater control over graded exposure
stimulus parameters as well as greater efficiency and economy in delivering the equivalent
of in vivo exposure within the therapist's office[2,3,4].

In the case of conventional virtual environment for acrophobia treatment, it was based on
over-costly devices or consisted of a low quality image in the realistic aspect. The goal of
this study was to develop inexpensive and more realistic virtual environment for exposure
therapy of acrophobia. It is based on inexpensive personal computer and it has two virtual

scenes which are constituted of the bungee-jump tower in the middle of the city and diving board in a swimming pool. The former includes the open lift surrounded by props beside a tower and the latter provides a view of lower diving boards and people who swim in the pool which allow the patient to feel realistic sense of heights.

2. Virtual Reality System Architecture

Software

Real-time virtual reality scene was designed with 3D modeling tools, Rhinoceros (Robert McNeel & Assoc.) and 3D Studio MAX(Kinetix). A simulation program was made with Visual C++ and DirectX 7.0 SDK(Software Development Kit) for real-time processing. 3D sound was added to the simulation for more immersiveness and the patient's height was designed for therapist to easily adjust.

Hardware

The virtual environment system for this study consists of a stereoscopic Head-Mounted Display (HMD) (ProView(tm) XL50, Kaiser Elector-Optics Inc., 1204H X 768V, 50 degree diagonal), an electro magnetic head tracker (FASTRAK, Polhemus, Inc.), 3D sound system. Real-time imagery was generated based on DirectX 3D accelerator (Elsa Inc., ErasorX graphic card), and it was executed on a Pentium-III 450MHz personal computer (128MB RAM).

3. Virtual environment scene

One of the advantages of virtual reality is that it is possible to make situation which is impossible or nonexistent in the real world. In other words, most fearful situation could be designed although there are little opportunities to come in contact with it in the real world. We construct two virtual environment scenes for treating acrophobia. One is a bungee-jump tower in a city, another is a diving board in swimming pool.

Bungee-jump tower in a city

A steel-frame building was constructed in the middle of the city. it was located after the model of Bungee-Jump building. The lift opened in every direction is added next to the frame. It can go up and down between 1st and 50th floor. The steel-frame building in the central area of a town can augment the fear of heights when the subject takes the lift. In order to increase reality, a road is lined with trees and cars are made to move away on the road.

Diving boards in a swimming pool

Diving boards were placed beside a swimming pool where people were swimming. The diving boards have 6 levels from 5 meters to 25 meters. A patient can be placed at any level. When that patient places at higher level, he can see the lower diving board. For the purpose of the more sense of presence, we let avatars walk around, swim and make a noise under the diving board.

4. Results

In this study, virtual environments for acrophobia treatment were developed focused on realistic visual and immersive environment. One is a bungee-jump tower in the mid-town, the other is diving board in swimming pool. Figure 1 is a snapshot that the patient was placed at 50th floor and looked lower scene that cars run on the road and trees are lined up. Figure 2 shows that the patient stands at level 4, looks at lower diving boards and swimming avatars.

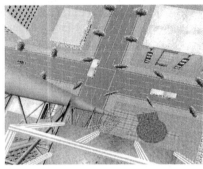 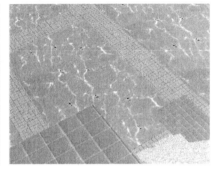

Fig. 1 Virtual Environment of Bungee-jump tower   **Fig. 2** Virtual Environment of diving board

Acknowledgments

This study was funded by the National Research Laboratory(NRL) Program at Korea Institute of Science & Technology Evaluation and Planning

5. References

[1] American Psychiatric Association, "Diagnostic and Statistical Manual of Mental Disorders(4th ed, rev)", Washington
[2] Strickland, D., Hodges, L. F., North, M. M., & Weghorst, S. "Overcoming Phobias by Virtual Exposure", Communications of the ACM, 1997, 40(8)
[3] Rothbaum, B. O., Hodges, L. F., Kooper, R., Opdyke, D., Williford, J. S., & North, M. "Virtual Reality Graded Exposure in the Treatment of Acrophobia: A Case Report. Behavior Therapy", 1995, 26, 547-554
[4] Rothabum, B. O., Hodges, L. F., Kooper, R., Opdyke, D., Williford, J. S., & North, M. "The efficacy of virtual reality graded exposure in the treatment of acrophobia" American Journal of Psychiatry, 1995, 152, 626-628

Medicine Meets Virtual Reality 2001
J.D. Westwood et al. (Eds.)
IOS Press, 2001

An endoscopic navigation system

Carsten Kübler, Jörg Raczkowsky and Heinz Wörn

*University of Karlsruhe (TH), Institute for Process Control and Robotics,
Kaiserstr. 12, 76128 Karlsruhe, Germany
{kuebler, rkowsky, woern }@ira.uka.de*

Abstract. Endoscopy is an important procedure for the diagnostic and therapy of various pathologies. We develop extensive and automated systems for this field. Due to application of these new systems, a patient is subject to considerably less strains, as opposed to prevailing commercial systems. The capability of such instruments, unlike the presently used systems, to independently follow anatomical peculiarities of the body means also a reduced risk of complications for a patient. A further advantage is that difficult to access regions deep inside the body, like the small intestine or peripheral parts of the bronchial tubes, can thus be reached. We use a complex navigation system for our new endoscopic system.

1. Introduction

Today there are several commercial localization systems for endoscopes which are denoted as navigation systems [1]. These localization systems displays the tip of a rigid endoscope in a preoperative acquired 3D-CT or 3D-MR-scan. The scans can be visualized 2D/3D and regions of interest can be preoperative marked and visualized. A simple navigation system for flexible endoscopes was developed to automate the endoscopy [2]. This system supports the physician to control the motion of a new tip driven endoscope in the colon and to automate the insertion of an endoscope.

The control for our endoscopic system is made automatic with a 6D-localisation system, a camera and contact sensors. This makes it possible for the physician to control the endoscope via a human-machine interface without using his own force, and to avoid many problems of today and future development, e.g., looping of the supply tube of an endoscope for the large intestine. The endoscope is driven in accordance with a new driving concept on the basis of fluid actuators or a magnetic probe [3].

2. Modelling

By fusion of all the sensor data in a relational data model, a model of the body inside by means of supplementary image processing. Amongst other things, it make possible to do a quick postoperative checkup. The relational model has been developed specially for endoscopy. In addition, the physician can intraoperatively see with this model what parts inside the body have already been examined. In this way, a complete examination of, e.g., bronchi can easily be proved.

Our navigation system consists of a module to generate a 3D-model of the examined region. This model is generated from the information of the relational data model and a general model of the examined region. The physician is able to mark a region in the 3D-model and the endoscope is automatically guided from the navigation system to the region.

3. System architecture

We use a modern PC workstation for our navigation system (see fig. 1). This system is used to store endoscopic video images combined with 6D-localization of the electromagnetic localization system. A raid system with two IDE harddisks is able to write the continuous stream of 21MB/s to a file.

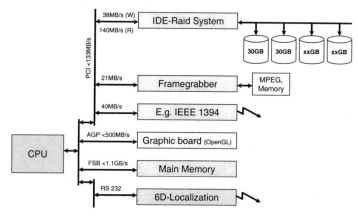

Figure 1: System architecture

The visualization of camera path in combination with video images is presented in fig. 2. The aim of the navigation system is to generate a 3D-modell of the tube (see fig. 3) and to find a marked region in spite of the motion of the examined tube in the body. The preconditions for reconstruction are a calibrated endoscope and an accurate 6D-localization system.

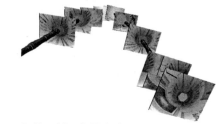

Figure 2: Combined 6D information and video images

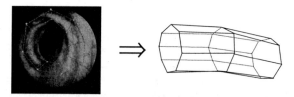

Figure 3: 3D reconstruction

4. Results

A few image filters to navigate a tip driven endoscope are already described in [4]. We need several more image filters in our navigation system which are adapted to endoscopic images. The output of the optical flow filter is presented in fig. 4. The optical flow image points out the pixels which are the dark center of the surrounding. The result was calculated out of 150 different directions for every pixel (see fig. 5). The advantage of this method is compared with the standard laplace filter.

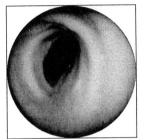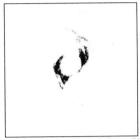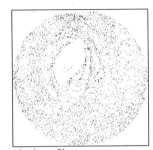

Figure 4: Endoscopic image, optical flow filter, laplace filter

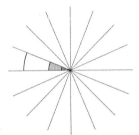

Figure 5: Optical flow - 16 directions per pixel

Acknowledgement

This work is performed at the IPR, Prof. H. Wörn. The research is being funded by the Ministry for Science, Research and Arts of Baden-Württemberg.

References

[1] Gunkel A.R., Thumfart W.F., Freysinger W., "Computerunterstützte 3D-Navigations-systeme - Überblick und Standortbestimmung", HNO 2/2000 48, Springer-Verlag, Page 75–90.

[2] Krishnan S.M., Kumar S. Yap C.J., Kassim M.I., Goh P.M.Y., "Computer-Assisted Intelligent Endoscopy". Proceedings of the 13th International Congress and Exhibition for Computer Assisted Radiology and Surgery - CARS'99, Page 156-160.

[3] Kübler C., Raczkowsky J., Wörn H., "Endoscopic Robots". Proceedings of the Third International Conference for Medical Image Computing and Computer-Assisted Intervention - MICCAI 2000, Page 949-955.

[4] Phee et al. "Automation of Colonoscopy Part II: Visual-Control Aspects". In: IEEE Engineering in Medicine and Biology 3 (1998), Page.81-88.

Medicine Meets Virtual Reality 2001
J.D. Westwood et al. (Eds.)
IOS Press, 2001

The Virtual Brain Project –
development of a neurosurgical simulator

Ole Vilhelm Larsen*, Jens Haase**, Lasse Riis Østergaard*, Kim Vang Hansen*, Henning Nielsen*

* Department of Medical Informatics and Image Analysis, Aalborg University, Denmark
** Department of Neurosurgery, Aalborg Hospital, Denmark

Abstract: As a joined project between Aalborg University and Aalborg Hospital Denmark, a neuro-surgical simulator is being developed. In this paper the objective of the project is outlined and an overview of the research activities within the project is given. Focus is on 3D modelling of the brain, deformable models and the development of two demonstrators, including one for training of punctuation of ventricle using visual and haptic feedback.

1. Background

The use of simulators in education and training has been known for many years in areas such as air and space pilot training and training for military vehicles [1]. In recent years, work within surgery simulation has also been reported. The BDI (Boston Dynamics Inc.) surgical simulator allows the user to control a virtual needle and a thread to perform a simulated end-to-end anastomosi [2]. Examples of other surgical simulators are the Karlsruhe Endoscopic Surgery Trainer [3] and the Epidaure project at INRIA [4].

Neurosurgical procedures of high complexity involve technical- and very refined surgical skills. Such skills are traditionally slowly developed over years of clinical practice. Continuous rehearsal of the surgical details results in basic surgical manipulations becoming automatisms. Surgical interventions are performed needing less "mental awareness", making the surgery safer. It is becoming increasingly difficult for young neurosurgeons to get the necessary practice. Inspired by the success of flight simulators, neurosurgery simulation seems to provide an alternative as a means of rehearsing surgical procedures.

The Virtual Brain Project is a national Danish collaboration between Aalborg University and Aalborg Hospital aimed at developing surgery simulation systems for neurosurgery for both educational and preoperative planning purposes. This paper gives an overview of the major activities undertaken by the project in the ongoing process of developing a simulator.

2. Neurosurgical simulation

The neurosurgical simulator being developed is directed towards both educational and preoperative purposes.

The educational system is targeted at young surgeons during their years of basic training. The system should allow for the surgeon to rehearse the sequence of steps in a given surgical procedure and to rehearse individual steps until perfection. Each step requires extensive skills in hand-eye coordination and coordination between different surgical tools. If the simulator is to be flexible it must be able to operate on different difficulty levels. At the bottom level, surgical procedures are made of standard steps with no complications added during surgery and at the top level several complications such as bleedings can occur during simulation. Just as in computer games, the surgeon advances through the different levels based on the performance at the previous level. It is considered important that the user can continuously perform a kind of self-test to measure his increase in surgery performance. Therefore for each step an expert must specify the correct performance and a score should be computed based on the difference between the correct action and the one performed by the young surgeon. Surgery simulation will initially focus on single users but holds the possibility to allow for simulation performed by a team of surgeons and nurses working together on the same patient. Simulation for educational purpose can be done on 3D models of a standard brain.

The preoperative system is designed to help the skilled surgeon in planning the surgical procedure prior to surgery on a real patient. This requires a patient specific 3D model of the brain. With such a model it is possible to plan the size and location of the skull opening and the trajectories to take to get to the target area. One of the very difficult tasks involved in surgery planning today is the mental construction of 3D structures of the brain based on a set of 2D slices. Surgery simulation will allow for a much more realistic and detailed assessment of the structures waiting to be discovered during surgery.

For both the educational and the preoperative system it is considered very important that the user is provided with both a visual and a haptic feedback.

3. 3D Modelling

The core of the simulator is a 3D model of the brain. We have decided to focus on modelling the brain surface, the cerebral vasculature and the tissue types i.e. gray matter, white matter and CSF. The goal is patient specific modelling and therefore emphasis has been placed on developing automatic procedures.

Based on proton density (PD) weighted magnetic resonance (MR) images, brain surface extraction is performed [5], which removes non-brain tissue. An example of the obtainable results is given in Figure 1a and 1b.

The result from the brain surface extraction (brain-only volume) is used as input to an unsupervised classification algorithm by which the brain is segmented into gray matter, white matter and CSF. The algorithm is a fuzzy c-means clustering algorithm [6], which iteratively subdivides the set of all voxels into 3 clusters, one for each tissue type, based on the intensity values in co-registered T1, T2 and PD MR images. In Figure 1c an example of a segmented slice is given and in Figure 1d a surface model of the cortical gray matter is shown.

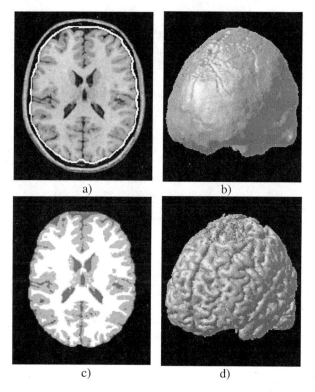

Figure 1: a) PD MR image with the contour of a brain surface extraction b) 3D surface of a brain surface extraction c) Result of fuzzy c-means segmentation into gray matter, white matter and CSF
d) 3D surface of cortical gray matter

The vasculature of the human brain has been given special attention since a large subset of neurosurgical procedures are related to malformations of the blood vessels. Furthermore, in any brain surgery great care must be taken not to get close to the major blood vessels in order not to damage the blood supply to the brain tissue.

Even though special angiographic imaging modalities exist for enhancing the blood vessels it has been decided to build the model of the vasculature on standard proton density weighted MR images. These images have been acquired using spin-echo whereby the blood vessels appear as dark structures. Currently, we have access to more than 150 data sets.

At present, special focus has been given to the internal carotid arteries, the middle cerebral arteries with all their branches, the proximal part of the anterior cerebral arteries, the anterior communicating artery, the vertebral arteries, the basilar artery, and the posterior cerebral arteries. Veins and sinuses have been disregarded.

The approach taken for modelling the vasculature utilizes general knowledge about the shape and size of the cerebral vasculature and is divided into multiscale vessel enhancement filtering, centre-line extraction, and boundary modelling [8].

To improve the discrimination between blood vessels and other tissue a filtering method that enhances dark tubular structures is used as a pre-processing step [9].

The purpose of the centre-line extraction process is to roughly estimate the centre-line of the vessel-tree involving both segmentation, and skeletonization. The skeleton is split into line segments with end points corresponding to branching points and termination points. The boundary modelling is currently carried out by simply generating cylinders around the skeleton segments. In Figure 2 results of the filtering and the 3D modelling of the vessels are shown.

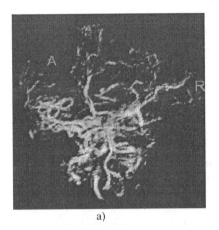 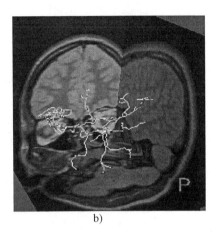

a)   b)

Figure 2: a) Volume rendered view of filtering result, b) 3D surface models

To improve segmentation of the vessels when doing patient specific modelling we are currently developing a statistical probability anatomy map (SPAM) for the above-mentioned bloodvessels. The cerebral vasculature has been extracted from more than 150 subjects using the approach described above. For each subject an expert identified the vessels.

The data is from the ICBM database [9] and is registered in Talairach space so data can be joined directly in a probability map. Apart from giving valuable documentation of the variability of the human cerebral vasculature, the SPAM will be used to improve the modelling process in the future by adding a priori information.

4. Deformable models

Surgery simulation is to a large extent manipulations of the 3D model of the brain. The fundamental requirements of a surgery simulator are modelling of deformations, cutting in tissue and also the ability to calculate a force feedback sensation. Neurosurgery simulation requires a mathematical model of the geometric and elastic properties of the entire brain. The challenge is to obtain both real-time deformation and high accuracy.

It can be argued that the following requirements are important in the development of deformable models of human tissue:

1. The deformations should be physically realistic.
2. The models should allow for cutting.
3. Haptic feedback
4. Fast calculation of deformations to allow for real-time simulations

To obtain the most realistic simulation, the model must approximate the physical tissue as well as possible and the deformations should be as similar to deformations of real tissue as possible. The elastic model should be both visual and haptic convincing.

If cutting should be performed, surface based models can not be used, since these models are empty inside and a cut will not open up for any underlying tissue. Cutting requires volumetric models of the tissue.

The Finite Element Method (FEM), which produces local mesh-based models, has been used for different types of surgery simulation, i.e. the liver [4], and the gal bladder [3].

Real-time simulation is a very challenging requirement; it requires speed-up algorithms, pre-calculations or simplified models. Methods using explicit inversion of the stiffness matrix in order to obtain interactive deformations have already been demonstrated [10]. Also extensive use of pre-calculation on a simplified model of liver has been used [4]. This, however, implies that the possibilities of topological changes such as cutting are lost.

We have decided to allow for a differentiation of the spatial and temporal accuracy in different parts of the model [11]. The differentiation is obtained by applying a dynamic FE sub-model with high accuracy to the area around the target point and a static FE sub-model with less accuracy for the remaining parts. The area with high accuracy is manually pointed out by the user as a special Region-Of-Interest, ROI. The different models are integrated into one FE model for the brain using a well-known technique called Condensation [12].

Experimental work has been conducted to evaluate the effect of having areas with different accuracy. Based on a set of MR slices a full dynamic FE mesh consisting of 578 nodes was generated for the entire brain. Furthermore, a condensed version consisting of only 200 nodes was constructed. Assuming that the full dynamic system calculates the correct deformation, it is possible to measure the spatial difference between the results of a deformation. The spatial difference is measured as the Euclidean distance between all common nodes in the models. Tests have shown that for the condensed version a frame rate of 35 could be obtained and deformations gave rise to a max error of 1.7 mm. The judgement of the neurosurgical staff of the Virtual Brain project was that the speed was sufficient to allow for a perception of real-time deformation and that the deformations themselves were looking realistic.

To allow for calculating of both deformation and haptic feedback we have started to use iterative methods for solving the FE model. The direct inversion of the matrix gives accurate deformations where as the iterative methods only converge towards the right deformation. More iterations give a more accurate result but a slower frame rate. Choosing a suitable number of iterations is a trade off between fast deformations and accuracy. Preliminary results using iterative methods and including haptic feedback look promising.

Both the visual and the haptic feedback are very computational demanding and with high, but limited, computer power any realistic modelling becomes a trade off between visual feedback and haptic feedback. We are currently investigating if any of the inputs is dominating. Studies documented in the literature show that for normal persons visual inputs dominate haptic input [13]. The nature of a surgeon's skill however gives rise to expectations that it might be different for surgeons. Experiments are currently being done.

5. Demonstrator

Due to the complexity of implementing a complete simulator, an intermediary step, the demonstrator unit has been developed. The unit serves as test-bed for bringing the research results within 3D modelling and deformable models together and for establishing the interaction with the user. The test-bed has also proven to be a good tool in the very important dialog between surgeons and engineers.

A demonstrator has been build around the Dextroscope Virtual Reality system from Volume Interaction. Dextroscope provides good VR immersion, in particular a more intuitive user interface compared to the traditional screen and mouse setup. The demonstrator includes a framework for choosing different surgical procedures, each procedure being broken down in a number of steps, each of which can be simulated individually. It also provides procedures for 3D visualisation and manipulation of the initial MR data, e.g. stepping through individual slices, user controlled reslicing, surface rendering etc. Several surgical tools have been implemented; a drilling device for creating an opening in the skull, scalpel for cutting in tissue, spatulas for pushing brain tissue around and ultrasound aspirators for removal of soft tissue. The system is currently limited to using only one tool at any given time. The current choice of tools is controlled through a 3D menu. The tools can interact freely with the brain model.

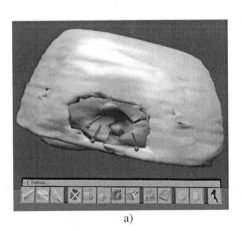
a)

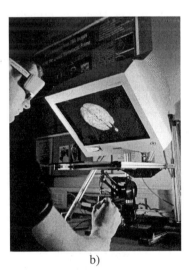
b)

Figure 3: a) Screen shot from the demonstrator, retraction of brain tissue to gain access to a tumour.
b) Simulator set-up including stereovision and haptic feedback.

In its current implementation, only a simple brain model containing skull, brain tissue and a tumour is available. See Figure 3a for a screen dump from a training session where a surgeon is pushing tissue to gain access to a tumour.

For surgery simulation to be any near the real experience it is necessary that the surgeon can feel the forces involved in the interaction between the instruments and the skull, brain, etc. A new demonstrator is currently being developed based upon a VR display system from ReachIn, which allows for haptic feedback. It utilizes a Phantom 1.0 force-feedback device which defines a 13cm*18 cm*21cm space where a stylus can be moved around with six degrees of freedom and give the user a haptic feedback with three degrees of freedom. The purpose of this demonstrator is to simulate the punctuation of the ventricle. Based on the 3D model of the brain, the system simulates the resistance from the needle penetration. During tissue penetration the reaction force is computed according to the different tissue types that the needle is penetrating. The visual perception of the depth of the needle and the change in the resistance force alert the surgeon that the target is reached. Figure 3b. shows the use of the demonstrator with haptic feedback.

6. Conclusion

The Virtual Brain Project is aimed at developing surgery simulation for neurosurgical procedures. Focus is on patient specific 3D models, deformable models and demonstrator systems with both visual and haptic feedback. Due to the huge complexity of the human brain and the level of accuracy required for neurosurgery, general simulation with high realism is years into the future awaiting a further rise in computer power. Simpler versions in terms of level of details developed for specific surgical procedures, but still with good educational effect, will become available within the next 1-2 years.

7. References

1. B.F. Goldiez, History of Networked Simulations. In: T.L. Clarke (Eds), Distributed Interactive Simulation Systems for Simulation and Training in the Aerospace Environment. SPIE Optical Engineering Press, 1995, pp 39-58.
2. R. O'Toole et al., Assessing Skill and Learning in Surgeons and Medical Students Using Force Feedback Surgical Simulator, Proceedings of the First International Conference on Medical Image Computing and Computer-Assisted Intervention MICCAI'98, LNCS 1496, pp 899-909, 1998.
3. U. Kuhn et al , The Karlsruhe Endoscopic Surgery Trainer - A Virtual Reality" based Training Systemfor Minimal Invasive Surgery, Computer Assisted Radiology, 1996.
4. S. Cotin and H. Delingette and N. Ayache, Volumetric Deformable Models for Simulation of Laparoscopic Surgery, in Computer Assisted Radiology, 1996.
5. S. Sandor and R. Leahy, Surface-Based Labeling of Cortical Anatomy Using a Deformable Atlas, IEEE Transactions on Medical Imaging, vol. 16, no. 1, pp. 41-54, 1997.
6. J.C. Bezdek, L.O. Hall, and L.P. Clarke, Review of MR image segmentation techniques using pattern recognition, Medical Physics, vol. 20, no. 4, pp. 1033-1048, 1993.
7. A.F. Frangi, W.J. Niessen, K.L. Vincken, and M.A. Viergever, Multiscale Vessel Enhancement Filtering, Proceedings of the First International Conference on Medical Image Computing and Computer-Assisted Intervention MICCAI'98, LNCS 1496, pp. 130-137, 1998.
8. L.R. Østergaard, O.V. Larsen, J. Haase, F. Van Meer, A.C. Evans , and D.L. Collins, Knowledge-based Extraction of Cerebral Vasculature from Anatomical MRI, Medical Imaging, February 17-23, 2001, San Diego, California, USA.
9. J.C. Mazziotta, A.W. Toga, A.C. Evans, P. Fox, and J. Lancaster, A probabilistic atlas of the human brain: theory and rationale for its development, NeuroImage, vol. 2, no. 2, pp. 89-101, 1995.
10. M. Bro-Nielsen, Finite element modeling in Surgery Simulation, Journal of the IEEE, vol 86, no 3, pp. 490-503, 1998.
11. Using Region-of-interest based Finite Element Modelling for Brain-Surgery Simulation, Kim Vang Hansen, Ole Vilhelm Larsen, Proceedings of the First International Conference on Medical Image Computing and Computer-Assisted Intervention MICCAI'98, LNCS 1496, pp 305-316, 1998.
12. Robert D Cook and David S. Malkus and Michael E. Plesha, Concepts and Applications of Finite Element Analysis, third edition, John Wiley & Sons, 1989.
13. M.A. Srinivasan and C. Basdogan, Haptics in virtual environments : taxonomy, research status, and challenges, Computers and Graphics (Special Issue on "Haptic Displays in Virtual Environments), Vol 21, no 4, 1997.

Medicine Meets Virtual Reality 2001
J.D. Westwood et al. (Eds.)
IOS Press, 2001

An Open and Flexible Framework for Computer Aided Surgical Training

Anders Larsson

Surgical Science AB, Medicinaregatan 3A, 413 46 Gothenburg, Sweden

Abstract

During the past year we have developed a new surgical skills training application called LapSim. We intend to describe the design, architecture and concepts of the software framework we have developed concurrently with the application. The framework is based on the concept of a classroom with students and teachers. Students, courses and results are stored in a centralized database and can be retrieved for review or modification. The students can also monitor their progress relative to other students or experts.

1 Introduction

This paper presents the design and architecture of the framework we have developed during the past year as part of the LapSim surgical skills training application. The LapSim project is designed to fill the educational need of junior surgeons or surgeons who are approaching minimally invasive techniques for the first time.

2 Architecture

We modeled the framework after a classroom model, a number of training systems are made available in a classroom. The students attend a course their teacher has designed. The teacher is able to manage students in the system and design courses. Courses are divided into two parts, a training part and an exam part. The training part of a course is a set of ordered tasks that the students have to perform. The teacher can set thresholds on the results that the students have to achieve before they can move on to the next task. The structure of the exam is very similar to the training program, the difference is that if the student does not reach the goals set by the teacher for a specific task they fail the entire exam and must ask for a second chance. When the exam has been passed the student have completed the course.

2.1 Database

To implement the classroom model we store all information in a centralized database. The database is implemented using a Standard Query Language (SQL) compliant Database Management System (DBMS) [2]. In our case we have chosen the PostgreSQL relational DBMS. The classroom model is implemented using a set of tables described in SQL statements on the database server. SQL is also used by the framework to query the database for students, results and course information.

2.2 Graphical User Interface

Since our approach is intended to be open and flexible to future changes of hardware platform or operative system we chose to build the GUI of our framework using the Java programming language [1] and its associated set of libraries and tools. The GUI is divided into two parts, the student mode and the more advanced teacher mode.

2.2.1 Student GUI

The student GUI contains all information that is necessary for the student. It enables the student to select a course from a list of the courses the student is registered on. When the student has selected a course he or she can train or try the exam, the latter is only available if the student has completed the training program.

2.2.2 Teacher GUI

The teacher needs to be able to perform administrative tasks, these tasks include managing the students and designing and trying out courses and exams. When managing students the teacher uses the GUI to add and remove students in the database and assign them to courses. Groups of students can be created allowing easier and faster management. The training program is created by selecting one of the tasks that is available in the application, the task is then added to the schedule. The order and number of tasks can be changed, each task in the schedule can also be customized. The teacher can change the parameters interactively for each task. When the parameters are changed the results are immediately shown in the configuration view. The teacher can try out the task with the current set of parameters. Thresholds can be set for each task, this means that the student must achieve results within the thresholds before they can advance to the next task. Thresholds are also used in the exam part of a course, if the student does not achieve the levels of performance required by the threshold settings he or she will fail the course.

2.3 Visualization

To accommodate realistic and fast graphics we have chosen to use OpenGL [4] as our development library. To describe surface properties and visual effects, we have implemented a simple language. This gives us the benefit of being able to change most visual aspects of the simulation without having to change the source code of the application.

2.4 Simulation

Each task is divided into two separate components, a few Java classes and a simulation component which is implemented in C++ [3]. The Java classes are used for connectivity between the framework and the C++ code as well as providing a configuration GUI for the task. The simulation component is programmed in the C++ language and compiled into native machine dependent instructions. This is necessary for obtaining maximum speed from the simulation. The simulation itself is done using a multi threaded design, which utilizes both processors. One processor handles the simulation logic, rendering and all auxiliary tasks such as the GUI. The second processor is dedicated to force feedback computations. This design is necessary since force feedback has high computational demands. The computational load stems from the fact that the system needs to update the forces at a frequency of 1kHz. This high update frequency is required for a realistic tactile feedback.

3 Results and Conclusions

The framework has proven to be flexible and powerful. The entire user interface needs no porting at all when one changes to a platform already supported by Java. The framework has been tested during a validation study. During the study the LapSim application was used for training a group of medical students. The training program was conducted during five weeks last autumn. After having completed the training period the students were evaluated on a pig model.

References

[1] Ken Arnold, James Gosling, and David Holmes. *The Java Programming Language.* Addison-Wesley, 3rd edition, 2000.

[2] Ramez Elmasri and Shamkant B. Navathe. *Fundamentals of Database Systems.* Benjamin-Cummings, 2nd edition, 1994.

[3] B. Stroustrup. *The C++ Programming Language.* Addison-Wesley, 3rd edition, 1997.

[4] Mason Woo, OpenGL Architectural Review Board, Jackie Neider, Tom Davis, and Dave Shreiner. *The OpenGL Programming Guide, The Official Guide to Learning OpenGL Version 1.2.* Addison-Wesley, 3rd edition, 1999.

Medicine Meets Virtual Reality 2001
J.D. Westwood et al. (Eds.)
IOS Press, 2001

Intracorporeal Suturing and Knot Tying in Surgical Simulation

Anders Larsson

Surgical Science AB, Medicinaregatan 3A, 413 46 Gothenburg, Sweden

Abstract

Intracorporeal suturing and knot tying is one of the most difficult tasks to perform during minimally invasive surgery. To master these tasks the student requires extensive training in a real or simulated environment. Realistic simulation of suturing and knot tying is a challenging task, the dynamic behaviors of the needle and thread are complicated to calculate efficiently in real time. We present our approach to simulated training of intracorporeal suturing and knot tying as well as our method for performance assessment. Different algorithms for physical modeling of suture thread dynamics are examined and evaluated.

1 Introduction

With the introduction of minimally invasive techniques in surgery new forms of training for junior surgeons and more experienced practitioners of conventional surgery have become necessary. Many of the minimally invasive techniques such as laparoscopy and artroscopy uses a camera image displayed on a monitor to give visual feedback to the surgeon. This makes computer simulation a tractable form of education for minimally invasive techniques. Some tasks such as suturing and knot tying are especially difficult when done minimally invasive. Two graspers or needle drivers are inserted in ports. One grasper brings with a suture needle with an attached piece of thread. The surgeon performs suturing by placing stitches, after the stitch has been placed the surgeon must tie a knot using the loose end of the thread and the needle end. During this maneuver the surgeon performs intricate movements with the instrument in order to wind up the thread on the instrument and forming a knot that is tight and secure. This complex task is extremely difficult and requires extensive training. This paper describes how we have tried to model this complex task in a computer simulation.

2 Background

We have developed a surgical skills training application that contains a number of different tasks which explain and teach basic skills, for instance, spatial navigation, camera handling.

Also more advanced tasks like suturing and knot tying are included. However, these tasks require very sophisticated simulation methods to behave and feel realistic. During the past year we have evaluated and implemented several different methods for simulation of suturing and knot tying. We intend to describe these and give directions for more detailed study.

3   Previous Work

Surgical simulation is a new and exiting area of research and education and not much has been published regarding simulation of suturing and knot tying. In computer graphics several related areas are studied. Here we can get ideas that carry more or less directly over to surgical simulation. For instance, modeling hair [6, 3, 11], cables [5] and cloth [2, 1, 10].

4   Methods

We have based our simulation on the mass spring method common in cloth simulation [2]. The idea is that we imagine our garment or thread in this case to be built by small point masses or particles, connected to each other with springs. This is nice since point masses do not have inertia and other properties found in rigid bodies. Each mass point is described by its mass m and a position x. On each particle gravity and other forces act which we sum up and denote F.

We describe the thread by a vector x of N points $x_i = [x_i, y_i, z_i] \in R^3$, where $[x_i, y_i, z_i]$ are the coordinates of x_i. We think of x_1 as the beginning of the thread, x_N as the end, and x_i is connected to x_{i+1}. Further each point has a mass vector $m_i = [m_i, m_i, m_i] \in R^3$ and we let M denote the $3N \times 3N$ mass matrix with diagonal $[m_1, m_1, m_1, m_2, \ldots m_n]$. The motion of a thread is described by the second order ordinary differential equation

$$\ddot{x} = M^{-1}F(x, \dot{x}). \tag{1}$$

For the numerical solution of this differential equation it is convenient to introduce the velocity $v = \dot{x}$ as an extra unknown and write the second order equation in first order form

$$\begin{bmatrix} \dot{x} \\ \dot{v} \end{bmatrix} = \begin{bmatrix} v \\ M^{-1}F(x, v) \end{bmatrix}. \tag{2}$$

By solving this system of equations each time step we get the motion of the simulated thread. Since this is an ordinary differential equation we must integrate it. There are two common methods, explicit and implicit integration described below.

4.1   Explicit Integration

The easiest form of integrator to implement is the forward Euler method which is an explicit method. The forward Euler method takes the form

$$\delta x = \delta t v, \quad \delta v = \delta t F(x, v) \tag{3}$$

Note that these expressions can be directly evaluated without solving any equations, hence the name explicit. Unfortunately the Euler method is not very accurate. We have used a fourth order Runge-Kutta integrator [9] for our explicit integration. We noticed that the system became much more stable and less visual artifacts was seen when we replaced the standard Euler with the Runge-Kutta method.

The mass-spring systems are dependent on the strength of the springs to hold the system together. When modeling suture thread it is difficult not to get a rubber like thread. This is due to the fact that for the system to remain stable we cannot set arbitrary strong spring forces between the particles. If we increase the spring strength the system of equations become stiff and difficult to solve with an explicit integrator. Therefore we have used the explicit method in situations where soft tissues and vessels have been modeled. Provot [10] has presented a method that tries to correct the problem with low spring coefficients by using a correction step after the integration has taken place. After each integration step the method finds the springs which are over-elongated and by moving the particles connected to those springs together the method removes the stretch from the system. We have implemented the method and it performs very well, but the convergence properties of the method is not known. We suspect it can be difficult to integrate the post modification step in a situation where we have complex interaction between the suture thread and objects. In those cases it is important that the particles are in contact with the surface and it does not seem easy to maintain contact constraints when using post integration position correction.

4.2   Implicit Integration

Some differential equations are what is called stiff equations. Explicit methods does not handle stiff equations very well unless we take short time steps, unfortunately this does mean that the simulation will become very slow. To counter this we can use implicit methods [9] the benefit is that we get greater stability and can take much larger steps. Baraff and Witkin presented a paper at SIGGRAPH '98 [1] that used implicit integration to achieve stable and fast simulation of complex garments. This method has since been used in commercial packages such as Alias Wavefronts Maya cloth.

When using the implicit method by Baraff we use the "backward Euler" method. The backward Euler method takes the form

$$\delta x = \delta t(v + \delta v), \quad \delta v = \delta t F(x + \delta x, v + \delta v) \tag{4}$$

Here the unknown δx and δv occur on the right hand side and thus a system of equations need to be solved to obtain δx and δv. To solve the system of equations in the backward Euler method, we approximate the nonlinear equations with linear equations using Taylors formula as follows

$$F(x + \delta x, v + \delta v) = F(x, v) + \frac{\partial F}{\partial x}(x, v)\delta x + \frac{\partial F}{\partial v}(x, v)\delta v. \tag{5}$$

Substituting this expression and $\delta x = \delta t(v + \delta v)$ into $\delta v = \delta t F(x + \delta x, v + \delta v)$ gives the equation

$$\left(I - \delta t M^{-1} \frac{\partial F}{\partial v} - \delta t^2 M^{-1} \frac{\partial F}{\partial x} \right) \delta v = \delta t M^{-1} \left(F + \delta t \frac{\partial F}{\partial x} v \right), \tag{6}$$

with the obvious simplified notation. This is a linear system of equations of the form

$$A \delta v = b, \tag{7}$$

where A and b are defined by the expressions (6). This linear system can be solved efficiently using an iterative method, for instance the conjugate gradient method. We have implemented the implicit method and it performs well for our application, the system is solved with few iterations and by exploiting the sparse structure of the matrices we achieve real-time frame rates. The added advantage is that the system behaves more naturally due to the stiffer springs the implicit method enables us to use. We are confident that using implicit methods is the best method for modeling suture threads and similar stiff materials. Unfortunately the method is not trivial to implement and very difficult to debug, a paper by Macri [7] gives a very good explanation of Baraff's method, we refer the interested reader to Macri's and Baraff's papers for more information on the implicit method.

4.3 Collision Detection

When performing simulation it is necessary to take collisions into account. In the case of a suture thread there are complex interactions between the thread and instruments and also the thread itself during knot tying. We have used hierarchical bounding boxes to perform fast culling and collision detection. The boxes are also used to find candidate thread segments for self intersection. The candidates are collected and a closest distance between them are calculated. If the distance is beneath a small threshold we insert an extra spring force between those two segments, note that it is important to continuously track how the colliding segments approach, if we don't do this the thin thread can fall through it self during the time step. When the suture thread collides with a surface or an object we restrict the movement of the thread in the penetrating direction but otherwise it can move freely across or from the surface. Sometimes it is necessary to constrain a point on the thread to a surface or an object such as the needle.

Constraining a particle to a point is done by giving the particle infinite mass, this locks the particle in its current position. Surface constraints are done in the same way, since the mass is described in three dimensions $m_i = [m_i, m_i, m_i] \in R^3$ we can easily control in which direction the particle can accelerate, refer to Baraff's paper [1] for more information. Further information on collision detection can be found in [3, 11, 6].

4.4 Rendering

The standard Phong shading model implemented in OpenGL is not suited well for rendering thin suture thread. Tube like objects are best rendered using an anisotropic shading model, which takes into account that some objects or materials have surface properties that scatter incoming light differently depending on the incoming light direction. Examples of such shading models are described in Poulin and Fournier's paper [8] and by Ken-ichi and Yoshiaki's paper [6]. We use an anisotropic lighting model calculated for each particle. The thread is then rendered by connecting each particle with a line segment. The line segments are shaded using the color we compute using our shading model.

4.5   Knot Detection

When training how to tie a knot it is important that the students learn the right instrument movements. After the student has finished the knot the system should ideally try to evaluate if the shape of the knot is correct or not. Our method breaks up the knot tying process into a sequence of moves and configurations that must be completed, after all steps are completed the knot is detected as correct. It would be nice to have an algorithm that could compare two different knots and tell us if they are equivalent but that is very difficult to calculate. Grzeszczuk et al [4] published a paper on an algorithm which does simplification of mathematical knots, unfortunately it takes several days to simplify a knot and therefore it is not feasible to use it for our purposes.

5   Results

We have concluded that the best results are obtained using implicit methods and in particular the one described by Baraff [1] and by Macri [7]. The method has proven to be stable and accurate and yields good results. The drawback is its mathematical complexity and its difficult implementation. The explicit methods are suitable for soft objects that is not dependent on stiff springs. The main benefit of the explicit methods are their simplicity. The forward Euler method is easy to integrate with collision detection and post particle modifications such as Provot's [10].

6   Conclusion

We have presented the different methods we evaluated and implemented as part of the research for our surgical skills training application LapSim. The implicit method described by Baraff [1] has been used successfully as the simulation behind our suture and knot-tying exercises and we have used the explicit method with a Runge-Kutta solver for simulating a soft blood vessel in LapSim.

References

[1] David Baraff and Andrew Witkin. Large steps in cloth simulation. *Proceedings of SIG-GRAPH 98*, pages 43–54, July 1998. ISBN 0-89791-999-8. Held in Orlando, Florida.

[2] David E. Breen, Donald H. House, and Phillip H. Getto. A particle-based computational model of cloth draping behavior. *Scientific Visualization of Physical Phenomena (Proceedings of CG International '91)*, pages 113–134, 1991.

[3] Agnes Daldegan, Nadia Magnenat Thalmann, Tsuneya Kurihara, and Daniel Thalmann. An integrated system for modeling, animating and rendering hair. *Computer Graphics Forum (Eurographics '93)*, 12(3):211–221, 1993. Held in Oxford, UK.

[4] Robert P. Grzezczuk, Milana Huang, and Louis H. Kauffman. Physically-based stochastic simplification of mathematical knots. *IEEE Transactions on Visualization and Computer Graphics*, 3(3):262–272, July–September 1997.

[5] Elke Hergenrther and Patrick Dhne. Real-time virtual cables bsased on kinematic simulation. In *WSCG '2000*, February 2000.

[6] Ken ichi Anjyo, Yoshiaki Usami, and Tsuneya Kurihara. A simple method for extracting the natural beauty of hair. *Computer Graphics (Proceedings of SIGGRAPH 92)*, 26(2):111–120, July 1992. ISBN 0-201-51585-7. Held in Chicago, Illinois.

[7] Dean P. Macri. Real-time cloth. In *Game Developers Conference 2000*, 2000.

[8] Pierre Poulin and Alain Fournier. A model for anisotropic reflection. *Computer Graphics*, 24(4):273–282, August 1990.

[9] William H. Press, Brian P. Flannery, Saul A. Teukolsky, and William T. Vetterling. *Numerical Recipes: The Art of Scientific Computing*. Cambridge University Press, Cambridge (UK) and New York, 2nd edition, 1992.

[10] Xavier Provot. Deformation constraints in a mass-spring model to describe rigid cloth behavior. *Graphics Interface '95*, pages 147–154, May 1995. ISBN 0-9695338-4-5.

[11] N. M. Thalmann, S. Carion, M. Courchesne, P. Volino, and Y. Wu. Virtual clothes, hair and skin for beautiful top models. *Computer Graphics International 1996*, 1996.

Medicine Meets Virtual Reality 2001
J.D. Westwood et al. (Eds.)
IOS Press, 2001

Automatic Skeleton Generation for Visualizing 3D, Time-dependent Fluid Flows: Application to the Virtual Aneurysm

Daren Lee, Daniel J. Valentino[†], Gary R. Duckwiler[†], Walter J. Karplus

Department of Computer Sciences
Department of Radiological Sciences[†]
University of California, Los Angeles 90095

{dalee@cs.ucla.edu, djv@ucla.edu,
gduckwiler@mednet.ucla.edu, karplus@cs.ucla.edu}

Abstract

Intracranial aneurysms are the primary cause of non-traumatic subarachnoid hemorrhage. Difficulties in identifying which aneurysms will grow and rupture arise because the physicians lack important anatomic and hemodynamic information. Through simulation, this data can be captured, but visualization of large simulated data sets becomes cumbersome, often resulting in visual clutter and ambiguity. To address these visualization issues, we developed an algorithm that extracts a skeleton of the patterns in 3D, time-dependent blood flow. The algorithm decomposes the blood flow into "bare-bones" components that can be visualized individually or superimposed together to formulate an understanding of the flow patterns in the aneurysm.

1 Introduction

Intracranial aneurysms are sacculations arising from a weakened portion of a cerebral artery. Identifying which aneurysms will grow and rupture is quite difficult. Difficulties arise because the vital aneurysm anatomic and hemodynamic data needed for decision making is often impossible to obtain with medical imaging techniques. Computational fluid dynamics systems have been developed to simulate this blood flow in aneurysms. Visualization of the large, complex volumes of data generated by these simulations is a highly intensive, interactive, and iterative process. Extracting and selecting interesting features in the data is often a very time-consuming process [11]. Insightful interpretations can be reached but require much visualization knowledge on the physician's part.

In our prior work we designed a simulation of brain hemodynamics and developed a system for visualizing blood flow, the Virtual Aneurysm [4]. In this work we extend our virtual-reality environment to address the visualization issues. The goal is to decompose the flow into components that share common behavior. These "bare-bones" components can then be analyzed individually or superimposed together to formulate an understanding of the blood flow patterns in the aneurysm. With this global understanding in mind, the physician can then perform a more effective detailed analysis of local behavior with other visualization tools. By providing this important anatomic and blood flow data to the physician, more informative treatment decisions can be made.

1.1 Related Work

Mathematical approaches have been proposed that visualize the vector fields of fluid flow. Helman and Hesselink [5, 6, 7] developed a method that analyzes critical points, to construct a flow topology. The 2D application of this method works well in general time-independent and time-dependent cases but the 3D application is limited to time-independent flow topology around a surface body. Ford [3] used critical points to estimate the coefficients of nonlinear differential equations to model the flow. Once these nonlinear models are known, critical flow lines can be visualized. This method is shown to work for 2D, time-independent cases but is not easily extended to 3D, time-dependent data.

Other research has concentrated on extracting the structural topology or skeleton of objects. Blum, whose motivation was the physiology of visual perception, introduced the concept of a skeleton and the medial axis transformation [2]. Montanari [8, 9] developed a completely analytical procedure for finding the skeleton based on Blum's medial axis transformation. Montanari's work, however, was intended for shapes extracted from 2D images. The concept of the skeleton was extended to 3D with thinning, a process which removes points that do not change the topology of the object [1, 10]. In this way, the 3D object is thinned until a skeleton remains. This approach is useful for continuous, volumetric data.

2 Skeleton Generation

A pathline is the trajectory of a massless particle released in the flow. By seeding many pathlines in the field, the flow patterns can be visualized. In 3D, however, using too many lines results in visual clutter and finding seed points that lead to descriptive lines is difficult [11]. Our approach analyzes these particle paths and reduces them to a characteristic representation or skeleton of the flow field.

The aim of the algorithm is to reduce the visual complexity of the pathlines while retaining the structure and information of the original data. To retain the overall structure, the global behavior of the pathlines needs to be taken into account. To reduce the visual complexity, the local behavior of the pathlines needs to be considered.

Our algorithm decomposes pathlines into logical groups of similar behavior and has two phases, global and local reduction. In both phases, two key features are used to identify pathline similarity — shape similarity and spatial locality. For example, pathlines that traverse similar paths and are close together tend to exhibit similar behavior.

The first point of a pathline is defined as the starting or seed position of a pathline. The last point of a pathline is defined as the terminating or final position of a pathline. The end points of a pathline is defined as both the first and last point of a pathline. The path length of a pathline is the distance the pathline traverses.

2.1 Global Reduction

Pathlines that are globally similar start and end in nearby areas and have similar shape. The spatial locality of pathlines is determined by analyzing the relative position of the end points. The shape similarity is determined by analyzing the path length, a rough descriptor of shape. The last points of the pathlines are grouped together to provide an initial global clustering. This clustering is then locally refined using a region growing technique that clusters together pathlines with similar path lengths and end points.

The global clustering algorithm used for the grouping of the pathline last points must not assume a fixed number of clusters since the number of flow groups is not known a priori and can change with every seed configuration. Schreiber's Voronoi diagram clustering method [12] meets this requirement and overcomes many of the disadvantages of the conventional k-means algorithm. The algorithm sequentially inserts a new cluster point in the Voronoi region with the largest error. At each iteration, the region with the largest error is subdivided into two regions and the Vonoroi diagram is updated. The insertion of new clusters continues until termination requirements are met. Hence, Schreiber's algorithm can adaptively create clusters based on properties of the data set.

For our global clustering of the last positions of the pathlines, the cluster error is given by the sum of the squared errors (SSE) using Euclidean distance. The clustering terminates when the current SSE becomes larger than the previous iteration's SSE. This indicates that the region with the current largest error has been subdivided erroneously. In this way, we achieve a local minimization of cluster error.

2.2   Local Reduction

The Voronoi clustering provides groupings where each cluster has pathlines with similar last points. To further refine the groupings, a region growing technique is used to check the starting positions and shape of the pathlines to ensure local similarity.

For each of the clusters generated by the Voronoi algorithm, we apply the region growing technique. The region growing algorithm starts with a random base pathline and checks all its closest neighbors for similarity. The similar neighbors are marked for group membership and then the region growing technique is recursively applied to each similar neighbor. When no more similar neighbors are found, a new pathline is chosen as the base object and the process is repeated for the next grouping. The algorithm terminates when all the pathlines have been assigned a grouping.

We define two pathlines to be similar if their end points and shapes are similar. The end points of two pathlines are defined to be similar if their distance between their corresponding end point is within an acceptable threshold. The shape of two pathlines is defined to be similar if the path lengths are within an acceptable threshold.

2.3   Region Growing Thresholds

The performance of our skeleton algorithm depends heavily on the region growing thresholds. Too small of a threshold creates many compact groupings; too large of a threshold creates groups with extremely varying behavior. Therefore, to generate reasonable groupings, the thresholds should take into account the distributions of the pathlines in each Voronoi group.

The spatial and shape similarity thresholds are based on the fan-like distribution of pathlines shown in Figure 1. For the fan distribution, we define an ideal clustering to be the three-pronged grouping, shown in Figure 1b, where each prong covers a third of the spanned area. We approximate the spanned area by calculating the group's standard deviation, σ. For a normal distribution, 2σ from the mean accounts for roughly 95% of the samples. To achieve our idealized three-pronged grouping, we use thresholds of $\frac{2}{3}\sigma_p^i$ and $\frac{2}{3}\sigma_s^i$, where σ_p^i is the standard deviation of the last points and σ_s^i is the path length standard deviation of the ith Voronoi group.

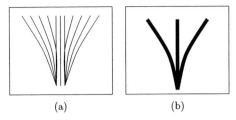

(a)   (b)

Figure 1: (a) Fan-like distribution of pathlines and (b) ideal three-pronged groups.

3   Experimental Results

We evaluated our algorithm by analyzing the effect of varying the position and path length thresholds. In each experiment, the pathlines were seeded in the same inlet vessel with the same 32x32 planar configuration for a total of 1089 pathlines. The pathlines were integrated over a basilar aneurysm blood field that was simulated using a model created from real patient data using pulsatile flow. The pathlines were distributed in all areas of the aneurysm with complex flow patterns. The seven threshold levels chosen were $\frac{1}{6}\sigma$, $\frac{1}{3}\sigma$, $\frac{1}{2}\sigma$, $\frac{2}{3}\sigma$, $\frac{5}{6}\sigma$, σ, and $\frac{7}{6}\sigma$. Two sets of experiments were run, one to evaluate the position threshold and another to evaluate the path length threshold. To test the effect of the position threshold, the path length threshold was held constant at $\frac{2}{3}\sigma_s$ while the position threshold was varied among the seven levels. To test the effect of the path length threshold, the position threshold was held constant at $\frac{2}{3}\sigma_p$ while the path length threshold was varied among the seven levels.

For each run, the Voronoi groups generated were identical. The number of members of each region growing group created was calculated and ordered from greatest to least. The first 9 groups for the position and path length thresholds are graphed in Figures 2a and 2b. The percentage of the total 1089 pathlines the first 9 groups represent are given in Table 1.

Total percentages for σ thresholds							
Set	$\frac{1}{6}\sigma$	$\frac{1}{3}\sigma$	$\frac{1}{2}\sigma$	$\frac{2}{3}\sigma$	$\frac{5}{6}\sigma$	σ	$\frac{7}{6}\sigma$
σ_p: % Total	49.2%	72.4%	84.7%	91.3%	96.3%	97.6%	98.2%
σ_s: % Total	69.8%	77.4%	88.2%	91.3%	95.7%	96.1%	96.1%

Table 1: Total percentage of the original 1089 pathlines the first 9 groups represent for the σ_p and σ_s thresholds.

In addition to the numeric data collected, screen images of each region growing group were captured. An example of the screen captures is shown in Figure 3. Based on visual inspection, we compared the screen captures for similarity. If the groupings had the same overall size, shape, and density and identical flow patterns could be inferred from the images, the images were marked as similar. The results of this visual inspection for different levels of threshold are given in Table 2 and 3.

4   Discussion

Our skeleton algorithm decomposes large, complex pathlines into logical groups of behaviors. The difficulty is choosing threshold levels that produce quality groupings. As shown in Table 1, smaller thresholds yield more compact groups and consequently the largest 9 groups

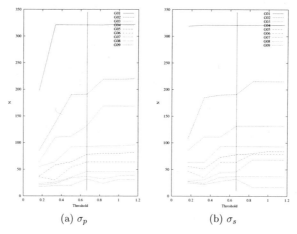

(a) σ_p (b) σ_s

Figure 2: Number of members (N) of largest 9 groups versus (a) position threshold σ_p and (b) path length threshold σ_s. The midline in both graphs represents the base $\frac{2}{3}\sigma$ thresholds.

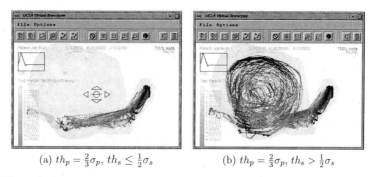

(a) $th_p = \frac{2}{3}\sigma_p$, $th_s \leq \frac{1}{2}\sigma_s$ (b) $th_p = \frac{2}{3}\sigma_p$, $th_s > \frac{1}{2}\sigma_s$

Figure 3: Screen captures showing (a) inlet-outlet flow and (b) swirling flow with inlet-outlet behavior for different levels of σ_s.

have less coverage of the original data. From our data and threshold levels chosen, σ_p has a greater effect than σ_s. As shown in Figure 2, before the base threshold of $\frac{2}{3}\sigma$, the change in σ_p causes more fluctuation than σ_s, especially for the first 3 groups which contain the majority of pathlines. As we increase the thresholds beyond the base $\frac{2}{3}\sigma$, overall the groupings stabilize. A closer inspection reveals that some of the groups stabilize before the base threshold and some after, an indication that the $\frac{2}{3}\sigma$ threshold may not be general enough.

From a visual point of view, changing the σ_p threshold causes much more variation in the similarity, as shown in Tables 2 and 3. The impact of the smallest σ_s level particularly stands out as it decomposes the largest group of the other levels into 3 distinct components. On the other hand, changing σ_s results in more consistent and stable visual similarity.

A stable grouping size, however, does not always translate into a quality visual representation. Consider, the screen captures in Figure 3. Each of the groupings are stable for the same number of threshold levels. We see, however, that they represent different patterns. Figure 3a strictly captures the inlet flow moving toward the outlet vessel whereas Figure

Visual Group Similarity for σ_p							
Group	$\frac{1}{6}\sigma_p$	$\frac{1}{3}\sigma_p$	$\frac{1}{2}\sigma_p$	$\frac{2}{3}\sigma_p$	$\frac{5}{6}\sigma_p$	σ_p	$\frac{7}{6}\sigma_p$
1	@	#	#	#	#	#	#
2	*	@	@	@	#	#	#
3	*	@	@	#	#	#	#
4	*	@	#	#	#	#	#
5	*	#	@	#	#	#	#
6	*	@	@	#	#	#	#
7	*	#	@	#	#	#	#
8	@	@	*	#	#	#	#
9	*	@	@	@	#	#	#

Table 2: The region growing groups were visually inspected and compared for the σ_p levels. Groups with the same symbol indicate visual similarity.

Visual Group Similarity for σ_s							
Group	$\frac{1}{6}\sigma_s$	$\frac{1}{3}\sigma_s$	$\frac{1}{2}\sigma_s$	$\frac{2}{3}\sigma_s$	$\frac{5}{6}\sigma_s$	σ_s	$\frac{7}{6}\sigma_s$
1	#	#	#	#	#	#	#
2	#	#	#	#	@	@	@
3	@	@	@	#	#	#	#
4	@	@	#	#	#	#	#
5	@	#	#	#	#	#	#
6	*	*	@	@	#	#	#
7	*	@	@	@	#	#	#
8	@	#	#	#	#	#	#
9	*	@	@	@	#	#	#

Table 3: The region growing groups were visually inspected and compared for the σ_s levels. Groups with the same symbol indicate visual similarity.

3b captures the swirling pattern within the aneurysm sac in addition to the inlet-outlet flow. To be as accurate as possible, our algorithm should decompose this behavior into two distinct patterns.

The experimental results indicate that, while the algorithm shows promise, the region growing thresholds need to be improved. As we have shown, our single threshold of $\frac{2}{3}\sigma$ is not general enough. Since the quality of the groupings varies with the threshold, an adaptive approach can be adopted to choose the best fit. Criteria for the best fit need to be considered carefully since, as we have seen, the best numeric representation is not always the best visual representation.

5　Conclusion

We presented an algorithm that simplifies the visual representation of pathlines while retaining the structure and information of the original data. Our algorithm decomposes pathlines into logical groups through a global clustering step using Voronoi techniques followed by a local refinement step using a region growing technique. While our algorithm shows promising results, the quality of the groupings can be improved. From the experimental results, it was shown that an adaptive thresholding technique needs to be included in the region growing to produce higher quality groupings.

Our algorithm filters and processes the flow data to generate the blood flow patterns automatically for the physician. By using our system, physicians will be able to interpret and understand complex 3D time-dependent blood flows more quickly and effective, without having to endure the time-consuming process of manually sifting through the data.

References

[1] Bertrand, G. & Aktouf, Z. (1994). Three-dimensional Thinning Algorithm using SubFields. In R.A. Melter & A.Y. Wu (Eds.), *Proceedings of the Vision Geometry III Conference* (pp. 113-124). SPIE–The International Society for Optical Engineering.

[2] Blum, H. (1967). A Transformation for Extracting New Descriptors of Shape. In W. Wathen-Dunn (Ed.), *Models for the Perception of Speech and Visual Form* (pp. 362-379). Cambridge: The M.I.T. Press.

[3] Ford, R.M. & Strickland, R.N. (1994). Nonlinear Models for Representation, Compression, and Visualization of Fluid Flow Images and Velocimetry Data. In L. O'Conner (Ed.), *IEEE Workshop on Visualization and Machine Vision* (pp.1-12). Los Alamitos, California: IEEE Computer Society Press.

[4] Harreld, M.R., Valentino, D.J., and Karplus, W.J. (1996). The Virtual Aneurysm: Virtual reality in endovascular therapy. In S.J. Weghorst, H.B. Sieburg, K.S. Morgan (Eds.), *Proceedings of Medicine Meets Virtual Reality 4* (pp.12-20). Amsterdam, Netherlands: IOS Press.

[5] Helman, J.L. & Hesselink, L. (1991). Visualizing Vector Field Topology in Fluid Flows. *IEEE Computer Graphics and Applications*, **11**(3), 36-46.

[6] Helman, J.L. & Hesselink, L. (1990). Surface Representations of Two- and Three-Dimensional Fluid Flow Topology. In A. Kaufman (Ed.), *Proceedings of the First IEEE Conference on Visualization* (pp.6-13). Los Alamitos, California: IEEE Computer Society Press.

[7] Helman, J.L. & Hesselink, L. (1989). Representation and Display of Vector Field Topology in Fluid Flow Data Sets. In G.M. Nielson & B. Shriver (Eds.), *Visualization in Scientific Computing* (pp.61-73). Los Alamitos, California: IEEE Computer Society Press.

[8] Montanari, U. (1968). A Method for Obtaining Skeletons Using a Quasi-Euclidean Distance. *Journal of the Association for Computing Machinery*, **15**(4), 600-624.

[9] Montanari, U. (1969). Continuous Skeletons from Digitized Images. *Journal of the Association for Computing Machinery*, **16**(4), 534-549.

[10] Palágyi, K. & Kuba, A. (1999). Directional 3D Thinning Using 8 Subiterations. In G. Bertrand, M. Couprie, L. Perroton (Eds.), *Proceedings of the 1999 8th Discrete Geometry for Computer Imagery Conference* (pp.325-36). Berlin, Germany: Springer-Verlag.

[11] Post, F.H. & van Wijk, J.J. (1994). Visual representation of vector fields. In L. Rosenblum, R.A. Earnshaw, J. Encarnação, H. Hagen, A. Kaufman, S. Klimenko, G. Nielson, F. Post, and D. Thalmann (Eds.), *Scientific Visualization: Advances and Challenges* (pp. 367-390). London: Academic Press.

[12] Schreiber, T. (1991). A Voronoi Diagram Based Adaptive K-Means-Type Clustering Algorithm for Multidimensional Weighted Data. In H. Bieri and H. Noltemeier (Eds.), *Computational Geometry – Methods, Algorithms, and Applications*, Lecture Notes in Computer Science 553 (pp. 265-275). Berlin: Springer-Verlag.

Medicine Meets Virtual Reality 2001
J.D. Westwood et al. (Eds.)
IOS Press, 2001

A computer-based simulator for diagnostic peritoneal lavage

Alan Liu
Christoph Kaufmann
Thomas Ritchie
{aliu|ckaufmann|tritchie}@simcen.usuhs.mil

Surgical Simulation Laboratory
National Capital Area Medical Simulation Center
Uniformed Services University of the Health Sciences
4301 Jones Bridge Road, Bethesda MD 20814, USA
http://www.simcen.usuhs.mil

Abstract. Diagnostic peritoneal lavage (DPL) is an emergency diagnostic procedure performed when intra-abdominal bleeding secondary to trauma is suspected. This procedure is part of the surgical skills section of the Advanced Trauma Life Support course. DPL is traditionally taught using anesthetized animals or cadavers. For reasons described below, these alternatives are not ideal. We have developed a computer-based diagnostic peritoneal lavage simulator. Our system addresses the shortcomings of the traditional method. We have used our system to teach ATLS®. Preliminary results suggests that our system is effective.

1. Introduction

The Advanced Trauma Life Support (ATLS®) course trains doctors in optimal assessment and resuscitation techniques for the seriously injured patient. ATLS® is recommended for all doctors caring for patients with serious injury. An average of 19,000 doctors in over 30 countries are trained annually in ATLS® [1]. This course is taught to all fourth year medical students at our university. The ATLS® course includes a surgical skills component. Students are taught tube thoracostomy, surgical airway, pericardiocentesis, and diagnostic peritoneal lavage. These skills are taught using cadavers or anesthetized animals (i.e. wet models). Groups of up to four students learn on each model.

Wet models have limitations. They are single use resources. For example, procedures requiring incisions can be performed at most once in a specific anatomic location. The same location cannot be reused for the next student. In addition, students who have made a mistake cannot redo the incorrect step. Cadavers are expensive, and can be difficult to procure. Most require refrigerated storage, and must be thawed prior to use. They do not have the physiology of live patients. Anesthetized animals do not have the same anatomy as humans. This can be a problem when teaching ATLS® skills such as pericardiocentesis [2]. Animal specimens are individually inexpensive, but require separate maintenance facilities, and staff to manage their care and feeding. Both the latter items may be costly. Finally, the use of animals and cadavers for medical education may raise ethical concerns.

In a previous paper [2], we described our work in exploring alternatives to wet models. Diagnostic peritoneal lavage (DPL) was not discussed. In this paper, we extend our work by describing a computer-based simulator for teaching DPL in ATLS®. A brief description of the procedure is given below. Section 2 describes our system in more detail. Section 3 describes our preliminary findings. Section 4 discusses the implications of our work. Finally, section 5 summarizes the key points of our paper.

DPL is performed when intra-abdominal bleeding secondary to trauma is suspected. The procedure is performed when alternative diagnostic methods such as computerized tomography (CT) or ultrasound imaging are unavailable, or when the patient's condition does not allow them to be performed. The DPL procedure involves several steps. First, the appropriate site is selected and a small incision made after local anesthesia. The incision minimizes drag on the catheter at a later step. A cannula is inserted in the incision and is used to penetrate the midline fascia in the abdominal wall. During insertion, the surgeon feels a sudden give or "pop" as the cannula passes through the fascia. Care must be taken not to insert the cannula too deeply and perforate the bowel. A flexible guidewire is passed through the cannula. The cannula is then removed and a catheter threaded over the guidewire. The guidewire is then removed. As a preliminary test, a syringe fitted on the catheter is used for aspiration. If gross blood is detected, bleeding is confirmed. If no blood is aspirated, the syringe is removed. Saline solution is introduced into the abdominal cavity through the catheter. The solution is then drained and send for laboratory analysis.

DPL is normally taught on anesthetized animals. In the following section, we present a computer-based system that provides an alternative for current practice.

2. Method

Our system consists of a desktop computer system and a commercially available haptic interface. The computer has 128 Mb of memory, a Pentium // 300Mhz CPU, and a Gloria Elsa Synergy graphics card. The computer uses the Windows NT operating system. OpenGL is used to access the graphics hardware. The haptic interface is the CathSim AccuTouch device manufactured by HT Medical Systems. Fig. 2 illustrates. The device contains a needle carrier. The needle carrier has a three degree-of-freedom (DOF) orientation sensor. Pitch, yaw,

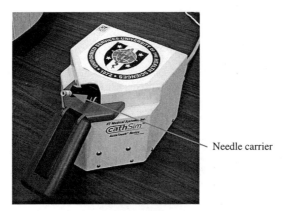 Needle carrier

Fig. 1: Haptic interface device.

and depth of insertion can be detected. The carrier also provides a one DOF passive haptic feedback. As the user pushes or pulls the carrier, resistance can be felt. The degree of resistance is controllable. By dynamically controlling the degree of resistance, it is possible to simulate the sensation of a needle piercing through various layers of tissue. Encoders located co-axial to the needle carrier permit guidewires, cannulas, and catheters to be detected. Our system uses the haptic interface to simulate the effect of inserting the cannula and other DPL instruments in the abdomen.

The system is initialized with a cannula in the needle carrier. When the program begins, the student is presented with a list representing the steps in the DPL procedure. Fig. 2 illustrates. Items on the list have been randomized. The student is required to know the correct sequence. The system does not proceed until the correct next step is chosen. Incorrect choices are recorded and reported at the end of the simulation. When a correct action is selected, the system displays a model of the human abdomen. The student is then prompted to perform the action. We describe each step in more detail.

Select site and make incision. The system displays an external view of the abdomen. The student uses the mouse to click on the correct location. Several regions with different degrees of desirability can be defined. For example, if the student clicks on an area normally reserved for individuals with pelvic fracture, the system reports that fact. A correct choice permits the student to proceed to the next step. Fig. 3 (top left) illustrates.

Insert cannula. The system displays an image of a cannula over the abdomen. The student controls the image with the haptic device. As the cannula is inserted, the system adjusts the resistance on the haptic device. The student feels an effect similar to passing a cannula through layers of abdominal tissue. The characteristic "pop" of the needle passing through the fascia is simulated by an abrupt decrease in resistance at the appropriate depth. During insertion, the student's entry angle, location, and depth of insertion is compared with instructor-defined optimal

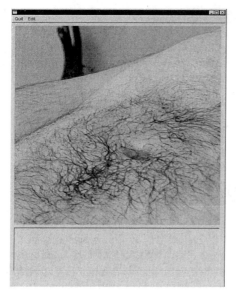

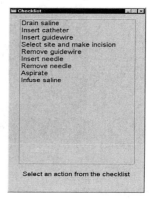

Fig. 2: Simulator user interface. The right window contains a checklist of
actions. The left window permits individual actions to be performed.

values. Excessive deviation (also instructor defined) is reported as an error, and the
student is asked to try again. Fig. 3 (top right) illustrates.

Insert guidewire. With the cannula inserted, the student inserts the guidewire.
The system displays the image of a guidewire over the cannula. An encoder in the
shaft of the needle carrier detects the guidewire's passage. The guidewire's image
updates accordingly when this occurs. The system reports an error if the guidewire
has been inserted too deeply, or not deeply enough. Fig. 3 (middle left) illustrates.

Remove cannula. An important precaution during DPL is not to lose direct
control of the guidewire. As the cannula is being removed, its position relative to
the guidewire is monitored. If the guidewire slips into the cannula, an error is
reported by the system.

Insert catheter and remove guidewire. An image of the catheter is displayed.
The student inserts the catheter over the guidewire and into the needle carrier. The
system tracks the catheter's movement and updates the image accordingly. As with
the previous step, loss of control over the guidewire generates an error message.
Fig. 3 (middle right) illustrates.

Aspirate. An image of a syringe attached to the catheter is displayed. The user
starts aspiration by clicking on a button on the screen. Depending on the system
configuration, this step may draw either gross blood, or no blood is extracted. The
student is prompted for the correct action based on the image shown. By default,
the system randomly displays gross blood half the time. The instructor can
override and force a positive or negative outcome as desired. If gross blood and the
correct student response is obtained, the system bypasses the remainder of the

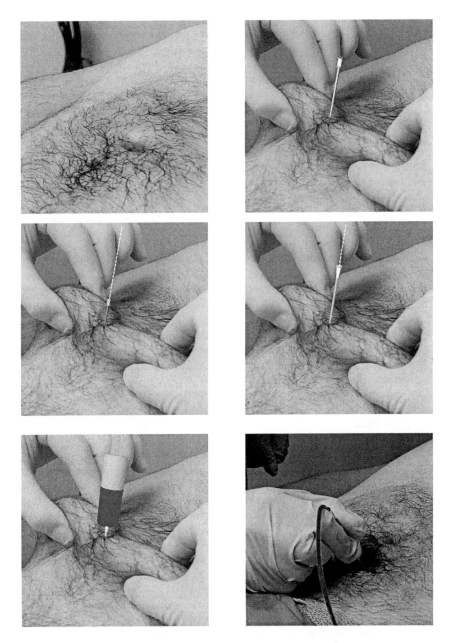

Fig. 3: Screen display from different steps of the simulation. Top left: site selection. Top right: Cannula insertion. Middle left: Guidewire insertion. Middle right: Catheter insertion. Bottom left: Gross blood detected on aspiration. Bottom right: Saline drain with a possible positive result.

simulation and generates a report of the student's performance. Fig. 3 (bottom left) illustrates.

Infuse and drain saline. If gross blood is not present, the student infuses saline through the catheter and drains the result. The system does not provide an analysis of the drained fluid. Instead, the system randomly displays either clear or red fluid being drained. The student is prompted to comment on the likely outcome of the procedure based on the image shown. As with the previous step, the instructor may override the randomization. Fig. 3 (bottom right) illustrates

Report generation. The simulator concludes by generating a summary of the student's performance. Each step corresponds to one section of the report. In each section, errors encountered for that step are reported.

3. Preliminary results

Permission was obtained to investigate teaching an ATLS® course using alternatives to wet models. DPL was taught using the computer-based system described in this paper. The course was attended by a group of six surgery residents and three staff surgeons, each of whom had previously taken the ATLS® course. A survey was conducted after the course. Students were asked to rate individual components of the course on a scale of 0 (poor) to 3 (very good). Of the nine students, seven rated the DPL component as 3 (very good), and two rated it as 2 (good). The average was 2.8. This compared favorably with the other components in the surgical skills section.

4. Discussion

Computer-based simulators have several advantages over wet models. Simulators can incorporate anatomically correct models. They do not bear signs of previous usage and can be deployed repeatedly. Unlike cadavers, simulators can be programmed to provide the correct physiological response. More importantly, their responses can be altered to suit the lesson being taught. Computer-based simulators do not have significant maintenance or storage costs. They do not require laboratory or clinical facilities for deployment.

Simulators have some disadvantages. The initial cost may be high, making their purchase less attractive. However, the availability of powerful personal computers at decreasing prices may ameliorate this. For example, the hardware cost of our DPL simulator is less than $7,000. In addition, different kinds of simulations can be run on the same hardware.

Simulators at present do not have the same degree of realism as wet models. For example, it is very difficult to simulate realistic bleeding. Simulating real-time tissue deformation due to cutting and other forces is non-trival. In addition, the ability to reproduce tactile forces is limited.

The preliminary results presented are encouraging. They suggest that the DPL simulator is useful in teaching this skill. However, the study involves a small sample, and does not compare our system with the use of wet models. The study also did not determine the specific contribution of our simulator to the overall success of the DPL session. Additional, more detailed studies are being planned.

5. Conclusion

We described a computer-based system for teaching DPL. Our system has several advantages over wet models. They include: reusability, having the correct anatomy and physiology, and low operating cost. We have used our simulator as part of an ATLS® course. A postcourse survey suggests that the DPL simulator may have value in teaching this surgical skill.

6. Acknowledgments

The authors gratefully acknowledge the assistance of the Association of Military Surgeons of the United States (AMSUS), and HT Medical Systems. The authors would also like to acknowledge LT Scott Zakaluzny for his assistance in acquiring the abdomen model used in our simulator.

7. References

[1]   American College of Surgeons Committee on Trauma, "Advanced Trauma Life Support® for Doctors", 6th edition, Chicago, IL (1997).

[2]   Kaufmann C., Zakaluzny S., Liu A., "First Steps in Eliminating the Need for Animals and Cadavers.", *MICCAI 2000*.

[3]   Ursino M., Tasto P.D.J.L., Nguyen B.H., Cunningham R., Merril, G.L. "CathSim: an intravascular catheterization simulator on a PC"., *Medicine Meets Virtual Reality. Convergence of Physical and Informational Technologies: Options for a New Era in Healthcare.* pp. 360-6, 1999.

Medicine Meets Virtual Reality 2001
J.D. Westwood et al. (Eds.)
IOS Press, 2001

Effects of Geared Motor Characteristics on Tactile Perception of Tissue Stiffness

Jeff Longnion +, Jacob Rosen+, PhD,
Mika Sinanan++, MD, PhD, Blake Hannaford+, PhD,

++ *Department of Electrical Engineering, Box 352500*
+ *Department of Surgery, Box 356410*
University of Washington
Seattle, WA, 98195, USA

Abstract
Endoscopic haptic surgical devices have shown promise in addressing the loss of tactile sensation associated with minimally invasive surgery. However, these devices must be capable of generating forces and torques similar to those applied on the tissue with a standard endoscopic tool. Geared motors are a possible solution for actuation; however; they possess mechanical characteristics that could potentially interfere with tactile perception of tissue qualities. The aim of the current research was to determine how the characteristics of a geared motor suitable for a haptic surgical device affect a user's perception of stiffness. The experiment involved six blindfolded subjects who were asked to discriminate the stiffness of six distinct silicone rubber samples whose mechanical properties are similar to those of soft tissue. Using a novel testing device whose dimensions approximated those of an endoscopic grasper, each subject palpated 30 permutations of sample pairs for each of three types of mechanical loads; the motor (friction and inertia), a flywheel (with the same inertia as motor), and a control (no significant mechanical interference). One factor ANOVA of the error scores and palpation time showed that no significant difference existed among error scores, but mean palpation time for the control was significantly less than for the other two methods. These results indicated that the mechanical characteristics of a geared motor chosen for application in a haptic surgical device did not interfere with the subjects' perception of the silicone samples' stiffness, but these characteristics may significantly affect the energy expenditure and time required for tissue palpation. Therefore, before geared motors can be considered for use in haptic surgical devices, consideration should be given to factors such as palpation speed and fatigue.

1. Introduction

Shorter hospital stays, decreased probability of infection, and minimal scarring are just a few of the many advantages associated with minimally invasive surgical techniques. Nevertheless, in exchange for these advantages, surgeons have typically been forced to use endoscopic surgical tools that convey only a fraction of the tactile information received with open surgical techniques [1,2]. Because tactile information regarding tissue properties, such as stiffness, is critical to the diagnosis of a full range of pathologies, a great deal of effort has been devoted to increasing tactile sensation [3]. Certainly, one of the more promising solutions to this problem, is the development of force-feedback endoscopic surgical devices. Previous research with a direct drive haptic surgical device has demonstrated the ability to relay tactile information between the grasping and handle ends of a teleoperated endoscopic grasper [4]. Nevertheless, in order to perform surgical tasks, these devices must be capable of producing forces and torques similar to those applied by surgeons using regular endoscopic instruments. One promising means of actuation is a geared motor, which offers a compact and efficient means of producing the necessary torque.

Although a high gear ratio ensures sufficient torque output from the motors, it also introduces undesirable effects such as friction forces, inertial effects, and gear cogging, which may limit a user's ability to perceive the characteristics of material being grasped by the device. These problems associated with a geared motor interference are not new, and efforts have been made to reduce these effects using control algorithms and force sensing. However these solution lead to added costs and challenging stability problems. Furthermore, the effects of the geared motor characteristics on perception of tissue properties are unknown, and this information is critical to determining the feasibility of using geared motors in haptic surgical devices.

The objective of this study was to test the effects of geared motor characteristics on perception of tissue stiffness and in particular to:

- Determine if a geared motor suitable for use in an endoscopic surgical tool produces motor characteristics that impair perception of stiffness.
- Examine how geared motor characteristics effect tissue palpation and perception of tissue stiffness.
- Begin exploring which characteristics are responsible for decreased perception.

2. Tools & Methods

2.1 Geared Motor Selection

A geared motor used in a hand-held haptic surgical device must be as physically small and lightweight as possible while still maintaining sufficient torque production capacity. Additionally, as friction force and inertia increase by the square of the motor's gear ratio it is important to minimize this value. Although, the motor selected for this experiment was only used as an open-circuited mechanical load, it was selected according to these design constraints. Based on kinematics analysis for a typical endoscopic grasper and measurements performed during minimally invasive surgery, a maximum continuous torque output of 1.5 Nm is required of the actuator. The maximum allowable motor weight was limited to 0.5 Kg. A number of geared motors were compared according to their total weight, maximum torque production, and gear ratio. The motor that most accurately satisfied the desired design constraints was a Maxon 70 Watt DC Motor with a 23:1 planetary gearhead (Fig 1, dark circle).

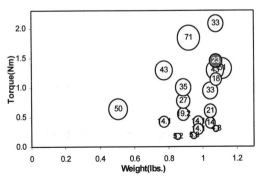

Figure 1: Geared Motor Comparison: Max Continuous Torque Vs. Weight Vs. Gear Ratio (gear ratio denoted by size of circles and numerical value)

2.2 Testing Device Design

The testing device included pliers with a grasping surface area of 103 mm² and lever arm lengths of 6.48 and 3.54 cm for handle and grasping finger loops respectively. These dimensions were chosen to approximate the equivalent dimensions of a typical endoscopic tool (Fig. 2). One finger loop was attached directly to the stationary based and the second finger-loop was attached to the base trough a shaft and a ball bearing. The modular design of the device allowed the use of a variety of shafted loads including a geared motor and a flywheel (Fig. 3). The adjustable flywheel was designed to match the reflected inertia of the motor shaft through the gear head.

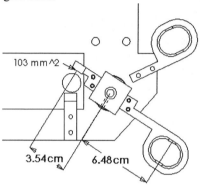

Figure 2: Top View of the Device Palpating a Silicone Rubber Sample

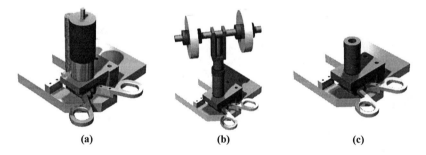

(a)   (b)   (c)

Figure 3: Different Configurations of Testing Device: (a) Geared motor (b) Flywheel (c) Control

2.3 Silicone Rubber Samples

Six silicone rubber materials were used as part of the experimental protocol. The Silicone materials compliance characteristics were controlled by the percentage (weight) of catalyst used during manufacturing. All the Silicone materials were shaped as a cylinder with a diameter of 14.7 mm and a length of 150 mm with the same color and texture. A detailed description of the mechanical properties of these materials was reported in [3]. In general the materials had an exponential stress-compression ratio under uniaxial compression (Eq. 1) conditions with an α and β parameters similar to soft tissue (Eq. 1)

$$K(\lambda) = \frac{dT}{d\lambda} = \alpha\beta e^{\alpha(1-\lambda)} \qquad (1)$$

where α and β are the material parameters, λ is the compression length-ratio, T is the uniaxial compression stress, and K is the material stiffness.

The six silicone rubber samples were evenly graded as measured by stress length-ratio characteristics; this makes them ideal for the purpose of the subjective testing experiment.

2.4 Experimental Protocol

The experimental protocol included six blindfolded subjects that were asked to rank the stiffness of silicone rubber samples using three testing devices. The experimental protocol included two step: (1) for each testing device the subject first used the testing device to palpate each sample in order from 1 to 6 (2) The subject was then blindfolded and randomly presented all 30 possible permutations of sample pairs. For each pairing, each subject was allowed to palpate the first silicone sample with out any time limit. The subject was then allowed to palpate the second sample of the pair until he or she decided which sample was stiffer. The time of palpation for the first and second sample along with the choice for the stiffer sample were recorded for each permutation. The protocol was repeated three times using three testing methods: (1) the device with the motor (inertia and friction); (2) the device with the flywheel (matched inertia), and (3) the device alone (control). The order of methods was varied for each of the six subjects in order to eliminate biasing. Due to experimental setup and the ability of a user to subjectively sense what method was being used, it was not possible to blind the subjects or the testers from knowledge of the method being tested.

2.5 Analysis

In the analysis of the experimental data, a number of variables were chosen as potentially indicative of discernability; these included the following.

- **Error Score (ES)-** For each permutation, if the pair was incorrectly discriminated, an error score was assigned according to the numerical difference in the samples. For example, an incorrect discrimination of sample 5 and sample 2 would receive an error score of 3. If no mistake was made an error score of zero was assigned.
- **Total Palpation Time (TPT)-** This is the sum of the first and second squeezing time for each permutation. A longer total palpation time might indicate a greater difficulty in palpation as well as an increased difficulty in discriminating between a pair of samples.
- **Second Palpation Time (SPT)-** This is the time that the subject spent manipulating the second sample. If a subject spends an extended period of time squeezing the second sample, the SPT might be an indicator of discrimination difficulty.
- **Time Ratio (TR)-** This is the second palpation time divided by the first palpation time. The use of this statistic is intended to eliminate the time variations of different squeezing techniques. A smaller ratio might indicate easier sample discrimination.

By comparing the first, second, and third methods tested, these variables were analyzed to determine if any learning had occurred. Specifically, one-factor analysis of variance (ANOVA) was utilized to determine if learning effects might be present in the ES, TPT, SPT, and TR.

In a similar fashion, ANOVA was utilized to determine whether the type of method (Control, Flywheel, or Motor) had a significant effect on ES, TPT, SPT, and TR. In general, a one-factor ANOVA test was used, but in some cases a two-way ANOVA was performed as well to determine if a difference existed between the subjects. Furthermore, in cases where ANOVA indicated significant differences among means, Scheffe's Method for post hoc analysis was utilized to determine which means were different.

3. Results

3.1 Minimal Learning Effect

When the first, second, and third methods were compared using a single-factor ANOVA, there was no significant difference between the mean of the error scores. In fact, ANOVA showed that none of the variables observed (ES, TPT, SPT, TR) were affected by learning from method to method. Furthermore, a comparison of error score versus trial number indicates that no noticeable learning can be seen both within each method and between the methods.

3.2 Negligible Method Type Effect

In general, subjects were able to discriminate the samples equally well regardless of testing method type (Fig. 4). The overall discrimination success rate was 84 %, with the control, flywheel, and motor having success rates of 83%, 86%, and 84% respectively. ANOVA demonstrated that the method type had no significance for error score or time ratio (See Fig. 4). However, the analysis did reveal that TPT and SPT were both significantly effected by the testing method (p = .002 and p = .03 respectively). Further analysis with Scheffe's method showed that, in both cases, the mean palpation time of the control method was significantly ($\alpha < 0.05$) less than for the other two methods.

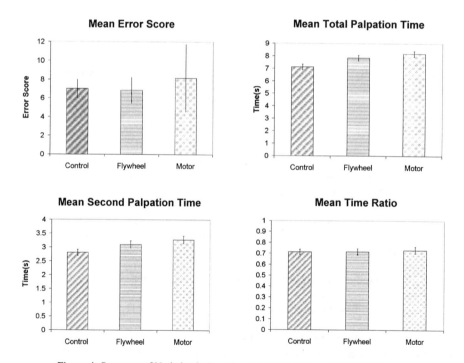

Figure 4: Summary of Variation in Experimental Variables across Method Type

3.3 Significant Difference Among Subjects

A two-way ANOVA revealed that error scores were significantly different for each subject and that a significant interaction existed between the subject and the testing methods. In fact, similar results were seen with the remaining variables (TPT, SPT, RT). Though, in general, low correlation existed between variables, it was found that subjects who spent less time palpating generally had a lower error score ($r^2 = .57$). A comparison of the normalized experimental variables for each subject is included in Figure 5.

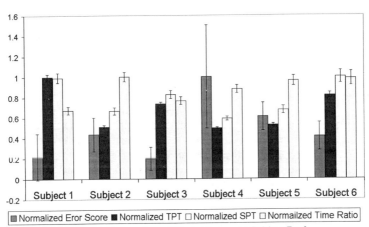

Figure 5: Comparison of Variables across Subject Pool

3.4 Subjective Observations

Although no specific instructions were given as to how the subjects should palpate the tissue, many of the subjects adopted a similar technique. Rate and accuracy varied greatly from subject to subject, however all subjects would generally palpate each sample repetitively. Most subjects would accelerate the pliers to a closed position and then hold it temporarily stationary before returning to an open position. For the cases where mechanical loads were present, subjects were observed to expend more effort in opening and closing the pliers.

4. Discussion and Conclusions

Many of the findings of this experiment were unexpected. Subjects were able to discriminate between the stiffness of the sample pairs more accurately than had been expected. Furthermore, none of the test variables demonstrated any significant difference between the flywheel and motor in perceiving the stiffness of the tested materials. Nevertheless, a number of potentially valuable conclusions may be drawn from this experiment.

As the method was varied between the control, flywheel, and motor, neither the error score nor discrimination percentage indicated any significant difference in a subject's ability to correctly discriminate the stiffness of the sample pairs. Thus, it appears that the motor characteristics of the geared motor chosen for this experiment were not able to significantly impair stiffness perception. If one considers a simplified model for the forces being applied during palpation, these findings make intuitive sense. The forces felt by the subject are described by the following relationship:

$$M = I\ddot{\theta} + B\dot{\theta} + K(\theta) \qquad (2)$$

where θ is the angular position of the pliers, $K(\theta)$ is a moment related to the deflection of the sample, B is proportional to the friction in the shaft, I represents the inertia of the device, and M is the moment experienced by the subject. When squeezing, most subjects would squeeze the silicone rubber to a certain point and then hold the pliers relatively stable. In this quasi-static state, the angular velocity and acceleration become less significant. Thus, it makes sense that in most of the experiments, subjects were able to sense tissue stiffness regardless of the motors friction and inertia.

In analyzing all of the experimental metrics, only the palpation time (both SPT and TPT) of the control was significantly less than the palpation time for the flywheel and motor. Certainly, as closing and opening involve both angular velocity and acceleration, the time and energy needed to repetitively palpate a tissue increase with friction and inertia. Thus, this slight but significant increase in palpation time for the flywheel and motor methods may be a result of this phenomenon.

In conclusion, it appears that the perception of stiffness is not significantly effected by the mechanical characteristics of the geared motor chosen for this experiment, but these characteristics may effect the time and energy exertion necessary for tissue palpation. Thus, although it may be possible to consider geared motors for use in haptic surgical devices, other factors, such as user fatigue and speed require consideration.

5. Acknowledgements

This research was made possible by the University of Washington Honors Program Scholarship, the Bill and Melinda Gates Honors Endowment Scholarship, and a major grant from WRF Capital. Also, this work was supported by a major grant from United States Surgical, a Division of Tyco-Healthcare, Inc. to the University of Washington, USSC Center for Videoendoscopic Surgery.

References

[1] K.T. denBoer , Herder , W. Sjoerdsma , Meijer , Gouma , Stassen. 'Sensitivity of laparoscopic dissectors,' Surgical Endoscopy, Volume 013, Issue 09, pp 869-87.

[2] F. Lai, R.D. Howe, P. Millman, S. Sur. 'Frame Mapping and Motion Constraint Effects on Task Performance in Endoscopic Surgery.' Proceedings of the ASME Dynamic Systems and Control Division, DSC- Vol. 67, Nashville, 1999.

[3] B. Hannaford, J. Trujillo, M. Sinanan, M. Moreyra, J. Rosen, J. Brown, R. Lueschke, M. MacFarlane, 'Computerized Endoscopic Surgical Grasper,' Proceedings, MMVR-98 (Medicine Meets Virtual Reality), San Diego, January 1998.

[4] J. Rosen, B. Hannaford, M. MacFarlane, M. Sinanan, 'Force Controlled and Teleoperated Endoscopic Grasper for Minimally Invasive Surgery - Experimental Performance Evaluation,' IEEE Transactions on Biomedical Engineering, vol. 46, pp. 1212-1221, October 1999.

Medicine Meets Virtual Reality 2001
J.D. Westwood et al. (Eds.)
IOS Press, 2001

A Virtual Reality Simulator for Bone Marrow Harvest for Pediatric Transplant

Liliane dos Santos Machado[1]
Andre Nebel de Mello[2]
Roseli de Deus Lopes[1]
Vicente Odone Filho[2]
Marcelo Knorich Zuffo[1]

[1] *Laboratório de Sistemas Integráveis - Universidade de São Paulo*
Av. Prof Luciano Gualberto, 158 travessa 3 Cidade Universitária
São Paulo - SP, 05508-900
{liliane, roseli, mkzuffo}@lsi.usp.br

[2] *Instituto da Criança*
Hospital da Clínicas da Faculdade de Medicina da Universidade de São Paulo
nebel@ajato.com.br, vicenteof@icr.hcnet.usp.br

Abstract. Bone marrow transplant is a relatively new procedure to treat recently considered incurable diseases. One important part of the procedure is the process of harvesting the donor bone marrow. We are developing a virtual reality simulator for bone marrow harvest that integrates interactive stereo visualization and force feedback techniques. The main objective is to offer a low cost virtual reality system to boost current adopted training methodologies for bone marrow harvesting.

1. Introduction

Bone marrow transplant, despite commonly held perceptions, is not a usual surgery. Basically, the bone marrow transplant consists of an infusion of healthy cells, capable of generating identical copies of themselves and producing blood cells. This process is completed by an intravenous reinfusion. The most complicated part of the bone marrow transplant is the process of harvesting the donor bone marrow. This invasive procedure is relatively simple, but the success of the procedure will depend on the physician's dexterity and his ability to manipulate the needle.

Virtual reality has been used with significant results in many critical mission medical applications, which demands intense decision making from physicians and mistakes are not allowed. The use of virtual reality techniques are beneficial in cases where a mistake could have a physical or emotional impact on the patient by helping to simulate procedures and surgical training. The possibility of producing a sense of touch, pressure and force for the physician is the main advantage using this technology, improving its medical performance.

In this project, we are proposing a virtual reality system for medical training in bone marrow harvest from children. This system should generate the force, pressure and touch sensations involved in the bone marrow harvest proceeding, giving to the physician the conditions to learn and improve this practice. The bone marrow harvest is a blind procedure, since physicians cannot see the internal patient anatomy. In our case we are providing a training tool which incorporate stereoscopic view of the human part of interest.

Our goal is to support the teaching and training of the physicians in this modality, providing competence to novice physicians, better quality for patient's attendance and better rehabilitation for bone marrow donors.

This project has been developed in joint cooperation with the Instituto da Criança (Children's Institute) of Hospital das Clínicas da Faculdade de Medicina da Universidade de São Paulo and counts on physicians experience and abilities to describe the bone marrow harvest procedure and test the proposed system.

2. The Bone Marrow Transplant

The bone marrow is a soft fatty tissue that is found inside bones that produces blood cells. The bone marrow from chest, skull, hip, ribs and spine, contain cells that can generate all family of blood cells of the human body. These cells (Figure 1a) includes the white cells (leukocyte) which protect the body against infections and the red cells (erythrocytes) which transport oxygen and remove the impurity from organs and tissues, and finally the platelets which act in the blood coagulation.

Some references [1] indicate that 95% of the total blood cells production into the human body is originated from the bone marrow and the rest in the liver and spleen. Some of the produced cells originated in the bone marrow are introduced directly in the blood, while some migrate to peripheral tissues to become lymphocytes. All blood cells had maturation stages and all mature blood cells are originated from key cells in the bone marrow.

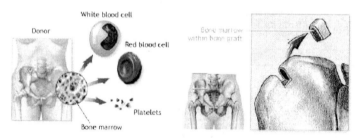

Figure 1. (a) Bone marrow and blood cells. (b) Bone marrow from the hip (iliac crest).
(obtained from www.adam.com).

The bone marrow transplant is a relatively new medical procedure to treat recently considered incurable diseases. The first success transplant was made in 1968, and since then has been a current procedure for patients with leukemia, aplastic anemia, lymphomas, multiple myelomas, disturbs in the immunology system and in some solid tumors such as the breast cancer and ovarian cancer [2]. Bone marrow transplants prolong the life of patients who might otherwise die. As with all major organ transplants, however, it is difficult to find bone marrow donors, and the cost of the transplant is relatively high. The hospitalization period is three to six weeks. During this time, patients are isolated and under strict monitoring because of the increased risk of infection. It takes about six months to a year for the immune system fully recovers from this procedure.

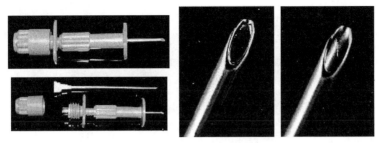

Figure 2. The Illinois syringe for bone marrow harvest.

The process to extract he bone marrow is made through many material aspirations from the iliac crest (Figure 1b) bone marrow (sometimes it includes the sternum bone also) from the donator under general anesthesia. The extraction is made through serial aspirations from the bone marrow using a thick needle and syringe (Figure 2); the total amount of material to be collected is around 200 ml. The bone marrow is filtered, treated, and transplanted immediately, sometimes it's frozen and stored for later use. The procedure is a blind procedure without any visual feedback except the external view of the donor, the physician need to feel the skin and bone levels trespassed by the needle to the bone marrow and then start the material aspiration. The patient will receive the bone marrow on a procedure similar to a blood transfusion.

The whole procedure apparently is quite simple, but from the physician point of view it demands great ability, which will offer a better recovery to the donator and less pos-harvesting pain.

3. Motivation

Surgical simulations for medical training using virtual reality technology are being a research topic for many medical modalities [3][4][5][6]. Despite it seems to be a simple transplant apparently, the bone marrow transplant is a high precision invasive procedure. The Instituto da Criança (Children's Institute) of Hospital das Clínicas of São Paulo realize on average 15 procedures every year. Currently the only training procedure available for novice surgeons is training with guinea pigs, real procedure observation and further supervision by trained surgeons in real procedures.

We intend to support the teaching and training of the physicians in this modality, allowing a better rehabilitation for bone marrow donors providing competence to novice physicians.

4. Proposed System

The proposed system is based on a "fish tank" [7] like semi-immersive virtual reality system where two surgeons (the tutor and the trainee) can share the same stereoscopic view of the bone marrow harvest procedure simulation. A high end PC Pentium III with stereo support board including a time-multiplexed Stereo Graphics Crystal Eyes shutter glasses [8] and a Phantom Desktop haptic device composes our simulator. Figure 3 shows the current available platform to the tests.

The haptic senses motion in 6 degrees of freedom providing realistic sense of touch. The trainee can feel the point of the virtual needle in all axes, and track its orientation (pitch, roll and yaw) like when manipulating a real needle.

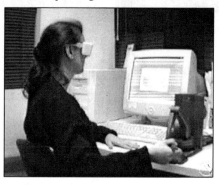

Figure 3. The system platform.

The system runs on a Windows NT workstation and was developed on C++, OpenGL and the Ghost API [9][10]. The simulator consists in a force feedback virtual interactive model of tissue layers from the pelvis region and its hardness and texture characteristics. Figure 4 describes these tissue layers.

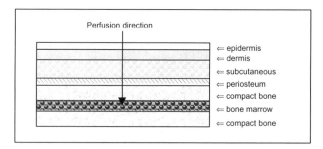

Figure 4. The perfusion tissue layers.

5. Results

The simulator objective is the training of novice physicians in the process of harvesting the bone marrow. Using a virtual syringe with a tactile feedback (simulated in the Phantom Desktop) the physician can penetrate thought the several tissue layers feeling the transitions among tissues, as well as feeling the texture associated to each layer.

Based on a subjective approach and based on the sensitive feelings from physicians we modeled the several physical properties of the tissues in the iliac crest in the following layers:

- Epidermis: approximately 2mm thick, elastic and slippery tissue;
- Dermis: approximately 7mm thick, elastic tissue;
- Subcutaneous: approximately 4mm thick, soft and non-resistant tissue;
- Periosteum: approximately 2mm thick, resistant, slippery, lubricated and smooth tissue.
- Compact bone: approximately 5mm thick, hard and resistant tissue;
- Bone marrow: approximately 10mm thick, soft tissue, without resistance.

A touch model was created with the layers described above for initial tests. Nowadays we are working on a second haptic model with consists on a 3D anatomy of the pelvis region. To this model the several external tissue layers are being compounded. In this case we will offer two kinds of simulations blind oriented and blindness oriented. In the blindness oriented simulations novice physician will be able to be visually assisted by a stereoscopic view of the anatomy having a better special understanding of the whole procedure.

6. Conclusions and Future Work

In this paper we proposed a basic simulator for bone marrow harvest for transplant. This simulator has being implemented using the Phantom Desktop force-feedback haptic system and the Ghost API. Using the features offered by the Phantom Desktop we modeled subjectively the tissue layers (crossed during the perfusion process) to achieve the bone marrow. Preliminary evaluation of the simulator by physicians indicates that the system has a potential use for the training of such procedures.

Further research directions are related to a better objective modeling of the tissue layers. We are also doing the modeling of the 3D anatomy of this body region of interest, in order to offer a better simulation environment to the physicians. Further evaluations would be possible using the blind procedure that is closer to real procedures.

Another future research direction is related with the modeling of the 3D signature of this procedure and the level of deep perfusion of the needle in order to measure objectively the quality of the procedure. In this case we would like to store, recognize and measure the spatial procedure signature in order to compare and evaluate it with "good" procedures.

7. Acknowledgements

This project is funded by Fundação de Amparo à Pesquisa do Estado de São Paulo, grant # 99/01583-0, with additional support from RECOPE/FINEP – "Visualização na Engenharia". Thanks to Anelise Stein for helping us to generate the 3D model.

References

[1] I.M. Roitt et al., Imunology. Mosby, 3th ed, 1993.
[2] Oncolink. URL from the Cancer Center at the University of Pennsylvania (USA).http://cancer.med.upenn.edu/specialty/med_onc/bmt/
[3] C.Basdogan, "Simulating minimally invasive surgical procedures in virtual environments: From tissue mechanics to simulation and training", notes from tutorial presented on Medicine Meets Virtual Reality 2000, March 2000.
[4] Burdea, G.; Patounakis, G.; Popescu, V.; Weiss, R.E.; "Virtual reality Training for the Diagnosis of Prostate Cancer"; IEEE Virtual Reality Annual International Symposium Proceedings, March 1999, pp190-197.
[5] Peifer, J. Eye Surgery Simulation. Biomedical Interactive Technology Center. In http://www.bitc.gatech.edu/bitcprojects/eyes_sim/eye_surg_sim.html
[6] M.A. Sagar, D. Bullivant, G.D. Mallinson, P.J. Hunter, I. Hunter. A Virtual Environment and Model of The Eye for Surgical Simulation. In Computer Graphics, Proceedings of SIGGRAPH'94, pages 205-212, 1994.
[7] K. Pimentel and K. Teixeira, Virtual reality - through the new looking glass, 2.ed. McGraw-Hill, 1995.
[8] Stereographics, Developer Handbook, StereoGraphics Corp., 1997.
[9] Ghost SDK Programmer's Guide Version 3.0. Sensable Technologies Inc., March 1999.
[10] Ghost API Reference Version 3.0. Sensable Technologies Inc., March 2000

Medicine Meets Virtual Reality 2001
J.D. Westwood et al. (Eds.)
IOS Press, 2001

Using Immersive VR as a Tool for Preoperative Planning for Minimally Invasive Donor Nephrectomy

Michael J. Mastrangelo Jr., MD[1]; James D. Hoskins, BS[1]; Mathew Nicholls, MD, PhD[4];
Larry C. Munch, MD[2]; Thomas D. Johnston MD[3]; K. Sudhaker Reddy, MD[3];
Dinesh Ranjan, MD[3]; Wayne O. Witzke[1]; Adrian Park, MD[1]

[1] *Division of General Surgery*
[2] *Division of Urology*
[3] *Division of Transplantation*
[4] *Department of Orthopedic Surgery*
Department of Surgery, University of Kentucky College of Medicine
800 Rose Street, Room C345, Lexington, KY 40536

Abstract: For surgeons approaching minimally invasive donor nephrectomy it is important to identify variant anatomy preoperatively since this anatomy can vary significantly from patient to patient. The goal of this operation is to preserve the architecture and function of the organ so it can be transplanted and function successfully. The ability of the surgeon to navigate through an individual patient's anatomy in a virtual three-dimensional (3D) immersive environment augments understanding of anatomical relationships particular to that individual patient and facilitates conveying that information to other physicians and students. Utilizing automated 3D reconstruction of high contrast computed tomography (CT) scan files viewed in this way, surgeons reported a better preoperative understanding of the anatomical variations and encountered fewer surprises at the time of surgery.

1. Introduction

The ability to manipulate 3D models and to view anatomy from different perspectives is especially useful in minimal access surgery where preoperative planning, patient positioning and port placement are paramount to success. CT scans with intravenous contrast medium are generally used for preoperative anatomical and vascular evaluation of potential kidney donors.[1] These studies are interpreted by physicians who assess the 3D relationship of the various organs, vasculature and surrounding tissue from sequential two-dimensional (2D) images. The interpretation of any anomalies is usually conveyed to other physicians in written form or discussed while viewing static 2D images. A significant problem with this method is the inherent conceptual limitation of conveying or teaching 3D relationships via 2D images. The usefulness of 3D representation of these scans has been well documented.[2][3][4]

2. Methods and Materials

This problem was addressed utilizing immersive 3D representation. Amira Software (Template Graphics Software Inc.) is an automated package that produces accurate and useful models in minutes and runs on a standard personal computer (PC). Other commercially available applications require manual painting of individual slices by engineers or trained technicians, resulting in reported turnaround times up to 72 hours.[5] The software accomplishes this by constructing isosurfaces from like threshold values and avoids the bias of a technician. Multiple models constructed at varying threshold windows can be displayed on the ImmersaDesk (Fakespace Systems Inc.). This allows groups of physicians and students to navigate and orient themselves in an uncluttered model, with fewer surfaces represented, before advancing to greater detail.

We researched and documented the utility of a commercially available computer application and its use in an immersive 3-D environment in order to overcome the limitations of 2D images. Amira software has the capability to interpret 2D slice data from CTs, magnetic resonance imaging (MRIs) and TIF files to construct isosurface 3-D structures from high contrast images.

The image data were collected on a Siemens Somatom Plus 4 CT scanner using IV contrast and 2 mm slice thickness to create high-resolution CT images through the abdomen in the region of the kidneys. These data were exported directly from the CT console to a Siemens MagicView 300 console as DICOM (Digital Imaging and Communications in Medicine) format so as to preserve data image details such as in-plane resolution, slice spacing/orientation, patient data, and relevant scanner parameters. The data were then archived from the MagicView 300 console onto removable storage media in DICOM format. The data are subsequently loaded and processed on a workstation with Amira. Rapid image segmentation was accomplished by taking advantage of the high signal of the renal vasculature in the contrast enhanced CT images. The signal from vasculature is much higher than adjacent tissues allowing for image segmentation based on signal threshold values. Once the threshold is chosen, the Amira software calculates and renders a 3-D isosurface based on all the image values at or above the selected threshold. Cropping reduced the size of the cubic target area to only that region that provided pertinent information for the primary task. Cropping also allowed much finer tuning of threshold levels to yield all of the information the data set could provide about the particular area of interest.

A true surface was then created from the isosurface and saved as an open inventor format file that is ported directly to the Immersadesk. The projected model on the Immersadesk was then viewed and its orientation in space controlled and altered in real-time by the reviewing surgeons. In this manner a view from any necessary angle in any required magnification could be obtained. Navigation through structure walls to view the inner-space of organs or vessels was also possible. Figure 1 shows an overview of the aorta, branching vessels and both kidneys.

Figure 1: Overview of aorta with arterial branches. Left renal vein with an early bifurcation and a large anomalous gonadal vein.

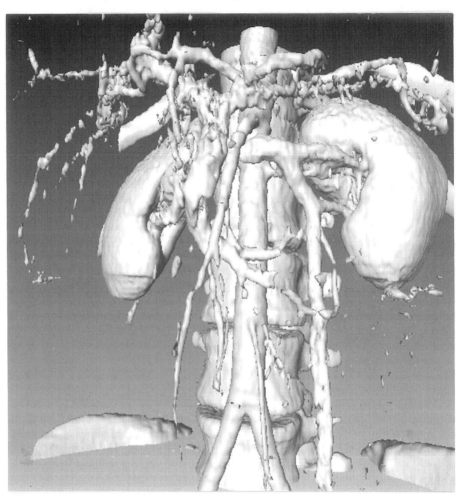

3. Results

This preoperative tool aided the surgeons in several ways. Isosurfaces were created in less than 60 seconds resulting in no delay for access to the information. The surgeons were better prepared for surgery because they had more precise information about the operative site. There were fewer unexpected structures so it was felt that surgery proceeded more quickly an efficiently.

Figure 2 : Non-visualized lumbar vein (160 density threshold).

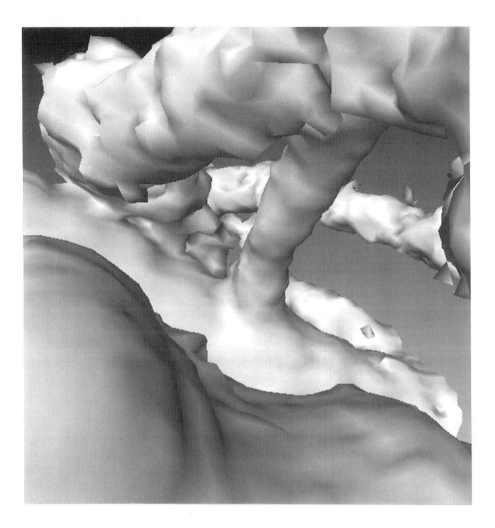

    Some structures that were difficult to identify and visualize with 2D CT alone were more apparent using the Amira reconstruction process. The branching and termination points of vessels were also more readily identified by surgeons. An example of this is the large anomalous left gonadal vein and early bifurcation of the left renal vein illustrated in figure 1. Although identified on 2D CT, the relationship of these structures was more readily understood and conveyed utilizing the 3D models. Three dimensional representations of anatomical relationships have been shown to facilitate teaching.[6][7]

Deep or less prominent structures are often obscured by more prominent or overlying structures. This is overcome by the ability to navigate in 3D space to a particular area and the ability to vary the amount of information projected by adjusting the threshold density levels. This is demonstrated in Figures 2 and 3 that are magnified views of a more finite area. Figure 2 shows the area behind the left renal vein that often contains lumbar veins contributing to the back of the left renal vein. This image is gated at a high threshold that demonstrates dominant structures. The image in figure 3 shows the same view gated at a lower threshold (90 instead of 160) to demonstrate less prominent structures. At this threshold a large lumbar vein, not seen in figure 2, is readily identified contributing to the left renal vein in figure 3. These lumbar veins are generally not identifiable in routine 2D CT images or standard 3D reconstructions.

Figure 3: Visualized lumbar vein contributing to the left renal vein (90 density threshold).

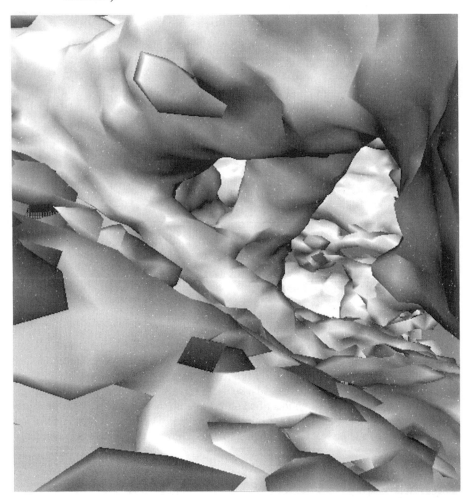

Viewing the 3-dimensional models on the ImmersaDesk allowed the surgeon the capability of actually navigating 360 degrees around or along the axis of a vessel resulting in a better understanding of its architecture. Amira is intuitive enough that physicians were able to learn to operate it without the need of a technician. This allowed the surgeons to control the view, resulting in efficient use of their time.

Relevant views of structures that might be useful for future research and publications were saved as graphics files or sent immediately to the surgeon's printer.

4. Future Directions

Isosurfaces of real human anatomy can be saved in 3-D modeling formats and incorporated in ongoing MIS procedure simulations on the ImmersaDesk. This is an excellent way to create models of specific patient's anatomy and have it available for rapid inclusion in the MIS simulator. Medical students would have the ability to observe abnormal or exceptional anatomy in patients they will be exposed to in their PBL sessions and rounds. They could better understanding anatomical interactions and navigate through a completely realistic model of a specific patient with the option of removing and/or making any degree translucent structures or tissue that might be hindering their view.

5. Discussion

Initial results of this pilot study suggest that this is an effective environment for evaluation and teaching. The combination of the Amira software and the ImmersaDesk provides a useful, accurate platform for evaluating CT scan data prior to laparoscopic donor nephrectomy. Immesive 3D representation of this data also augments the conveyance of information for telemedicine teaching and consultation as identified in previous studies.[8] An ongoing prospective trial is underway to validate its usefulness as a diagnostic tool and its potential for improving preoperative planning for laparoscopic donor nephrectomy.

References

[1]   AH. Dachman, GM Newmark, MT Mitchell, ES Woodle, Helical CT examination of
       potential kidney donors. AJR Am J. Roentgenol. Jul 171 (1), (1998), 193-200.
[2]   PA. Smith, EK Fishman, Three-dimensional CT angiography: Renal applications.
       Semin. Ultrasound CT MR. Oct. 19(5), (1998), 413-24.
[3]   BW. Lindgren, T. Demos, R. Marsan, H. Posniak, B. Kostro, D. Calvert, D. Hatch
       R. Flanigan, D. Steinmuller, R. Lewis, Renal computer tomography with 3-
       dimensional angiography and simultaneous measurement of plasma contrast
       clearance reduce the invasiveness and cost of evaluating living renal donor
       candidates. Transplantation Jan 27; 61(2), (1996), 219-23.
[4]   DM. Coll, BR Herts, WJ. Davros, RG. Uzzo, AC. Novick, Preoperative use of 3-D
       volume rendering to demonstrate renal tumors and renal anatomy, Radiographics
       Mar-Apr. 20(2), (2000), 431-8.
[5]   L. Lerner, H Henriques, R. Harris, Interactive 3-Dimensional Computerized Tomography

Reconstruction in the Evaluation of the Living Renal Donor, J. Urology 161, (1999) 403-407.

[6]   S. Gorbis, RC. Hallgren, Visualization technology in medical education, J. Am. Osteopath. Assoc. 99(4), (1999), 211-4.

[7]   GL. Nieder, JN Scott, MD Anderson, Using Quick Time virtual reality objects in computer-assisted instruction of gross anatomy. Clin. Anat. 13(4), (2000), 287-93.

[8]   B. Pham, J. Yearwood, Delivery and interactive processing of visual data for a cooperative telemedicine environment. Telemed. J. Summer 6(2), (2000), 261-8.

Medicine Meets Virtual Reality 2001
J.D. Westwood et al. (Eds.)
IOS Press, 2001

Virtual Eye Muscle Surgery
Based Upon Biomechanical Models

Herwig Mayr

*Department of Software Engineering for Medicine, Upper Austrian
Polytechnic University, Hauptstr. 117, A-4232 Hagenberg, Austria*

Abstract. *Within our research project "SEE-KID", a Software Engineering Environment for Knowledge-based Interactive Eye Motility Diagnostics, we focus on virtual reality training for the surgery of human eye muscles of - mostly - children age 1 to 3. Our report gives details on the sound integration of biomechanical muscle data into our virtual reality models in order to evaluate the quality of specific techniques for eye motility surgery regarding real-world pathologies. We illustrate the usefulness of our software system describing some of the possible medical applications, like optimized transposition surgery of the musculus obliquus superior.*

1 Introduction

SEE-KID, our *Software Engineering Environment for Knowledge-based Interactive Eye Motility Diagnostics*, is an ongoing project, partially funded by the Austrian ministry of science and the research fund of the national chamber of commerce, the goal of which is to extend the current capabilities of our 3D VR modeler for the human eye, its orbita and its muscles, to enable common surgical eye muscle operations (transposition, shortening, splitting, etc.) in a graphic interactive way that is familiar to an experienced surgeon.

Additionally, the system can be used for education and training purposes, because by means of extensive possibilities for parameterization of the human eye model, every common pathological case of human eye motility can be modeled - and subsequently tried to correct. Using modern capabilities of VR systems, a surgeon can simulate a pathological behavior pre-operatively, and subsequently develop the most appropriate surgery by applying virtual surgical operations onto the VR model, relying on appropriate surgery best practices stored in a knowledge base, if available.

2 Abstraction of a Functional Eye Model

In order to create a full biomechanical model of the human eye and not just detailed images from different directions, our research work concentrates on the development of a functional model of the human eye that can be visualized in acceptable quality, but is additionally suitable for exploring the motility of the eye and can serve as a basis for medical surgery of the eye muscles. Our goal is to explicitly stress the mathematical-geometrical background of eye motility in order to analyze the possibilities and limits of modeling the eye muscle surgery process. In doing so, the medical surgeon shall be enabled to gain insight into specific pathological problems and to experimentally train and optimize his surgery techniques.

For a suitable representation of a functional eye motility model, the following medical components of the eye (or, in case of analyzing stereoscopic behavior, both eyes) are modeled together with their interaction capabilities (see Fig. 1):

- head, bulbus, orbita,
- the four straight eye muscles:
- the two oblique eye muscles:
- the objects constraining the muscles (pulleys, trochlea, etc.).

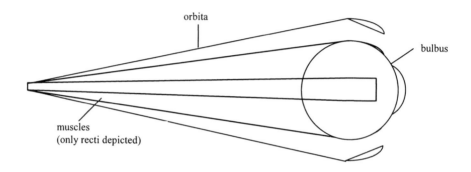

Fig. 1: Functional abstraction of the human eye

3 The SEE-KID System

3.1 State of the Art in Eye Motility Surgery

Technical modeling of human eye muscles using multi-body dynamics is already available at a high level (cf., e.g., [7], [9]). However, only few approaches to the medical interpretation of technically gathered data can be found in literature. Mostly, medical interpretations have been made using statistical methods based upon a large number of patient data (e.g. by Simonsz [12]). Such interpretations only allow the detection of pathological classes and describing their characteristics. The analysis of the causes of the pathology is restricted to hypo- or hyper-functioning of muscles or groups of muscles. Anatomical factors, i.e. biomechanical deficiencies of a patient and subsequent recommendations for eye muscle surgery, can not be gained directly from such statistical interpretations.

In the same way, the technical models described in [3], [9], [11] do not allow a well-founded interpretation of the medical results. These models rather focus on a realistic, anatomic visualization of human eye motility, and generally do not support surgery actions.

3.2 Incremental Development of the SEE-KID System

Model-based eye muscle surgery has been performed at the hospital "Barmherzige Brüder" in Linz, Austria, by Siegfried Priglinger since 1978. Several surgery techniques have been developed or refined by Dr. Priglinger, e.g.,

- a torque-reducing operation that splits straight muscles into a Y-shape in order to reduce nystagmus and squinting,

- reinforcement of oblique muscles using a similar splitting surgery,
- weakening of oblique muscles by a controlled backward transposition (so-called "polarization" of the oblique muscles).

The main advantage of our SEE-KID system is that it combines available biomechanical models with practically proven surgery processes in the way they are performed on a real patient. For the first time it combines a sound mathematical model with appropriate surgery processes in the area of eye motility correction. Fig. 2 depicts the layout of our current prototypic system; for details on the underlying concepts we refer to [5] and [10].

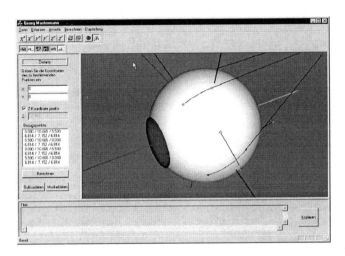

Fig. 2: Screenshot of our system for visualizing human eye muscle pathologies

4 Models Within SEE-KID

The focus of our clinical simulation system SEE-KID is to build a dynamic, interactive biomechanical simulation, comprising geometric, dynamic and kinematic models of the human eye.

4.1 Geometrical Model, Visualization

The geometrical model of SEE-KID implements the constrained 3D orientation of the eyeball within the orbita. Taking into consideration that kinematics of ocular movements follow well defined geometrical laws, we need to analyze and define the properties of our model according to these laws. Eye movements in 3D space involve translations as well as rotations. The geometrical model of SEE-KID will only focus on the rotational aspects of eye movements, so we assume a head-fixed coordinate system and refer to eye movement and eye position as a rotational property of the eyeball (see also [4]).

The oculomotor system restricts the rotation of the eyeball and optimizes movements during saccades. These restrictions are known as Listing's and Donder's laws [4]. The SEE-KID model calculates Listing's plane by splitting every saccade into two rotations from source position to primary position and then from primary position to destination position. Using this method, Listing's law is obeyed throughout the trajectory (see Fig. 3), and Listing's plane can be visualized.

4.2 Dynamic Behavior Model – Muscle Force Prediction

This part of the model deals with the simulation of the oculomotor system of the human eye. The dynamic behavior model therefore needs to simulate force production of all 6 eye muscles. The SEE-KID system uses a general muscle force prediction model, which is then parameterized for every single eye muscle. Thus, this model comprises 6 instances of autonomous muscle models, each developing force which in turn is applied through the biomechanical model. The main research work in this field consists of finding a proper muscle contraction model, fitting the properties of extraocular muscles. Since eye muscles are physiologically related to muscles of the limb, existing models can be evaluated and adapted. The focus of our work lies in modeling musculotendon actuators, which consist of an active, force-producing part (the muscle itself) and a passive element (tendon), applying force to the eyeball.

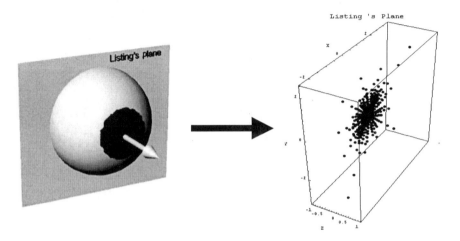

Fig. 3: Projection of quaternion vectors defining Listing's plane

The SEE-KID system adopts an extended Hill-type model, originally developed by Zajac (see [13]), refined and implemented by Brown [1]. This muscle model was developed for use in a hierarchical framework for skeletal dynamics simulation. The simulated muscles are represented by realistic physiological properties, controlled by an arbitrary set of activation commands, ranging from pre-recorded EMG data to dynamic, feedback-driven reflex models. The SEE-KID system uses latter issue to apply muscle driven eye orientation. Due to the model's architecture it is possible to identify properties that correlate with the physiology of extraocular muscles.

Brown's model enables user defined muscle building by aggregating parameterized muscle fiber types into muscle blocks including recruitable motor units. A given muscle then exists, as already explained, of three interacting elements: the contractile element, a series elastic element, and a muscle mass (see Fig. 4). The contractile element and series elastic element, both act on the muscle mass, which has inertial properties to prevent instabilities from arising within the muscle. The contractile element, in effect, consists of as many smaller contractile elements as are defined by the number of motor units, each of which has a passive parallel elastic element, an individually defined firing frequency, and force-length-velocity relationships as determined by the fiber type properties. The parallel elastic element includes a small viscosity for the purpose of stability [2].

Modified Hill-type model

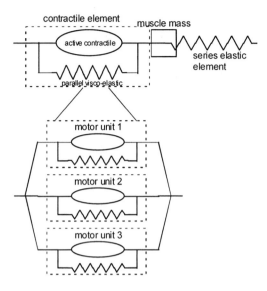

Fig. 4. Basic elements of the muscle model [2]

Each muscle block takes as input parameters activation and musculotendon path length at given time. Activation can be preset at fixed levels directly, or replaced with other systems in order to simulate a neural controller mechanism. The output of the muscle block is the produced force at a given time, activation and length.

4.3 Biomechanical Model

As explained in the previous section, the biomechanical model is responsible for the correct transformation between muscle simulation and geometrical representation. Rotation of the eyeball is caused by contracting muscles which extort torque at the muscle's insertion. Therefore, the biomechanical model accounts for geometrical properties of the extraocular muscles, like path ways, insertion points and pulleys (see [8]). These biomechanical properties notably influence the way muscles act on the eyeball. Thus, the biomechanical model is responsible for the exactness and clinical relevancy of the whole system, because it considers physiologic and anatomic constraints in order to combine other participating models in the system.

Saccades can be modeled as combined rotations about arbitrary axes defined by the extraocular muscles. Another important implication in this context is the modeling of pulleys which extend our initial definition. A pulley consists of a ring or sleeve of collagen, elastin and smooth muscle, encircling an extra-ocular muscle, and coupled to the orbital wall (see [8]). Muscle actions differ in conventional and pulley models. According to this extended model the functional origin of a muscle is introduced and refines the definition of the axis of rotation for a muscle (see Fig. 5).

Our future work will concentrate on embedding the pulley model in our current biomechanical model for the SEE-KID system in order to produce clinically relevant simulations. A biomechanical model including pulleys was implemented by Miller (see [6]).

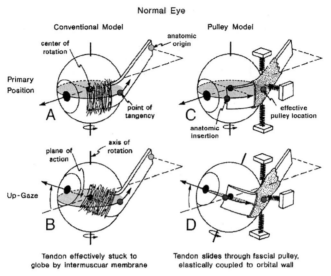

Fig. 5: Influence of pulleys onto muscle force direction [8]

5 Sample Applications for SEE-KID

5.1 Muscle Shortening Regarding an Appropriate Unreel-Strain

The *unreel-strain* is that section of the muscle that follows the curvature of the bulbus from the insertion of the muscle to its point of tangency (i.e. that point where the muscle strain leaves the surface of the bulbus). When a muscle contracts, the length of the unreel-strain is reduced, whereas the point of tangency remains more or less unchanged. This implies that the torque of a muscle remains approximately constant as long as the unreel-strain has a length greater than zero.

In SEE-KID, for each transposition of an insertion of a muscle (and particularly for each shortening) the alteration of the unreel-length of the muscle is continuously re-calculated and visualized. Infeasible transpositions (leading to an unreel-length of 0) immediately issue a warning and can only be performed by a surgeon through overruling the recommendations of SEE-KID (or are not allowed at all).

5.2 Torque-Reducing Transposition of the Musculus Obliquus Superior

Since the musculus obliquus superior is guided onto the bulbus via the trochlea, all theoretically possible points of tangency form a circle upon the lateral area of the bulbus, the so-called "tangent circle". In order to avoid an unreel-length of 0 for the musculus obliquus superior (see the previous chapter), the insertion of the muscle has to be placed outside of the tangent circle.

If the insertion of the musculus obliquus superior is located in such a way that the muscle force direction does not pass through the Z-axis (this generally indicates a pathological case), the muscle issues an irritating torque around the Z-axis. In order to minimize this torque, the surgeon has to displace the insertion of musculus obliquus superior in such a way that a minimum deviance from the Z-axis is achieved. This torque-reducing transposition is supported by algorithmical and graphical means in SEE-KID, additionally enabling maximizing of unreel-length.

5.3 Suitability for Telesurgery

Our SEE-KID system relies on common standards for communication and visualization. Therefore it can be used jointly over the internet thus enabling medical tele-training and tele-education. Additionally it supports one aspect of internet medicine by enabling distance surgery to simultaneously support a real surgery. In the same way, decentralized patient data and surgery process recommendations can be accessed by our system.

SEE-KID will primarily be used as a medical training and education system for medical surgeons at the "Barmherzige Brüder" hospital in Linz, Austria. Ophthalmologists will be able to access the system via the Internet and can in this way exchange experience and get surgery recommendations from the eye motility surgery experts at the hospital. When the system has reached full functionality, it will be offered to interested hospitals and surgeons for a nominal fee.

Literature

[1] Brown, I.E., Cheng, E.J., and Loeb, G.E. (1999). Measured and Modeled Properties of Mammalian Skeletal Muscle: I. The effects of post-activation potentiation on the time course and velocity dependencies of force production. J Musc Res Cell Motil. Vol 20: 443-456.

[2] Cheng, E., Brown, I., Loeb, J. (1999). Matlab-Muscle Model. http://brain.phgy.queensu.ca/muscle_model

[3] Demer, J.L., Miller, J.M., Poukens, V., Vinters, H.V., Glasgow, B.J. (1995). Evidence for Fibromuscular Pulleys of the Recti Extraocular Muscles. Invest. Ophtalm. & Vis. Sc., Vol. 36, No., 6, 1125 - 1136

[4] Haslwanter, T. (1995). Mathematics of Three-dimensional Eye Rotations. Vision, Res. Vol. 35, No. 12, 1727 – 1739

[5] Mayr, H., Jacak, W., Priglinger, S., (1996). Computer-aided Preparation of Eye Surgery (in German). In E. E. Dittel, P. Kopacek (eds.). Proc. 3.Jahrestagung EDV im Krankenhaus, pp. 60 - 73, Schriftenreihe der Abteilung für System- und Automatisierungstechnik, Wissenschaftliche Landesakademie für Niederösterreich, Krems, Österreich, Mai 1996.

[6] Miller, J.M. (1995). Software Review: Program Simulates Orbit Gaze Mechanics, Ophthalmology World News, Nr.12, 1995.

[7] Miller, J.M. (1995). Orbit™ 1.5 Gaze Mechanics Simulation User's Manual No. Eidactics; Suite 404; 1450 Greenwich Street; San Francisco, CA 94109; USA.

[8] Miller, J.M., Demer, J.L. (1999). Clinical Applications Of Computer Models For Strabismus. In eds Rosenbaum, A and Santiago, AP, Clinical Strabismus Management. cty Philadelphia, pub W. B. Saunders.

[9] Miller, J.M., Robinson D.A. (1984). A Model of the Mechanics of Binocular Alignment. Comput. and Biomed. Res., Vol. 17, No. 12, 436 - 470

[10] Priglinger, S., Jacak, W., Mayr, H., (1997). Ein Softwaresystem zur Vorbereitung von Augenoperationen (in German). Proc. MEDEVA '97, Schloss Hagenberg, Österreich.

[11] Robinson, D.A. (1975). A Quantitative Analysis of Extraocular Muscle Cooperation and Squint. Invest. Ophthalmol. 14, 801 ff.

[12] Simonsz, H.J. (1989). The Mechanics of Squint Surgery. Habilitationsschrift des Fachbereiches Humanmedizin der Justus-Liebig-Universität Gießen, Deutschland, Acta Strabologica

[13] Zajac, F.E. (1989). Muscle and tendon: Properties, models, scaling and application to biomechanics and motor control. Crit. Rev. Biomed. Engng. Vol. 17: 359-411.

Medicine Meets Virtual Reality 2001
J.D. Westwood et al. (Eds.)
IOS Press, 2001

Development of an International Net-Based Medical Information System for Advanced Surgical Education

A. Mehrabi, H. Schwarzer, Ch. Herfarth, F. Kallinowski

Department of Surgery, University of Heidelberg
Im Neuenheimer Feld 110, 69120 Heidelberg, Germany
e-mail: arianeb_mehrabi@med.uni-heidelberg.de

Introduction

Advanced medical education, access to specific knowledge and attending international congresses is limited by mobility barriers and scarce financial resources (Gawad et al., 1998). Our department started a project called „alumni med-live" being sponsored by the German Ministry for Cooperation and the German Service for Foreign Education. This project combines the care for medical graduates (alumni) with the possibilities offered by modern information technology to present medical lectures digitally. In the „med-live series" there are by now over 2000 lectures available on over 75 CDs (Kallinowski et al., 1998a). Since June 2000, access is gained to a database via the internet (www.med-live.de).

Lectures and interactive multimedia medical courses are available (Mehrabi et al., 2000a). The inherent complexity of medical knowledge (Mehrabi et al., 2000b) as well as the profound visual orientation pose special requirements on internet-based information systems. These requirements are summed up in table 1.

Table 1: Requirements of an internet-based medical information system
- breaking up multimedia documents into single units that are stored independently
- platform dependent presentation of multimedia documents over the internet
- minding the knowledge and experience of the user
- putting together new presentations from different matching units
- editing the documents via the internet without prior computer knowledge

In order to meet these requirements the multimedia information needs to be split into smaller units and to be stored in a database. A three-level database architecture was developed based on a component-based document model (Schwarzer et al., 1999) and put into practice with the help of ObjectStore and Weblogic Commerce Server. After the database was started under www.med-live.de the logic behind the above mentioned requirements became obvious. Some points will still need to be realized in the future due to limited resources available now. At present there are about ten days worth of medical information available over the net. This equals 100,000 documents with 3.5 GB of information. This information shall be added to every 30 days. In the course of the next 12 months an addition of at least 40 days is planned. This new platform for publication is available for all medical fields. Lectures, video-clips and all other forms of audio-visual medical contributions can be distributed world-wide.

On June 17th 2000 a cooperation of 303 professors of 53 university hospitals and academic clinics was formed to constitute the virtual faculty of medicine. At present it represents 35 different medical fields. The plenary assembly has chosen a structure that combines efficient work with democratic control. The goal of the virtual faculty of medicine is to ensure the quality of the integrated lectures. The assembly is composed of different fields. They elect a speaker, advisory boards and a secretary that together form the dean's office of the virtual faculty. An elected president supervises the management which also puts itself up for election on a regular basis. Only members of the virtual faculty are authorized to comment on and supervise the quality of the contributions. Only positively rated contributions remain in the published content.

Basic and advanced education in medicine is also characterized by multiple economic and technical interdependences (Kallinowski et al., 1998b). The foundation of the virtual faculty for medicine makes it possible for members of the medical profession to advance education not only nationwide but also in foreign countries. Of about 1400 university professors in Germany over 20 percent have in a first sweep agreed to take an active part in the virtual faculty. This number has increased by about 350 candidate members in the past three months. Another 300 people have already indicated their interest in staying informed on the process. The assembly decided to remain open to cooperation of interested individuals from all over the world. Right now colleagues in Austria and Switzerland are involved. About one third of the contributions are in English.

Interaction between users and authors

The „alumni.med-live" project forms ties for alumnis worldwide with their home universities. The graduates are addressed in contact-events involving them with the present work. These contact events promote requests for new contents of information that are then put together by the authors and certified by the virtual faculty. The laboratory for computer-based training (CBT) then implements this material in the database that is simultaneously advanced to the highest technical standard. Of course authors can independently publish new results in their respective fields of study. The publication of such a lecture is possible at any time so that the database is continuously updated. Accepted contributions are also evaluated by the users. In this way we are for the first time able to ensure the quality of education. In the long run it can be determined whether a contribution addressed a large number of people and whether the users were satisfied with its contents. The number of people addressed can be derived from counting the number of people accessing the program as well as the time-span which they spend inside certain parts of the program. Upon leaving the program, the user can evaluate the value and quality of the information offered. Thus, a score can be formed that determines the target group that uses the offered information. The quality of education can be monitored which may in the long run enhance the quality of advanced education and medical treatment (Kallinowski et al., 2000). As a positive effect the information offered can be adjusted to the knowledge and experience of the user (table 1). The concept has been tested in Asia, the Middle East and South America with satisfying results.

Future developments

It is difficult to foresee the future of a development that takes place at an explosive rate. It is already possible to offer each user „his" individual program. This happens when he chooses from a pool of provided digitalized educational paths. The distribution is limited by the number of channels available but the fastest networks and modern satellite transmission will soon make waiting periods something of the past.

Considering the estimated amount of data it will soon be necessary to submit incoming contributions automatically to members of the different fields for certification. This calls for additional interaction between authors and the database. This way several authors of different fields will at different locations work together to meet a specific request. Technical developments to allow such a cooperative working environment are expected. The result could completely change traditional forms of advanced education. The information age will in this regard be another noticeable help in facilitating daily-life.

References

Gawad K. A., Mehrabi A., Staff Ch., Blöchle C., Izbicki J. R., Kallinowski F., Broelsch C. E. Multimedia CD-ROM: Ein neues Medium zur Verbesserung der Wissensvermittlung. Langenbecks Arch Chir Suppl II S. 880-881, 1998

Kallinowski F., Mehrabi A., Schwarzer H., Herfarth Ch. Entwicklung einer multimedialen CD-ROM-Reihe zur Verbesserung der chirurgischen Aus- und Weiterbildung. Langenbecks Arch Chir Suppl II S. 885-887, 1998a

Kallinowski F, Eitel F. Neue Ansätze der chirurgischen Aus- und Weiterbildung. Chirurg 69: 1323, 1998b

Kallinowski F., Mehrabi A., Schwarzer H., Herfarth Ch. Computer-basierte Trainingssysteme - Eine neue Methode zur Aufklärung des Patienten im chirurgischen Alltag In: LEARNTEC 2000, Beck U., Sommer W. (Hrsg.) Band 2 S. 901-905, 2000

Mehrabi A., Ruggiero S., Schwarzer H., Fritz Th., Herfarth Ch., Kallinowski F. Innovativer Weg zur Verbesserung der Aus- und Weiterbildung in der Chirurgie durch CBT am Beispiel der CD-ROM "Distale Radiusfraktur" In: LEARNTEC 2000, Beck U., Sommer W. (Hrsg.) Band 2 S. 907-916, 2000a

Mehrabi A, Glückstein C, Benner A, Hashemi B, Herfarth C, Kallinowski F. A new way for surgical education - Development and evaluation of a computer-based training module. Comput Biol Med 30: 97 - 109, 2000b

Schwarzer H, Mehrabi A, Wetter T, Kallinowski F. A component-based approach to authoring, interaction modeling and reuse of multimedia resources in a web-based training system. In: Victor N, Blettner M, Edler L, Haux R, Knaup-Gregori P, Pritsch M, Wahrendorf J, Windeler J, Ziegler S (Hrsg.) Medical Informatics, Biostatistics and Epidemiology for Efficient Health Care and Medical Research. Meidzinische Informatik, Biometrie und Epidemiologie 85: Urban und Vogel, 1999

Medicine Meets Virtual Reality 2001
J.D. Westwood et al. (Eds.)
IOS Press, 2001

Virtual Reality Based Surgical Assistance and Training System For Long Duration Space Missions

Kevin Montgomery PhD; Guillaume Thonier; Michael Stephanides MD;
Stephen Schendel MD DDS

1. National Biocomputation Center, 701A Welch Road Suite 1128, Stanford, CA 94305
2. Department of Computer Science, Stanford, CA 94305

Abstract. Access to medical care during long duration space missions is extremely important. Numerous unanticipated medical problems will need to be addressed promptly and efficiently. Although telemedicine provides a convenient tool for remote diagnosis and treatment, it is impractical due to the long delay between data transmission and reception to Earth.

While a well-trained surgeon-internist-astronaut would be an essential addition to the crew, the vast number of potential medical problems necessitate instant access to computerized, skill-enhancing and diagnostic tools. A functional prototype of a virtual reality based surgical training and assistance tool was created at our center, using low-power, small, lightweight components that would be easy to transport on a space mission. The system consists of a tracked, head-mounted display, a computer system, and a number of tracked surgical instruments. The software provides a real-time surgical simulation system with integrated monitoring and information retrieval and a voice input/output subsystem.

Initial medical content for the system has been created, comprising craniofacial, hand, inner ear, and general anatomy, as well as information on a number of surgical procedures and techniques. One surgical specialty in particular, microsurgery, was provided as a full simulation due to its long training requirements, significant impact on result due to experience, and likelihood for need. However, the system is easily adapted to realistically simulate a large number of other surgical procedures. By providing a general system for surgical simulation and assistance, the astronaut-surgeon can maintain their skills, acquire new specialty skills, and use tools for computer-based surgical planning and assistance to minimize overall crew and mission risk.

1 INTRODUCTION

NASA's current plans for a manned mission to Mars in 2025 involve a journey between 120-180 days to reach the planet, between 200-600 days on the surface, followed by a 120-180 return trip[9,10,24]. The crew size would be between 4-6 crewmembers, of which one would be designated as a Chief Medical Officer (CMO). This surgeon-internist-astronaut would be responsible for the well-being of the other crewmembers and, in the case of a medical emergency, the entire mission may be their responsibility.

In order to perform their job, the CMO on such a long-duration mission will need to maintain surgical skills in absence of real cases and, when an accident occurs, may need to acquire new, specialized surgical skills, plan a surgery, and have assistance performing surgery. Moreover, should the CMO be the injured party, a crewmember with limited medical training may need to perform advanced medical care, perhaps involving surgery.

Specific problems that are anticipated include intra-abdominal emergencies, fractures (due to trauma exacerbated by bone demineralization), radiation effects (Immuno-suppression/infection and cancer). The risks associated with these conditions include decreased performance of crewmember, loss of crewmember, and/or mission failure.

In light of these challenges, a number of alternatives to having a single trained surgeon have been discussed. Telemedicine is largely ineffective due to the long distance between the Earth and Mars. It takes from 7 to 22 minutes for light to reach Earth and return to Mars. Moreover, blackout periods of up to 30 days are anticipated when the two planets are on opposite sides of the Sun. Due to these drawbacks, it is clear that an autonomous crew on such a mission will be a requirement. Another alternative would be to have many crewmembers trained for surgery, but therein lies a tradeoff with the size of the crew- on such a mission, there may be many tasks to perform beyond maintaining crew health. Finally, robotic surgery, although promising for longer-term exploration, will be unavailable for some time due to the complexities in replicating a surgeon's skill.

The skills required of the CMO will include those in general medicine, intensive care, and surgery. Basic surgical skills include aseptic techniques, dissection, suturing, among others. Advanced skills include speed, optimal exposure, anatomy knowledge, and knowledge of procedures (indications, approach, complications and management, and postoperative care). However, some specialized skills will require extensive preflight training and in-flight maintenance.

One example of a specialized surgical skill, microsurgery, involves the reconstruction of tissues, such as reattaching a severed or crushed finger, under a microscope. This often requires the surgeon to suture blood vessels and nerves that are less than 1mm in size. While the loss of one or more fingers could clearly limit performance of the affected crewmember, the procedure requires a great deal of training and this level of training directly impacts outcome (The average rate of successful microsurgical procedures increases from 79% to 96% as surgeons gain clinical experience). In order to develop this specialized surgical skill, the surgeon must dedicate 6 months of time toward learning the technique and also continually practice their skills over time to maintain proficiency. While this is one example of a specialized skill, the time commitment for skills acquisition and maintenance, multiplied by many unique specialty surgical skills, demonstrates that the CMO will not be able to be an expert in everything.

For these reasons, the CMO astronaut/surgeon requires a system for skill maintenance and acquisition, as well as for surgical planning and assistance. Additional benefits of such surgical simulators[1-8,12,13,15-18,20,22-23,25] would be the ability to present the surgeon with different scenarios (anatomical variations such as gender, size, etc, diseases/trauma and conditions, and gravity/operating environmental differences), quantify performance and simulate the surgical result, and provide for faster training[11,14,19,21] both preflight and during the mission. Additional benefits of this generalized sensor input and display system include eliminating the need for separate monitors, displays and lightboxes, as well as providing a generally useful platform for augmented reality display and interaction. For example, such a system would also be useful for overlay of wiring diagrams on equipment, intercrew communication, telepresence for inspection of hazardous locations, as well as countermeasures for depression and other psychological affects of long-duration spaceflight. The requirements of such a system are that it have low power consumption, small size, and low weight (mass).

2 MATERIALS AND METHODS

A functional, usable prototype of an augmented reality surgical training tool was created at our center, using small, lightweight, low-power computer components that would be easy to transport on a space mission. The system consists of a see-through head-mounted computer display (HMD, Sony Glasstron PLM-S700), a tracking device (Ascension Technologies pcBird electromagnetic tracker), computer system (Sony Vaio or desktop system), and

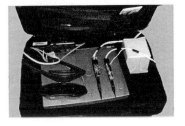

tracked surgical instruments (microsurgical forceps, Osteomed Corp, etc). Interaction with the system is provided through voice input (DragonSystems NaturallySpeaking) and speech synthesis (Microsoft Speech).

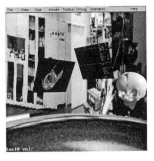

The system produces computer-generated imagery overlaid onto the real world, including virtual "hanging windows" for information display (CT/MR scans, vital signs, live endoscopic video, step-by-step instructions, dictation/communication screens), 3-D models of anatomy, and other information (for example, the projected trajectory of a drill) to assist the surgeon during a procedure. In addition, virtual patient models can be brought up within the environment for surgical skills training.

This system uses common off-the-shelf hardware and can be easily modified to use improved head-mounted displays, trackers, and computer systems as they become available. Instead, we have sought to provide a hardware/platform independent application and are focusing on refining the user interface and functionality for surgical assistance. The system component cost of this prototype is roughly $15,000, it's weight under 15 lbs., and power consumption under 60 watts.

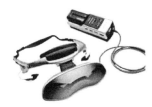

2.1 Software

Custom software was developed using C++ and the OpenGL, GLUT, and GLUI graphics libraries. This software provides for rapid information access and display, as well as a full surgical simulation engine capable of soft-tissue modeling supporting haptic interactions.

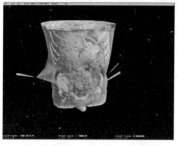

It communicates with the tracking devices mounted on the HMD and surgical instruments and with networked haptic devices, captures live video sources from a framegrabber (FlashBus MV Pro, Integral Technologies) for endoscopic video acquisition, and displays this information within the environment. When in training mode, the user can also bring up patient-specific anatomical models and interact with them using the tracked surgical instruments and/or haptic devices and our soft-tissue modeling engine.

2.2 Content

Currently, a number of medical content modules have been produced for the system. These include craniofacial anatomy and surgical technique, hand anatomy, inner ear anatomy, dental anatomy, and simulators for surgical anastomosis and other simple procedures. An ongoing related project (the *iAnatomy* project) seeks to collect and collate information on every piece of human anatomy and every surgical technique and currently has access to ophthalmic anatomy, hand anatomy, and general anatomical dissection.

Microsurgery training was used as the first example, but the system has been adapted to realistically simulate a number of other surgical procedures. The user interacts with 3D computer generated soft tissues, in this case blood vessels, and virtual sutures that obey the laws of physics and deform like real vessels. Anatomical variations can be introduced (different sized vessels, different orientations, end-to-side anastomosis, etc) and can be performed over and over again at any magnification or operating conditions (Earth gravity, zero gravity, Mars gravity) and provides a number of metrics quantifying the surgeon's performance.

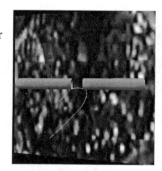

3 RESULTS

Functionally, the system provides a reasonable and useful system with fast response and adequate graphics refresh rate. The ability for the user to bring up important information (vital signs, CT data, etc) by voice command was found to be extremely intuitive. The use of real surgical instruments for training, as well as for intraoperative use, also

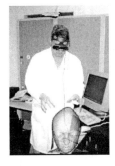

contribute to ease of use and low learning curve requirements of the system. Computer generated soft tissues deform and respond to instrument manipulation as real life tissues. In the specific case of microsurgical anastomosis, the lack of tactile feedback from the vessels does not significantly affect the overall experience. The program is easy to use since the interaction with the vessels happens through real microsurgery instruments, with the user looking at a stereo image of vessels as if viewed through the microscope.

Real-time graphics performance of the system was found to be limited with the PC-based platform and especially challenging due to minimal hardware acceleration provided on small footprint portable computers (laptops). Despite this lack of hardware graphics acceleration, 6 frames per second were realized on the Sony Vaio platform and was found to be mainly limited to graphics fill-rate. A second development system (PentiumIII 550MHz with Oxygen GVX1) attains 15 frames per second, even when capturing live video off-screen and rendering it as a texture. Performance of the mass-spring simulation engine on this platform, while complex to analyze in detail, was also adequate at this display rate for 30,000-50,000 element geometries in this prototype system.

4 DISCUSSION

The effect of working in the virtual environment approximates that of working on real patients in the operating room and is comparable to existing methods of training. During long duration space flights, a system similar to the one we developed could provide the hands-on experience necessary to perform a complicated procedure.

While the current HMD is usable, we anticipate the need for higher resolution head-mounted displays in the near term and anxiously await new technologies such as retinal scanning displays, holographic optical elements, among others, which promise significantly improved resolution and dynamic range. In addition, improvements in tracking will also be welcome and we anticipate moving to more precise optical tracking methods before testing the system intraoperatively.

The graphics and computational performance of the current system is anticipated to continue to increase in accordance with Moore's Law (performance doubling roughly every 18 months) and will yield a system easily capable of providing real-time imagery and simulation by the time of the first long-duration mission. In anticipation, continuing work on the system will produce a usable and highly integrated tool for medical officers in space or medical professionals on the ground.

In addition to computing and graphics performance, moving from a briefcase-sized unit to a handheld-sized computer unit worn on the belt would make the system even more usable. In initial discussions with palm-sized computing vendors (Tiqit),

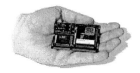

computation power appears tractable in the near term, while graphics power will take somewhat longer to develop. In either case however, computing and graphics performance in this form factor is projected to be adequate and commercially available within 10 years.

As for the simulation engine, the refinement of the physical properties and interactions between soft tissues such as skin, subcutaneous fat and muscles will lead to an even more realistic simulation environment. Simulation of blood and integration of on-line, interactive computational fluid dynamics will allow for comparison of different vascular interventions, should the be required. Similarly, adding more biomechanical modeling and simulation tools will also allow for predictive modeling of osteotomies and orthopedic interventions.

The content of the system is being increased as well. In addition to the anatomy and surgical technique content already underway, easy access to an electronic medical record of the patient will be required. Finally, as the content and functionality of the system increases, the need for improved and intelligent user interfaces will become more important.

5 ACKNOWLEDGEMENTS

This work was supported under the NASA grant NAS-NCC2-1010 (Stephen Schendel, PI). Many individuals contributed to this project and deserve special mention, including Joel Brown, Cynthia Bruyns, Benjamin Lerman, Frederic Mazzella, Simon Wildermuth and Jean-Claude Latombe.

6 REFERENCES

[1] Barde C, "Simulation Modeling of the Colon," First International Symposium on Endoscopy Simulation, World Congresses of Gastroenterology, Sydney, 1990.

[2] Bostrom M, Singh SK, Wiley CW, "Design of An Interactive Lumbar Puncture Simulator with Tactile Feedback," IEEE Annual Virtual Reality Symposium, p. 429-435, 1993.

[3] Bro-Nielsen M, Helfrick D, Glass B, Zeng X, Connacher H, "VR simulation of abdominal traumas surgery", MMVR98, IOS Press, p 117-123, 1998.

[4] Bro-Nielsen M, J.L. Tasto, R. Cunningham, and G.L. Merril, "PreOp Endoscopic Simulator: A PC-Based Immersive Training System", Medicine Meets Virtual Reality 7 (MMVR-7), San Francisco, California, IOS Press, 1999

[5] Colgate JE, Grafing PE, Stanley, MC, Schenkel G, "Implementation of Stiff Virtual Walls in Force-Reflection Interfaces," IEEE Annual Virtual Reality Symposium, p. 202-208, 1993.

[6] Cover SA, N. F. Ezquerra, J. F. O'Brien, et. al. "Interactively Deformable Models for Surgery Simulation," IEEE: Computer Graphics and Applications, v13(6)., pp. 68-75, November 1993.

[7] De S, Srinivasan MA, "Thin walled models for haptic and graphical rendering of soft tissues in surgical simulations", Medicine Meets Virtual Reality 7 (MMVR-7), IOS Press, p94-99, 1999.

[8] Gillies D, Haritsis A, Williams C, "Computer Simulation for Teaching Endoscopic Procedures," Endoscopy, 24, 1992.

[9] Hamilton, D.R., "Medical Selection Criteria for Exploration Mission Crews", SmartSystems 2000, Houston, TX, Sept 2000.

[10] Janney, R.P., Armstrong, C.W., Stepaniak, "Medical Training Issues and Skill Mix for Exploration Missions", SmartSystems2000, Houston, TX, Sept 2000.

[11] Johnston, R, Bhoyrul, S, Way, L, "Assessing a virtual reality surgical skills simulator", Studies in Health Technology and Informatics, v29, p608-617, 1996.

[12] Lorenson W, and Cline H, "Marching Cubes: A 3D High Resolution Surface Extraction Algorithm," Computer Graphics, 21, 4, p. 163-169, 1987.

[13] Millman PA, Stanley M, Colgate JE, "Design of a High Performance Haptic Interface to Virtual Environments," IEEE Annual Virtual Reality Symposium, p. 216-222, 1993.

[14] O'Toole, RV, Polayter, RR, Krummel TM, "Measuring and developing suturing technique with a virtual reality surgical simulator", J Am Coll Surg, v189, p114-127, 1999.

[15] Peifer J, et al., "Virtual Environment for Eye Surgery Simulation," Medicine Meets Virtual Reality II, IOS Press, 1994.

[16] Pieper S, et al., "A virtual environment system for simulation of leg surgery," Stereoscopic Displays and Applications II, SPIE Electronic Imaging, San Jose, CA, 1991.

[17] Poon A, Williams C, Gillies D, "The Use of Three-Dimensional Dynamic and Kinematic Modeling in the Design of a Colonoscopy Simulator," New Trends in Computer Graphics, Springer Verlag, 1988.

[18] Sagar MA, Bullivant D, Mallinson GD, Hunder PJ, Hunter, "Virtual Environment and Model of the Eye for Surgical Simulation," Computer Graphics Proceedings, p. 205-212, 1994.

[19] Satava, R.M., "Medical Applications of Virtual Reality", J Med Systems v19, p275-280, 1996.

[20] Stredney D, "Virtual Simulations: Why We Need Pretty Pictures," Medicine Meets Virtual Reality I, IOS Press, 1992.

[21] Taffinder, N, Sutton, C, Fishwick, RJ, McManus IC, Darzi, A, "Validation of virtual reality to teach and assess psychomotor skills in laparoscopic Surgery: results from randomized controlled studies using the MIST VR laparoscopic simulator", Studies in Health Technology and Informatics, v50, p124-130, 1998.

[22] Tendick F, Downes M, Cavusoglu CM, Gantert W, Way LW, "Development of virtual environments for training skills and reducing errors in laparoscopic surgery", Proceedings of Surgical-Assist Systems, SPIE, p 36-44, 1998.

[23] Tseng CS, Lee YY, Chan YP, Wu SS, Chiu AW, "A PC-based surgical simulator for laparoscopic surgery, MMVR98, IOS press, p115-160, 1998

[24] Wear, M.L., Marshburn, T., Billica, R.D., "Medical Risk Assessment for Mars Missions", SmartSystems 2000, Houston, TX, Sept 2000.

[25] Wiet G, Yasgel R, Stredney D, et al., "A Volumetric Approach to Virtual Simulation of Functional Endoscopic Sinus Surgery," Medicine Meets Virtual Reality 6, IOS Press 1997.

322

Medicine Meets Virtual Reality 2001
J.D. Westwood et al. (Eds.)
IOS Press, 2001

Military Medical Modeling and Simulation In The 21ST Century

Gerald Moses, Ph.D.
HQ, U.S. Army Medical Research and Materiel Command
Telemedicine and Advanced Technology Research Center
Fort Detrick, Maryland

J. Harvey Magee
SHERIKON, Inc., HQ, U.S. Army Medical and Research Materiel Command
Telemedicine and Advanced Technology Research Center
Fort Detrick, Maryland

John J. Bauer, MD
HQ, U.S. Army Medical Research and Materiel Command
Telemedicine and Advanced Technology Research Center
Fort Detrick, Maryland

Robert Leitch MBE RGN
HQ, U.S. Army Medical Research and Materiel Command
Telemedicine and Advanced Technology Research Center
Fort Detrick, Maryland

Abstract. As we enter the 21st century, military medicine struggles with critical issues. One of the most important issues is how to train medical personnel in peace for the realities of war. In April, 1998, The General Accounting Office (GAO) reported, "Military medical personnel have almost no chance during peacetime to practice battlefield trauma care skills. As a result, physicians both within and outside the Department of Defense (DOD) believe that military medical personnel are not prepared to provide trauma care to the severely injured soldiers in wartime. With some of today's training methods disappearing, the challenge of providing both initial; and sustainment training for almost 100,000 military medical personnel is becoming insurmountable. The "training gap" is huge and impediments to training are mounting. For example, restrictions on animal use are increasing and the cost of conducting live mass casualty exercises is prohibitive. Many medical simulation visionaries believe that four categories of medical simulation are emerging to address these challenges. These categories include PC-based multimedia, digital mannequins, virtual workbenches, and total immersion virtual reality (TIVR). The use of simulation training can provide a risk=free realistic learning environment for the spectrum of medical skills training, from buddy-aid to trauma surgery procedures. This will, in turn, enhance limited hands on training opportunities and revolutionize the way we train in peace to deliver medicine in war. High-fidelity modeling will permit manufacturers to prototype new devices before manufacture. Also, engineers will be able to test a device for themselves in a variety of simulated anatomical representations, permitting them to "practice medicine".

Military Medicine Struggles to Train Personnel

Now that we have entered the 21st century, in the wake of downsizing and restrained resources, military medicine struggles with a number of issues critical to its future. One of the most important is how we train in peace for the realities of conflict. This is not a new problem. Ever since military medicine took to the field of battle, physicians, nurses and medics have struggled to retain their essential combat medical skills and to train their acolytes in peace. During the Vietnam War, the United States developed what appeared, to many, to be the technological solution to the problems of combat casualty care: the helicopter medical evacuation on demand. But experience showed that the helicopter alone was not sufficient to reduce the mortality rate. The key was -- and still remains -- the expertly trained medic at every level of care.

Thirty years later, the US military faces the same challenge. In April 1998, the General Accounting Office (GAO)[1] reported, "military medical personnel have almost no chance during peacetime to practice battlefield trauma care skills. As a result, physicians both within and outside the Department of Defense (DOD) believe that military medical personnel are not prepared to provide trauma care to the severely injured soldiers in wartime, which could result in loss of lives and limbs." This issue is even the more critical in the contemporary world where the expectations of society and the war fighter are higher than ever, their tolerance for casualties lower and the nature of operations more complex.

The same GAO report also noted, "These [referring to DOD and GAO reports on medical operations during the Gulf War] reports highlighted that many military medical personnel, including physicians, nurses, and corpsmen, had either never treated trauma patients or had no recent experience."[2]

Congressional awareness of these factors led to the enactment of legislation in 1996 requiring DOD to implement a demonstration program to provide trauma training for military medical personnel through one or more public or nonprofit hospitals.

The GAO identified a number of other issues. Two of the most critical deal with the large numbers of personnel requiring training and the lack of formal training opportunities for them.

With respect to the large numbers of personnel requiring training, the report said, "Another issue concerns the ability of the civilian centers to train large numbers of military medical personnel...Currently [1997 data], the total number of active duty military medical personnel is about 100,000."[3] Incidentally, these numbers do not even include the military reserves! The GAO noted "Another wartime medical training issue is how such training might be handled in the reserves..."[4]

As to lack of formal training, the GAO reported "After physicians complete residency training, no formal DOD or service hands-on program exists for sustaining trauma care skills...Enlisted medical personnel such as combat medics and field corpsmen, receive initial medical readiness training in both basic military and life support skills." [5] The GAO report describes this entry level training, then states "However, the medics do not receive hands-on trauma experience at a hospital or on board an ambulance...Before deployment, both military physicians and enlisted medical personnel are required to take courses on combat casualty care...These courses consist of classroom instruction, animal laboratories, and field training and include the principles of trauma life support. These courses also do not provide hands-on exposure to actual trauma patients."[6]

Those engaged with the health care industry are familiar with the "see-one, do-one, teach-one" model of training used for decades. If patients were aware of the myriad pressures in training, they may be more apt to favor a "see-me, do-somebody else" approach.

The need to provide medical skills training is now recognized at the highest levels of Congress as a major factor in maintaining medical readiness. Military medical personnel must obtain -- and sustain -- procedural skills for treating combat casualties. This has led to many approaches to achieve the goal: enlisting the skills and experience found in Emergency Medical Systems (EMS) and trauma centers, Advanced Trauma Life

Support (ATLS) training, Special Forces advanced training, e.g., Operational Emergency Medical Support (OEMS), various military unit level initiatives.

Formal training methods used to teach skills needed for combat trauma care involve classroom instruction, video presentations, animal laboratory training, various computer-based programs including interactive CD-ROM, and exposure of military medical personnel to trauma patients in civilian hospitals. The treatment of civilian casualties provides some valuable lessons of trauma care but does not provide the realistic replication of combat specific wounds, battlefield environmental stressors, or battlefield unique problems concerning logistics and triage.

However, providing initial and sustainment training to almost 100,000 active duty military medical personnel is becoming insurmountable. The "training gap" is huge, and impediments to training are mounting. Restrictions on animal use are increasing; costs of conducting live mass casualty exercises are prohibitive. Third party payors are resistant to reimburse for medical training, and ethical considerations may surface surrounding the practice of trauma training in inner city Level 1 Trauma Centers by training on indigent minority populations.

There are several primary contributors to this widening gap. First, the types and ranges of injuries seen in war are different to those seen in peace, even in trauma centers of major cities. Second, both the austere combat environment and the limited resources with which wartime casualties are managed are different than in peace. Third, the sheer numbers of personnel to be trained far outweigh the resources available to train them.

Simulation May Provide the Answer
PC-Based Interactive Multimedia Training Systems

The information age is revolutionizing everyone's ability to communicate with speed and high quality multimedia capabilities, and this offers both opportunity and challenge. Training aids now have the capability to "wow" audiences with quality presentations, yet we are even further challenged to develop training media to deliver training that is both realistic and affordable.

PC-based multimedia systems are relatively inexpensive in comparison to other categories. They can be more readily deployed to locations anywhere. Once the programming refinements are worked out, they will be shown to be consistent and ideal for individual training.

At present, there are inconsistent standards, complicating the possibility of using them for Continuing Medical Education certification. There is a requirement for policy direction, and while policy is not in itself negative, the fact remains that the medical educational community has not yet addressed these issues fully. For example, with respect to certification, how does a trainee or his / her institution know what level of quality assurance went into developing a particular product?

An example of development in this area is the Simulation Technologies for Advanced Trauma Care (STATCARE), under development by Research Triangle Institute (RTI) under Cooperative Agreement DAMD17-99-2-9046 with the U.S. Army Medical Research Materiel Command. This work is being done under the Dual Use Science and Technology Award. STATCARE is managed by the TATRC, Ft. Detrick, Maryland.

Targeted toward Emergency Medical Technician (EMT) and paramedic training, STATCARE Trauma Patient Simulator (TPS) is a real-time, physiologically accurate, 3D VR simulator for emergency care training. Its physiology responds to trauma and treatment by the trainee. It has configurable scenarios and patients (scenes, trauma, injuries, gender, ethnicity). Patient care skill sets & procedures are scaleable. It has natural caregiver-patient voice interaction (spoken dialog, level-of-consciousness behavior), as well as integrated courseware, distance learning, and reference materials

Digitally-Enhanced Mannequins

At present, digitally enhanced mannequins are complex devices and expensive as well. They are limited to stand-alone capability. To exploit their technical capability, mannequins need integration into a training system. Military and commercial development is taking place in this area. Research and development efforts to enhance mannequin capabilities are positive, as well as efforts to developing training systems.

Considerable research has been conducted in the past decade or more, and the mannequin devices have become more robust in their capability. Digital mannequins are now full-body patient simulators controlled by mathematical models of physiology and pharmacology, offering great flexibility for instructional use. The market is competitive, which, over time, should drive unit prices down as manufacturers are able to reduce costs of production. They are quite suitable for team training.

In addition to development of the mannequins themselves, significant development is also taking place to systematize approaches to training. For example, Dr. David M Gaba, M.D., and his team at the Veterans Administration Palo Alto Health Care System, have developed a Medical Simulation Center in which many medical crisis situations can be simulated. They have applied lessons learned about crisis management behavior from aviation simulation and have developed approaches for Crisis Resource Management (CRM) in health care. Dr. Gaba discusses this in Crisis Management in Anesthesiology, published in 1994[7], dealing with gaps in training and operational culture in health care. Under a congressionally funded program, and overall guidance of the TATRC at the USAMRMC, the US Army Simulation, Training and Instrumentation (USASTRICOM) is the Program Manager for the Combat Trauma Patient Simulation (CTPS) program, which is developing a training system based upon a digitized mannequin. The vendor is Medical Education Technologies, Inc. As an indication of progress in this area, Sergeant Major James N. Lansing notes in Military Medical Technology, "The Army National Guard is answering the challenge of exploiting the potential of state-of-the-art mannequins by adding distance learning to the educational mix. A resulting proof-of-concept teaches front-line medics how to perform invasive procedures that can prevent costly on-the-job training in combat."[8]

Virtual Workbenches

This is an area of rapid technological development. Some individual medical procedures, e.g., intravenous insertion of a needle, are now possible to simulate. Virtual workbenches are ideal for practice of minimally invasive procedures.

Virtual workbenches are limited by their stand-alone capability, and haptic feedback capability is limited by current technology.

An example of virtual workbench development is the Endoscopic Surgical Simulator being developed by HT Medical Systems, Inc. under Cooperative Agreement DAMD17-99-2-9031, and is managed by the TATRC, Ft. Detrick, Maryland. The prototype ureteroscopic simulator integrates technologies that push the boundaries in computer-based real-time simulation. Technologies include computer models that represent the physics of collisions and resulting deformation during interaction of various medical devices as well as real-time physiologic modeling of tissue trauma. The prototype, first demonstrated April 30, 2000 in Atlanta at the American Urologic Association conference, allowed users to manipulate a proxy ureteroscope within a tactile feedback interface device and visualize, in both simulated video and fluoroscopic views, the ureters and the calyx of the kidney.

Total Immersion Virtual Reality

TIVR development is in its infancy, but it holds promise to create the most realistic simulation environment. In addition to providing a location in which clinical procedures can be simulated, it also creates an atmosphere in which the "sights and sounds of war" – even smells -- can be simulated.

Future development depends upon the ability of several technologies to reproduce realistic haptic feedback to the trainee. Also, TIVR requires the greatest investment in development time and money.

Research on TIVR for training in support of the Medical Simulation Training Initiative (MSTI) is already underway with the Center for Innovative Minimally Invasive Therapy (CIMIT) in Boston, MA, under the auspices of a U.S. Department of the Army Cooperative Agreement DAMD 17-99-2-9001.

Strategic Plan for Simulation Training

The GAO clearly recommended the need for a strategic plan, with goals, identified actions, and appropriate milestones for achievement. "[Combat] trauma care training is essential for DOD to successfully fulfill its wartime medical mission. The lack of priority for combat trauma care training led individual surgeons, military treatment facilities, and combat units to attempt to meet trauma care training needs on their own. Command support for these individual efforts has been difficult to sustain because DOD currently has no clear goals or strategy for trauma care training as it relates to medical readiness."[9]

Single Agency Integration of Research Efforts

Recognizing that many diverse simulation efforts were taking place in a disjointed fashion, TATRC sponsored an Integrated Research Team (IRT) meeting for Medical Modeling and Simulation (MM&S) in February 2000, co-hosted by the U.S. Army Medical Research Materiel Command (USAMRMC) and U.S. Army Simulation, Training, and Instrumentation Command (USASTRICOM). The complexity of the effort to unify and focus current divergent research efforts in medical modeling and simulation required a process like an IRT meeting. Materiel developers, combat developers and representatives of several other government agencies provided their perspectives of the importance of modeling and simulation to address current military medical training and education issues. Early in the proceedings, the conferees recognized the likelihood that MM&S will have wider application to peacetime military and civilian healthcare. Also, two categories of researchers rendered presentations: researchers currently managed by TATRC, and researchers in several categories of simulation who are exploring next-generation technologies for potential submission.

The IRT was unique in that it enabled many key players to come together *early* in the process to identify military medical training needs and to assist in developing a strategy to address them.

Three recommendations were supported by Major General Parker, Commanding General, USAMRMC: (1) Conduct further development of a fully integrated, tech-based investment strategy for MM&S, in direct support of the Joint Warfighter Science & Technology Plan; (2) Conduct follow-on IRTs to structure appropriate Integrated Product Teams and devise best methods of leveraging consortium involvement; (3) Designate TATRC as the Command oversight agent for the management of MM&S research.

Enabling Technologies

A limiting factor to the use of simulations for medical training has been the lack of fundamental science to permit realistic representations of medical procedures as a basis for simulation. If we are to provide training realistically and to do so cost-effectively, we must develop underlying
enabling technologies as part of a long-term, strategy. This strategy must address tissue modeling, haptics integration, physiological representations and overall systems architecture.

Domain Expert Cooperation

Success in this effort can occur only through continuing coordinated efforts among domain experts in their own fields, e.g., medical personnel working side by side with engineers, computer scientists and designers and managers, to make an end product that is useful and valuable for the intended customer.

Virtual reality (VR) simulation has been identified in both the Joint Science and Technology Plan for Telemedicine (approved by Armed Services Board of Research and Materiel, 1998) and the Joint Warfighter Science and Technology Plan as a primary approach for increasing individual medical skills proficiency trauma training in the military.

Given the limited funds that are available, and the scope of science that must be addressed, we must make efficient use of collaborations to prevent aimless research. With a programmatic approach, multiple institutions can develop applications specific simulations, using a Common Anatomic Modeling Language (CAML). This will integrate efforts within bioengineering, medicine, manufacturing, and the Department of Defense (DOD). When developed, these enabling technologies and the Total Immersion Virtual Reality (TIVR) environment can provide a cost-effective foundation of realism that is essential for both initial and sustainment medical proficiency training.

Summary

If we are to radically improve military trauma training and close the widening training gap in military medicine, we must develop both technology and learning systems. A visionary strategic plan is essential and must be based squarely on solid medical science. It must enhance integration of efforts underway. It must be implemented through a reasoned, disciplined, systematic, science based R&D approach. Within the framework of its broad, over-arching Medical Modeling and Simulation (MM&S) strategy, the Telemedicine and Advanced Technology Research Center (TATRC), Headquarters U.S. Army Medical Research and Materiel Command have taken the lead.

References

[1] GAO/NSIAD-98-75, *Medical Readiness,* p 2.
[2] GAO/NSIAD-98-75, *Medical Readiness,* p 2.
[3] GAO/NSIAD-98-75, *Medical Readiness,* p 7
[4] GAO/NSIAD-98-75, *Medical Readiness,* p 8

[5] GAO/NSIAD-98-75, *Medical Readiness*, p 14
[6] GAO/NSIAD-98-75, *Medical Readiness*, p 15
[7] Fish, K. J., Gaba, D. M., Howard, S. K.: <u>Crisis Management in Anesthesiology</u>, Churchill Livingstone, New York, 1994
[8] Lansing, J.N. (2000), Training at technology's crossroads. <u>Military Medical Technology, 4,</u> 6-7.
[9] GAO/NSIAD-98-75, *Medical Readiness*, p 44

Medicine Meets Virtual Reality 2001
J.D. Westwood et al. (Eds.)
IOS Press, 2001

New Graphics Models for PC Based Ocular Surgery Simulator

Nobuhiko MUKAI[1], Masayuki HARADA[1], Katsunobu MUROI[1], Taiichi HIKICHI[2], and
Akitoshi YOSHIDA[2]

[1] *Information Technology R&D Center, Mitsubishi Electric Corporation*
5-1-1 Ofuna, Kamakura, Kanagawa, 247-8501, JAPAN
E-mails: [mukai, haradam, muroi]@isl.melco.co.jp
[2] *Department of Opthalmology, Asahikawa Medical College*
2-1, Midorigaoka-higashi, Asahikawa, 078-8307, JAPAN
E-mails: [hikichi, pyoshida]@asahikawa-med.ac.jp

High-end graphics workstations (GWS) have been used for surgical simulators utilizing Computer Graphics (CG) and Virtual Reality (VR) technologies. This is because the simulators need lots of computing power, mainly for collision detection among objects modeled as a set of polygons. In this paper, we propose to use mathematical functions to model objects for collision detection. However, for graphic display we continue to use polygonal representation. Using the new model, we have developed a PC based ocular surgery simulator, which creates realistic surgery image in real-time. The computation time was found to be much lower than that in the conventional method.

1. Introduction

These days, many medical simulators have been developed with CG and VR technologies [1, 2, 3]. These simulators are very useful and important because some of the diseases are unique to human being and there is no better alternate method for surgeons to practice and improve their skills. We also had developed an ocular surgery simulator based on high-end GWS, with which ophthalmologists can get training for vitreous surgery [4, 5, 6]. With the system, surgeons can get a stereo view of the surgery image through binoculars that simulate ocular surgery microscope. During the surgery, they use two surgical instruments with both their hands; one is a light guide that illuminates the interior of the eye, and the other is a surgical instrument such as vitreous cutter, peeler, or forceps. Haptic devices are used for these virtual surgery instruments so that they can feel force feedback of the surgery. Surgeons use two foot-switches also; one is a microscope pedal, by which they can change the microscope position, focus, zoom ratio, and so forth. The other is a vitreous cutter pedal, by which they can control the aspiration power of core vitrectomy (a method of extracting vitreous humor out of the eye using vitreous cutter). With this vitreous surgery simulator, opthalmologists can get training for *pre-retinal membrane*, which is a case where a membrane proliferates on the center of the retina.

The membrane is like a thin, soft, small paper sticking to the retina. Care should be taken during the membrane removal so that the surgical instrument should not penetrate the retina

2. Purpose

High-end GWS has enough computing and graphics powers to create realistic surgery images in real-time. However, it is too expensive compared to Personal Computer (PC), which has become very popular. Therefore, we have decided to develop a PC based ocular surgery simulator by decreasing the requirement of computing power. We have also decided to develop another simulation case *sub-retinal membrane*, since only the former case is not enough for the training.

Sub-retinal membrane is a disease, where some part of the retina swells and a membrane proliferates under the retina. In this case, the surgery steps involved are as the following:

1) A surgical instrument called *sub-retinal cannula* is inserted into the eye and pricked into the swollen part of the retina.
2) Balanced Salt Solution (BSS) is injected under the swollen retina so that the part of the retina is expanded to make room for easier removal of the membrane.
3) Using another instrument *sub-retinal forceps,* the membrane is removed out of the swollen retina.
4) Irrigation is performed with Sulfur HexaFluoride gas (SF6) instead of BSS. With this irrigation, the gas is injected into the eye through a thin pipe called *irrigation cannula* and expands gradually like a soap bubble, pushing all BSS out of the eye thorough another instrument called *flute needle.*
5) Contact lens is changed from BSS irrigation lens to the gas one so that the surgeon can get a clear view of the eye and assess whether the surgery has succeeded or not.

For the simulation of these surgery steps, lots of collision detection among different objects is required such as collision detection between the retina and the surgical instrument in the step 1) and the collision detection between the retina and the gas bubble in the step 4). Usually, many intersection calculations are needed between polygons (which constructs the retina) and a line (which represents the surgical instrument), or among polygons (which constructs the retina and the gas bubble).

Our scope of work is to develop a PC based real-time ocular surgery simulator for the simulation of sub-retinal membrane, using new graphics model of objects.

3. Methods

3.1 New Model Concept

Collision detection between polygons and a line, or among polygons requires many intersection calculations. Intersection calculations are computation intensive and the number of intersection calculations increases with total number of polygons. However, if the objects are modeled as mathematical functions, the required number of intersection calculations is much less compared to the other case. Therefore, the calculation time is much less compared to the conventional method with polygonal model. However for graphic display, we use polygonal model because drawing hardware requires polygons to generate CG images.

3.2 Retina Model

In the case of sub-retinal membrane, the center part of the retina swells like a small hill. The swollen retina is depicted as shown in Fig.1 although it is a little bit exaggerated.

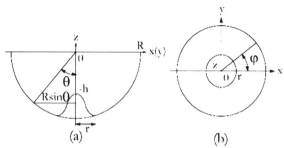

Fig.1 Swollen retina model

The posterior part of the retina including the swollen part is defined as the following.

$$F(x, y, z) = (R \sin \theta \cos \phi, R \sin \theta \sin \phi, - R \cos \theta) \qquad \text{if } R \sin \theta > r$$
$$= (R \sin \theta \cos \phi, R \sin \theta \sin \phi, - R \cos \theta + h(\cos \eta + 1)) \text{ if } R \sin \theta \le r$$
$$\text{where, } 0 \le \theta \le \pi / 2, \ 0 \le \phi \le 2\pi, \ \eta = (R \sin \theta / r)\pi, \ 0 \le \eta \le \pi \ (\text{for } R \sin \theta \le r) \qquad \text{(Eq.1)}$$

For the graphics model, polygons constructing the retina are created by the following algorithm:

```
for (j = 0; j ≤ N; j++) {
    for (i = 0; i ≤ M; i++) {
        φ = i * dφ;  θ = j * dθ;  x[i, j] = R sin θ cos φ;  y[i, j] = R sin θ sin φ;
        if (R sin θ > r) z[i, j] = −R cos θ;
        else z[i, j] = −R cos θ + h(cos((R sin θ / r)π) + 1);
    } }
for (k = 0, j = 0; j < N; j++) {
    for (i = 0; i = M; i++) {
        P[k, 0] = jM + i;  P[k,1] = (j + 1)M + i;
        P[k,2] = (j + 1)M + (i + 1)%M;  P[k,3] = jM + (i + 1)%M;  k++;
    } }
where, M : polygon number along φ direction, N : polygon number along θ direction
        M(N − 1): the number of total polygons, dφ = 2π / M, dθ = (π / 2) / N;
        P[k,l]: index number of polygon creating quadrangle, 0 ≤ k < M(N − 1), l = 0,1,2,3
        A%B : reminder of A divided by B
```

Fig.2 Algorithm for creating retina graphics model

The normal vector of the membrane at each vertex is calculated as shown in Fig.3 and Fig.4. In Fig.4, the swollen part of the retina is placed at the center of the eye so that this part of the eyeground can be considered as a flat plane and $\eta=0$ and $\eta=\pi$ represents the top and the bottom of the hill respectively. Usually, normal vector at a vertex is calculated as the average of the normal vectors of its adjacent polygons. With this algorithm shown in Fig.3, the normal vector at each vertex is directly calculated without calculating the normal vectors of adjacent polygons

```
for (j = 0; j ≤ N; j++) {
    for (i = 0; i ≤ M; i++) {
        φ = i * dφ;  θ = j * dθ;
        if (R sin θ > r) { nx[i, j] = − sin θ cos φ; ny[i, j] = − sin θ sin φ; nz[i, j] = − cos θ; }
        else { η = (R sin θ) / r  // in case of R sin θ ≤ r
            if (0 ≤ η ≤ π / 2) {
                nx[i, j] = sin(η / 2) cos φ;  ny[i, j] = sin(η / 2) sin φ; nz[i, j] = cos(η / 2);  }
            else {  // in case of π/2 < η ≤ π
                nx[i, j] = sin((π − η)/2) cos φ; ny[i, j] = sin((π − η) / 2) sin φ;
                nz[i, j] = cos((π − η) / 2);  }
} }
```

Fig.3 Calculation of normal vector

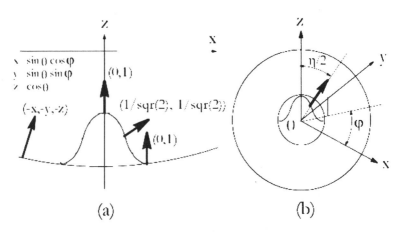

(a)   (b)

Fig.4 Nomal vector of swollen retina model

In Fig.5, the point (x, y, z) is the tip of the surgical instrument. With the mathematical function model, the collision detection between the swollen retina and the surgical instrument can be determined as the following.

From (Eq.1), $z = −R \cos \theta + h(\cos \eta + 1) \cong −R + h(\cos \eta + 1)$ because $\theta \cong 0$. Therefore,

$$\eta = \cos^{-1}((R + z)/h - 1) \tag{Eq.2}$$

Also, from (Eq.1), $\eta = (R\sin\theta / r)\pi$. Then, $(R\sin\theta / r)\pi = \eta = \cos^{-1}((R+z)/h - 1)$.

As a result, $R\sin\theta = (r/\pi)\cos^{-1}((R+z)/h - 1)$. Here, notice that $R\sin\theta = \sqrt{(x^2 + y^2)}$ if the tip of the instrument is on the swollen retina. The collision detection algorithm is described in Fig.6.

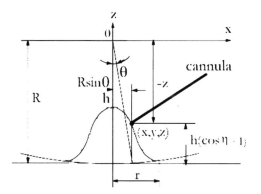

Fig.5 Distance relationship of swollen retina model

if $(-R \le z \le -R + h)\{$

     $R\sin\theta = (r/\pi)\cos^{-1}((R+z)/h - 1);$

     if $(R\sin\theta \ge \sqrt{(x^2 + y^2)})$ (x, y, z) is inside of the swollen retina; $\}$

Otherwise (x, y, z) is outside of the swollen retina;

Fig.6 Algorithm of collision detection with swollen retina model

By pushing the swollen retina with the instrument, the retina is deformed at the intersection and its vertex position moves to (x, y, z), which is the tip position of the instrument.

3.3 Gas Bubble Model

In the step 4) of the **section 2**, when SF6 gas is injected into the eye through irrigation cannula, a gas bubble is created at the tip of the instrument and the bubble expands to fill the inside of the retina with SF6. The gas bubble expands to the size of the retina and never expands beyond the eye size. The insertion position of the instrument is biased from the center of the eye. Therefore, the shape of the gas bubble should be controlled not to exceed the eye size.

     In Fig.7, the eye and the gas bubble are depicted. The center of the eyeball is placed at the origin $(0,0,0)$. However, the center of the gas bubble is biased from the origin and is placed at $C(cx, cy, cz)$. Suppose that $P(px, py, pz)$ is one point on the gas bubble. The line segment that passes through $C(cx, cy, cz)$ and $P(px, py, pz)$ is,

$$x = (px - cx)t + cx, \quad y = (py - cy)t + cy, \quad z = (pz - cz)t + cz, \quad 0 \le t \le 1 \qquad (\text{Eq.3})$$

Also, the intersection point $Q(qx, qy, qz)$ is on the line segment and on the eye so that,

$$qx = (px - cx)t + cx, \quad qy = (py - cy)t + cy, \quad qz = (pz - cz)t + cz, \quad 0 \le t \le 1 \qquad \text{(Eq.4)}$$

$$(qx)^2 + (qy)^2 + (qz)^2 = R^2 \qquad \text{(Eq.5)}$$

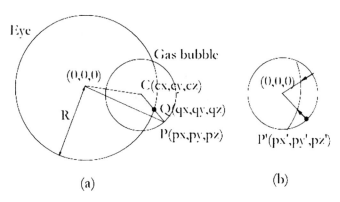

Fig.7 Gas bubble model

With (Eq.4) and (Eq.5), the intersection $Q(qx, qy, qz)$ is solved and the length $|CP|$ and $|CQ|$ are calculated. Then, let us consider the modeling coordinate of the gas bubble (See Fig.7 (b)). In the modeling coordinate, the center of the gas bubble is placed at the origin of the modeling coordinate. Let us $P'(px', py', pz')$ as the modeling coordinate of $P(px, py, pz)$. By shrinking the modeling coordinate of the gas bubble, which exceeds the eye size, by $|CQ| / |CP|$, the gas bubble can be fit to the inside of the eye.

4. Results and Conclusion

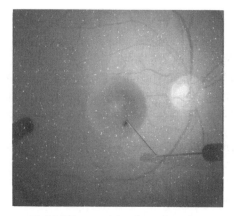

Fig8. Pricking cannula into the swollen retina

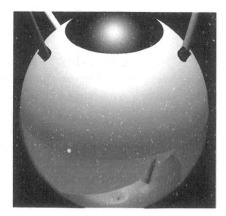

Fig 9. Gas injection

In Fig.8, the surgeon is trying to prick the sub-retinal cannula into the swollen part of the retina. There is a membrane inside of the swollen retina. Notice that the surgeon has a light guide with his/her left hand so that the right part of the eyeground is illuminated. Fig.9 shows the gas injection. The gas bubble is injected from the irrigation cannula, which is biased form the center of the eye. The gas bubble expands from the left side to the right side until it fits to the inside of the eye. The bubble size never exceeds the eye size. In the figure, the right hand instrument is partly hidden by the expanding gas bubble.

By defining the graphics models with both polygons and mathematical functions, not only real-time image drawing but also real-time collision detection has been achieved. For the collision detection between the retina and the surgical instrument, many intersection calculations are needed, if the objects are represented by conventional polygonal model. However, if the objects are modeled as mathematical function, just one calculation is sufficient to judge whether the tip position of the instrument is inside the swollen retina or not. When the retina is constructed of 1,600 polygons, collision detection time with conventional model using polygons was found to be $7.2ms$. On the other hand, it was just $2\mu s$ with the new model. That is, our proposed method is 3,600 times faster than the conventional one. As a result, some CPU power can be assigned to another job such as coordinate transformation, clipping, and drawing.

We have succeeded in developing a PC based real-time ocular surgery simulator. It is already being used by several opthalmologists and they evaluate that the quality of graphics image and the response time are good enough for their training, and also user interface of the simulator is almost the same as that of real surgeries.

References

[1] Suzuki N., Hattori A., Takatsu A., Kumano T., Ikemoto A. Adachi Y., and Uchiyama A., "Virtual Surgery System using Deformable Organ Models and Force Feedback System with Three Fingers", Lecture Notes in Computer Science, Vol.1496, pp. 397-403, 1998

[2] Neumann P.F., Sader L.L, and Gieser J., "Virtual Reality Vitrectomy Simulator", Lecture Notes in Computer Science, Vol.1496, pp.910-917, 1998

[3] Schill M.A., Gibson S. F. F., Bender H. J., and Männer R., "Biomechanical Simulation of the Vitreous Humor in the Eye using an Enhanced Chain Mail Algorithm, Lectures Notes in Computer Science, Vol.1496, pp.679-687, 1998

[4] Mukai N., Harada M., Muroi K., Terada T., Hikichi T., and Yoshida A., "Vitreous Surgery Simulator System", JJME, Vol.37, p.282, 1999

[5] Mukai N., Harada M., Muroi K., and Terada T., "Ocular Surgery Simulator System", Mitsubishi Electric Technical Report, Vol.73, No.11, pp.34-37, 1999

[6] Harada M., Mukai N., and Muroi K., "Membrane Peeling Model for Ocular Surgery Simulator", Proceedings of the Virtual Reality Society of Japan Fifth Annual Conference, pp.421-424, 2000

Medicine Meets Virtual Reality 2001
J.D. Westwood et al. (Eds.)
IOS Press, 2001

LAHYSTOTRAIN
Development and Evaluation of a complex
Training System for Hysteroscopy

Wolfgang K. MÜLLER-WITTIG[1], Dipl.-Inform, Alex BISLER[1], Dipl.-Inform.,
Uli BOCKHOLT[1], Dipl.-Math., Jose Luis LOS ARCOS[2], PhD,
Peter OPPELT[3], MD, Jan STÄHLER[3], MD, Gerrit VOSS[1],Dipl.-Inform.
[1] *Fraunhofer-Institut für Graphische Datenverarbeitung (Fraunhofer-IGD)*
Department Visualization & Virtual Reality
Rundeturmstraße 6, D-64283 Darmstadt, Germany
Phone: +49-6151-155277, Fax: +49-6151-155196
E-mail: {vossg\bockholt\muellerw}@igd.fhg.de
URL: http://www.igd.fhg.de/www/igd-a4
[2] *Foundation LABEIN, Information Technologies Department,*
Zamudio, Spain
[3] *Universitäts-Frauenklinik Frankfurt*
Zentrum für minimal-invasive Operationen, Frankfurt, Germany

Hysteroscopy has already become an irreplaceable method in gynaecoloic diagnosis and therapy. In the diagnostic case the hysteroscope with a 30° optic is insert transvaginally, in the therapeutic case the resctoscope with a 12° optic is used. The endoscoppic intervention requires special surgical skills for endoscope handling and remote instrument control. To acquire these skills currently hands-on training in clinical praxis has become standard, which is linked with higher danger for the women. To overcome current drawbacks of traditional training methods the European project LAHYSTOTRAIN was set up, that tries to combine Virtual Reality (VR), Multimedia (MM) technology, and Intelligent Tutoring Systems (ITS) to develop an alternative training system for hysteroscopic interventions.

The first prototype of the LAHYSTOTRAIN demonstrator has been shown on several European conferences. An evaluation of the system was performed, with the idea, to collect feedback and impressions, that should be considered in further developments. This paper presents the LAHYSTOTRAIN prototype and the results of these evaluations.

1. Motivation

The use of VR Techniques in endoscopic training is a challenging and promising task. Especially for the endoscopic uterus intervention, where no training possibilities like cadaver studies exist, there is a high demand for simulators with the aim to maximize quality control and to minimize the risk for the patient. While several groups are working on the simulation of laparoscopic gynaecology [1,2], the current focus of the

LAHYSTOTRAIN project is the simulation of hysteroscopic interventions. It is a European project conceived to establish a complex training system combining Multimedia, Intelligent Tutoring and Virtual Reality Techniques [3].

2. Tools & Methods

The first prototype developed in the project is a Training System for hysteroscopy. The training starts with a web-based Multimedia Course, where theoretical aspects of hysteroscopy are considered. This course includes theoretical aspects of hysteroscopy reaching from the preparation of the intervention (setting up the patient, choosing the appropriate instruments) to complication management strategies. The trainee proves his understanding by passing an exam, which qualifies him for the VR Simulator, where practical skill training is performed.

The VR Simulator is combined with an Intelligent Tutoring System choosing the appropriate training scenario, monitoring the session, detecting errors, and giving explanations. For the training of diagnostic procedures a database of several cases was set up including pathologies, like polyps, an intracervical adhesion, atrophic mucosa, uterus septus and uterus subseptus (c.f. Figure 1). After a session the trainee has to specify the detected pathology in the annexed questioner.

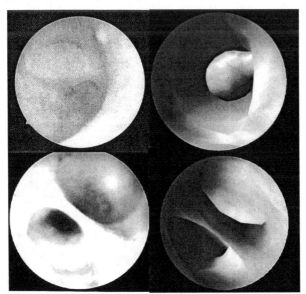

Figure 1: Comparison of real endoscopic images (l.) and modelled pathologies (r.)

The hysteroscopic intervention is also well suited for simulation of therapeutic interventions, because here endoscope and tools are combined in one single instrument - the resectoscope. Only position, orientation and the opening angle of the resectoscope have to be registered. For the simulation of the resectoscope the instruments of KARL STORZ GmbH are integrated into the "Laparoscopic Interface" from Immersion Cooperation. The trainee handles the original instrument and moves the simulated electrodes, used for resection of pathologic tissue, along the resectoscope´s axis. To describe the manipulation of the virtual situs simulation algorithms for tissue deformation and cutting are integrated into the simulation system [4][5].

3. Evaluation

Two different kinds of evaluation are performed concerning the training simulator. One is the personal evaluation of the trainee's session, the other one is a global evaluation with the idea to collect feedback and impressions of the first prototype.

To perform the personal evaluation of a training session the VR simulator is combined with and Intelligent Tutoring System (ITS). This ITS evaluates the following issues during the training session:

1. How good is the navigation of the endoscope? How is the visibility of the therapeutic target in the endoscopic output?
2. Has the intervention been performed in an appropriate time?
3. Are there all the pathologies identified correctly?
4. If cutting was performed, how matches the virtual cut with the optimal predefined cut?

The data for these endoscopic aspects are collected and analyzed by the affiliated Intelligent Tutoring System. The trainee gets a score like evaluation of his session. Only if he has proven his skills he can pass over to the next level.

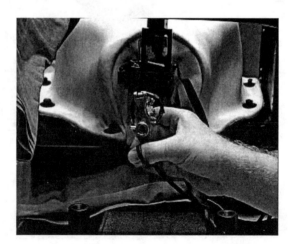

Figure 2: Setup of the training simulator

For a global evaluation of the Training System the Hysteroscopy Simulator was presented on the leading European gynaecology conferences and was tested by a large audience reaching from medical students to experienced surgeons (c.f. Figure 3). 33 of them filled out an evaluation sheet where feedback about the prototype and the training concept was collected. The evaluation sheet was structured into four groups with the following topics:

- Realism of the simulator
- Handling of the instruments
- Application domains of the simulator
- Integration possibilities into the medical curriculum

4. Results

The evaluation of the training simulator showed the following results:

- Most of the asked physicians (72 %) can image to learn surgical procedures via VR based training simulators like this, 51 % had the feeling to handle a real instrument but only 9 % characterized the realism of the virtual anatomic structures as "good".
- The realization of the endoscope simulation including the handling of the optics is characterized as well suited for training from 52 % of the asked gynecologists.
- According to the gynaecologists a VR training simulator like this can be used to supplement in
  - Training of the medical stuff during surgical and genaecological educationa (82 %)
  - Training of medical students (76 %)
  - Learning of anatomy (69 %)
  57% think of the VR simulator as a possible tool that could be used for quality enhancement.
- More than 80% estimate the hysteroscopy simulator as an innovative approach for revolutionizing endoscopic education, they think that medical education can be improved with a system like that and they can imagine an integration of the system into the medical standard curriculum.

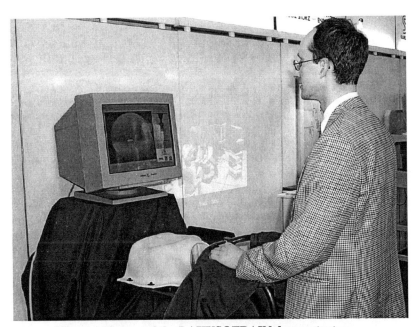

Figure 3: Set-up of the LAHYSOTRAIN demonstrator

5. Conclusions

The Evaluation of the prototype showed that VR Simulation is accepted and strongly demanded for medical education of a broad majority. Critically assessed was the realism of the simulated anatomy and pathology. More effort should enter into texture generation and illumination of the virtual situs. The intuitiveness of the instrument handling got a predominantly positive feedback. Particular the use of the original instrument handles and the simulation of the optic are emphasized.

The LAHYSTOTRAIN concept of combining intelligent tutor, VR, WWW, and multimedia shows that the complete educational process can be covered considering the individual training level of the trainee. The next steps in the development of the simulator are integration of force feedback and further evaluation in Hysterosocopy Training Courses. This concept has general applicability to other medical specialties.

Acknowledgments

The European Commission under the Joint Call orchestrated by the Educational Multimedia Taskforce funds this project. We thank Prof. Dr. h.c. Dr.-Ing. José L. Encarnação and Prof. Dr. med. M. Kaufmann for providing the environment in which this work was possible. We also thank all our colleagues and students at our laboratory, especially Berit Klahsen, Mario Becker and Albert Schäffer. Without their work we would not have been able to achieve the results presented herein.

References

[1]   Székely, G. et al. *Virtual Reality Based Surgery Simulation for Endoscopic Gynaecology*, Proceedings of Medicine Meets Virtual Reality, pp. 351-357, San Francisco, 1999

[2]   Çakmak, H.K., Kühnapfel, U.: *The "Karlsruhe Endoscopic Surgery Trainer" for minimally invasive surgery in gynaecology*, 13th Internat. Congress on Computer Assisted Radiology and Surgery (CARS '99), Paris, 1999

[3]   Voss, G., Bockholt U., Los Arcos JL. Müller W, Oppelt P., Stähler J., LAHYSTOTRAIN, *Intelligent Training System for Laparoscopy and Hysteroscopy*, Proceedings of Medicine Meets Virtual Reality, pp. 359-364, Imperial Beach CA, 2000

[4]   Bockholt, U., Müller W., Voß, G., Ecke, U., Klimek L. *Realtime Simulation of Tissue Deformation for the Nasal Endoscopy Simulator (NES)* in: Computer Aided Surgery, Journal of Image Guided Surgery (Ed. R. Bucholz), John Wiley & Soms, Inc., November 1999

[5]   Voss, G., Hahn J., Müller W., Lindeman R. *Virtual Cutting of Anatomical Structures*, Proceedings of Medicine Meets Virtual Reality, pp. 381-383, San Francisco, 1999

Medicine Meets Virtual Reality 2001
J.D. Westwood et al. (Eds.)
IOS Press, 2001

MEDNET: A Medical Simulation Network Grand Challenge

Michael D. Myjak, M.S.
The Virtual Workshop, Inc.
P.O. Box 98 Titusville, FL 32781
<*mmyjak@virtualworkshop.com*>

Joseph Rosen, M.D.
Dartmouth Hitchcock Medical Center
One Medical Center Drive, Lebanon, NH 03756
<*Joseph.M.Rosen@Hitchcock.ORG*>

Keywords: Advanced Distributed Simulation (ADS) DIS Telemedicine HLA

Abstract - The need to improve war-fighter training led to significant advancements in simulator technology. Now, simulator technology is ready to be applied to a new challenge: an evolutionary approach to training military medical personnel that will result in improved combat casualty care. With the exception of the introduction of helicopter evacuation support during the Korean War, changes in combat casualty care have not significantly altered the percentage of wounded soldiers lost in combat since World War II. The introduction of battlefield simulator training has improved strategic planning and combat readiness. It is time to apply these same tools to improve medical planning, military medical readiness and execution of casualty care.

1. MEDNET - An Overview

The MEDical simulation NETwork (MEDNET) is envisioned as a comprehensive simulation system that can be used to augment combat casualty care, support civilian medical training, and to provide just-in-time basic first-aid training in the event of terrorist attack. Viewed as a "Grand Challenge" for improving military medical readiness and combat casualty care, MEDNET is anticipated to become a fully integrated part of the overall strategic training mission of military medical personnel.

The challenge before us is the integration of a number of existing and evolving simulation and medical technologies. The concepts behind MEDNET are based on the blending of Advanced Distributed Simulation (ADS) technology and modern, emerging telemedical technology. ADS technology includes enhanced Distributed Interactive Simulation (DIS), as well as constructive and live simulation capabilities. In support of

ADS, the Institute for Electrical and Electronics Engineers recently approved a simulation interface standard [IEEE 1516] known as the High Level Architecture (HLA). The HLA is sponsored by the Defense Modeling and Simulation Office (DMSO).

Based on the HLA standard, MEDNET could enable the simulation of any number of events and environments including, but not limited to, civilian patients, wounded combatants, patient surroundings, and the various echelons of care. In addition, MEDNET could leverage Internet technologies to incorporate a "virtual clinician" to provide support in diagnosis and disbursement of general medical knowledge to both medical and non-medical military or civilian personnel.

To date, biological weapons have not been used. However, in the unlikely event of a widespread biological threat such as unforeseen terrorist activity or a natural outbreak of disease, having MEDNET available to provide assistance to non-medical personnel may save a significant number of lives. Biological weapons are strategic in nature, and often spread well beyond their intended target (i.e., the Dandelion Effect). Should a biological threat occur, quarantine measures will no doubt be implemented and communications media (e.g., telephone, radio and networking services) will become critical assets in fighting such terrorist activities. MEDNET, perhaps as an extension to the Health Alert Network, can play a role in supporting the transmission and communication of medical information and operations to combat the biological threat over a widely distributed communications network.

Recent advances in World Wide Web technologies and applications, continuous performance improvement in computing and communications hardware, and the continued evolution of the Internet-2 and Next Generation Internet indicate that future bandwidth will be available to support and sustain a geographically dispersed, distributed simulation system. In the following sections, we will describe the various components of MEDNET.

2. The Components of MEDNET

The concept for MEDNET is based on existing distributed and reconfigurable simulation system technology suitable for both individual and team training. The primary components of MEDNET include the ADS system (the core of MEDNET) and infrastructure, the virtual patient simulator, a fully immersive 3D rendering system, an injury catalog database incorporating a comprehensive library of known branched-physiological scenarios, and an adaptive intelligent interface module called the Virtual Clinician Assistant.

Using the components of MEDNET, future civilian and military medical personnel will be able to educate and train in a synthetic environment (e.g., surgical theater, urban street accident, battlefield, rural area, etc.), triage and treat virtual injuries, and seek expert guidance, all from within the virtual environment of MEDNET. Whether from a portal on the World Wide Web to a fully immersive virtual environment, MEDNET will be capable of offering a wide range of educational and training capabilities. The Grand Challenge of

MEDNET is to provide this vast array of capabilities in a cohesive system that also supports differing levels of detail.

At one end of the spectrum is MEDNET's Web Portal Interface. Through this interface, MEDNET has the capability of providing basic first aid information to a broad constituency, such as the general public. In an operational setting, MEDNET has the capability to support JIT communications and operations support. In instances of terrorist attack, hundreds of thousands of people are going to want to know where to turn for general first aid information, assistance, or quarantine rules in the event of a biological threat. In the latter example, we now know that local and regional hospitals and trauma centers become quickly overloaded when the number of injured reach O(100). In fact, a recent simulation (a socratic dialogue) sponsored by the Institute for Security Technology Studies at Dartmouth last July indicated that health officials may be unable to triage the vast majority of the injured public. Further, as the first responders are the second to fall, the system is expected to collapse rapidly. Then where will people turn for basic information and first aid? The answer is the Internet. And where on the Internet will they be able to find up-to-the-minute information in an on-going crisis? MEDNET.

At the other end of the spectrum is MEDNET's fully immersive environment. In its fully immersive capability, a virtual reality (VR) cave would be constructed around modern data-grade video graphics projectors, suspended from the ceiling and displaying on four surrounding walls. The expectation of this system is that this simulated "synthetic" environment will render a 360-degree field of view that fully immerses the participant(s).

In the center of this rendered space resides a table (a high definition volumetric display) that will present the virtual patient image to the interactors. This display presents a stereoscopic image that appears as a scale model resting on a table, gurney, or litter. The interactor(s) may view this image from any angle: by walking around the table or by leaning over it to gain perspective from various azimuths and altitudes. Perhaps of particular interest are the data fusion capabilities of this display, which integrates graphical or multi-dimensional datasets with the virtual patient display. A true synthesis of MRI, 3D ultrasound, or other CT data can be used to "morph" the virtual patent to simulate a particular patient condition. When merged and morphed with data from the Visible Human Project, a true-to-life rendering is produced. But the grand challenge goes even further: simulating the entire patient: electro- mechanically, chemically, biologically, etc.

3. The Virtual Patient Simulator

At the center of the MEDNET synthetic environment will be the high fidelity Virtual Patient Simulator or VPS. The VPS is the subsystem responsible for modeling and rendering the human patient form in considerable detail. The core of the human model used by MEDNET could initially be constructed using a blend of ADS technology developed by the U.S. Department of Defense and the Visible Human project from the

National Institute of Health. However, there is little reason to stop there. There are many systems and processes that can be modeled, both independently and in synchronicity with other systems. Theoretically, this could take us down to the operational level of DNA, or as high a level as bedside manner JIT Training. The challenge is both research-oriented and educational.

There are many ways in which a human patient simulator could be used. For example, scenario-specific data for a virtual patient simulation could be initially drawn from a physiological patient database. Then mathematical behavioral models contained within the injury catalog would be selected to create a scenario-specific medical event, possibly from stored Magnetic Resonance Imaging (MRI) data sets. These displays will be superimposed on the digitized Visible Human and "*morphed*" as appropriate onto a standard human model. Visual or *polygonalized* data collected from the National Library of Medicine's Visible Human project can then provide a texture mapped overlay to generate quite realistic imagery. In another example, the virtual patient-generated image might contain generic ADS entity models. It may be possible to extend this presentation (such as in a learning environment) by synchronizing and registering a live data fed and superimposing it with the simulated patient. Given that live patient information is being collected (e.g., x-ray mapping) and displayed in the surgical theater today, this part of the challenge is the next logical step.

In most technical training environments, immediate assessment and feedback on performance can greatly enhance the task acquisition process.

Initial VPS systems will likely be a composite simulation system (a blend of live, real-time and constructive simulation technology) utilizing an aggregation of both low and high fidelity modeling techniques. Low fidelity modeling will be accomplished using constructive simulation techniques. When aggregated with virtual simulations, the VPS will be used to manage the majority of the patient's sub-systems in a logical and coherent fashion. High fidelity modeling that requires a high-degree of interaction will be accomplished strictly using real-time distributed interactive simulation techniques. Today, multi-processor-based systems are capable of providing the high-degree of interaction and fidelity required to train a clinician or medical corpsman. What's missing is the human patient simulation.

4. The Haptic Interface

Human-computer interaction has historically consisted of limited interaction with visual displays of iconic and character data on a two-dimensional screen. Networked Virtual Environments (Net-VEs) offer an alternative interaction paradigm in which users are no longer simply external observers of data but are active participants with their data in a 4D virtual world. Within the Net-VE, force sensation plays an important role in recognition of 4D objects and our interaction with them. The hardware and software technology involved in the creation of interactive virtual environments such as MEDNET is still relatively new, however, haptic devices are already available in commercial-off-the-shelf form.

A high fidelity haptic simulation of surface contact presents a demanding technical challenge in the design of force reflecting Net-VEs. In fact, the creation and quantification of the characteristics of each of MEDNET's application components is a research task in itself. One of the main objectives of the MEDNET Grand Challenge is to stimulate research. This includes the identification and quantification of representative force sensations by an interactor in the 4D synthetic environment.

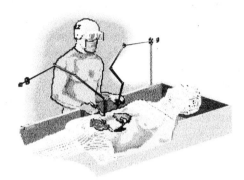

Figure 1 High-Fidelity MEDNET Simulator Configured for Surgical Training.

Surrounding the volumetric display within MEDNET will be a set of haptic (tactile/force-feedback) interaction· tools.   These tools that comprise a technology assessment will permit the interactor to reach out, touch and *feel* the VPS. The haptic systems in MEDNET that permit the interactor to touch, feel, and otherwise "physically" interact with the VPS will lead to evaluation and characterization of the fidelity necessary in haptic devices and the human factors associated with tactile and force-feedback systems in medical simulation applications.

High fidelity, distributed interactive simulation techniques will provide for adequate *man-in-the-loop* interaction and response times.   Although direct feedback to the interactor will be provided for by the haptic system, interaction and rendering will be controlled by the distributed Net-VE. Entity-to-interactor interaction will encompass various surgical tools and simulated telemedical instruments.   Additional techniques can be programmed into the MEDNET system as new tools are added to support a variety of training and educational tasks.

5.   Three and Dour Dimensional Displays

In many applications, the understanding and interpretation of visual images are inherent parts of the problem solving process. Examples in medical imagery range from diagnostic radiology and fluid-structure interaction to problems involving operator-assisted telerobotics. In MEDNET, the computer can be used to perform image, data, and knowledge processing in a way that is aligned with an understanding of the user.

Pseudo-holographic display systems can enhance our understanding and interpretation of visual images. They also provide for more realistic imagery. For the interactors, this display system can enhance interaction with the virtual patient simulation and further the immersion effects. In addition, several different levels of medical clinicians can be trained using MEDNET's reconfigurable environment. Clinicians can perform physical assessment tasks and practice procedures.

The objective of these systems is to provide high-fidelity video stimuli to the trainee with a minimal amount of distortion. This can occur in the VR Cave, or through the desktop using LCD shutter glasses. This can enhance the realism associated with the actual simulated environment. While this appears feasible and sensible on the surface, little research has been done to verify training effectiveness, cost effectiveness, human factors, or the impact of display system types. Network performance and training effectiveness are particularly troublesome and limited. However, initial system prototypes do appear quite promising, and recent assessments by the Army Research Laboratory appear to support the claim that interactors using 3D visualization appear to perform at a superior level to those using only 2D visualization. Thus we have good evidence to believe that 4D interaction may indeed be superior still.

6. The Virtual Clinician Assistant

A significant amount of research has been conducted in developing techniques for embedded assessment for intelligent tutoring systems. This area focuses on the application and extension of real-time embedded assessment technology to casualty care. Today we believe that this level of assessment could now be integrated with modern knowledge-base technology and made available to the public at-large through the Web.

Consider that in most technical training environments, immediate assessment and feedback on performance can greatly enhance the acquisition process. This is especially true for procedural based applications (e.g., diagnostics, control procedures, etc.). When procedural errors are identified in real-time, it is easier for the learner to comprehend the context in which the error occurred. Often it is the situational variables that lead to a procedural error, hence corrective feedback in real-time aids in learning to avoid situationally induced errors.

The Virtual Clinician is the focus of research on the development of a prototype real-time intelligent embedded assessment module that would be integrated with MEDNET. This module would capture the procedural knowledge for a selected subset of diagnostic and/or operational activities. This involves knowledge engineering of selected procedures, development of the prototype knowledge model, and integration and testing with the Virtual Clinician interface. Further, timely information could be programmed into this interface to provide Just-In-Time training to public at-large.

One of the side benefits of a validated embedded assessment module is that it reduces the number of live assessment experts needed for training. The Virtual Clinician prototype will be structured so that it can be extended into a comprehensive model in the out-years of the MEDNET program. This is perhaps by far, the most visionary component of MEDNET.

A key element necessary to enhance many of the tools and models being developed is the need for an intelligent diagnostic aid. The intelligent diagnostic aid would exploit neural network technology, specifically back propagation neural networks, to provide expert diagnosis based on selected physiological scenario inputs. This type of expert systems approach is vital to the development of medic and physician-centered training. A fundamental reason for the importance of this type of system to the long-term goals of the MEDNET project is the same as for any expert system, the retention of expert knowledge.

Often the time between armed conflicts is lengthy. As a result, each time the military enters an armed conflict, it has a staff of physicians and medics with little or no direct experience in combat casualty care. The objective of the intelligent diagnostic aid within MEDNET is to create a system that can capture combat casualty diagnostic knowledge so that it is permanently archived and accessible during future training and conflicts. Later, this knowledge can moved into the civilian sector to aid in diagnostic training and emergency room care.

7. Conclusion

A grand challenge is a feat no one has attempted, but one in which we can see how it could be accomplished. MEDNET is one such grand challenge. This challenge will generate an immersive and highly adaptable virtual environment that will allow individual participants or teams to train simultaneously. The scenes presented within the MEDNET cave can change from a front line battlefield, through combat support hospital, all the way back to a remote hospital located in rural New Hampshire or urban Miami. Indeed, the entire continuum of support echelons can be modeled. Modeling treatment received prior to, during or after transportation, or post-operative care can be but one focus of MEDNET simulations. Situational awareness training garnered through each step in the design of the 21st century medical system will be supported.

This integrated use of MEDNET, coupled with the World Wide Web and Health Alert Network represents a training simulation of providing casualty care as a comprehensive and realistic simulation exercise. Further, as our communication infrastructures stabilize and evolve, there is every reason to believe that a training system such as MEDNET could also be used in an operational capacity. The MEDNET training environment will therefore be a knowledge delivery environment, enabling medical personnel to better understand and manage the toll exacted by casualties.

Medicine Meets Virtual Reality 2001
J.D. Westwood et al. (Eds.)
IOS Press, 2001

Laser-Pointing Endoscope System for Natural 3D Interface between Robotic Equipments and Surgeons

Yoshihiko NAKAMURA   Mitsuhiro HAYASHIBE

Department of Mechano-Informatics, University of Tokyo

7-3-1, Hongo, Bunkyoku, Tokyo 113-8656 Japan

Abstract

Precise measurements of reference points would be mandatory if robotic equipments would be introduced in operation rooms. We develop a real-time laser-pointing endoscope using an optical galvano scanner and a 955fps high-speed camera. This system provides the scanned 3D image of the liver under the endoscopic surgery and a touch screen interface so that surgeons can intuitively indicate points of interest with precise 3D position. Some results of in-vivo experiments on a liver of pig are shown to verify the effectiveness of the proposed.

1   Introduction

Surgeons in endoscopic surgery have developed the skill to manipulate their hands relying on the two dimensional image on the video monitor. It requires more efforts to get the skill and more mental tension at operations. Stereo image presentation has become available as technology. However, it is still controversy which is more comfortable and informative for surgeons to have a stereo image or a monocular image twice as clear as the stereo image since the available intensity of light source and the rate of transparency of endoscopic optics are limited and have to be shared for stereo imaging. The 3D information seems less important for surgeons or can be compensated by surgeons with their skills and experiences even with a monocular image. However, the 3D information has not been integrated efficiently in surgical robot systems.

Technical advance of minimally invasive surgery introduces more and more equipped environments[1]. Master-slave robotic systems have recently been introduced in operation rooms. Da Vinci (Intuitive Surgical Inc.[2]) and Zeus (Computer Motion Inc.[3]) have been applied for endoscopic cardiac surgery and laparoscopic surgery. The surgeons are now able to control two arms in the patient body with two master devices outside at a distance. Even in these systems, the interface between the robotic systems and surgeons are only a straightforward one, where the human interface is still limited to direct manipulation between master and slave robotics devices.

Minimally invasive surgery with robotic systems would be technologically improved if surgeons are provided with the 3D shape of internal geometry and the 3D coordinates of point of interest in an intuitive manner. Being integrated with a real time interface, such technology would make a significant difference in the operational environments. Surgeons could easily reach the point of interest in the monitor screen, toward which the robot should move, with high precision in endoscopic surgery including robotic system.

In this paper, we develop the laser-pointing endoscope system with a laser light source, a 2D optical galvano scanner, and a 955fps high-speed camera. We also propose a touch screen interface so that surgeons can intuitively indicate points of interest on the 2D screen.

2   Intra-Operative 3D Geometric Registration and Interface

Improvement of human interface is certainly essential in technological issues of minimally invasive surgery. In this paper, we make use of active control of a laser marker as a doctor's interface with surgical equipments. Triangulation with the laser projection system and an endoscopic camera measures the 3D coordinates of the laser point-marker[4] [5]. This system finds its clinical applications in a broader sense of human interface such as :

(1) *it in-situ* 3D point registration from 2D image

When a target point of operation is visible in a monocular endoscopic image, a surgeon would reach the point with a slave robot by carefully moving the master equipment in the depth direction with the help of visual information such as the unfocussedness and the deformation due to touch. Even with binocular endoscopic images, it is still not too intuitive for a surgeon to perceive precise 3D geometry. This is why a surgeon has to keep his/her mental tension in using the master-slave robotic systems.   With the laser-pointing endoscope we propose in this paper, a surgeon might

touch the point of interest on a monocular endoscopic image of a touch screen. Then, the controlled laser marker will immediately point the point of interest. After a confirmation, the total system of equipments obtains the precise 3D coordinates of the point of the surgeon's interest as illustrated in Fig.1. This information would be used in various different ways. In a simple but aggressive scenario, the surgeon might use a command to move a forceps to a point 5 mm above the point carefully avoiding touches with any parts of the body based on the 3D map inside the body, which is also captured by the controlled laser marker. In a rather conventional scenario, the information would be used for navigation, by reporting the surgeon when the forceps comes close to the point, and even warning him/her when it does with an excessive speed.

(2) *it in-situ* 3D shape recovery from 2D image

In tele-surgery or tele-medicine, an expert doctor in distance may wish to know the 3D shape and size of a particular area to make any medical decisions. Such information is valuable also for local surgeons. Indicating the area on a touch screen, the doctor and/or surgeon would interactively activate the laser-pointing endoscope for scanning the area. Being combined with the ultra-violet light-emitting technology, the laser-pointing endoscope could be used to locally illuminate and find the dye absorbing areas. For instance, Fig.2 shows the picture of marked liver at the range which is decided from touch screen in in-vivo experiment.

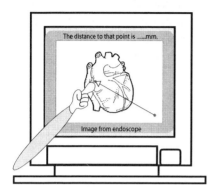

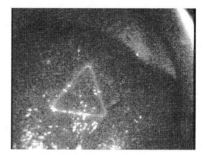

Fig. 1 Touch Screen Interface   **Fig. 2 Marking on the liver**

(3) *it in-situ* interpretation of pre-operative data due to deformation

The precise anatomical data of a patient is accessible using CT or MRI. The data is usually evaluated in the pre-operative conferences to discuss and plan the surgical procedures. One of current issues is how to utilize such data in the operation room. The CT or MRI data shows geometrical inconsistency with the deformation due to the change of patient's body postures. For deformation, a surgeon has to develop the imagination to map the pre-surgical date onto the deformed one. If we scan the organ *in-situ* using the laser-pointing endoscope, we compute and estimate its internal deformation using the scanned data.

3   Laser Pointing Endoscope

The prototype as shown in Fig.3 was developed using a laser light source, a galvano scanner, two cameras of different standards and a LCD monitor with touch screen interface. Being controlled by the mirrors of galvano scanner, a laser spot is projected inside the patient's body through an endoscope. We used a closed loop controlled galvano scanner (General Scanning Inc.: G120DT), which responds up to 1kHz of the input signal. The laser spot is captured by a 955 fps high-speed camera (DALSA Inc.) and an image capture/processing board (Viper-Digital (CORECO Inc.): 256 X 256 pixels in 256 gray scale). Due to the gray scale image of high speed camera, It is not suitable for the surgeon to be provided. Therefore, being split by a beam-splitting prism, color images are captured by an NTSC CCD camera and presented to the surgeon as illustrated in Fig.4. Information from high speed camera is used only for 3D geometric information of organs. The 3D coordinates of reference points are reconstructed from the tracked 2D data by the image capture/processing board and the input angle signals to the 2D laser scanner.

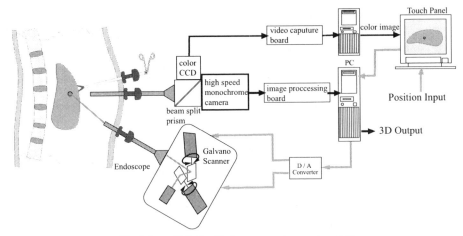

Fig. 3 Laser Pointing Endoscope: system components

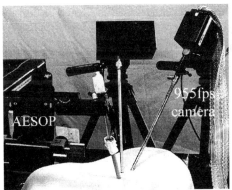

Fig. 4 Developed prototype

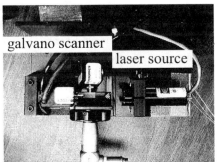

Fig.5 Combined Endoscope with laser scanner

4 Experiments

4.1 3D Pointing Interface

In the current endoscopic surgery, surgeons have to mentally extract necessary information from the image of endoscope. In other words, they must judge the distance and the size of object using their sense. The surgeons would feel less tired if they were released from the mental load.

The 3D pointing interface works as follows:

(1) the surgeon toughes the screen of endoscopic image at a point of interest.

(2) the laser marker is controlled using the galvano scanner so that its position in the endoscopic image converges to the point of interest.

(3) Once converged, the 3D coordinates in the camera frame of the point of reference are recovered.

We tested the interface and measurements in in-vivo experiments on the liver of a pig. This system could provide the surgeon with the 3D coordinates of the point of interest in real-time. The response time from the touch on screen to the output of 3D coordinates was approximately 0.5 second. We will share the trace data that shows how the laser spot were controlled and converged to the target point on the liver.

Fig.5 shows the trace of 3D coordinates while the laser marker converges to the point of reference on the liver of pig.

The touch screen interface assists a surgeon to intuitively indicate the point of interest on the 2D monitor screen (NTSC). The galvano scanner actively controls the laser spot inside the patient to locate it in the 2D monitor screen (NTSC) at the indicated point by the surgeon. And this system is realized by high speed tracking (955fps) and laser control using differential vector in the image. In every frame, differential vector between present laser point and destination is calculated. And laser beam is projected to the direction of the differential vector according to its size until the difference has turned into subthreshold.

As the swing angle of laser beam per frame is large, the time to converge is short. However, if the swing angle is larger, the image processing time takes more due to the larger area of investigation. This issue brings trade-off between the swing angle and the investigation area. To dicrease the loss time, we made an optimal adjustment. In the case of maximum swing angle, laser mark in the next frame would be captured at the edge in the investigation area as illustrated in Fig.7.

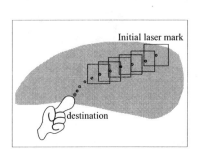

Fig. 6 Convergence in the endoscopic image   Fig. 7 The 3D trace of laser mark on the liver

4.2   Scanning 3D Shape

The human skin was successfully scanned, though the contrast of image was weak due to tissue absorption and diffusion. In order to investigate the optical conditions, we scanned the 3D shape of pig's liver in in-vivo experiments as shown in Fig.8. Even with the wet and shinny surface condition, it was possible to obtain the positional data using a semiconductor laser light source. The laser power was 15mW. We scanned the area of 20cm square and obtained the 4000 points data. Sampling time took 1.2ms for each point, and the total measuring time was approximately 5.0 seconds. The 3D data was rediscribed in Virtual Reality Modeling Language 2.0. The shape of liver is easily percieved by general www browser with VRML plug-in software. Fig.9 and Fig.10 show the reconstructed 3D VRML image of the scanned liver in in-vivo experiment.

The obtained information could be used, for example, for the local surgeon to provide the robotic equipment controller with a reference point, or for the remote mentoring doctors to numerically measure the location, length, and/or area of interest inside the patient's body.

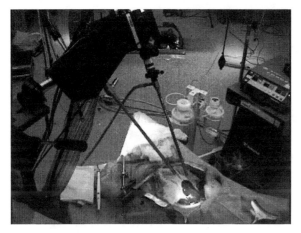

Fig. 8 Scanning liver at the in-vivo Experiment

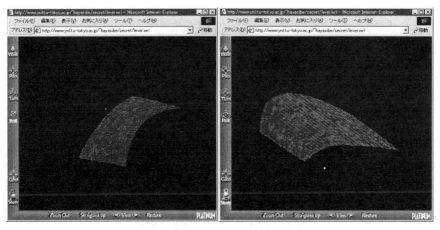

Fig. 9 Reconstructed 3D VRML data of liver

5   Conclusion

The conclusion of this paper is summarized in the following four points:

(1) The concept of laser-pointing endoscope was proposed.

(2) The laser-pointing endoscope provides the surgeons with a natural 3D interface, which was designed and fabricated using a touch screen and a high-speed camera

(3) The laser-pointing endoscope can obtain the intra-operative geometric information of the internal surface in laparoscopic surgery. An in-vivo measurement of pig's liver was carried out and used for reconstruction of 3D surface model.

(4) The preliminary in-vivo experiments cleanly support the functionality of the laser-pointing endoscope. The in-vivo 3D measurements would be useful to use the pre-operative geometric information such as CT and MRI images into the operation room, taking account of the deformation.

Acknowledgements

This work was supported in part through "Development of Surgical Robotic System" (PI:Prof. MD. Takayuki TSUJI) under the Research for the Future Program, the Japan Society for the Promotion of Science, and through "Telecommunications Advancemment Organization of Japan" (PI: Prof. Mamoru MITSUISHI).

References

[1] Marc O. Schurr: "Robotic Devices for Advanced Endoscopic Surgical Procedures,"
Journal of the Robotics Society of Japan, Vol.18 No.1, pp.16-19, (2000).

[2] G S.Guthart: "The Intuitive Telesurgery System," Proceedings of the IEEE International Conference on Robotics and Automation, pp.618-621, (2000).

[3] Computer Motion Inc., "Internet Home Page", http://www.computermotion.com.

[4] S.Baba, H.Kawakami and Y.Nakamura: "Laser pointing endoscope for Minimally Invasive Surgery," Proceedings of Robomech'99, 1P2-10-009, (1999).

[5] Y.Nakamura, M.Hayashibe: "Real-Time Laser-Pointing Endoscope Using Galvano Scanner and 955fps High Speed Camera," Proceedings of the Computer Assisted Orthopaedic Surgery, pp.267-269, (2000).

[6] H.Zuang, K.Wang, and Z.S.Roth: "Simultaneous Calibration of a Robot and a Hand-Mounded Camera, " IEEE Trans. on Robotics and Automation, Vol.11 No.5, pp.649-660, (1995).

Medicine Meets Virtual Reality 2001
J.D. Westwood et al. (Eds.)
IOS Press, 2001

Robotic Stabilization that Assists Cardiac Surgery on Beating Hearts

Yoshihiko NAKAMURA   Kosuke KISHI

Department of Mechano-Informatics

University of Tokyo

7-3-1, Hongo, Bunkyoku, Tokyo 113-8656 Japan

Abstract

Minimally Invasive Direct Coronary Artery Bypass (MIDCAB) requires surgeons the precision of hand skill and the mental concentration, since it needs to work on beating hearts. We propose a surgical robot system that compensates motions of organs during operations. The motion canceling robot system consists of three technologies: visual synchronization, motion synchronization and master-slave control. In this paper, we verify the effectiveness of the prototype system by in-vivo experiment.

1 Introduction

Minimally Invasive Direct Coronary Artery Bypass (MIDCAB) is paid an attention to as minimally invasive procedure of the cardiovascular surgery region. Conventional procedures of the coronary artery bypass surgery incise most of the thorax, and use a heart-lung machine. The MIDCAB was developed to make the incision minimum like Figure.1, and not to damage the respiratory function. In addition, the chance of complications such as cerebral infarction and aorta dissociation is reduced, since the extra corporeal circulation using a heart-lung machine is not adopted. It is another advantage that there is no degradation of erythrocyte by extracorporeal circulation [1][2].

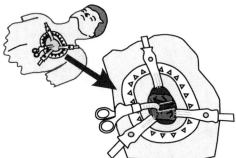

Fig. 1 Minimally invasive direct coronary artery bypass

Minimally invasive cardiac surgery such as direct coronary artery bypass or endoscopic coronary artery bypass requires surgeons of the precision of hand skill and the mental concentration. The request becomes even harder if it is to be done on beating hearts in order to minimize patients' damage. Recently, though the master-slave robotic surgical systems such as da Vinci (Intuitive Surgical Inc.) and Zeus (Computer Motion Inc.) are developed for the practical use [3][4], the difficulty of the surgery on the beating heart has not been solved. We propose a master-slave robotic surgical environment for surgeons that compensates the motion of organs during operations, especially that of beating hearts.

2 Robotic Heartbeat Synchronization

We would like to propose the motion compensation technology with which a surgeon sees the stationary image of the point of interest on a monitor screen and, relying on the image, manipulates the master device reaching the slave robotic device for the point of interest. In reality, the point of interest is on the beating heart. The slave robotic device moves in synchronization with the heartbeat and changes its relative position to the point of interest according to the motion of the manipulated master device.

We call the motion compensation technology the *"Heartbeat Synchronization"* which consists of three technical elements: *Visual Synchronization, Motion Synchronization,* and *Master-Slave control.*

Visual synchronization provides the stationary image of the point of reference, while *motion synchronization* moves the slave robotic device in accordance with the heart beat and keeps it relatively stationary to the point. In *master-slave control*, the motion of the master device is transferred to the slave robotic device and controls the relative position of the slave robotic device to the point of interest. The overall system is illustrated in Figure 2.

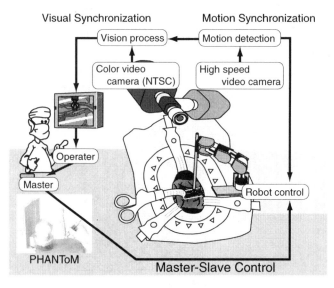

Fig. 2 Heartbeart Synchronization

3   Components

3.1   Master-Slave Robotic Devices

3.1.1 Slave device

The current design of slave robotic device has four degrees of freedom being driven by small integrated actuators (YASUKAWA Electric), each consisting of a brashless AC motors, a harmonic drive reducer, and an optical rotary encoder. The slave robotic device has the kinematic design as shown in Figure 3, which is intended to be used fixed on the oval frame (approximately 20cm X 15cm) that is commonly used in the MIDCAB (see Figure 1) to maintain the access window and to fix devices such as mechanical stabilizers.

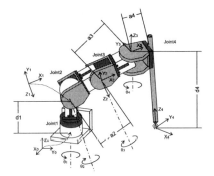

Fig. 3 Slave Robotic Device

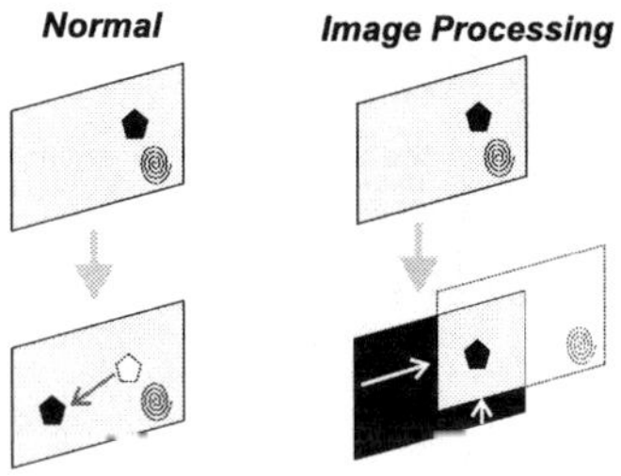

Fig. 4 Tracking and image rendering
for visual synchronization

3.1.2 Master device

As the master device, we adopted the Phantom Desktop (SensAble Technologies, Inc.), which has six-axes joint measurements and three axes of haptic force feedback. The force feedback function is not currently used in our system. The haptic sensation could be used to feedback the force interaction at the endpoint of the slave robotic device, or to establish haptic communication between the surgeon and the assisting surgical navigation system.

3.2   Visual Synchronization

Visual synchronization implies to provide surgeons with the stationary image of the moving point of reference on the beating heart. The image processing system tracks the point of reference and continuously obtains its position on the image. The image is cut out from the image memory and relocated so that the point of reference always remains in the same position on the monitor screen. The similar function was used in camcorders to reduce image disturbances due to hand vibration using gyro sensors or by simple digital image processing. Combining the function with the image tracking, the tracking reliability and time of computation are the critical issues to challenge. The scheme is illustrated in Figure 4.

We previously used a single color NTSC camera for tracking and image rendering using image processing boards such as Tacking Vision (Fujitsu) and IP5000 (Hitachi) [5]. It worked fine for visual synchronization, though the stability of motion detection was not excellent and the update rate of motion is limited by the NTSC standard (the flame rate of 30Hz, the field rate of 60Hz), which resulted in the low accuracy of motion synchronization which we discuss in the next subsection.

In the new prototype system, we adopted two different CCD video cameras; a color NTSC camera and a monochrome high-speed camera (Dalsa: model CA-D6, 955 fps, 256 X 256 pixels). The motion of the point of reference is tracked and measured using the high speed camera and an image capture/processing board (Coreco: Viper-Digital), while the image of the NTSC camera is used for rendering. The color image is cut from the image memory according to the position measured using the high speed camera. This image processing is done by IP5000 (Hitachi).

The two cameras were integrated using a half-mirror prism into a dual-head video camera to share a common view as shown in Figure 5. The two cameras use a single zoom lens for 35 mm MF single lens reflex camera, which was selected because of its long flange-back length.

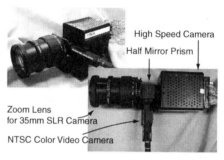

Fig. 5 A dual-head video camera for visual synchronization

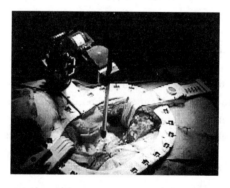

Fig. 6   In-vivo experiments for motion synchronization

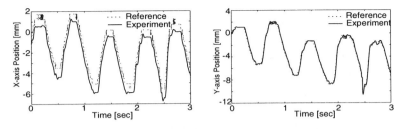

Fig. 7 Motion Stabilization System Response

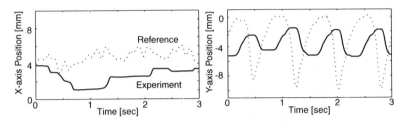

Fig. 8 Responses of motion synchronization with a NTSC camera

3.3 Motion Synchronization

The measured position of the point of reference on the beating heart is now used as feedback signal to control the endeffector of slave robotic device relatively to the point of reference. We established near 1ms visual feedback control system using the high speed camera. The slave robotic devise moves with the motion of reference point. Therefore, the slave robotic devise is seen stationary in the rendered monitor image as well as the point of reference.

The experimental verification of motion synchronization was successfully conducted in-vivo for a pig as seen in Figure 6. Figure 7 shows the data of experiment, where the X and Y axes are those in the image plane of the camera. Small and almost constant errors remained in X axis, since it was a direction that the gravity effect appeared. The errors were afterward removed with a simple gravity compensation algorithm implemented in the controller. For the reference of readers, the data of similar experiments, that was previously done using a NTSC camera only, is shown in Figure 8. The comparison of Figures 7 and 8 clearly shows that the near 1 ms visual feedback control is surprisingly effective to synchronize the slave robot motion with the heartbeat.

4 Experiments of Heartbeat Synchronization

As seen in Figure 9, a laser point was projected on a paper underneath the oval frame window to which the slave robot was fixed. The laser point was projected from a laser pointer oscillating under the paper at the frequency of approximately 1.5Hz. The measured motion of the laser point was used for the visual and motion synchronizations. At the same time, an operator manipulated the master device

(Phantom desktop) while watching the synchronized image. The command signal was transmitted from the master to the slave robotic device and additively combined with the vibrating laser point measurement. We had seen the slave robot vibrating fairly complex, if we had seen it directly. On the contrary, we saw on the monitor screen the slave robot quietly moving toward the stationary point of reference.

The results of experiments are graphically shown in Figure 10. The bottom two graphs are those of the motion of master device. The middle two graphs show the vibration of laser point measured using the high speed camera. The top two graphs are of the combined motion of the slave robotic device, where the solid line shows the real motion of the slave device, while the broken line indicates the combined reference signal.

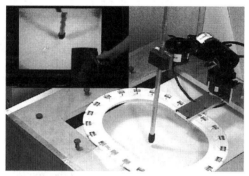

Fig. 9 Oscillating laser point and the synchronization system

5   Conclusions

The results of this paper are summarized in the following four points:

(1) The concept of the heartbeat synchronization for minimally invasive cardiac surgery was introduced.

(2) The visual and motion synchronization technologies were developed, which   were made possible by adopting a 955 fps high speed camera.

(3) Through in-vivo experiments, we confirmed the functionality of the visual and motion synchronization.

(4) The heartbeat synchronization system was prototyped integrating the visual and motion synchronization technologies into the master-slave robot system. Experiments in an artificial environment clearly verified the effectiveness of the system.

Acknowledgements

This work was supported in part through "Development of Surgical Robotic System" (PI:Prof. MD. Takayuki TSUJI) under the Research for the Future Program, the Japan Society for the Promotion of Science, and through "Telecommunications Advancemment Organization of Japan" (PI: Prof. Mamoru MITSUISHI).

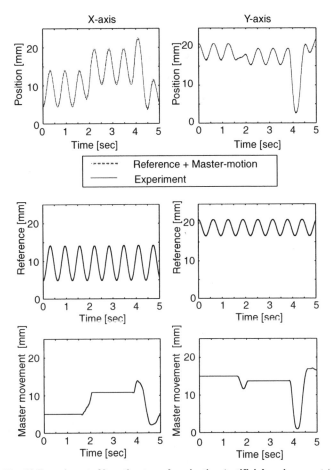

Fig. 10 Experiment of heartbeat synchronization (artificial environments)

References

[1] S.Kitamura: "Coronary artery reconstructive surgery," Heart, Vol.30 No.8, pp.539-pp.540(1988).

[2] T.Ohtsuka: "Minimally Invasive Cardiac Surgery: Background, Current Status, Future and Application of Robotic Technology," Journal of the robotics society of Japan, Vol.18 No.1, pp.12-15(2000)

[3] G S.Guthart: "The Intuitive Telesurgery System," Proceedings of the IEEE International Conference on Robotics and Automation, pp.618-621(2000).

[4] H.Reichenspurner, R.Damiano, M.Mack, D.Boehm, H.Gulbins, C.Detter, B.Meiser, R.Elgass and B.Reichart : "Use of the voice-controlled and computer-assisted surgical system ZEUS for endoscopic coronary artery bypass grafting," J Thorac Cardiovasc Surg, Vol.118 No.1, pp.11-16(1999).

[5] H.KAWAKAMI: "Motion-Cancelling Robot System for Minimally Invasive Cardiac Surgery," Journal of the robotics society of Japan, Vol.18 No.6, pp.115-pp.123(2000).

[6] S.Usui, K.Itou and K.Mita:"The base of the biomedical signal processing," Ohm Co., (1985).

Medicine Meets Virtual Reality 2001
J.D. Westwood et al. (Eds.)
IOS Press, 2001

4D Visible and Palpable Simulation Using Dynamic Pressure Model Based on Cardiac Morphology

Megumi Nakao[1], Masaru Komori[2], Tetsuya Matsuda[1], Takashi Takahashi[2]

[1]Graduate school of informatics, Kyoto University,
[2]Department of Medical Informatics, Kyoto University Hospital
Address: Sakyou, Kyoto, 606-8507, Japan
E-mail: meg@kuhp.kyoto-u.ac.jp

Abstract: A goal of this work is proposal and construction of *ActiveHeart System*: a simulation environment that enables anyone to see and touch heart beat in real time. In this paper, a method to express real-time graphic and haptic behaviour of a beating heart is mentioned. The data for the beating heart model was obtained from ECG-gated 3D MRI of a normal volunteer. The elastic information was assumed as a uniform value with clinically experienced elasticity. Using a real-time 3D graphics and a haptic device, a simulation environment of the beating heart was designed and implemented. After the construction, some cardiovascular surgeons evaluated the implemented system. Its visualization and beating expression were scored excellent, but some details in haptic expression were remained to be improved. Finally, for more realistic cardiovascular surgical simulation, future development of the method is discussed.

Keywords: Cardiac Simulation, Haptics, Interactive Visualization, Medical Education

1. Introduction

As a result of wide spread of a virtual reality in the medical field, novel studies that focus on tactile sense appeared. [1] A system to reconstruct haptics of in vivo organs can perform more realistic analyses and simulations like virtual surgery. [2][3][4] And recent days, there is also a remarkable work that aim to acquire elasticity of in vivo organs no invasively with Magnetic Resonance Elastography technique and represents tactile sense of internal organs such as liver and thigh. [5] It is meaningful that these studies aim at simulations and tactile sense reproduction of static organs for static dataset using theoretical phisical models.

On the other hand, haptic information during a cardiovascular surgery is very important for diagnosis and design of surgical strategies. Therefore, a system that simulates the motion of cardiac muscles and valves with tactile sense allows medical students and surgeons to learn palpation objectively. But it has been difficult to measure morphological information of entire cardiac cycle, because the heart is an active organ and has dynamic motion. In addition, study of cardiac dynamics requires analysis of multi-dimensional variables and complex parameters. Therefore few studies have ever tried to describe and simulate tactile sense of beating heart based on in vivo datasets.

2. Purpose

Considering above requirements of palpable cardiac simulation for medical education and surgical training, a main goal of this study is proposal and construction of the ActiveHeart System: a simulation environment that enables anyone to see and touch heartbeats in real time. To begin with, this paper provides a method to describe dynamic pressure of heart based on time series cardiac morphology. Based on this beating heart model, using a personal computer and a haptic device, a novel simulation environment of beating heart is designed and implemented. This simulation of the beating heart with haptic device enables medical students and surgeons to learn tactile sense of heartbeat, and contributes to medical education and surgical training.

3. Methods

The datasets for the beating heart model was obtained from ECG-gated 3D MRI of a normal volunteer. The whole data consist of time series 15 chest volumetric data for one cardiac cycle, and after extracting the region of heart, we have acquired the morphological beating heart data. The most important point to construct haptic simulation environment of beating heart is how to generate appropriate force from time series volumetric data. This work classified tactile expression of beating heart to static model and dynamic model. It is because the tactile sense of cardiac dynamics consists of active pressure by the heartbeats and passive stress by pushing its surface.

To describe dynamic force, collision detection and force calculation approach are required. This work proposes an original space mapping method to describe these procedures. This method aims to completely register a real world to virtual space generated by volume data and performs realistic force feedback with concise procedures. In addition, this space mapping methodology can also give a solution to beating expression and realize a specific algorithm to describe active pressure. In this force model, it supposes that the user is touching the surface of cardiac muscle and active force is returned during cardiac diastole, because active pressure is mainly generated by the motion of the cardiac muscle during cardiac diastole, not by the blood pressure during systole.

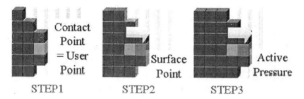

Figure1. This figure illustrates the method of active force generation by the myocardial motion during diastole. The elastic information was assumed as a uniform value with clinically experienced elasticity.

4. Results

Tactile expression of the beating heart is provided through a PHANToM haptic device after smoothing force values. Calculation time to generate real-time volume image is another problem when constructing 4D visible simulation environment. This work solved this problem by processing rendering procedure on volume rendering hardware. As a result of the implement, realistic calculation time was achieved to operate rotating, cutting and zoom in/out interactively while the heart object is beating. Figure2 illustrates constructed ActiveHeart System: 4D visible and palpable simulation environment of beating heart.

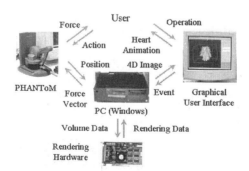

Figure2. The Overview of ActiveHeart System. This system has graphic and haptic processes and each procedure achieves optimal performance by parallel computing. These two processes are also controlled synchronously each other by the system main process.

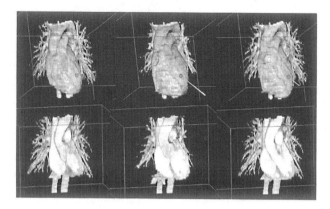

Figure3. 4D visible and palpable simulation of the beating heart. Upper images: haptic expression of the heartbeat. User point is described as a sphere image and line images show generated dynamic force vector. Lower images: real time visualization of inner organs and blood flow.

Finally, a qualitative evaluation was applied to the ActiveHeart System with some cardiovascular surgeons. According to this evaluation, the graphic performance of this system is high and provides interactive reference platform to analyse optional inner organs. As for haptics, this system attains realistic tactile sense of the heartbeat. But some details in haptic expression were remained to be improved, because this system only supports single haptic interface and so on. For visible and palpable educational system for various heart diseases, we are now developing the interface and adding heart pressure to this system. In the near future, we believe this system will be available for medical education for palpation and basic surgical training in procedures such as intra-cardiac catheter ablation.

5. Conclusions

This work provided dynamic force description about active pressure and passive stress based on cardiac morphology. Using model, graphic and force feedback algorithm was described and implemented as ActiveHeart system using rendering hardware and haptic interface. System processes by parallel computing were also developed to optimise and synchronize graphics and haptics. Consequently, constructed simulation environment performed realistic tactile sense reproduction and real time visualization of beating heart.

References

[1] Paul J.Gorman, Andreas H.Meier, M.Krummel, "Computer Assited Learning and Training", Computer Aided Surgery vol.5, p120-127, 2000
[2] Karl D. Reinig, Charles G. Rush, Helen L. Pelster; "Real-Time Visually and Haptically Accurate Surgical Simulation", Proceedings of Medicine Meets Virtual Reality 4, 1996
[3] J. Berkley, S. Weghorst, H. Gladstone, G. Gaugi, D. Berg, M. Ganter, "Banded Matrix Approach to Finite Element Modelling for Soft Tissue Simulation", Virtual Reality, 1999
[4] Naoki Suzuki, Asaki Hattori, Takeshi Ezumi, Akihiko Uchiyama et al; "Simulator for virtual surgery using deformable organ models and force feedback system", Proceedings of Medicine Meets Virtual Reality 7, 1999
[5] M.Suga, T.Matsuda, T.Takahashi et al; "Sensible Human Projects: Haptic Mondeling and Surgical Simulation Based on Measurements of Practical Patients with MR Elastography -Measurement of Elastic Modulus", Proceedings of Medicine Meets Virtual Reality2000, p334-340, 2000
[6] Megumi Nakao, Masaru Komori, Tetsuya Matsuda, Takashi Takahashi; "ActiveHeart: 4D Visible and Palpable Simulation Environment of Beating Heart", Proceedings of the Sixth International Conference on Virtual Systems and Multi Media, p448-455, 2000

Medicine Meets Virtual Reality 2001
J.D. Westwood et al. (Eds.)
IOS Press, 2001

The Representation of Blood Flow in Endourologic Surgical Simulations

Peter OPPENHEIMER, Arnab GUPTA, Suzanne WEGHORST
Human Interface Technology Laboratory, Washington Technology Center
University of Washington, Seattle, WA 98195

Robert SWEET, James PORTER
Dept. of Urology, University of Washington, Seattle, WA 98195

Abstract. An image-based approach has been developed to represent bleeding in a simulator for transurethral resection of prostate (TURP). While previous attempts have simulated bleeding over tissue surfaces or in blood vessels, our approach focused on the macroscopic visualization of bleeding in a fluid environment. TURP is an ideal procedure for simulation-based training because of the dynamic environment and the variety of flow patterns it presents. The first step in the development of the simulator was the generation of blood flow movies which consisted of capturing videos of bleeding vessels *in vitro*, processing them to separate the actual blood from the background anatomy and organizing the movies into a parametric database. During the running of the simulation, resection of prostate tissue systematically triggers bleeding events and the playback of a blood flow movie. The blood flow movie is texture mapped onto a virtual surface that is positioned oriented, morphed, composited and looped into the virtual scene.

1. Introduction

Simulating bleeding poses a big challenge in surgical simulation. We have developed an image-based representation of blood flow for use in the simulation of transurethral surgery. In addition to providing added realism, it will allow the training surgeon to practice responding appropriately to the challenges of hemostasis (control of bleeding) under a variety of different fluid flow conditions at various skill levels.

While previous representations of dynamic blood flow have modeled bleeding over tissue surfaces [2] or flow at the micro-scale (e.g. within blood vessels) [4], our work focuses on the macroscopic visualization of blood being discharged in a fluid environment. Our image-based approach uses captured video sequences of blood flow as source data sets that are positioned, oriented, composited, morphed and looped into an existing virtual model of the anatomy.

Our system simulates the bleeding that takes place during transurethral resection of the prostate (TURP). The surgical approach consists of placing an endoscope in the urethra and resecting prostate tissue with loop electrocautery. During the resection process, bleeding vessels and sinuses in the prostate are exposed and the resulting blood flow is either stopped by applying the loop on the source and coagulating, or resecting it by cutting another prostate chip over the area. The operative area during this procedure is continuously irrigated with a clear fluid that flows from a source coaxial to the scope. The irrigation keeps the area of resection distended and free of blood and debris. This gives the surgeon visibility to resect the prostate adenoma and to coagulate bleeding vessels.

There is a clinical need for a TURP simulator in the urology community. Performing TURP is an essential skill that needs to be in every urologist's armamentarium, yet the ability to perform one well is a dying art. This is primarily due to the emergence of medical management as front line therapy for symptoms associated with bladder outlet obstruction. TURP still remains the gold standard. The number of TURPs that residents do during their residency has diminished substantially. Urologists in practice are doing fewer and fewer procedures and are in danger of weakening their skill.

TURP is an excellent model for representing blood flow in transurethral surgical simulators. The complexity and dynamic nature of the procedure combined with its relatively simple anatomy also make TURP an ideal procedure to simulate. Furthermore, it is an excellent model for simulating bleeding in a number of fluid flow states. The procedure is performed in a fluid environment, and therefore blood flow is not constrained to adhere to the tissue surface.

Interactive TURP simulations have been described by Ballaro et. al. [1], and Gomes et. al. [3]. Gomes et. al. describes a series of red dots that emanate from the cut. It is essential for training surgeons performing TURP to learn the art of hemostasis. Accurate simulation of bleeding has been a limiting factor.

2. Materials and Methods

The steps used to represent blood flow are as follows. Prior to running the simulation we generated a blood flow movie database. This was accomplished in three steps.
1) Video capture of blood flow "movies"
2) Image processing to separate the blood image from its background.
3) Organization of the movies into a parametric database.

During the running of the simulation, the blood flow movies are rendered through:
1) The triggering of a bleeding event during the simulation task.
2) The mapping of the blood flow movies onto a virtual surface that is positioned oriented, morphed, composited and looped into the virtual scene.

2.1 Video capture of anatomical tissue and blood flow "movies"

In vivo and *in vitro* approaches were used to capture video sequences of anatomical tissue and blood flow during TURP. The *in vivo* approach consisted of extracting images from actual TURP procedures performed in the OR. A virtual model of the transurethral passage, the prostate, and the bladder was texture mapped with images captured during a panoramic sweep of the surgical arena from an actual cystoscopic inspection. This approach was similar to the one used in the cholecystectomy simulator previously developed in our lab [6]. When capturing images of blood *in vivo*, we found that unconstrained camera movement and difficulty in distinguishing the blood from the tissue and resecting loop during image processing made the resulting blood flow movies unsuitable. This attempt led us to take an *in vitro* approach to capturing bleeder movies of the lower genitourinary tract as well as providing us with an understanding of the flow patterns to be captured.

The *in vitro* apparatus consisted of a surgical rubber glove bladder with a plastic funnel pelvic support connected to a black rubber tubing urethra sealed with an 10-mm laparoscopic port (see figure 1). Though not anatomically accurate, the relative heights and lengths of the components were calibrated to reproduce physiologic fluid flow properties of an actual TURP. Our specifications were as follows:

1)	Glove height above urethral-tubing:	30 cm
2)	Length of urethral-tubing	60 cm
3)	Diameter of urethral-tubing	10 mm

Blood flow was simulated by injecting red dye mixed with glycerol into the urethral-tubing wall using a 60cc syringe and 18-25 gauge angiocatheters. A Circon/ACMI® 28 French continuous flow resectoscope with xenon light source and a single-chip camera, were used to capture video images of the resulting blood flow under various fluid conditions with a digital video recorder. A 3-liter bag of water was hung 100cm above the urethral tubing and run through the resectoscope to provide inflow irrigation.

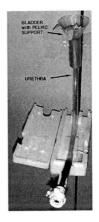

Figure 1. *in vitro* apparatus for capturing blood flow movies

2.2 Image process to separate the blood image from its background

Adobe Photoshop® and Premiere® were used to create opacity maps for the frames of the blood flow movies. The opacity map corresponding to a given source frame is a frame that is white where there is blood foreground and black were there is urethral rubber tubing background. Grey values indicate partially opaque blood. This opacity map is used to composite the blood flow movie into the simulator in a way that renders only the blood and not the rubber tubing.

2.3 Organization of the movies into a parametric database

We have created a library of blood flow movie clips that are categorized based on the following characteristics:
(1) Severity of bleeding
(2) Orientation within anatomy
(3) Level of irrigation inflow
(4) Level of irrigation outflow
Specific bleeding vessels as well as a general "red hazing" of the field were treated as separate but related phenomena Video clips of various degrees of "red haze" were obtained separately.

2.3a Severity*:* After studying the *in vivo* footage, it was determined that the wide spectrum of bleeding vessels encountered during TURP can be broken down into three types of blood flow. To get an intuitive feel of the flow occurring in each of these vessels, we examine the velocity components that play a dominant role. Here we assume that the velocity profile of flow within the urethra has a 3-dimensional parabolic shape. No-slip condition at the wall allows for zero velocity of particles near the resection bed. Along the center of the tube, where inertial forces of the wall are lowest, velocity of particles is highest.

Vector representation of the velocity of blood particles emanating from the resection bed can be resolved into x-, y- and z-components (figure 2). To get an intuitive feel of the flow occurring in each of the "severity" levels, we examined the velocity components that played a dominant role. In a type 1 vessel, referred to as a "trailer", the bleeding was the least severe and the initial motion of the blood particles was dominated by the normal and tangential velocity components. A type 2 vessel, referred to as a "oozer", was of moderate severity and the initial motion of the blood particles was dominated by the axial, normal and tangential velocity components. A type 3 vessel we referred to as a "gusher". It represents the most severe form of bleeding from a vessel or sinus. Here, the initial motion of the blood particles is dominated by axial and normal velocity components (Figure 3). Type 0 bleeding was a bleeder that disappeared with increased irrigant flow. Type 4 bleeding was referred to as "red out".

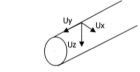

x-component → *tangential velocity* (U_x)
y-component → *axial velocity* (U_y)
z-component → *normal velocity* (U_z)

Figure 2. Vector representation of the velocity of blood particles

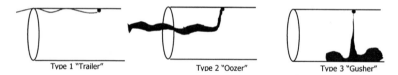

Type 1 "Trailer"   Type 2 "Oozer"   Type 3 "Gusher"

Figure 3-demonstrates 3 types of bleeding observed during actual TURP.

2.3b Orientation: To take into account the effect of the position of blood vessels on bleeding, separate video clips of a given bleeding vessel were shot coming from the roof, the floor, the 2 o'clock and the 4 o'clock orientations. These clips can be mirror-imaged.

2.3c Amount of irrigant inflow: Separate movie clips were taken of a given bleeder under 4 different inflow states which will correlate with the inflow desired by the resectionist. Level 0 corresponds to no inflow ranging up to level 3, which corresponds to high flow inflow irrigation.

2.3d Amount of irrigant outflow: The above clips were taken each with outflow either on or off.

2.4 The triggering of a bleeding event during the simulation task.

During the performance of the simulated resection task, the resection loop collides with the polygonal prostate surface model. This cuts a chip off the prostate leaving a raw newly resected surface (bed). A randomly generated number of bleeding sites (0-4) is attached to the resection bed. The severity of the bleeders is also randomly generated. The probability distributions are based on a predetermined skill level. Application of the resection loop with coagulation current successfully at the bleeder site removes the bleeder. Alternatively, one may resect the bleeder.

2.5 The mapping of the blood flow movie onto a virtual surface that is positioned, oriented, morphed, composited and looped into the virtual scene.

Each of the bleeders described above is rendered as a blood flow movie texture-mapped onto a "bleeder surface". The surface is attached to the bleeder site and oriented perpendicular to the axes of the resection bed. (See figure 4 below) Additionally, the bleeder surface may be morphed to conform to the anatomy of the opposite wall of the urethra. Each successive frame of the blood flow movie is mapped sequentially onto the bleeder surface and may be looped if necessary. As bleeders are allowed to bleed, red haze movies accelerate accordingly by means of a feedback mechanism where the blood discharge is tracked and used to modulate the opacity of the visual field.

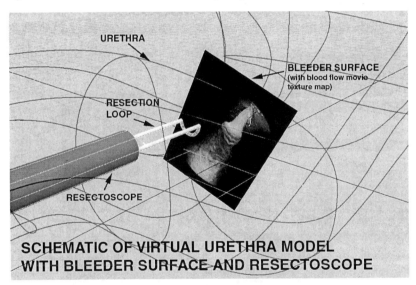

Figure 4.

3.Results

The following images are a result of our approach to representing blood flow.

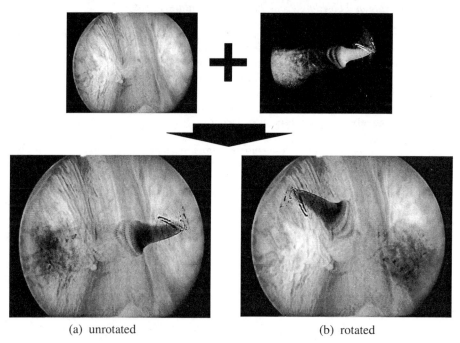

(a) unrotated   (b) rotated

Figure 5. Blood Flow Movie Surface Composited into Virtual Urethra

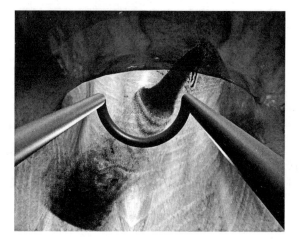

Figure 6. Scene from TURP Simulation with Blood Flow Movie

4. Future Directions

Like Yamaguchi et al [6], we intend to apply computational fluid dynamic models by mapping these blood flow movies onto a surface generated by parallel flow-lines along the genitourinary tract. We will take into account the relative convexity/concavity of the opposite wall of the prostate as resection takes place.

These techniques have cross-procedural potential that can be applied to other endourologic procedures such as laparoscopic nephrectomy, ureteroscopic procedures, cystoscopy/stent placement, percutaneous nephrolithotomy, and other transurethral procedures.

Eventually we hope to generalize our approach to blood flow representation to include non-fluid environments as well. In that case we will need to map a larger library of blood flow movies onto deformable projection surfaces as well as use hydrostatic modeling to visualize the surface of the blood relative to the underlying tissue.

5. Conclusion

By using video footage of simulated bleeding we succeed in effectively representing the diffusive characteristics of blood in a fluid environment without investing on the computational time that would be necessary if a particle-based modeling approach were used. Advances in computer performance and the ability to stream video to texture memory, enabled this image based approach to blood flow representation

References

[1] Ballaro A, et. al. "A computer generated interactive transurethral prostatic resection simulator." *J Urol* 1999 Nov;162(5):1633-5
[2] Basdogan C et. al. "Simulation of tissue cutting and bleeding for laparoscopic surgery using auxiliary surfaces." *Stud Health Technol Inform.* 62:38-44 (1999)
[3] Gomes MP et. al. "A computer-assisted training/monitoring system for TURP structure and design." *IEEE Trans Inf Technol Biomed* 1999 Dec;3(4):242-51
[4] Harreld MR, et. al. "The virtual aneurysm: virtual reality in endovascular therapy." *Proceedings of MMVR Conference.* 13-20 (1996)
[5] Oppenheimer P, et. al. "Laparoscopic Surgical Simulator and Port Placement Study." *Proceedings of MMVR Conference.* 233-35 (2000)
[6] Yamaguchi T, et. al. "Computational visualization of cardiovascular blood flow." *Proceedings of MMVR Conference.* 703-712 (1996)

372

Medicine Meets Virtual Reality 2001
J.D. Westwood et al. (Eds.)
IOS Press, 2001

An Experiment on Fear of Public Speaking in Virtual Reality

D-P. Pertaub[1], M. Slater[1] and C. Barker[2]

Department of Computer Science, University College London, Gower Street,
WC1E 6BT, United Kingdom[1]

Department of Psychology, University College London[2]

Abstract. Can virtual reality exposure therapy be used to treat people with social phobia? To answer this question it is vital to know if people will respond to virtual humans (avatars) in a virtual social setting in the same way they would to real humans. If someone is extremely anxious with real people, will they also be anxious when faced with simulated people, despite knowing that the avatars are computer generated? In [17] we described a small pilot study that placed 10 people before a virtual audience. The purpose was to assess the extent to which social anxiety, specifically fear of public speaking, was induced by the virtual audience and the extent of influence of degree of immersion (head mounted display or desktop monitor. The current paper describes a follow up study conducted with 40 subjects and the results clearly show that not only is social anxiety induced by the audience, but the degree of anxiety experienced is directly related to the type of virtual audience feedback the speaker receives. In particular, a hostile negative audience scenario was found to generate strong affect in speakers, regardless of whether or not they normally suffered from fear of public speaking.

1 Introduction

Social phobia is a prevalent and disabling anxiety disorder [1]. People who suffer from social phobia fear, and if possible avoid, one or more social performance situations. One common example of social phobia is fear of public speaking. This can be particularly difficult for the sufferer as presentation giving is crucial to many responsible jobs and thus fear of public speaking can have a serious impact on an individual's career prospects.

Cognitive-behaviour therapy is the leading psychological treatment for phobias. It typically involves systematic exposure to feared situations ('exposure therapy') and the use of cognitive techniques to help patients identify and challenge anxiety-related negative thoughts. Avoidance behaviour is overcome in the course of the exposure sessions, where patients note that their anxiety attenuates with prolonged exposure to the stimulus, a process known as habituation.

Virtual reality can be used in exposure therapy to substitute an artificially created and controlled stimulus for the real one. An increasing number of case studies and anecdotal reports claim success for treating a wide range of specific phobias, such as fear of heights, fear of flying and fear of spiders [2, 3, 4, 5, 6, 7, 8]. While there have been many published studies of the application of virtual reality to specific phobias, to our knowledge there is only one concerning social phobias [9]. In contrast to that study, which used a virtual lecture theatre with a large audience, we concentrated on a small seminar type setting. Rather than conducting therapy, we were interested in the prior question of whether a speaker's anxiety response depends on the type of feedback received from a virtual audience. If appropriate affect is generated by the experience of speaking to a small group of avatars, it would suggest that virtual reality can be successfully deployed in the treatment of other social phobias. Studying small groups will help us to understand the design parameters for creating successful synthetic social encounters.

Three different virtual audiences were developed (negative, positive and static) and an experiment was conducted to explore whether the type of audience would influence the emotional response of the speaker. Details of the experiment are described in Section 2. A summary of the between-groups results and the written comments as well as a report of the debriefing sessions is given in Section 4. Conclusions are presented in Section 5. A more in-depth description of the experiment and formal statistical results are left to another paper [10].

2 Experiment

2.1 Experiment Design

Forty three subjects were recruited for the experiment, but three sets of results were discarded because of incomplete data. All subjects gave at least two talks to a virtual audience. Audience type was one factor in the experiment. Subjects were randomly assigned to one of three groups, distinguished by the type of virtual audience they spoke to first. Subjects who gave their first talk to either the negative or the positive audience gave their second talk to the other animated audience. Subjects who spoke to the static audience gave their second talk to the static audience again. The second factor was immersion, or the mode of delivery of the virtual environment (full stereo head-mounted display or desktop monitor).

If only the results of the first talk are considered, the design is a between-groups experiment. All the results together can be thought of as a within-groups design.

2.2 Scenario

The virtual audience consisted of a group of eight formally dressed male avatars, seated in a semicircle around a table. In order to foster the illusion of life, the avatars continuously exhibited small twitching movements, blinking and shifting about in their chairs. Two animated audience scenarios were scripted, designed to model the behaviour and reactions of a friendly, appreciative audience and a hostile, unreceptive audience. Facial animations, direction of gaze, body posture and short animations were selected to convey as unambiguous an evaluative message as possible, and the choice of responses was aided by reference to the literature on non-verbal communication [11, 12, 13]. Each audience scenario consisted of a set of ten major audience responses. The distributive properties of the DIVE virtual environment [14] were exploited to allow an unseen operator to listen to the talks and trigger the next response in the sequence at appropriate points in the speech. The operator could also play a selection of audio recordings of audience comments at any time during the talk.

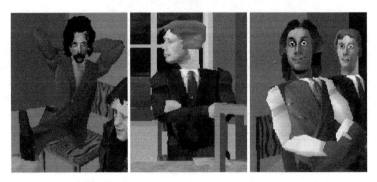

Figure 1. Various postures and facial expressions communicate listener attitudes. From left to right: an audience member puts his feet on the table with arms behind head indicating extreme relation and dominance. Closed upper arm posture communicates disagreement [11] while large smiles and plenty of eye contact suggest interest and an affinity for the speaker [12]. Crossed legs do not consistently convey either positive or negative attitudes to the speaker.

2.3 Method

Subjects were students or members of staff at University College London. Each subject came into the Department of Computer Science twice, with an interval of a couple of days between the visits. On the first occasion, subjects completed the Personal Report of Confidence as a Speaker (PRCS) [15] and the Fear of Negative Evaluation [16] questionnaires. The PRCS provides a measure of general public speaking anxiety. Subjects were instructed to prepare a five minute talk for presentation at the next visit. They were told they would give the same presentation twice, to a computer generated virtual audience. They were informed that the talk might be recorded for later analysis. No details of the workings of the system were provided.

On the day of the talks, subjects using the head mounted display stood in an empty darkened room while giving their talk. Subjects using the 21 inch desktop monitor sat alone in the same darkened room. All subjects were fitted with a microphone and head-phones. A concealed operator sat at a remote terminal and played a pre-recorded invitation to begin speaking. At appropriate intervals, the operator triggered the next in a pre-determined sequence of ten animated audience responses. In the case of the static audience, the operator simply monitored the talk. A warning was played 30 seconds from the end and an audio clip told the speaker to stop after 5 minutes. At the end of each talk, subjects were taken to a different room and asked to complete questionnaires asking them about the experience.

All subjects gave at least two talks. Subjects who gave their second talk to the negative audience were asked to give a short third talk, this time to the positive audience again. For ethical reasons we wanted the last experience to be a pleasant one. No data was collected for this talk.

3 Variables

There were three main response variables, two designed to assess the degree of self-reported anxiety generated by the experience of giving the talk and another to measure the speaker's assessment of their performance. The first was a modified form of the Personal Report of Confidence of a Public Speaker (MPRCS), altered to refer to the talk just given. A checklist of 9 anxiety symptoms (sweating, discomfort in stomach, heart palpitations, tremors, nerves/feelings of being scared, tightness in chest, tenseness, loss of balance, tenseness) provided a second response variable (Somatic). The third variable (self-rating) was the subject's own assessment of their performance, rated on a scale from 0 to 100 where 0 indicated complete dissatisfaction and 100 indicated complete satisfaction with their talk.

4 Results

4.1 Statistical Results

The results from the between groups design are discussed in depth in [10]. A short summary for each of the main response variables of the main findings follows.

Modified PRCS. The MPRCS is a measure of the anxiety experienced by the subject when speaking to the virtual audience. A logistic regression analysis was performed on the data for post-talk MPRCS. The best fitting regression model found included the two main factors (immersion, audience type) and positive correlation between the PRCS measured prior to all talks and MPRCS, measured after the talk. The group that spoke to the negative audience had a significantly higher MPRCS than the other groups (positive or static audiences). Interestingly, the slope of the regression line of MRPCS on prior PRCS was significantly different between the audience types. For the positive and static audiences there was a positive slope, but for the negative audience the slope was not significantly different from 0. This means that the prior PRCS cannot predict the post PRCS when the audience faced by the subject was negative.

Somatic and Self-Rating. For the response variable Somatic, a logistic regression analysis found only audience type and prior PRCS to be significant. The negative audience group exhibited by far the highest level of somatic response, while the positive and static audience groups had lower response levels with no significant difference between them. A normal regression model was performed on self-rating and both prior PRCS and audience type were significant. There was no significant difference between positive and negative audience results for self rating. Self rating would appear to be lower if the audience is animated.

4.2 Debriefing session and written reports

After each talk, subjects were asked to write down any comments about the talk they had just given, and were prompted to mention the best and worst aspects of the speech. At the end of the experiment, subjects were invited to expand upon these comments and draw comparisons between the different audience conditions they had experienced. These debriefing sessions afforded us an opportunity to obtain a deeper and richer picture of the sessions than was possible with the written questionnaire entries.

It was clear from the outset that almost all subjects were treating the experiment as a serious opportunity to give a talk. Their assumption was that their role was to try and win the audience over, a plan that seemed reasonable despite the fact they were facing a virtual audience.

4.2.1 Animated audience group comments

For the most part, the affect generated was appropriate to the type of audience response, but there were clearly some idiosyncratic reactions amongst the subjects. All subjects speaking to an animated audience were successfully able to decode the valence of the audience response. Due to the stereotyped nature of some of the responses, several subjects (7) reported a sense of amusement when the audience reacted, although a number of these subjects admitted that the amusement was paired with feelings of tension and nervousness.

Twelve subjects reported that although they knew the audiences were not real, the experiences felt like giving a real presentation in many significant respects. Similarities included heightened anxiety just before the talks, emotional reactions to the audience while speaking and the use of presentation strategies to attempt to connect with the audience. Subjects made the following comments:

'You get involved in a situation, it doesn't matter whether it's real or not. I needed to try to convince them.'

'The emotions were similar. Before I gave the talk I felt exactly as I would feel in the department. I had cold hands and I was sweating!'

'It felt a lot like a presentation, like the ones that I give in the department. I approached it in the same way as a real presentation. I jotted down notes the night before..'.

The negative audience was capable of generating very strong speaker emotions, regardless of whether it was encountered at the first talk or at the second. Subjects repeatedly reported they could find no way to 'bring back' the audience when the avatar listeners lost interest. Some subjects interpreted their incapacity to influence the audience as a failure on their part as a speaker. Many reported feelings of confusion or disorientation and a tendency to forget what they wanted to say. Six subjects described the experience as very disturbing or disconcerting. Five subjects commented they would have walked out of the room if they had received a response like that from a real audience. One subject mentioned that it was immensely satisfying to be able to survive the audience. Another confided that the thought 'My talk is boring' kept reverberating inside his head. Other subjects commented:

'It felt really bad. I couldn't just ignore them. I had to talk to them and tell them to sit up and pay attention. Especially the man on the left who put his head in his hands; I had to ask him to sit up and listen.... I entered a negative feedback loop where I would receive bad responses from the audience and my performance would get even worse.... I was performing really badly and that doesn't normally happen.'

'I was upset, really thrown. I totally lost my train of thought. They weren't looking at me and I didn't know what to do. Should I start again? I was very frustrated. I felt I had no connection to them. They weren't looking at me. I just forgot what I was talking about.'

'The first audience was terrible. They were really disturbing. From the beginning they were uninterested and it really put you off..... I couldn't say everything I wanted to say.'

The pattern of subject response to the positive audience scenario was much less homogenous. Some subjects clearly took heart from the enthusiastic response of their listeners. One subject recalled *'It was clear that one audience was really positive and interested in what I was saying and it made you feel like telling them what you know.'* Another noted *'I felt great. Finally nobody was interrupting me. Being a woman, people keep interrupting you in talks much more... But here I felt people were there to listen to me.'* One commented *'They were staring at me. They loved you unconditionally, you could say anything, you didn't have to work'.* However nine subjects felt that the positive audience responses were very exaggerated and became off-putting and distracting. Two commented that it lacked the challenge and the audience 'buzz' of the negative scenario.

Ten people explicitly claimed that the negative audience was the more realistic of the two. One subject summed up this view when she said *'I found the first* (positive) *audience fairly unconvincing; they all sat up straight and stared at me with these moronic grins and made comments like 'wonderful' at inappropriate moments'.* Six subjects stressed that the timing of audience responses seemed to be a determining factor. One explained that it was very off-putting to be congratulated when they began to make an important point, rather than after it.

4.2.2 Static audience group comments

All subjects speaking to the static audience commented on how stiff and unresponsive the audience was. This was especially the case with the desktop condition, where subjects talked to what was effectively a static image of an audience. One subject reported that *'it was more like talking to a mirror than to a real audience. There was no sense of satisfaction because there was no feedback, I didn't know if they liked it or not... It felt like a real practice presentation. I tend to practice speaking to a wall. This was slightly more real'.* Subjects also had a tendency to be more critical of the appearance of the avatars; the subject's written responses for the static audience were full of suggestions on how the look of the computer characters could be improved. Most subjects felt that their second talk was better than the first, perhaps unsurprising as they were giving the same talk twice to the same static audience.

4.2.3 Discussion

Both the statistical results and the debriefing sessions clearly show the anxiety provoking effect of the negative audience scenario. An intriguing result is the claim that the negative audience was more realistic than the positive one. Both audiences featured exaggerated reactions and were subject to the same delays in triggering responses. But in real seminar settings, encouraging comments and gestures tend to occur at very specific points during a talk - the end of phrases, units of information or other characteristic segments of speech. Very short response intervals govern these feedback mechanisms. The negative audience did not listen and did not have to obey these conversation facilitating conventions. It was realistic but at the same time unusual: In many societies, there tend to be few genuine overt displays of negative evaluation in social exchanges between adults [12]. That might account for part of the reason why the negative audience was found quite so disturbing.

5 Conclusions

These results confirm the results of our initial pilot study [16]. People responded to virtual seminar audiences much as they would respond to real audiences; they felt more at ease with a positive group of listeners and experienced considerable discomfort with an unpleasant, unforgiving audience. With the animated audience scenarios, and with the negative audience scenario in particular, there was sufficient co-presence to elicit strong affect in virtual speakers. Our findings indicate that virtual reality scenarios with computer generated characters could be of use in treating and investigating a range of social performance situations, but that the appropriate timing of avatar responses is critical to maintaining co-presence.

References

[1]   Kessler, R.C., McGonagle, K.A., Zhao, S., Nelson, C.B., Hughes, M., Eshleman, S., Wittchen, H.-U., and Kendler, K.S. (1994) Lifetime and 12-month prevalence of DSM-III-R Psychiatric Disorders in the United States, Archives of General Psychiatry, 51, 8-19.

[2]   Botella, C., Banos, R. M., Perpina, C., Villa, H., Alcaniz, M., Rey, A. (1998) Virtual Reality Treatment of Claustrophobia. Behaviour Research and Therapy 36(2):239-246, February 1998.

[3]   Carlin, A., Hoffman, H. G., Weghorst, S., (1997) Virtual reality and tactile augmentation in the treatment of spider phobia: a case report. Behaviour Research and Therapy 35, 153-158.

[4]   North, M. M., North S. M., Coble, J.R., (1998) Virtual Reality Therapy: An effective treatment for phobias, Virtual Environments in Clinical Psychology and Neuroscience, Studies in Health Technology and Informatics, Volume 58.

[5]   Rothbaum, B. O., Hodges, L. F., Kooper, R., Opdyke, D., Williford, J., North, M. M., (1995a) Effectiveness of Computer-Generated (Virtual Reality) Graded Exposure in the Treatment of Acrophobia. American Journal of Psychiatry, 152, 626-628.

[6]   Rothbaum, B. O., Hodges, L. F., Kooper, R., Opdyke, D., Williford, J., (1995b). Virtual reality graded exposure in the treatment of acrophobia: a case study. Behaviour Therapy. 26, 547-554.

[7]   Rothbaum, B. O., Hodges, L. F., Watson, B. A., Kessler, G. S., Opdyke, D. (1996) Virtual reality exposure therapy in the treatment of fear of flying: a case report. Behaviour Research and Therapy. 34, 477-481.

[8]   Strickland, D., Hodges, L., North, M., Weghorst, S., (1997) Overcoming Phobias by Virtual Exposure, Communications of the ACM, volume 40, p 34-40.

[9]   North, M. M., North S. M., Coble, J.R., (1998) Virtual Reality Therapy: An effective treatment for the fear of public speaking. International Journal of Virtual Reality Vol.3 No.2, 2-6.

[10]   Pertaub, D-P., Slater, M., Barker, C., (2000) An experiment on public speaking anxiety in response to three difference types of virtual audience.

[11]   Bull, P. (1987), Posture and Gesture, Oxford, Pergamon.

[12]   Argyle, M. (1988) Bodily Communication, Methuen & Co Ltd .

[13]   Mehrabian, A., (1968) Relationship of attitude to seated posture, orientation and distance. Journal of Consulting and Clinical Psychology 32:296-308.

[14]   Frecon, E. and Stenius, M. (1998) DIVE: A scaleable network architecture for distributed virtual environments, Distributed Systems Engineering Journal, 5(3), 91-100.

[15]   Paul, G. (1966) Insight vs. desensitization in psychotherapy. Stanford University Press.

[16]   Watson, D., Friend, R., (1969) Measurement of social-evaluative anxiety (FNE), Journal of Consulting and Clinical Psychology 33 448-457.

[17]   Slater, M., Pertaub, D-P., and A.Steed (1999) Public Speaking in Virtual Reality: Facing and Audience of Avatars, IEEE Computer Graphics and Applications, 19(2), March/April 1999, p6-9.

Medicine Meets Virtual Reality 2001
J.D. Westwood et al. (Eds.)
IOS Press, 2001

Exploring the Visible Human's Inner Organs with the VOXEL-MAN 3D Navigator

B. Pflesser[1], A. Petersik[1], A. Pommert[1], M. Riemer[1], R. Schubert[1], U. Tiede[1],
K. H. Höhne[1],
U. Schumacher[2], E. Richter[3]
[1]Institute of Mathematics and Computer Science in Medicine,
[2]Institute of Anatomy, [3]Dept. of Pediatric Radiology
University Hospital Eppendorf, Hamburg, Germany

Abstract. Improved rendering and segmentation techniques lead to a new quality of 3D reconstructions of the Visible Human. Using these we have implemented an interactive atlas of anatomy and radiology of the inner organs.

1. Introduction

Computer-based 3D models of the human body reported to date suffer from poor spatial resolution. The Visible Human project [1-3] has delivered high resolution cross-sectional images that are suited for generation of high-quality models. Yet none of the 3D models described to date reflect the quality of the original images. This is due to the fact that, for the majority of anatomical objects contained in the data, the cross-sectional images could not be converted into a set of coherent realistic surfaces. If, however, we succeed in converting all the detail into a 3D model, we gain an unsurpassed representation of human structure that opens new possibilities for learning anatomy and simulating interventions or radiological examinations. Using improved techniques for segmenting and modeling the 3D anatomy of the Visible Human data we achieve a nearly photorealistic computer based model. As a first application we have implemented an interactive 3D-Atlas of the anatomy and radiology of the inner organs.

2. Material and Methods

2.1. Data

Photographic cross-sectional images from the male Visible Human were used to create models of the head, neck, and torso as well as the corresponding inner organs. The original data set consists of 1871 photographic cross-sections with a slice distance of 1 mm. The cross-sections themselves have a spatial resolution of 1/3 mm. For the model of the inner organs, the resolution was reduced to 1mm for reasons of data storage and computing capacity. From 1049 such slices, an image volume of 573x330x1049 volume elements ("voxels") of 1 mm^3 was composed, where each voxel is represented by a set of red, green and blue intensities ("RGB-tuple"). The Visible Human data set also includes two sets of computer tomographic images of 1mm slice distance, one taken from the fresh, the other (like the photographic one) from the frozen cadaver. Both were transformed into an image volume congruent with the photographic one.

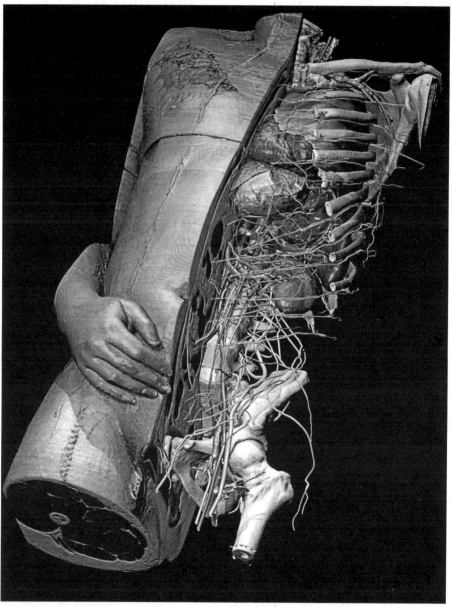

Fig. 1. High resolution 3D model derived from the Visible Human data set. The major organs were reconstructed from the cryosections thus exhibiting the original organ texture. Small vessels and nerves were implanted as artificial structures based on landmarks present in the image data

2.2. Segmentation

The image volume thus created was segmented with an interactive tool, which is an extension of an earlier development for RGB data [5]. It can be regarded as an "electronic sculpturing tool". On a cross-section, an expert "paints" a typical region of the organ under consideration. All voxels in the volume with similar RGB-tuples are then collected by the program to form a "mask". This mask usually needs to be refined by repeating this procedure in order to include the target organ completely. The resulting cluster in RGB space has an ellipsoid shape, due to the slight correlation of the colors; this cluster is then converted into the mathematical form of an ellipsoid, which facilitates subsequent computations. There are, of course, other regions with the same characterization present in the volume. If they are not connected to the target organ, it can be isolated easily; if not, 3D interactive cutting tools are used.

2.3. Graphic modeling

There are many anatomical constituents, such as nerves and small vessels, which are too small to be segmented adequately, but need to be included in a comprehensive anatomical model. For these, we have developed a modeling tool that allows us to include tube-like structures into the model. Ball-shaped markers of variable diameter are imposed by an expert onto the landmarks still visible on the cross-sections or on the 3D image; these markers are automatically connected to form tubes of varying diameter. Unlike the segmented objects, which are represented as sets of voxels, the modeled structures are represented as composed of small triangles.

2.4. Knowledge modeling

Each voxel of the thus generated *three-dimensional* objects is connected to a knowledge base containing object descriptions within the structure of a semantic network [4,6,7]. Different networks were created for the different views of systemic or topographic anatomy of the inner organs. Within the views, the anatomical constituents are linked by relations like *part of, has part, branching from* or *branching to*.

2.5. Visualization

The 3D visualization algorithm we have developed is characterized by the fact that it renders *surfaces* from *volume* data. This is different from the volume rendering typically used for visualizing the Visible Human data set. As in volume rendering, the program casts rays from an image plane onto the image volume in viewing direction. However, the rays stop at the first encountered object. Surface texture and surface inclination (important for proper computation of light reflection) are calculated from the RGB-tuples at the segmented border line. The decisive quality improvement is achieved by determining the object surfaces with a spatial resolution higher than the resolution of the original voxels. While such subvoxel resolution may be achieved easily by sampling with high rates in volume rendering, the determination of distinct adjacent *surfaces* in subvoxel resolution is a major problem that has been solved only recently [8]. This makes the high resolution visualization of distinct surfaces possible, which is the characteristic feature of our approach.

The objects modeled with the surface modeler are visualized with standard computer graphics methods within the context of the volume objects. The visualization program, an extended version of the VOXEL-MAN system [4], runs on UNIX workstations.

2.6.   Implementation

Because of the high resolution and the sophisticated algorithms, the computation of a single image may take several minutes, even on a high end workstation. The model is therefore being made available for interaction and exploration via precomputed "Intelligent QuickTime VR (QTVR) Movies" [9] called "scenes". In contrast to standard QTVR movies they contain label tracks pointing to the knowledge base. The Navigator viewing software based on this technique runs on high end personal computers.

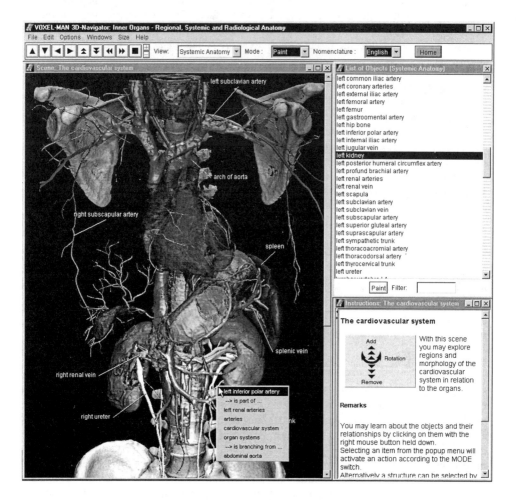

Fig. 2. User interface of the VOXEL-MAN 3D-Navigator. The user may rotate the scene and add/remove objects. He may interrogate by highlight organs by clicking on them in the scene or on their name in the List of Objects.

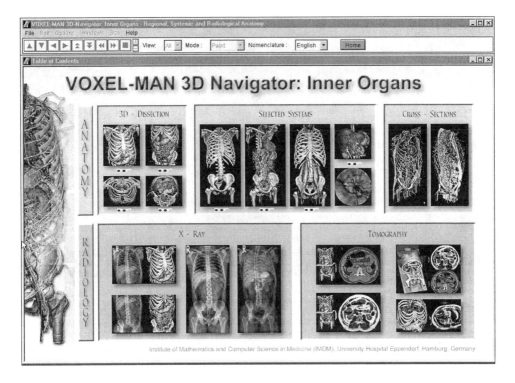

Fig. 3. Table of contents of the VOXEL-MAN 3D-Navigator: Inner Organs. The scenes may be selected by clicking on the icons.

2.7. Results

The VOXEL-MAN 3D-Navigator [10,11] contains about 650 three-dimensional anatomical objects, mostly of the thorax and the abdomen, including the nervous and the cardiovascular systems.

The material is organized as a set of 19 interactively explorable scenes (Fig. 3), each of which shows a special aspect of anatomy. The user's range of options includes inspection of anatomy from all directions, unveiling interior structures, and interrogation of objects (Fig. 2). Several of the scenes are additionally available in stereoscopic (red/green) format. The anatomical nomenclature is available in Latin, English, and German.

A special feature of the model involves the possibility of simulating radiological examinations (Fig. 4). Since the absorption values for every voxel are available in the original tomographic data, artificial X-ray images from any direction can be computed. Based on the information of the model, both the contributing anatomical structures and the extent of their contribution to the final absorption can be calculated. Similarly, the information present in cross-sectional radiological images (Computer Tomography, Magnetic Resonance Imaging, Ultrasound) can be clarified by presenting them in the corresponding 3D context. The integrated knowledge base allows the interrogation of the model from the viewpoints of regional and systemic anatomy as well as concerning the relation to the peritoneal cavity.

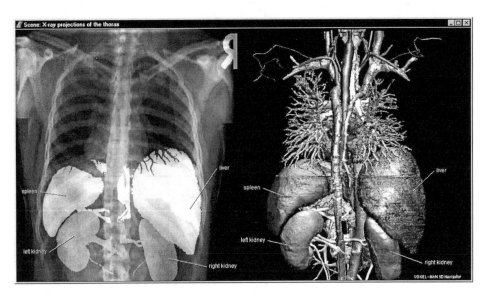

Fig. 4. Simulated X-rays. The X-ray manifestation of organs may be viewed parallel to the 3D-view.

3. Conclusions

We have implemented an interactive atlas of anatomy and radiology of the inner organs built from the Visible human data. With improved rendering and segmentation techniques we achieved a new quality of 3D reconstructions The presentation of these reconstructions in precomputed "Intelligent Quicktime VR Movies" with the Navigator viewing software leads, together with the integrated knowledge to a "self-explaining virtual body". Ist use as an interactive atlas of anatomy and radiology is only one of many possible applications.

4. References

1. V. Spitzer, M. J. Ackerman, A. L. Scherzinger, D. Whitlock, The visible human male: a technical report, J-Am-Med-Inform-Assoc 3(2) (1996) 118-130.
2. M. J. Ackerman, The Visible Human Project: a resource for anatomical visualization, Medinfo. 9 Pt 2 (1998) 1030-1032.
3. V. Spitzer, D. Whitlock, The Visible Human Data Set: the anatomical platform for human simulation. Anat-Rec. 253(2) (1998) 49-57.
4. K. H. Höhne, B. Pflesser, A. Pommert, M. Riemer, T. Schiemann, R. Schubert, U. Tiede, A new representation of knowledge concerning human anatomy and function,. Nature Med. 1(6) (1995) 506-511.
5. T. Schiemann, U. Tiede, K. H. Höhne, Segmentation of the Visible Human for high quality volume based visualization. *Med. Image Anal.* 1997; **1**(4):263-271.
6. R. Schubert, K. H. Höhne, A. Pommert, M. Riemer, T. Schiemann, U. Tiede, Spatial knowledge representation for visualization of human anatomy and function. In: H. H. Barrett, A. F.Gmitro, (eds.), IPMI 93. Proceedings of the 13th Conference on Information Processing in Medical Imaging; Springer-Verlag, Berlin Heidelberg 1993. Lecture Notes in Computer Science 687, pp. 168-181.
7. A. Pommert, R. Schubert, M. Riemer, T. Schiemann, U. Tiede, K. H. Höhne, Symbolic modeling of human anatomy for visualization and simulation. In: R. Robb (ed.), VBC

94. Proceedings of the Conference on Visualization in Biomedical Computing; SPIE Proceedings 2359. , 1991, pp. 412-423.

8. U. Tiede, T. Schiemann, K. H. Höhne. High quality rendering of attributed volume data. In: Ebert D, et al. (eds.), Vis 98. Proceedings of the Conference IEEE Visualization IEEE Computer Society Press; 1998. pp. 255-262.

9. R. Schubert, B. Pflesser, A. Pommert, K. Priesmeyer, M. Riemer, T. Schiemann, et al., Interactive volume visualization using "intelligent movies". In: J. D. Westwood et al. (eds.), MMVR 99. Proceedings of the Conference Medicine Meets Virtual Reality; IOS Press, Amsterdam, 1999. Studies in Health Technology and Informatics 62. pp. 321-327.

10. K. H. Höhne, B. Pflesser, A. Pommert, K. Priesmeyer, M. Riemer, T. Schiemann, R. Schubert, U. Tiede, H.-C. Frederking, S. Gehrmann, S. Noster, U. Schumacher, VOXEL-MAN 3D-Navigator: Inner Organs. Regional, Systemic and Radiological Anatomy, Springer-Verlag Electronic Media, Heidelberg, 2000. (3 CD-ROMs, ISBN 3-540-14759-4).

11. http://www.uke.uni-hamburg.de/navigator

5. Acknowledgements

We thank Victor Spitzer and David Whitlock (University of Colorado) and the National Library of Medicine for providing the Visible Human data set. We are also grateful to Jan Freudenberg, Sebastian Gehrmann, and Stefan Noster for substantially contributing to the segmentation work. The knowledge modeling work was supported by the German Research Council (DFG) grant # Ho 899/4-1.

Medicine Meets Virtual Reality 2001
J.D. Westwood et al. (Eds.)
IOS Press, 2001

Virtual Reality as an assessment tool

for arm motor deficits after brain

lesions

Lamberto PIRON*, Federica CENNI§, Paolo TONIN§ and Mauro DAM*

*Department of Neurology and Psychiatry University of Padova, via Giustiniani

5, 35100 Padova,§ Department of Neurorehabilitation San Camillo Hospital,

via Alberoni 70, 30011 Lido di Venezia, Italy

Abstract

The currently used assessment techniques for measuring neurological deficits are time consuming and may lack of sensibility and repeatability. Previous studies suggested that the cinematic analysis of the movement, might represent a reliable alternative instrument for documenting the degree of motor impairment. To verify this hypothesis we investigated motor/functional progress in 20 post-stroke patients, undergoing rehabilitation therapy, by means of a widely used clinical test (Fugl-Meyer scale), and by evaluating kinematics of arm motion. After rehabilitation therapy, velocity and duration of reaching movements significantly improved with respect to baseline values. Before and after rehabilitation there was a significant correlation between each cinematic parameter and the clinical scale scores. These results, suggests that the cinematic analysis of movement can be proposed as a precise and objective assessment tool to be used in clinical practice.

1. Introduction

Motor deficits and motor recovery after brain lesions are usually ascertained by rating scales. However, clinical measures should be very simple in order to avoid unacceptable inter observers variability, as a consequence they lack of sensitivity. The relevance of using more accurate and reliable methods is suggested by the findings of Whishaw et al in lesioned rats [1]. They demonstrated that animals utilized different motor strategies to complete a reaching task, depending on the extent and site of the lesion. These differences were not evident by observing rat's behavior but only by studying the detailed kinematics of limb movements. Although promising, the cinematic analysis of movement has been scarcely applied to patients with brain injuries, and its clinical suitability is far to be demonstrated [2]. The present investigation was undertaken in the attempt to verify if cinematic measures can be useful for quantifying motor deficits and for documenting motor recovery in patient with ischemic brain lesions [3, 4]. To this aim we have used a Virtual Reality (VR) based system.

2. Methods

We selected 20 subacute post-stroke patients, with mild to intermediate motor impairment of the arm, i.e. subscore of the Fugl-Meyer scale for the upper extremity (Fugl-Meyer UE) ranging from 30 to 60 [4]. There were 13 males and 7 females, mean age 55.7 ± 8.2. The ischemic lesion was localized in the territory of the right (12 cases) and left (8 cases) middle cerebra artery. The time interval between the vascular accident and the entry into the study was 8,2 ± 5.6 months. No patient had clinical evidence of cognitive impairments or of language disturbances interfering with verbal comprehension.

Patients underwent a four weeks rehabilitation program consisting of one hour of conventional rehabilitation therapy daily, five days per week.

Before and after therapy, the degree of motor impairment was evaluated with the Fugl-Meyer UE scale [5].

At entry into the study and at discharge, mean duration (sec), mean velocity (cm/sec), and the morphology of trajectories of 20 consecutive reaching movement were determined by means of a VR based system. This apparatus consisted of a PC workstation (Pentium II 350 MHz processor, with 128 MB of RAM, a 32MB video card and graphics accelerator), a high resolution LCD projector (1200 Ansi-Lumen), a 3D motion tracking system (Polhemus 3Space Fastrack, Vermont, U.S.A.), and a dedicated software for processing and representing the motor tasks and arm position data (Kinematix Expert learning System for rehabilitation, Kinematix. Inc. Massachusetts, U.S.A.). The movement recording system consisted of a magnetic receiver positioned on the object handled by the subject with the compromised arm. This sensor measured continuously the motion of the hand in the workspace. The static accuracy of the position signal was 0.76 mm RMS and 0.15 degrees RMS for orientation. Resolution is 0.0005 cms/cm. Latency was 4 msec unfiltered from the center of receiver measurement period to beginning of transfer from output port. The sampling rate was 120 Hz.

Patients performed a sequence of reaching task, i.e. moving an envelope from a homing position to a mailbox slot. The subjects were seated in front of the wall screen grasping the envelope where the magnetic receiver was positioned. The software created the virtual environment consisting of a handling (envelope) and a target (mailbox) object. Virtual handling object matched the real object held by the subject. The subject moved the real envelope, and observed on the screen the trajectory of the corresponding virtual object toward the virtual mailbox (Fig. 1). Once the required task was adequately completed, the system provided a rewarding signal.

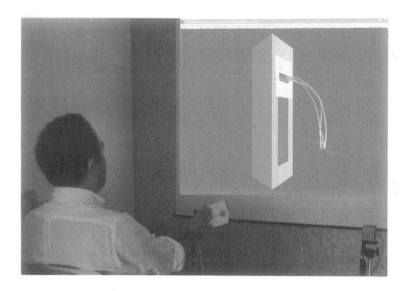

Fig.1

The Wilcoxon test was used to determine the statistical significance of the differences in the mean duration and velocity of reaching movements, before and after the therapy.

Correlation analysis (Spearman's was used to assess the relationship between duration or velocities and Fugl-Meyer UE scores, before and after therapy.

Statistical significance was considered at $p \leq 0.05$.

3. Results

None of the twenty patients reported side effects due to the interaction with the virtual environment. At discharge, mean duration and mean velocity of the reaching movements, performed with the affected arm, significantly changed. with respect to the values recorded at entry into the study (Fig. 2 A, B).

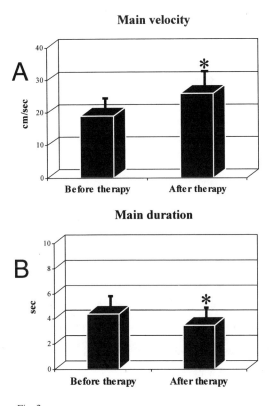

Fig. 2

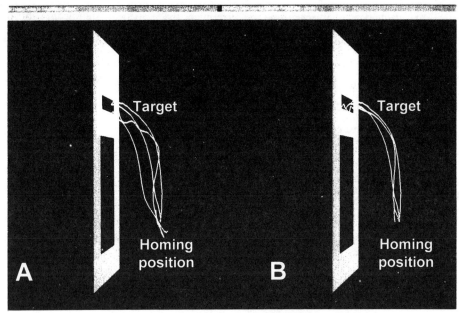

Fig. 3: **A** trajectories before therapy, **B** trajectories after therapy.

Mean duration and mean velocity improved from 4.4 ± 1.6 sec to 3.5 ± 1.7 sec, and from 19.6 ± 15 cm/sec to 26.3 ± 20 cm/sec, respectively.

Movement duration and velocities were significantly related to Fugl-Meyer UE scores before (ρ = -0.97, p < 0.01; ρ = 0.95, p < 0.01) and after VET therapy (ρ = -0.82, p < 0.01; ρ = 0.82, p < 0.01). Morphologic modifications of the reaching movements paralleled the improvements in velocity and duration in response to rehabilitation. Representative trajectories from a post-stroke a patient before and after therapy are shown in Fig. 3. Trajectories irregular and dispersed at entry into the study became straight and coherent at discharge.

4. Discussion

In this investigation, we have evaluated the clinical value of kinematics for characterizing upper arm motor impairments in post-stroke patients. We have studied the morphological features, velocity, duration of reaching movements performed with the compromised arm by means of a VR based system.

No patient complained of any discomfort caused by the interaction with the "non immersive virtual world" and easily familiarized with the experimental procedure. We observed that the mean duration and mean velocity of the reaching movements ameliorated in response to physical therapy; arm trajectories reassumed the prototypic appearance of those executed in absence of brain lesions. These results are consistent with previous observations showing that improvements of the cinematic characteristics of reaching or drawing circle tasks paralleled motor recovery in post stroke patients [6]. In this study we have also found that there was a significant correlation between mean duration and mean velocity of movements and the Fugl-Meyer UE scale scores. These results may suggest that the clinical evaluation scale and the cinematic analysis of movement may provide very similar information. However the latter method represents a quicker and more objective measure of motor system deficit than the former.

Several apparatus have been employed to measure kinematics or other movement characteristics in animal as well as in humans, including videotape recording and robotic devices [7]. However VR based systems may offer some potential advantages compared to the above methods. In fact, by modifying the complexity of the virtual scenarios and/or of the experimental setup, one may set a variety of reproducible tasks aimed to evaluate specific motor abilities [2]. For instance, patient's capacity to perform pronation/supination movements can be investigated by changing the position of the target (i.e., the orientation of mailbox slot, in our experimental setup). The characteristics of whole upper extremity motion can be derived by using magnetic receivers positioned on different part of the arm. All these data may be useful for setting rehabilitation exercises shaped to individual needs.

In conclusion the present study demonstrated that simple cinematic features of reaching movement a can be used for measuring the degree of motor impairment and of motor learning in post-stroke patients. In prospective, VR-based systems may provide detailed information about patient's motor system deficits that may be exploited in rehabilitation therapy.

References

1.   Whisaw IQ, Gorny B, Sarna J. Paw and limb use in skilled and spontaneous reaching after pyramidal tract, red nucleus and combined lesions in the rat: behavioral and

anatomical dissociations. Behav Brain Res 1998;93:167-183

2. Nudo RJ. Recovery after damage to motor cortical areas. Curr Opin Neurobiol 1999;9:740-747

3. Rose FD, Attree EA, Johnson DA. Virtual reality: an assistive technology in neurological rehabilitation. Curr Opin Neurol 1996:9:461-467

4. Wilson PN, Foreman N, Stanton D. Virtual reality, disability and rehabilitation. Disability and Rehabilitation 1997;19:213-220

5. Fugl-Meyer AR, Jaasko L, Leyman L, Olson S et al. The post-stroke hemiplegic patient. 1. A method for evaluation of physical performance. Scand J Rehab Med 1975;7:13-31

6. Holden M, Todorov E, Callahan J, Bizzi E. Virtual Environment training improves motor performance in two patients with stroke: case report. Neurology1999;23:57-67

7. Volpe BT, Krebs HI, Hogan N, Edelstein OTR et al. A novel approach to stroke rehabilitation: robot-aided sensorimotor stimulation. Neurology 2000;54:1938-1944

Medicine Meets Virtual Reality 2001
J.D. Westwood et al. (Eds.)
IOS Press, 2001

Multislice CT and Computational Fluid Dynamics: A new technique to visualize, analyze and simulate hemodynamics in aortic aneurysms and stentgrafts

D. Pless, D. T. Boll, J. Goerich, Th. R. Fleiter, R. Scharrer-Pamler, H.-J. Brambs

University of Ulm
Department of Diagnostic Imaging
Steinhoevelstrasse 9
89075 Ulm
Germany
+49(0)731/502-74 31
+49(0)731/502-66 92
daniela.pless@medizin.uni-ulm.de

The interest of this study is on analysing blood flow phenomena like velocity, pressure and wall shear stress in the aorta before and after treatment of abdominal aortic aneurysm by placement of an endovascular stentgraft to get a better estimation of risk of rupture of the aneurysm and to optimise the shape of the stentgrafts.

The blood flow simulation is based on Finite Element Method (FEM). After segmentation of geometry of the aorta from CT scans a three dimensional mesh is generated. Then blood flow is simulated by means of the Computational Fluid Dynamics Software (CFD).

1. Background/Problem

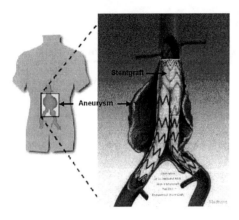

Figure 1. Abdominal Aortic Aneurysm (left) and endovascular stentgraft which prevents the aneurysm from further extension (right).

Abdominal Aortic Aneurysm, which is a focal enlargement of the abdominal aorta occurs among approximately 2% of the elderly population (fig. 1). The patho-physiology is only partially understood and most of the aneurysms are discovered incidentally during conventional abdominal ultrasound examinations because usually it do not cause any symptoms. The primary complication of abdominal aortic aneurysm is acute rupture, a frequently lethal event despite emergent surgical intervention. The technique of endovascular repair is a new catheter-based minimally invasive technique in which a prosthetic graft is introduced into the aortic lumen via the common femoral artery. In spite of quite good results there are still some drawbacks as migration or dislocation of the stentgraft as well as leakage and thrombosis. This new technique should help to understand the causes of these complications and to enable an individually optimised stent design for any patient to provide most adequate blood supply of the legs.

2. Methods & Tools

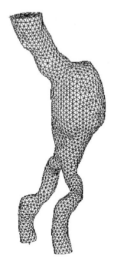

Figure 2.
Geometry of an abdominal aneurysm covered with a triangulated surface mesh.

The technique combines Multislice CT and flow simulation to visualize individual flow- and pressure-changes within aortic aneurysms and stentgrafts. The geometry of the aneurysm and the stentgraft, respectively is created out of a CT scan of the descending aorta including bifurcation. Therefore a segmentation soft-ware, which allows to separate the aorta from surrounding tissue is applied. After geometry creation an unstructured volume mesh consisting of about 100 000 cells is generated (fig. 2). The division of the volume into sub elements is needed for an adequate accuracy in flow calculation. Furthermore it is necessary to simplify the highly complex physiological process of blood flow without neglecting its most decisive characteristics to obtain a reliable and reproducible simulation. The steady and pulsatile simulations are carried out under consideration of Navier-Stokes equation. The aorta can be regarded as a tube with a diameter of 20-30 mm. Blood is treated as a newtonian fluid with laminar flow. For pulsatile flow a time dependent flow is generated by time shifted pressure profiles. Gravity is activated to approximate blood flow in upright position of patient.

3. Results

A reliable method for analysing individual changes of blood flow caused by aortic stentgrafts has been developed. The calculation enables visualization of velocity, turbulence, pressure and wall shear stress in a colorcoded three dimensional and animated way.

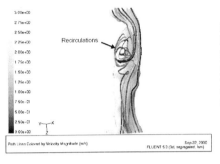

Figure 3.
Display of blood flow through an aneurysm as path lines colorcoded by velocity. The lighter the color of the path lines the higher the velocity.
In the aneurysm velocity is decreased and recirculations occur. The turbulences are the more distinctive the more the aneurysm shows sacciform shape.

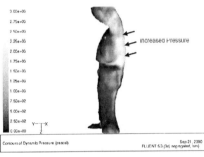

Figure 4.
Display of dynamic pressure to the wall of the aneurysm. At the back of the aneurysm sac an area of high pressure (arrows) is indicated. This correlates to the zone an aneurysm most frequently ruptures.
It showed that the more the shape of the aneurysm is sacciforme the more local pressure maxima occur.

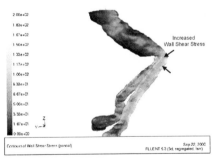

Figure 5.
Display of wall shear stress after placement of an endovascular stentgraft. In this case migration of the stentgraft lead to kinking of both stent legs. In the area of kinking Wall Shear Stress and Pressure are significantly higher. Further there is an increased wall shear stress and Pressure in the docked stent leg compared to the integrated leg.

4. Conclusions

The technique allows to simulate and visualize dynamic blood flow parameters before and after implantation of an aortic stentgraft non-invasively out of static computer-tomography datasets without additional time exposure and effort for the patient. In addition to the standard procedures it can help to estimate the risk of rupture of the aneurysm and the choice of the appropriate operation method and in the end an individually optimised stentgraft for each patient should be enabled.

Medicine Meets Virtual Reality 2001
J.D. Westwood et al. (Eds.)
IOS Press, 2001

The Effect of Simulator Use on Learning and Self-Assessment:
The Case of Stanford University's E-Pelvis Simulator

Carla M. Pugh, M.D., Sakti Srivastava, M.D., Richard Shavelson, Ph.D., Decker Walker, Ph.D., Teresa Cotner, Ph.D., Beth Scarloss, MS, Merry Kuo, MS, Chantal Rawn, BA, Parvati Dev, Ph.D., Thomas H. Krummel, M.D., and Leroy H. Heinrichs, M.D., Ph.D.

Stanford University Medical Media and Information Technology (SUMMIT)
Stanford University College of Medicine - 251 West Campus Dr. Suite 230
Stanford, California 94305-5466

1. Background

Proper clinical assessment of the female reproductive anatomy is one of the most difficult skills for students to learn. Not only is the exam technically complex, but many psychosocial issues are involved as well. Unlike physical examination of the chest wall, where the teacher can see what and where the student is touching, examination of the female pelvic anatomy does not afford this perspective. After the student has introduced his or her hand or fingers into the vaginal vault, the instructor cannot see the structures or anatomic region the student is touching. In addition, the instructor cannot intervene to guide the student's hand to the correct anatomic region or structure of interest. In our attempt to address the difficulties involved in teaching and assessing medical students learning proper clinical assessment of the female pelvis, we have developed a pelvic exam simulator, the E-Pelvis.

2. Methods & Tools

The E-Pelvis is a newly designed device that consists of a partial manikin – umbilicus to mid thigh – constructed in the likeness of an adult human female. The manikin is instrumented internally with several electronic sensors that communicate, indirectly, with a computer-generated interface for the purpose of immediate visual feedback. The device allows students and instructors to see which structures are being touched and how much pressure is being applied while the pelvic exam is being performed.

Eighty-seven medical students, fifty females and thirty-seven males, in an Introduction to Clinical Medicine course, participated in the study. Seventy-five students had no prior experience in performing pelvic exams. The remaining twelve had varying levels of experience with the exam ranging from observation at the patient's beside to actually performing the exam. The protocol consisted of a training phase, and an assessment phase. During the training phase, all of the students were shown a videotape of the exam. The students were then randomly divided into three groups, the simulator, manikin and control groups. The simulator group (n = 31) learned to perform the exam on the E-Pelvis simulator. The manikin group (n = 28) learned to perform the exam on a partial manikin without the feedback technology. The control group (n = 23) learned the concept of performing the exam with the aid of manikin parts (a cervix and uterus) and anatomical drawings.

The assessment phase occurred in two parts, the simulator assessment and the educator assessment. During the simulator assessment module, students from all three groups performed pelvic exams on three different simulators and then reported their findings in a written format. In the second part of the assessment phase, all students performed an exam on paid patient educators who simultaneously taught the exam while assessing the students' beginning skills, ending skills and rapport.

3. Results

The assessment forms completed by the paid patient educators included Likert scale ratings from 1 – 6 (poor – excellent). Data from these forms were coded and evaluated using SPSS statistical software. The results of the study showed that the students in the simulator and manikin groups were rated higher than the control group for their beginning skills scores, 3.8, 3.9 and 3.3 respectively, Figure 1. For the ending skills scores, the educators rated the simulator group higher than both the manikin and control group 5.3, 5.1 and 5.0 respectively, Figure 2. The simulator group was also rated highest on rapport when compared to the manikin and control groups 5.32, 5.2 and 4.7 respectively, Figure 3. Only the results for rapport were statistically significant, $p < .05$.

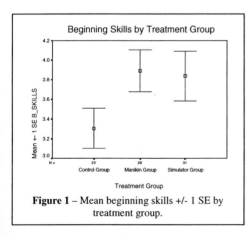

Figure 1 – Mean beginning skills +/- 1 SE by treatment group.

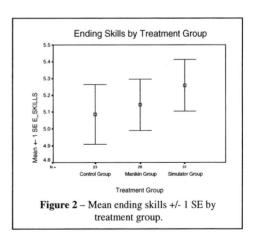

Figure 2 – Mean ending skills +/- 1 SE by treatment group.

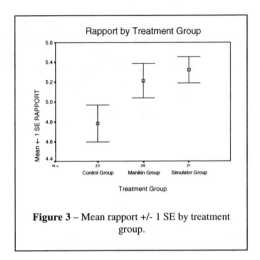

Figure 3 – Mean rapport +/- 1 SE by treatment
group.

4. Discussion

The findings show that the students in the simulator-trained group were rated significantly better on rapport when compared to their colleagues in the manikin and control group. Although we cannot be completely sure what this means, the qualitative data provides some insight into the possibilities underlying this phenomena. The video and audiotapes of the three different teaching sessions show that the student and instructor interactions were very different in these groups. In the control group, the students played more of a passive role as the instructor lectured and gave demonstrations. In the manikin group, the students and instructors interacted in a one-on-one fashion. In most cases, the instructor stood at the student's side, while the student was performing the exam, and played the role as a coach. The student readily depended on the instructor for feedback as apparent in the continuous questioning and affirmation that took place between the two individuals.

In the simulator group, the visual feedback allowed for a different interaction between the students and instructors than what was seen in the manikin and control groups. The instructors and students were able to see whether the exam was being done correctly or not, thus the role of the instructor changed somewhat. In most cases, the role of the instructor was one of confirmation. There was verbal confirmation induced by visual cues such as, "Okay, I see on the screen that you have successfully completed the exam." In addition, there was confirmation by witnessing the student repeat parts of the exam, assuring the student's that what had been done was done correctly. In many cases, the student and instructor would engage in an 'assessment on demand' interaction in which the instructor would ask the student to touch certain areas of importance. For example, the instructor might first ask the student if he or she felt comfortable with the exam and if the student said yes, the instructor would then ask the student to demonstrate palpation of the cervical os or the fundus.

The students in the simulator group also took part in the confirmation process with their classmates. When one student finished the exam, watching another student's performance provided some reassurance of equal experiences. The student-student interactions during this assurance process provided an opportunity for the students to teach one another, confirming what they had experienced while learning to perform the exam. This type of interaction allows for the use of feedback to enhance self-learning.[12]

The findings from the qualitative data show that the students in the simulator group may have had a superior learning experience when compared to their colleagues in the manikin and control group. The instantaneous feedback from the simulator, combined with affirmation of that knowledge from an instructor and the interaction with their classmates, may have resulted in increased confidence in their exam skills[3]. Having reached a certain level of confidence, the students probably entered the educator sessions more comfortable with their ability to do the exam. Although it is impossible to prove, this may have implications for the results reported by the educators in relation to the superior rating of the simulator group on rapport.

Overall, the results must be considered in light of the research methods used. Because the students had a very limited amount of time in the treatment groups they were not allowed to practice the exam to a point of maximum confidence. This limitation may have had some effect on the end results. Another methodological issue to consider is that all three treatment groups entered an assessment mode with the simulator before being evaluated by the educators. Meaning, the students in the control group had an opportunity to perform pelvic exams during the assessment mode, rendering a possible pre-test/ post-test effect on the beginning skills score reported by the educators. Also, the ending skills score provided by the patient educators, in part, is a measure of their own teaching in addition to a measure of the treatment condition effects. Despite these issues, the educator variables still have indications regarding use of the simulator as a teaching tool.

In using the beginning skills variable as an indicator of treatment group effectiveness, especially the effectiveness of the simulator as a teaching tool, these results show that with limited use, the simulator is an effective teaching modality. This is important to note considering that the addition of a computer interface to the learning environment for this exam has the potential to distract the learner and alter the learning experience[4].

The results also give insight into appropriateness of the skills learned on the simulator. Even with the time restrictions, which limited student learning during the treatment mode, the students in the simulator group still performed comparably well on their beginning and ending skills and significantly better on rapport, when compared to the manikin and control groups. In this case, what is not significant is equally as important as what is. It is important to note that the educators did not single students out in the simulator group as having worse beginning or ending exam skills when compared to their colleagues in the manikin and control groups. In fact, the educators rated the students in the simulator group significantly better on rapport. This implies that the skills learned on the simulator were helpful in their ability to perform the exam in a real-life situation.[5]

5. Conclusion

The addition of real-time visual feedback for medical students learning to perform female pelvic exams may provide a superior educational experience when compared to traditional learning modalities.

6. References

[1] D. Butler and P. Winne, Feedback and Self-Regulated Learning: A Theoretical Synthesis. Review of Educational Research 1995, 65(3):245-281.

[2] Bangert-Drowns, et al., The Instructional Effect of Feedback In Test-Like Events. Review of Educational Research 1991, 61:213-238

[3] A. Bandura and R. Walters, Social Learning and Personality Development. Holt, Rinehart and Winston, New York, New York, 1963, 44-67.

[4] R. Satava and S. Ellis, Human Interface Technology-An Essential Tool for the Modern Surgeon. Surg Endosc 1994 Jul;8(7):817-20.

[5] F. Rose and E. Attree et al., Training in Virtual Environments: Transfer to Real World Tasks and Equivelance to Real Task Training. Ergonomics 2000, Apr:43(4):494-511.

Medicine Meets Virtual Reality 2001
J.D. Westwood et al. (Eds.)
IOS Press, 2001

CompAc
Information System
for Traditional Chinese Medicine

Alexandra RADU[1], Cristina-Simona ALECU[2], Adina RACLARIU[2],
Lavinia NANU[3], Maria LOGHIN[2], Emilia STANCIU[2], Andrei NECULA[2],
Constantin IONESCU-TIRGOVISTE[4], Victor PATRUGAN[2]

[1] *Romanian Radio Broadcasting, 60-64 General Berthelot, Bucharest, Romania*
[2] *Software ITC SA, 167 Calea Floreasca, 72321 Bucharest, Romania*
[3] *Institute for Postgraduate Studies in Medicine and Pharmacy, Bucharest*
[4] *"N.Paulescu" Institute of Nutrition and Metabolic Diseases, Bucharest*

Abstract. The paper presents a system developed for the assistance of diagnosis and treatment in alternative medicine, based on traditional Chinese methods. The system named CompAc, is a result of an interdisciplinary cooperation and is designed for the physician, specialist in acupuncture. The Compac system allows the determination of the type of energetic imbalance starting from the clinical picture of the patient and establishing whether an organ or any of the viscera are affected. It allows also the indication of different variants of treatment. The diagnosis proposed by the system has to be confirmed by the physician and can be modified by him. The system is also useful for medical training.

1. Introduction

In the last years the methods of alternative medicine have become more important in the treatment of diseases. These methods are efficient, sure and useful, with positive results.

Treatment in Chinese Medicine is based on the following principles:

- the patient is considered as a whole (holistic concept);
- treatment is highly flexible and individualized.

Alternative Medicine conceives disease as an energetic imbalance resulting from an excess or deficiency of some functions in the positive (**Yang**) or negative (**Yin**) sense of an organ or system. The 153 syndromes taken into account in the system are differentiated on the basis of eight categories grouped in four oppositions: *Yin-Yang, Deficiency-Excess, Interior-Exterior, Cold-Heat*

2. System description

The CompAc system allows the determination of the type of energetic imbalance starting from the clinical picture of the patient and establishing whether an organ or any of the viscera are affected. The diagnosis algorithm is based on the comparison of the results of the clinical examination of the patient with the clinical patterns of the syndromes stored in a database. A score is calculated for each of the syndromes among which the system seeks to differentiate.

The system displays the first 5 syndromes, which best explain the symptomatology of the patient, in the decreasing order of the scores (figure 1). The precision of the diagnosis proposed by the system depends on the amount of information recorded from the patient. At any rate the diagnosis has to be confirmed by the physician and can be modified by him.

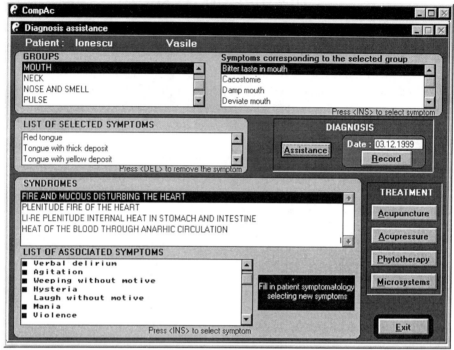

Figure 1. "Diagnosis assistance" screen

The system, based on a large amount of information from *acupuncture* [1][7], *acupressure* [5], *phytotherapy* [6] and *microsystems* (some zones of energetic projection of some organs or functions) [4][8] allows the indication of different variants of treatment. The information offered to the physician is completed by the display of anatomic (figure 2) or botanic charts.

In order to optimize the diagnosis, the system also provides information from fields related to acupuncture:

- chirology - the main types of palms are displayed (corresponding to the 5 elements: *metal, wood, fire, water, earth*) to help establish the **constitution** of the patient and the vulnerability of his channels ("meridians");
- characterological testing - by means of the BERGER and/or REQUENA criteria, the **psychosomatic type** [2] of the patient is determined.

The traditional Chinese chronoacupuncture methods Tzu Wu Liu Chu Liao Fa and Ling Kwei Ba Fa can also be used in the establishment of the point formulae, allowing optimization depending on the opening times [3][4].

The system can also be used for training. The **Theory** module allows the user the access consultative functions, offering information about the main notions used in Traditional Chinese Medicine (from the knowledge databases of the system): channels and points, syndromes, the five elements law, tongue examination, pulsology, microsystems, plants.

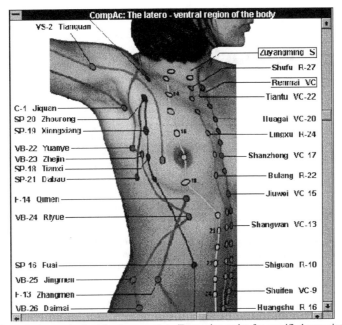

Figure 2. Anatomic chart for **Acupuncture** (Romanian codes for specified acupoints)

3. Conclusions

The system has been installed and is being tested at the *Institute for Postgraduate Studies in Medicine and Pharmacy* in Bucharest and in some clinics in Romania.

The **CompAc** system can be used in:

- medical practice
- medical research
- teaching of alternative medicine
- self-therapy through phytotherapy and acupressure.

The system's value consists in the great amount of information stored in the system's databases, the flexibility of the correlation between databases and the ease of use.

References

[1] *** Essentials of Chinese Acupuncture. Foreign Languages Press, Beijing, 1980.

[2] Y.Requena, Acupuncture et Psychologie - Pour une approche nouvelle de la psycho-somatique, Maloine, Paris, 1982

[3] H.Lu, The time-honored Chinese techniques of acupuncture, Acad.Orient.Herit., Vancouver, 1978.

[4] L.Tureanu, V.Tureanu, Microsystems, optimal times and extraordinary points in acupuncture, Ed. All, Bucuresti, 1994.

[5] S.Ivan, Acupressure, Bucuresti, 1992

[6] Z.Jinhuang, L.Ganzhong, Recent advances in Chinese herbal drugs - actions and uses, Science Press, Beijing, 1991.

[7] Chen Jing, Atlas anatomique des points d'acupuncture, Editions scientifique et technique du Shandong, Beijing, Chine, 1984.

[8] Y. Pesikov, S. Rybalko, Auricular Acupuncture. Clinical atlas, Three Dragons, Donetsk, Ukraine, 1994.

Medicine Meets Virtual Reality 2001
J.D. Westwood et al. (Eds.)
IOS Press, 2001

Force-feedback in Web-based Surgical Simulators

Mark Riding and Nigel W. John
Manchester Visualization Centre, University of Manchester
Manchester, United Kingdom

There is a growing requirement in the field of surgical training to allow trainees to practice procedures in a way that does not place patients in any risk. Computer based simulators allow students to gain experience and develop three-dimensional awareness in a safe and controlled environment. Typically systems that have been developed to perform this task are, due to their specialist nature, expensive to buy. With the increasing availability of Force-Feedback devices for the gaming market, is there now a cost-effective alternative for surgical simulations? In this paper we investigate the possibility of using such a device as a haptic input tool for surgical simulations.

1. Introduction

Previous work at the Manchester Visualization Centre (MVC) has resulted in the creation of innovative, low fidelity surgical simulators implemented using web technologies, in particular VRML (Virtual Reality Modelling language) [1-3]. The objective of the work detailed in this paper is to integrate a Force Feedback mouse with these simulators so that the trainee can experience haptic feedback when he/she inserts a needle, cannula, or other surgical appliance into the (virtual) body.

A web-based Lumbar Puncture simulator has been used for this work [1]. This simulator featured inter-object collision detection routines additional to VRML's built in avatar / scene detection routines. Initially there was no cost-effective force-feedback device that could be used in conjunction with a VRML scene to represent haptic effects so the two techniques used to provide the trainee with tactile cues were:

- to rely solely on graphical features of the Virtual Environment (visually correlated force/tactile feedback).
- to exploit auditory human sensory channel to cue contact and force exertion.

However, it was evident that a simple tactile feedback system could provide far more added value to the simulator.

There are commercial haptic devices available today. One of the most innovative developers of haptic devices is Immersion Corporation [4] and they have even produced advanced laparoscopic frames that are already being used by commercial surgical training products such as MIST/VR [5]. Immersion has also applied their technology to low-end devices and recently developed a mouse with haptic support. The mouse technology has been licensed to Logitech and is now widely available, called the Wingman Force-Feedback Mouse. With the arrival of this device, there is a cheap ($100) alternative to the more typical, and more expensive, haptic devices used in high fidelity surgical simulations. A software development kit (Feel Foundation Classes: FFC_SDK) is provided by

Immersion that allows force-feedback effects to be added to existing Windows C++ applications.

It is the development of a reusable technique to facilitate communication between VRML and this SDK that forms the basis of this work.

2. Method & Tools

The most obvious way to add extra functionality to a VRML scene is to make use of the External Authoring Interface (EAI). This approach could be taken to allow communication with the C++ force-feedback SDK, however applet security restrictions and the general complexity of combining so many different technologies make this approach somewhat less desirable.

Alternatively ParallelGraphics have released a Software Development Kit that allows the embedding of their Cortona VRML client as an ActiveX object into web pages and applications [6]. A programming interface is provided to give the embedding application access to the VRML scene's nodes, and to trap and create events within the scene. By embedding the Cortona client into a Microsoft Foundation Class (MFC) based application, we can directly incorporate the features from the FFC_SDK, and allow the VRML scene to interact indirectly with the force-feedback mouse.

This approach is certainly feasible, though not without cost, since we have lost the web deliverability and platform independence of a pure VRML implementation. These drawbacks are acceptable since the force-feedback mouse is only available for the Windows platform, and having a clean and usable implementation of force-feedback in VRML outweighs the requirements of web-deliverability.

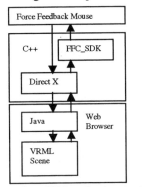

Figure 1: Java / EAI application structure   Figure 2. Cortona SDK-based application structure

3. Results

The force-feedback mouse is a two-degree of freedom device. Attempting to recreate haptic effects that have their basis in the three-dimensional world would be problematic at best. The simplistic interaction that is a feature of the simulations already developed lends itself well to this device though, since after first setting a needle's entry point to the body and angle of insertion, the actual insertion is along a straight path. To control motion along such a vector requires only one degree of freedom from an input device, and so, conversely the force-feedback mouse has a more than adequate range of motion for this particular application. In fact, effort must be made to ensure that we constrain device motion to movement along a single axis at the time of needle insertion.

The haptic effects offered by the force-feedback mouse include opposing or supporting forces in arbitrary directions, feelings of texture, and vibrations. Although the device is unable to completely restrict motion in a given direction, the subtle forces involved in the medical procedures simulated tend not to require such a degree of haptic feedback.

To tailor appropriate haptic effects for use in the simulator, medical input was sought. As part of the WebSET project [7] a range of haptic effects are being created with help and direction from medical personnel, to represent the sensations felt when inserting a needle through tissue appropriate for a lumbar puncture procedure. Collision detection code from previous versions was updated to detect when a needle entered skin tissue, ligaments, the spinal membrane (dura meter) or reached bone. Haptic effects can then be scheduled to play at the appropriate time, giving the simulator user the sense of force-feedback we are trying to achieve.

4. Conclusions

Two sets of conclusions can be drawn from this work, that of the suitability of the technology used to facilitate communication between VRML and the C++ FFC_SDK, and the suitability of the force-feedback mouse for use as a haptic input device in surgical simulations.

In the first case, although the technology employed worked adequately well, a better implementation would be one that was entirely web-deliverable. The Cortona SDK offers access to the VRML scene from a HTML and JavaScript interface, and a flavour of the FFC_SDK also takes the same approach. It is feasible that the two technologies could be combined to produce an online version of the simulator with haptic support, and work is ongoing in this area.

The second area of concern is less well defined however, and the suitability of the force-feedback mouse for use in surgical simulations, and indeed of low-fidelity simulations in general is a much bigger question, and one which cannot be adequately answered without further research.

5. Acknowledgements

The authors wish to thank Nick Phillips, Consultant Neurosurgeon at the Leeds General Infirmary, and the ICSM team at St Mary's hospital London, who have provided clinical guidance during the development of this work.

6. References

[1] N.W. John, M. Riding, "Surgical Simulators on the World Wide Web - This Must Be The Way Forward?", *Proceedings of UKVRSIG 99*, Salford, UK, September 1999.

[2] N. Phillips, N.W. John, "Web-based Surgical Simulation for Ventricular Catheterisation", *Neurosurgery: Official Journal of the Congress of Neurosurgical Surgeons*, Vol. 46, No. 4, pp933-937, April 2000.

[3] N.W. John, N. Phillips, "Surgical Simulators Using the WWW", *Proceedings of Medicine Meets Virtual Reality 2000*, Newport Beach, California, USA, January 2000.

[4] Immersion Corporation website: http://www.immersion.com

[5] http://www.vrweb.com

[6] Cortona VRML browser website: http://www.parallelgraphics.com/cortona/

[7] WebSET Project website: http://www.vmwc.org/projects/webset

Medicine Meets Virtual Reality 2001
J.D. Westwood et al. (Eds.)
IOS Press, 2001

A Survey Study for the Development of Virtual Reality Technologies in Orthopedics

Robert Riener[1] and Rainer Burgkart[2]

[1] Institute of Automatic Control Engineering and
[2] Clinic for Orthopaedics and Sport-Orthopaedics, Klinikum Rechts der Isar,
Technical University of Munich (TUM), 80290 Munich, Germany

Abstract. Virtual reality (VR) technologies have the potential to support medical education and training. In order to orient the development of medical VR applications towards the actual deficiencies and demands in orthopedics, we performed a survey among 56 orthopedic physicians. They were asked to provide information about the kind of physical joint evaluation tests which they perform most often, the importance of physical joint evaluation in comparison to alternative diagnostic methods, and their opinion about current medical education system as well as the prospects of VR applications in orthopedics. The main conclusion of this survey is that VR applications have the potential to improve the lacking medical education and orthopedic training, e.g. by improving the quality of joint evaluation methods, reducing the high number of unhealthy, risky and expensive alternative diagnostic procedures.

1. Introduction

Due to limited access to a greater pool of patients during single training blocks an effective training of medical students or young orthopedic physicians is difficult. There is almost no opportunity to simultaneously learn the small haptic, but clinically important, differences due to different grades of injury of the same anatomic structure (e.g. ligament lesion grade I to III). However, reliable and improved joint evaluation will become more and more important, also because of the fact that the number of joint affections has been significantly increasing in Germany within the last years (Fig. 1) [1]. Reasons for this are the aging population and new kinds of sports [2].

Therefore, a newly founded research group at TUM is developing virtual reality (VR) technologies for the education of medical students and for the training of physical joint evaluation in orthopedics [3-5]. Different VR approaches are under development, where the mechanical properties of a healthy or pathological joint (e.g., knee) are simulated and presented to the user by haptic, graphical, and acoustic displays. These virtual environments allow the user to train physical joint evaluation by inspection of the joint function, palpation of the joint tissue, and performing different clinical tests. Consequently, it has the potential to improve diagnostic training and therapeutic planning.

In order to orient the development of VR applications towards the actual deficiencies and demands in medical education and training, we performed a survey among orthopedic physicians in private practice.

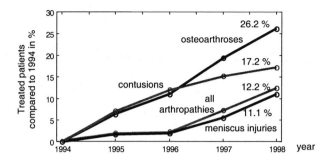

Figure 1: Increase of certain joint affections in Germany [1].

2. Methods

222 orthopedic physicians in private practice in the Munich area were asked to participate in this survey. A letter was sent to them containing a questionnaire and information about the current VR applications developed by this group. 56 physicians (25.2 %) filled out and sent back the questionnaire.

Information was requested about the number of treated patients, the frequency of affections in hip, knee, ankle, shoulder, elbow, and wrist joints, as well as the kind of clinical tests usually performed when evaluating the knee joint. Furthermore, the physicians should comment the importance of physical evaluation tests compared to other diagnostic methods (instrumented joint evaluation with arthrometers; arthroscopy; imaging techniques). Finally, they should express their opinion about the current medical education and training and the prospects of VR applications in orthopedics.

3. Results

The main results concerning the application of physical joint evaluation methods are:
- Physical joint evaluation is a very frequently performed task. The knee joint is diagnosed and treated most often, followed by ankle, shoulder, hip, elbow, and wrist joint.
- Frequent joint evaluation tests at the knee joint are flexion/extension/hyperextension movement and varus-valgus stress tests, the Lachman test, meniscus and drawer tests.
- Physical joint evaluation is indispensable to diagnose the correct joint affection and allow an optimal therapeutic planning (Fig. 2). Furthermore, it has the potential to avoid unnecessary invasive interventions (arthroscopy, open surgery) as well as expensive and/or unhealthy imaging techniques (X-Ray, CT, MRI).
- Instrumented knee joint evaluation with arthrometers (e.g., KT-1000) is no serious alternative. Only 10 % apply them. Most physicians were not convinced of them.

The physicians were also asked for their individual opinions about the current education and training system in orthopedics:
- Learning physical joint evaluation methods is time consuming and takes several years.
- 82 % agree that there is the need to improve orthopedic education and training (Fig. 2).
- More than the half believe that medical education and training can be improved by VR technologies. Another third (32 %) says that VR has the potential to do so.
- Two third wish to test or use a joint simulator, if they would have access to one (Fig. 2).
- Only a minority (9 %) thinks that a "technical training environment" will intimidate or frighten the medical user (Fig. 2).

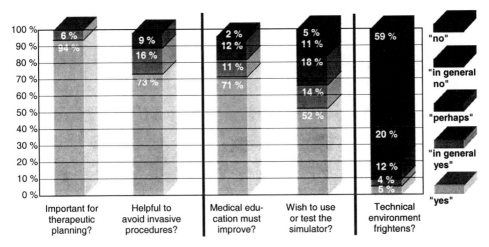

Figure 2: Some results of the survey performed among 56 orthopedic physicians in private practice. The survey took place in Munich, from March 1st till April 10th, 2000. (Towards 100 missing %: no response)

4. Discussion and Conclusion

Physical joint evaluation methods have an indispensable meaning in orthopedics, since they are easy to perform and no practical alternatives exist. Carefully performed evaluation tests have the potential to minimize the rather high percentage of diagnostic arthroscopic interventions (22 % of all knee arthroscopies in Germany are purely diagnostic [6]). This is important to reduce the risk of infections, compartment syndromes, and joint and nerve lesions.

Inaccurate or erroneous diagnoses also lead to the frequent use of unhealthy and/or expensive imaging techniques. There is the urgent necessity to reduce the high number of imaging procedures, for example by better clinical evaluation methods.

Most of the orthopedic physicians who participated in this survey agree that medical education and training has to be improved, since it is rather theoretical, time consuming and ineffective. The majority assumes that many VR applications have the potential to support future education and training of medical students and orthopedic physicians.

References

[1] Statistisches Bundesamt VIII A, Gesundheitsdaten, Krankenhausdiagnosestatistik, Statistisches Bundesamt, Wiesbaden (1994-1998).
[2] K. Steinbrück, Epidemiologie von Sportverletzungen - 25-Jahres-Analyse einer sportorthopädisch-traumatologischen Ambulanz. *Sportverletzung Sportschaden* 13, 1999, pp. 38-52.
[3] R. Riener, J. Hoogen, R. Burgkart, M. Buss, and G. Schmidt, Development of a Multi-Modal Virtual Human Knee Joint for Education and Training in Orthopaedics. Proc. of the 9th MMVR 2001, this volume.
[4] J. Hoogen, P. Kammermeier, and M. Buss, Multi-Modal Feedback and Rendering in Virtual Environment Systems. *Proc. of the RAAD'99 Conference*, Munich, Germany,1999, pp. 221-226.
[5] H. Baier, M. Buss, F. Freyberger, J. Hoogen, P. Kammermeier, and G. Schmidt, Distributed PC-Based Haptic, Visual and Acoustic telepresence system - Experiments in Virtual and Remote Environments. *Proc. of the IEEE VR'99*, Houston, Texas, USA, 1999, pp. 118 - 125.
[6] K. H. Kleimann, B. Markefka, and G. Holfelder, Potentialermittlung für Hüft- und Kniegelenkoperationen in Allgemeinkrankenhäusern der Bundesrepublik Deutschland. *Untersuchungsergebnisse des Marktforschungsinstituts Vector GmbH*, Oldenburg, 1995.

410

Medicine Meets Virtual Reality 2001
J.D. Westwood et al. (Eds.)
IOS Press, 2001

Development of a Multi-Modal Virtual Human Knee Joint for Education and Training in Orthopaedics

R. Riener[1], J. Hoogen[1], R. Burgkart[2], M. Buss[1], G. Schmidt[1]

[1]*Institute of Automatic Control Engineering and*
[2]*Clinic for Orthopaedics and Sport-Orthopaedics, Klinikum Rechts der Isar,*
Technical University of Munich (TUM), 80290 Munich, Germany

Abstract. Due to limited simultaneous access to a greater pool of patients an effective training of medical students or young orthopedic physicians is difficult. A knee joint simulator that comprises the properties of a healthy or pathological knee can support medical education and training. In this paper a mechatronic system is presented that provides visual, acoustic, and haptic (force) feedback so that it allows a user to touch and move a virtual shank, bones or muscles within the leg, and simultaneously observe the generated movement, feel the contact force, and hear sounds. These and further features enable the user to study and assess the properties of the knee, e.g. by testing the joint laxity and end-point stiffness in six degrees-of-motion (DOF) and by grasping and pulling at muscles, rupturing ligaments or changing muscle/ligament paths. Such a tool can support training of physical knee evaluation required for diagnosis and therapeutic planning, since any kind of pathology of any subject type can be tested at any time. Furthermore, it can provide a better understanding of functional anatomy, e.g. for the education of medical students.

1. Introduction

Injuries, diseases, and pre- and post-surgical properties of the knee joint can be evaluated by performing different kinds of clinical tests based on inspection, palpation and movement of the knee. These include passive movement tests in flexion/extension, varus/valgus (abduction/adduction), internal/external rotation, and anterior/posterior directions to determine mid-range laxity and end-point stiffness of the joint (Fig. 1). More specific tests exist to assess disruption of cruciate or collateral ligaments (e.g., Lachman test, anterior/posterior drawer tests, pivot shift tests) or injury of the menisci (e.g. McMurray test, Steinmann test).

A lot of experience is required to diagnose pathological joint properties. However, due to limited simultaneous access to a greater pool of patients an effective training of medical students or young orthopaedic physicians is difficult. Therefore, a newly founded research group at TUM is developing a multi-modal knee joint simulator that comprises the properties of a healthy or pathological knee joint and presents them to a user by visual, acoustic, and haptic (force) feedback. With this simulator any kind of pathology of any subject type can be tested at any time. Such a tool can support training of physical knee evaluation required for diagnosis and surgical planning. Furthermore, it can provide a better understanding of functional anatomy, e.g. for the education of medical students.

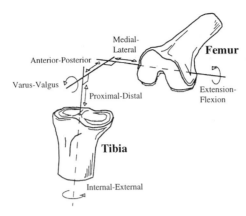

Figure 1: Knee joint definitions, adapted from [1].

2. Tools and Methods

2.1 The Three Modalities: Graphic, Acoustic and Haptic Display

The user can immerse into the virtual environment by using a visual, acoustic, and haptic display [2]. Visual feedback is provided by a SGI graphics workstation. At this state of the study objects were approximated by cylinders, cones, spheres, cubes using the openGL-based graphic library MAVERIK (Dept. of Computer Science, University of Manchester, UK). Fig. 2 shows the graphical representations in two different user modes.

The acoustic rendering is performed on a Sun Workstation (Solaris). Whenever a command is received from the dynamic knee model (e.g. after gaining certain thresholds), a specific sound sample is called from a set of different pre-recorded sounds and sent to a pair of speakers. This can be a sound uttered by the patient due to pain, or the sound that is produced by the articulating surfaces in the (pathological) knee joint.

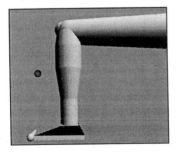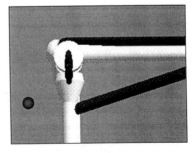

Figure 2: Symbolic graphical representation of the leg and internal anatomical structures in the "surface mode" (left) and "open-mode" (right), respectively. The small sphere represents the user's finger tip. Its location can be changed by moving the handle of a kinesthetic feedback device (Fig. 3).

Haptic (force) feedback to the hand of the user is provided by a 3D Desktop-Kinesthetic-Feedback-Device, DeKiFeD3 [2], [3], which exerts 3D forces up to 60 N (Fig. 3). These forces are measured by a 6 DOF force-torque sensor, in order to enable a force-control loop which runs at 1000 Hz. The position of the hand is recorded by angle encoders of the DeKiFeD3. Together with the actual object locations (shank, bones, muscles etc.) obtained from the model computations, the hand position serves as input to the haptic rendering algorithm (Fig. 4). The haptic rendering is comprised of a collision detection and a contact force computation, both running at 1000 Hz. Within a common object-fixed reference system a constraint-based God-object method [4] is performed to detect a collision between finger tip and the surface of one of the virtual objects. The contact force is computed on the basis of a linear-elastic spring model.

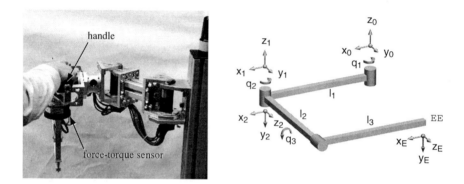

Figure 3: Desktop-Kinesthetic-Feedback-Device with three active DOF (DeKiFeD3) [3].

Different stiffness properties were taken into account for the various objects as well as for the posterior and anterior side of the shank (calf and shin, respectively). The direction of the contact force is computed as a vector normal to the surface of the virtual object. The computed contact force is fed into the dynamic knee model (equations of motion). The same amount of force but with a negative sign is fed into the DeKiFeD3. This "reaction force" serves as desired force for the DeKiFeD3 force control loop and makes the user "feel" the actual contact force (Fig. 4).

2.2. Implementation

The system runs on three processors: the haptic server (including haptic rendering process, knee model, and DeKiFeD3 force control) and the graphic and acoustic clients. The separation of the different processes was first proposed by Adachi, et al. [5]. Decoupling the haptic server from the graphic and acoustic client is important since the haptic control loop must run on a very high rate (1000 Hz) to achieve a high fidelity force display. In contrast, the graphic client runs at 30 Hz and the acoustic client receives only discrete signals indicating the beginning or end of a certain sound. Fig. 4 shows how the haptic, visual, and acoustic modalities interact with each other. Fig. 5 depicts an overview of the entire experimental setup.

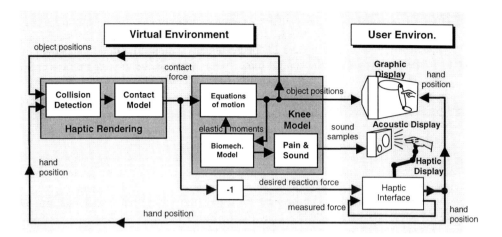

Figure 4: Virtual and user environment including the interaction of the haptic, visual, and acoustic modalities.

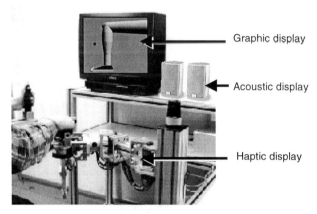

Graphic display

Acoustic display

Haptic display

Figure 5: Experimental setup

It can be switched between two modes. In the "surface mode" the user can see and touch the skin of the thigh, shank and foot. In the "open mode" it is possible to look under the skin and to observe and touch internal structures such as bones (tibia, fibula, femur, and patella), muscles (rectus femoris head of the quadriceps and short head of the biceps femoris), and ligaments (medial and lateral collateral ligament, patella tendon/ligament). The graphical representation has been represented by simple geometries which are only roughly approximated to real anatomical shapes.

3. Biomechanical Model

3.1. Leg Dynamics

The contact force causes the leg to move depending on its magnitude, direction, and contact location. The translational and rotational movement is computed by a system of six equations of motion. Input to the equations are three force components in anterior/posterior, lateral/medial, and proximal/distal direction and three moment components in flexion/extension, varus/valgus, and internal/external rotation. The three input forces are equal to the components of the contact force vector, whereas the three input moments are obtained by the cross product of the contact force vector and the vector connecting the contact point with the knee joint centre of rotation. The equations of motion are solved by an implicit Euler integration algorithm at 1000 Hz.

3.2. Viscoelastic Knee Model

Due to the anatomical structures surrounding the knee joint (ligaments, tendons, menisci, connective tissue, etc.) passive viscoelastic effects exist between shank and thigh. In the model, each translational and rotational degree of the lower leg is characterised by a specific viscous and elastic characteristic [6]. Data of passive elastic knee joint properties were taken from the literature and own measurements. The elastic moment in flexion/extension direction was modelled by a exponential function of the flexion/extension angle [7]. Piecewise polynomial functions were used to approximate the passive elastic characteristics in anterior/posterior, varus/valgus, and internal/external rotation so that the model agreed well with experimental data [8]. Analogously, the passive elastic force in medial/lateral direction was fit to data from [9]. The elastic properties in distal/proximal direction were modelled by a simple linear function with a relatively high stiffness, since there was no data found in the literature. Passive viscous effects (damping) were modelled by linear functions. To obtain a realistic pendulum movement, the damping coefficient for the viscous moment around flexion/extension was derived from passive pendulum tests [10]. Viscous and elastic forces and moments were fed into the equations of motion.

3.3. Additional Physiological Functions

With the knee simulator further knee functions can be evaluated. For example, for neurological tests the knee tendon reflex can be activated. To induce a reflex response, the contact has to occur in a certain region close to the patella tendon and the contact force and force gradient have to be above certain threshold values. Another function verified with the simulator is the palpation of the pulse. When touching the shank near the hollow of the knee, the pulse can be felt. To simulate an acoustic reaction of the patient due to pain an output sound is produced (e.g. "ouch") when either the contact force gradient or the elastic joint moment gains a particular threshold value. Joint sound as usually can be detected in certain diseases (e.g. arthritis) can also be produced when the shank is moved.

3.4. Grasping a Muscle

In the open mode a muscle can not only be touched, but also grasped (by turning a switch) and pulled similarly to a rubber tube (Fig. 6). During pulling the force that is provided to the operator's finger is equal to the vector sum of the passive elastic muscle forces, which act between the finger tip and the proximal and distal ends of the muscles. To compute the elastic forces, the muscle was considered as a series of linear elastic springs. Thus, the effective stiffness in the proximal or distal muscle part depends on its original length before pulling.

When pulling a muscle, the passive elastic muscle force not only generates a force feeling in the grasping finger but also causes the lower leg move.

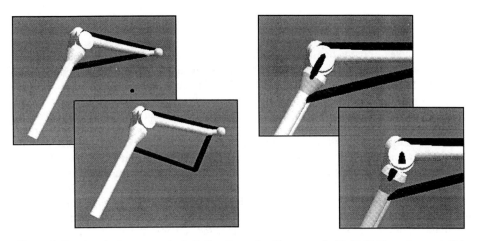

Figure 6: Functions in the open mode. Left: Grasping and pulling a muscle. Right: Cutting a ligament. Note that the representation of muscle shapes and paths (origins and insertions) is only symbolic and has not been adapted to real anatomical data.

3.5. Ligament Rupture

It is also possible to touch, grip (by turning a switch) and pull the medial collateral ligament until it ruptures at a certian threshold force (Fig. 6). This is represented in the graphical and haptic display: the user can see how the ligament splits into two pieces and feel how his arm jerks back as soon as the ligaments ruptures. The damaged ligament causes a change of the elastic characteristic in varus-valgus direction, which can be verified by the user when moving the tibia in medial direction.

4. Results and Discussion

With this knee simulator the user can assess the properties of the knee by testing the joint angular range of the lower leg, feel the joint laxity and end-point stiffness, or produce a pendulum movement in flexion/extension direction. Knee stability can be tested in anterior/posterior, medial/lateral, internal/external rotation, and varus/valgus directions. Rotational movements about the vertical shank axis can be generated by applying a force to the foot. Different parameter sets can be applied to represent the properties of a healthy and an injured knee joint. For diagnostic purposes additional tests can be performed such as activation of the knee tendon reflex and palpation of the pulse.

To simulate an acoustic reaction uttered by the patient due to pain an output sound is produced (e.g. "ouch") when either the contact force or the elastic joint moment gains particular threshold values. Additionally, in the open mode, muscles, bones, and ligaments can be touched and grasped. When pulling the muscle like rubber tubes the resulting movement of the shank can be observed while feeling the change in muscle tension due to changing muscle length. Muscle and ligament origins and insertions can be transferred and the resulting changes in the elastic joint properties can be assessed by moving the lower leg or touching the muscles.

The outstanding result of this study is that the quality of the force feedback is considerably good and the physiological properties of the simulated knee joint are rather realistic. This could be achieved by running the force control loop as well as the haptic rendering process at the high frequency of 1000 Hz. An important prerequisite for this was that the complex, highly non-linear, elastic properties of the knee joint could be well approximated by algebraic expressions. These reduced the computational effort significantly compared to more physiologically based knee models [10].

One problem of the presented simulator is the limited force and workspace of the DeKiFeD3 with respect to the leg dimensions of an adult human subject. Another problem is that only a 3 DOF point contact can be generated. In a future version a "CyberGrasp" device that is connected to a 6 DOF robot with a sufficiently large workspace will be used in order to avoid the mentioned problems and, thus, allow full performance of the knee joint simulator. Furthermore, the graphical representations of anatomical geometries will be improved by implementing anatomical data obtained from medical imaging techniques (CT and MRI). An advanced, further developed VR simulation environment as presented in this study will have the potential to provide a better understanding of human anatomy, functional anatomy, physiology, and pathology, and support the education of medical students and the training of physical joint evaluation.

5. Acknowlegements

The authors thank Kerstin Wendicke, Benno Zerlin, Hubert Baier, Jan Peters, and Matthias Henze for their support in this study. This work was supported in part by the German Research Foundation (DFG) within the collaborative research centre SFB 453 on "High-Fidelity Telepresence and Teleaction".

References

[1] S. L. Woo, G.A. Livesay, and B.A. Smith, Kinematics. In: Fu, Harner, Vince (eds.), Knee Surgery, Williams and Wilkins, Baltimore, 1994, pp. 173-187.

[2] J. Hoogen, P. Kammermeier, and M. Buss, Multi-Modal Feedback and Rendering in Virtual Environment Systems. *Proc. RAAD'99 Conference*, Munich, Germany, 1999, pp. 221-226.

[3] H. Baier, M. Buss, F. Freyberger, J. Hoogen, P. Kammermeier, and G. Schmidt, Distributed PC-Based Haptic, Visual and Acoustic telepresence system - Experiments in Virtual and Remote Environments. *Proceedings of the IEEE VR'99*, Houston, Texas, USA, 1999, pp. 118 - 125.

[4] C. B. Zilles and J.K. Salisbury, A Constraint-Based God-Object Method for Haptic Display. *Proc. ASME Haptic Interfaces for Virtual Environment and Teleoperator Systems*, Chicago, IL, Nov. 1994, pp. 146-150.

[5] Y. Adachi, T. Kumano and K. Ogino, Intermediate representation for stiff virtual objects. *Proc. IEEE Virtual Reality Ann. Int. Symposium* 1995, 203-210.

[6] J. Peters and R. Riener, A Real-Time Model of the Human Knee for a Virtual Orthopaedic Trainer. *Proceedings of the International Conference on Biomedical Engineering*, Singapore, December, 6-9, 2000, in press.

[7] K. L. Markolf, J. S. Mensch, and H. C. Amstutz, Stiffness and laxity of the knee – the contributions of the supporting structures. A quantitative in vitro study. *J. Bone Joint Surg. [Am]* 58 (1976) 583-594.

[8] R. Riener and T. Edrich, Identification of Passive Elastic Joint Moments in the Lower Extremities. *J. Biomechanics* 32 (1999) 539-544.

[9] R. L. Piziali, J. Rastegar, D. A. Nagel and D. J. Schurman, The Contribution of the Cruciate Ligaments to the Load Displacement Characteristic of the Human Knee Joint. *J. Biomech. Eng.*, 102 (1980) 277-283.

[10] R. Riener, J. Quintern, and G. Schmidt, Biomechanical model of the Human Knee Evaluated by Neuromuscular Stimulation. *J. Biomechanics* 29 (1996) 1157-1167.

Medicine Meets Virtual Reality 2001
J.D. Westwood et al. (Eds.)
IOS Press, 2001

Objective Laparoscopic Skills Assessments of Surgical Residents Using Hidden Markov Models Based on Haptic Information and Tool/Tissue Interactions

Jacob Rosen[+,*], Massimiliano Solazzo[++],
Blake Hannaford[+,**], Mika Sinanan[++,***]

[+] Department of Electrical Engineering, Box 352500
[++] Department of Surgery, Box 356410
University of Washington
Seattle, WA, 98195, USA

E-mail/ URL : [*]rosen@rcs.ee.washington.edu, [**]blake@u.washington.edu, http://rcs.ee.washington.edu/brl/
[***]mssurg@u.washington.edu, http://depts.washington.edu/cves/

ABSTRACT

Laparoscopic surgical skills evaluation of surgery residents is usually a subjective process, carried out in the operating room by senior surgeons. By its nature, this process is performed using fuzzy criteria. The objective of the current study was to develop and assess an objective laparoscopic surgical skill scale using Hidden Markov Models (HMM) based on haptic information, tool/tissue interactions and visual task decomposition. *Methods:* Eight subjects (six surgical trainees: first year surgical residents 2xR1, third year surgical residents 2xR3 fifth year surgical residents 2xR5; and two expert laparoscopic surgeons: 2xES) performed laparoscopic cholecystectomy following a specific 7 steps protocol on a pig. An instrumented laparoscopic grasper equipped with a three-axis force/torque sensor located at the proximal end with an additional force sensor located on the handle, was used to measure the forces and torques. The hand/tool interface force/torque data was synchronized with a video of the tool operative maneuvers. A synthesis of frame-by-frame video analysis was used to define 14 different types of tool/tissue interactions, each one associated with unique force/torque (F/T) signatures. HMMs were developed for each subject representing the surgical skills by defining the various tool/tissue interactions as states and the associated F/T signatures as observations. The statistical distance between the HMMs representing residents at different levels of their training and the HMMs of expert surgeons were calculated in order to generate a learning curve of selected steps during laparoscopic cholecystectomy. *Results:* Comparison of HMM's between groups showed significant differences between all skill levels, supporting the objective definition of a learning curve. The major differences between skill levels were: (i) magnitudes of F/T applied (ii) types of tool/tissue interactions used and the transition between them and (iii) time intervals spent in each tool/tissue interaction and the overall completion time. The objective HMM analysis showed that the greatest difference in performance was between R1 and R3 groups and then decreased as the level of expertise increased, suggesting that significant laparoscopic surgical capability develops between the first and the third years of their residency training. The power of the methodology using HMM for objective surgical skill assessment arises from the fact that it compiles enormous amount of data regarding different aspects of surgical skill into a very compact model that can be translated into a single number representing the distance from expert performance. Moreover, the methodology is not limited to *in-vivo* condition as demonstrated in the current study. It can be extended to other modalities such as measuring performance in surgical simulators and robotic systems.

1. Introduction

One of the paramount issues in surgical education is the evaluation of surgical skill. An accurate means of assessing surgical skill would allow surgical educators to evaluate the effectiveness of skills training, monitoring progress and learning curves of students and residents along the course of their study. Skill evaluation in surgery in general, and laparoscopic surgery in particular, is currently a *subjective* process, carried out in the operating room or performed off-line using a video tape by expert surgeons grading the performance of the student. By its nature, this process is performed using fuzzy criteria.

Surgical skills are accessible for analysis in three different environments : (1) open or minimally invasive surgery (MIS) utilizing traditional surgical tools and equipment, (2) a robotic system using a master/slave setup, and (3) a simulator utilizing a haptic device that generates force feedback in addition to a virtual reality graphic representation of the surgical scene. All of these systems have a human-machine interface. Through this interface, visual, kinematic, and dynamic information is flowing back and forth between the surgeon and the environment. The aim of the current research was to develop methodology to acquire and analyze information at the human/tool interface in order to quantitatively and objectively evaluate surgical skill and learning curves of MIS. The power of the proposed methodology is that it can be incorporated into any of the three environments.

The methodology developed in the current study was based on the Hidden Markov Modeling (HMM). HMMs were extensively developed in the area of speech recognition (for mathematical review see [1]). Based on the theory developed for speech recognition HMMs have become useful statistical tools in the fields of robotics, teleoperation [2, 3, 4], human manipulation actions, manufacturing, gesture recognition. They are also being applied to the recognition of facial expressions from video images, DNA and protein modeling, nuclear power plants, and detection of pulsar signals. These applications suggest that the HMMs have high potential to provide better models of the human operator in complex interactive tasks with machines.

2. Materials and Methods

2.1 Subjects and Protocol

Eight subjects (six general surgery residents: first year residents - 2xR1, third year residents 2xR3, fifth year residents - 2xR5 and two expert, attending laparoscopic surgeons - 2xES) each completed the experimental protocol. The protocol consisted of two phases. During the first phase, subjects watched a 45-minute video of the surgical procedure guided by a senior surgeon to standardize the technique of the procedure into 7 steps for purposes of the study.. Following this introduction in the second phase, each subject performed a laparoscopic cholecystectomy on a pig using using the force/torque sensing instrument. All surgical procedures and animal care were reviewed and approved by the Animal Care Committee of the University of Washington. Based on pilot data analysis, force/torque data from 3 steps of the laparoscopic cholecystectomy (positioning of the gallbladder - LC-1, exposure of the cystic duct - LC-2, and dissection of the gallbladder - LC-3) were recorded. During these steps the instrumented endoscopic tool was used with an atraumatic grasper, a Babcock grasper, and a curved dissector (Fig. 1c).

2.2 Experimental System Setup

During each procedure, information was collected from two sources: (*i*) force/torque data measured at the human/tool interface and (*ii*) visual information of the tool tip interacting with the tissues. The two sources of information were synchronized in time, displayed in real time using graphical user interface, and acquired simultaneously at a sampling rate of 30 Hz for off-line analysis. Two sets of sensors measured the F/T at the interface between the surgeons' hand and the endoscopic grasper handle (Fig 1a). The first sensor was a three-axis force/torque sensor (ATI-Mini model) which was mounted into the outer tube (proximal end) of a standard reusable 10-mm endoscopic grasper (Storz). The sensor was capable of simultaneously measuring the three components of force (F_x, F_y, F_z) and three components of torque (T_x, T_y, T_z) in a Cartesian frame (Fig. 1b). A second force sensor (Futek - FR1010) was mounted to the endoscopic grasper handle to permit the measurement of grasping force (F_g) applied by the surgeon's fingers on the instrument. For a detailed description of the system see [5, 6, 7]

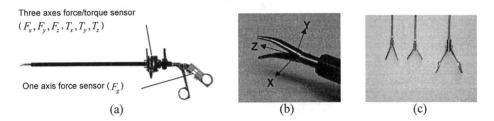

Three axes force/torque sensor
($F_x, F_y, F_z, T_x, T_y, T_z$)

One axis force sensor (F_g)

(a)   (b)   (c)

Figure 1: The instrumented endoscopic grasper: (a) The grasper with the three axis force/torque sensor implemented on the outer tube and a force sensor located on the instrument handle (b) The tool tip and X,Y,Z frame aligned with the three axis force/torque sensor (c) Tool tips used in the surgical procedure (from left to right): Atraumatic Grasper, Babcock grasper, Curved dissector.

2.3 Data Analysis

Two types of analysis were performed on the raw data: (*i*) Video Analysis, encoding the tool-tip/tissue interactions into states; and (*ii*) Hidden Markov Modeling (HMM), for modeling. The performance of surgeons at different level of their training (R1, R3, R5, ES) was then compared.

Video analysis was performed by two expert surgeons , reviewing thevideo of each surgical procedure step, frame by frame (NTSC - 30 frames per second). The encoding process used a library of 14 different discrete tool maneuvers in which the endoscopic tool was interacting with the tissue in a unique F/T pattern (Table 1). For example, in laparoscopic cholecystectomy, isolation of the cystic duct and artery (LC-2) involves performing repeated pushing and spreading (PS-SP - Table 1) maneuvers which in turn requires pushing forces mainly along the Z axis (F_z) and spreading forces (F_g) on the handle that form a characteristic pattern or signature. These 14 states can be grouped into three broader types (*I, II, III*) based on the number of movements performed simultaneously. Type *I* are fundamental maneuvers that include the idle state (moving the tool in space without touching any structures within the insufflated abdomen). The forces and torques used in idle state represent mainly the interaction of the trocar with the abdominal wall plus smaller gravitational and inertial forces. In the grasping and spreading states, compression and tension are applied to tissue by closing/opening the grasper handle. In the pushing state, compression is applied to tissue by moving the tool along the Z axis. For sweeping, the tool is placed in one position while rotating around the X and Y axes (trocar frame). Type *II* and type *III* states are defined as combinations of two or three Type I states (Table 2).

During the second step of the data analysis, Hidden Markov Models (HMM) and the methodology for evaluating surgical skill in laparoscopic surgery were develop. HMMs were selected for modeling the surgical procedure because their generic architecture fitted very well the nature of laparoscopic surgery task assessment. Moreover, the HMM mathematical formulation provided a very compact form that statistically summarized relatively complex tasks such as individual steps of a laparoscopic surgery procedure.

Type	State Name	State Acronym	Force / Torque Pattern						
			Fx	Fy	Fz	Tx	Ty	Tz	Fg
I	Idle	ID	*	*	*	*	*	*	*
	Grasping	GR							+
	Spreading	SP							-
	Pushing	PS			-				
	Sweeping	SW	+/-	+/-		+/-	+/-		
II	Grasping - Pulling	GR-PL			+				+
	Grasping - Pushing	GR-PS			-				+
	Grasping - Sweeping	GR-SW	+/-	+/-		+/-	+/-		+
	Pushing - Spreading	PS-SP			-				-
	Pushing - Sweeping	PS-SW	+/-	+/-	-	+/-	+/-		
	Sweeping - Spreading	SW-SP	+/-	+/-		+/-	+/-		-
III	Grasping - Pulling - Sweeping	GR-PL-SW	+/-	+/-	+	+/-	+/-		+
	Grasping -Pushing - Sweeping	GR-PS-SW	+/-	+/-	-	+/-	+/-		+
	Pushing - Sweeping - Spreading	PS-SW-SP	+/-	+/-	-	+/-	+/-		-

Table 1: Definition of tool/tissue interactions and the corresponding directions of forces and torques applied during MIS.

Each laparoscopic surgical step could be decomposed into a series of finite *states* defined by the way the surgeon is interacting with the tissues (Table 1). The surgeon could move from one state to another or stay in the same. Once the surgeon was interacting with the tissue in a specific state, a certain F/T signature was applied by the surgeon through the surgical tool to the tissue. These F/T signatures, each defined as an *observation,* was composed of seven components vector of data $(F_x, F_y, F_z, T_x, T_y, T_z, F_g)$. Since the F/T were continues stream of data distributed normally, each state could be defined by seven normal distributions functions chartered by a mean and a standard deviation ($N_i(\mu, \sigma)$ $i = 1...7$). Combining the 7 elements vector into joint multivariable distribution function $f(O)$ was done by using Eq. 1.

$$f(O) = \frac{1}{(\sqrt{2\pi})^N |\Sigma|^{1/2}} e^{-(O-\mu)'\Sigma^{-1}(O-\mu)/2}$$ (1)

where: O is the F/T observation vector; μ is the mean vector; Σ is the covariance matrix, and N is the observation vector size.

An example of the state analysis is given in Figure 2. The diagram describes the process of deconstructing a laparoscopic surgical procedure step. Circles in this diagram represented states and lines represented transitions between states. The F/T data - observation signals were not included in Fig. 2. The HMM is termed "hidden" due to the fact that tool/tissue interactions - the states - not included in the analysis and the only observed signals are the F/T data. Although any procedure step could be decomposed manually using a frame-by-frame video analysis, this is time consuming and unnecessary since the data can also be evaluated mathematically by the HMM once its parameters are optimized.

From the mathematical perspective, four elements should be defined in order to specify a HMM (λ) [23]: (*i*) the number of states in the model – N, (*ii*) the state transition probability distribution matrix – A, (*iii*) the observation symbol probability distribution matrix – B, and (*iv*) the initial state distribution vector– π. The HMM is then defined by the compact notation (7)

$$\lambda = (A, B, \pi)$$ (2)

Given the HMM architecture there are three basic problems of interest [1]: (*i*) The evaluation problem – Computing the probability (P) of the observation sequence given the model (λ) and the observation sequence (O).

$$\text{Given: } \begin{cases} \lambda = (A, B, \pi) \\ O = o_1, o_1, ..., o_T \end{cases} \qquad \text{Compute: } \{ P(O \mid \lambda) \qquad (3)$$

(*ii*) Uncover the hidden states – Computing the corresponding hidden state sequence (Q), given the observation sequence (O) and the model (λ).

$$\text{Given: } \begin{cases} \lambda = (A, B, \pi) \\ O = o_1, o_2, ..., o_T \end{cases} \qquad \text{Compute: } \{ Q = q_1, q_2, ..., q_T \qquad (4)$$

(*iii*) The training problem – Adjusting the model parameters (A, B, π) to maximize the probability (P) of the observation sequence (O).

$$\text{Given: } \{ \lambda = (A, B, \pi) \}; \text{ Adjust: } \{ A, B, \pi \text{ ; Maximize: } \{ P(O \mid \lambda) \qquad (5)$$

Using the given HMM architecture (Fig. 2a), HMMs were trained for each surgeon performing each step of the surgical procedure (8 HMM models, one for each surgeon performing one surgical procedure step). The skill level of each subject (R1, R3, R5) was evaluated based on the statistical distance between his/her HMMs and the expert surgeons (ES)

Given two HMMs λ_1 and λ_2 the statistical distances between them $D(\lambda_1, \lambda_2)$ and $D(\lambda_2, \lambda_1)$ were defined by Eq. 6

$$D(\lambda_1, \lambda_2) = \frac{1}{T_{O_2}} [\log P(O_2 \mid \lambda_1) - \log P(O_2 \mid \lambda_2)] \text{ ; } D(\lambda_2, \lambda_1) = \frac{1}{T_{O_1}} [\log P(O_1 \mid \lambda_1) - \log P(O_1 \mid \lambda_2)] \qquad (6)$$

$D(\lambda_1, \lambda_2)$ is a measure of how well model λ_1 matches observations generated by model λ_2 relative to how well model λ_2 matches observations generated by itself. Since $D(\lambda_1, \lambda_2)$ and $D(\lambda_2, \lambda_1)$ are nonsymmetrical, The natural expression of the symmetrical version is defined by Eq. 7.

$$D_S(\lambda_1, \lambda_2) = \frac{D(\lambda_1, \lambda_2) + D(\lambda_2, \lambda_1)}{2} \qquad (7)$$

In order to scale the statistical distance between the various groups (R1, R3, R5) and the expert surgeons (ES), for each surgical procedure the statistical distance between a certain group and the expert group ($D_S(\lambda_{Ri}, \lambda_{ESi})$) was normalized with respect to the distance between the two experts ($D_S(\lambda_{ES1}, \lambda_{ES2})$) - Eq. 8.

$$\overline{D}_S(\lambda_{Ri}, \lambda_{ESi}) = \frac{D(\lambda_{Ri}, \lambda_{ESi})}{D_S(\lambda_{ES1}, \lambda_{ES2})} \qquad (8)$$

The practical meaning of the normalized statistical distance ($\overline{D}_S(\lambda_{Ri}, \lambda_{ESi})$) is how far each subject is from performing like the sampled expert surgeons.

3. Results

The data analysis demonstrated several phenomena. First, expert and novice surgeons took different paths to reach the same goal. Each group utilized states and transitions not used by the other group. Secondly, studying the median completion time of the novice surgeon group and the expert surgeon group showed a significant difference between these groups ($p<0.05$). The surgical procedure's completion time was longer for the R1 by a factor of 1.5 to 4.8 when compared to the ES. The difference between R1 and ES was more profound in steps requiring higher dexterity and more complex skills compared to steps where a specific organ was placed in a specific position (e.g. positioning of the gallbladder). The main factor contributing to the significant difference in the completion times between R1 and ES was the time spent in the *idle* state. The R1 spent significantly more time in the idle state compare to the ES.

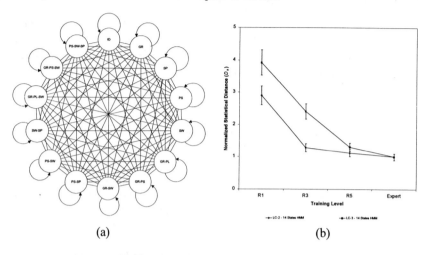

(a)   (b)

Figure 2: HMM Analysis - **(a)** HMM architecture defined by 14 fully connected state diagram (arrow heads of all the lines connected two states were omitted for simplifying the drawing) **(b)** The performance or "learning" curve of surgical residents while performing MIS - Normalized statistical distance between two different HMM architectures (continuous 14 state model, and discrete 4 state model) representing the performance of surgical residents(R1, R3, R5) at different year of training compared to experts surgeons

HMMs were developed foreach of the 8 subjects (and statistical distances were normalized ($\bar{D}_S$ - Eq. 8) between ES and R1 ,R3 ,R5 (Fig. 2b). The objective laparoscopic surgical skill learning curve showed significant differences between all skill levels (Fig.2b). The $\bar{D}_S$ value converged to a value of one exponentially as expertise increased although the highest gradient was between R1 and R3. This results suggest that surgical residents acquire a major portion of their laparoscopic surgical capabilities between the first and the third years of training. Calculating the $\bar{D}_S$ values for LC-1 (not plotted in Fig.2b) showed no significant difference between the groups. This is correlated with the F/T magnitude differentiation analysis between the R1 and ES. The practical meaning of that result is that a simple surgical maneuver such as LC-1 may not include sufficient haptic information to differentiate skill levels. On the other hand, more complex steps such as LC-2 and LC-3 do provide such information (Fig. 2b).

4. Discussion

Surgery with minimally invasive techniques is a complex task that requires a synthesis between visual and haptic information. Analyzing MIS in terms of these two sources of information is a key step towards developing objective criteria evaluating technicalperformance.. The power of this methodology is that it brings together thousands of observations through different aspect of a surgical procedure into a single, objectively-derived number. This number represents the probability that surgical performance for the subject under study approximates that of an expert.

The preliminary results expressed in this study suggest that HMMs derived from carefully standardized surgical tasks should allow objective quantification of skill based on the statistical distance between HMMs. Moreover, this methodology may be useful to determine if a surgical trainee's technical performance matches his or her peers.

Another facet of the HMM methodology for objective surgical skill assessment arises from the fact that it is not limited to the *in-vivo* conditions demonstrated in the current studybut could be extended to other modalities such as surgical simulators and robotic systems.

Acknowledgments

This work was supported by a major grant from United States Surgical, a Division of Tyco-Healthcare, Inc. to the University of Washington, USSC Center for Videoendoscopic Surgery.

References

[1]   Rabiner L.R., a Tutorial on hidden Markov models and selected application in speech recognition, Proceedings of the IEEE, Vol. 77, No. 2, Feb 1989.

[2]   B. Hannaford, P. Lee, "Hidden Markov Model Analysis of Force/Torque Information in Telemanipulation," Proceedings 1st International Symposium on Experimental Robotics, Montreal, June 1989.

[3]   B. Hannaford, P. Lee, "Hidden Markov Model of Force Torque Information in Telemanipulation," International Journal of Robotics Research, vol. 10, no. 5, pp. 528-539, 1991.

[4]   B. Hannaford, P. Lee, "Multi-Dimensional Hidden Markov Model of Telemanipulation Tasks with Varying Outcomes," Proceedings IEEE Intl. Conf. Systems Man and Cybernetics, Los Angeles, CA, Nov. 1990.

[5]   Rosen J., M. MacFarlane, C. Richards, B. Hannaford, C. Pellegrini, M. Sinanan, Surgeon/Endoscopic Tool Force-Torque Signatures In The Evaluation of Surgical Skills During Minimally Invasive Surgery, Studies in Health Technology and Informatics - Medicine Meets Virtual Reality, Vol. 62, pp. 290-296, January 1999.

[6]   Rosen J., C. Richards, B. Hannaford, M. Sinanan, Hidden Markov Models of Minimally Invasive Surgery, Studies in Health Technology and Informatics - Medicine Meets Virtual Reality, Vol. 70 pp. 279-285, January 2000.

[7]   Richards C., J. Rosen, B. Hannaford, M. MacFarlane, C. Pellegrini, M. Sinanan, Skills Evaluation in Minimally Invasive Surgery Using Force/Torque Signatures, Surgical Endoscopy

Medicine Meets Virtual Reality 2001
J.D. Westwood et al. (Eds.)
IOS Press, 2001

Digital trainer developed for robotic assisted cardiac surgery

Jan Sigurd Røtnes[1,2], Johannes Kaasa[1], Geir Westgaard[1],
Eivind Myrold Eriksen[1], Per Øyvind Hvidsten[1], Kyrre Strøm[1],
Vidar Sørhus[1], Yvon Halbwachs[1],Ole Jakob Elle[2], Erik Fosse[2]

1) *SimSurgery AS, email: j.s.rotnes@simsurgery.no*
   URL: www.simsurgery.no
2) *Interventional Centre, National Hospital, Rikshospitalet,*
   N-0027 Oslo, Norway, email: j.s.rotnes@klinmed.uio.no
   URL: www.rikshospitalet.no/intervensjon

Abstract: Robotic systems for cardiac surgery have been introduced in clinical trials to facilitate minimally invasive techniques. Widespread use of surgical robotics necessitates new training methods to improve skills and continue practicing as the robotic systems are frequently being upgraded. Today, robotic training is performed on expensive animal models. An integration of a digital trainer with the two present robotic systems applied in coronary artery bypass procedures on beating heart requires real time simulation of tissue mechanics, sutures, instruments and bleeding. However, it requires no extra haptic device, since the robotic master is the haptic apparatus itself. By developing new data structures and parametric geometry descriptions we have demonstrated the possibility of obtaining surgical simulation on a standard PC Linux system. This technology is beneficial when simulation is exploited over a network with limited bandwidth, especially when it comes to the handling of soft tissue dynamics.

1. Introduction

Minimal invasive, image guided therapy is one of the main trends in medicine today, either as interventional radiological techniques or as video-assisted surgery. This trend is facilitated by the development of information and image acquisition technologies and the combination of the two. In the treatment of some diseases, like gall-bladder disease, peripheral vascular disease or coronary disease, minimally invasive techniques are already applied to most cases. It is likely that this trend will continue when fully digitized imaging modalities further develops along with robotic technology. The new interventional procedures require quite different skills than conventional surgical techniques, thus, the need for facilitating the education and training process is very important. Virtual reality surgical training is an educational method ideal for image guided procedures. Simulator technology with appropriate tactile feedback from the instrument implies a training potential similar to animal and cadaver cases without the ethical and financial limitations

[1-3]. We have also experienced quite a challenge in keeping the heart of the animals beating throughout the training procedures.

The surgical procedure in coronary artery bypass surgery is now undergoing significant changes. The standard method until now has been operation on arrested heart through a sternotomy access. To avoid using an artificial heart-lung machine (and hence reduce potential adverse effects as brain lesions and reduce cost by omitting the pump) new off-pump minimally invasive techniques are introduced, with both sternotomy and more minimally invasive accesses. Surgical methods in these off-pump procedures require new skills because the operation is performed on beating-heart, and also because new instruments and techniques are required. Telemanipulation (robotic surgery) is one such beating-heart enabling technology. Controlling the robotic master devices requires significant training since the technology imposes both new possibilities and limitations.

To provide realism in surgical simulators with objects in the scene that exhibit physically correct behaviors - new geometric modeling techniques are necessary unless conventional techniques are applied on supercomputers with many processors [4]. Real-time simulation of a surgical procedure with speed and realism in its presentation requires models that include both the viscoelastically behaviors of organs together with the anchoring of the biologic structures. The practical constrain in simulator systems comprises appropriate modeling methods, computational power and haptic apparatus. In telemanipulating systems the latter is an integrated part of new technologies that would appreciate a digital simulator, thus the haptic system itself is not a challenge in our digital simulation development.

In this paper we report our experiences with parameterized geometric models integrated with tissue mechanical properties, a generic technology suitable for surgical digital simulators that we applied in the development of a digital simulator for robotic assisted cardiac surgery.

2. Material & Tools

A new company, SimSurgery™, was established as a joint venture between the Interventional Centre (Rikshospitalet-National Hospital of Norway) and The Mobile Media Company to develop core modeling technologies and products with focus on medical applications. The Interventional Centre [5] is a research and development department combining surgical, radiological and engineering methods to develop new minimally invasive procedures. In the robotic Zeus™ [6] program at the Interventional Centre (Figure 1), a project was established to develop a digital simulator for coronary anastomosis surgery, financed partly by governmental trust funds (SND and The Research Council of Norway).

The three major parts of the digital simulator are the geometric model, the physical model, and the tissue-tool interaction. The need for fast and realistic simulation of the dynamic behavior of the organs, together with a high level of interactivity, including cutting, grasping, and suturing, put strong requirements on the representation of the geometric and physical models. Most systems for surgical simulation apply polygon-based geometric models with either a finite element or spring-mass formulation of the physical model [7-9]. Implementation of a polygon-based geometrical model yields a large number of nodes that need to be included in the physical model, and thereby slowing down the simulation. A reduction of the resolution of the polygon mesh, however, will reduce the visual realism of the geometrical object. Furthermore, polygon-based modeling also entails great complexity with introduction of topology changes for instance when tissues are cut (operated on).

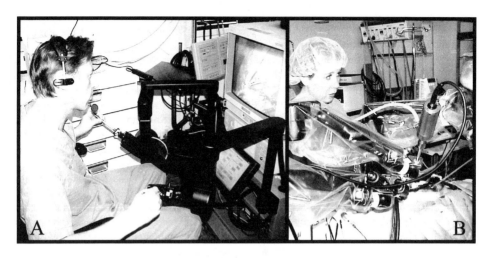

Figure 1 The master console (A) of the robotic system Zeus™ (B) from a coronary
beating-heart training session with a pig.

As for the physical model, the finite element model is a discrete formulation of a
continuum, and another method is the spring-mass model, which represents a division of
the physical object into particles (distributed masses) with springs connecting the particles.
The spring-mass model yields a simpler and more flexible model, and is therefore better
suited for on-line topological changes.

We wanted to develop a new geometric representation format combined with
appropriate data structures which model the intrinsic tissue properties and which
approximately exhibit physically correct behaviors as in the real viscoelastically anatomy.
First, we applied a Non-Uniform Rational B-Splines-like technology (NURBS), defined on
regular mesh, in hierarchical object-oriented data structures (Geometry Anchored
Geometries- GAGs, Norwegian patent, USA patent pending) for the geometric modeling.

The speed and realism of the simulation of interaction between a simple suture
model and a vessel geometry was very promising, but cutting hole in the geometric
representation (tissue) and thereby changing the topology for arbitrary cutting directions
entailed the need for an alternative to the GAGs technology. By implementing
parameterized surface representations defined on irregular mesh, we obtained larger
potentials in representation of local geometry, multiple smooth deformations, variable
smooth resolution and more efficient change of topology.

The elastodynamical properties of the tissue/vessels were simulated as control
points in the parameterized geometric structures, i.e. the control points of the geometrical
structures were defined as a subset of the particles in a spring-mass model. The suture
model was represented of elements of smooth, continuos geometrical structures.
Instruments, textures and other environment details were integrated by utilizing 3-D
graphic hardware. The geometrical model and the elastodynamical parameters of the
physical model were defined as a priori information from empirical observations of clinical
cases.

Linux was chosen as the operating system for the simulator. We have found Linux suitable as the operating system for a real-time system, interfaced with new fast graphic cards. The main advantage is its open-source availability. Unnecessary constrain could appear in a demanding real-time system without the freedom of modifying the operating system. Linux is also an ideal platform for remote maintenance and system update that we believe is important with increasing employment of simulators. Linux distributions often consist of complete developer packages for facile startup, thus, we see an increasing amount of nice creative software being developed. Linux allow parallel processor design. However, Linux still lack (September 2000) optimal hardware drivers especially with OpenGL calls.

3. Results

The parameterized geometries implemented on standard PC Linux system resulted in fast animation and realistic performance, due to the dramatically more efficient method of data structuring and data handling. The more complex the 3-D model was, the more efficient the modeling became, as compared to tasks solved with more conventional 3-D polygon-based methods. In our prototype (September 2000) the suture model was integrated with our new data structure for dynamical three dimensional (3D) geometries comprising a simulated Internal Mammary Artery (IMA) and the Left Anterior Descending coronary artery (LAD) (Figure 2). Interaction between structures modeled with different geometric representations, like the suture penetrating the vessel walls appeared realistic, but involved new technical solutions. The necessary computational power for realistic appearance and real-time interaction (30 frames/sec) between the suture model and the modeled arteries was much lower than what was available on the simulator with one Pentium III processor (700 MHz). A result we found very promising for solving more demanding computational tasks e.g. to simulate knot tying.

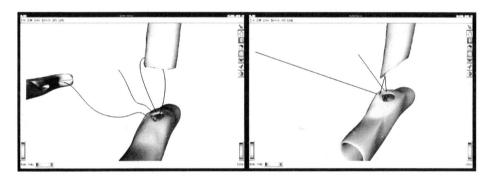

Figure 2. Two examples of single frames (A and B) from 30 frames/sec sequences where the simulated suture pull the simulated Internal Mammary Artery (IMA) towards the Left Anterior Descending coronary artery (LAD).

The software models were resolution independent, thereby enabling structures to appear simple when viewed from far away, and to expose complex details when viewed up close. This increased the potential efficiency of complex interactive applications such as surgical simulators (Figure 3).

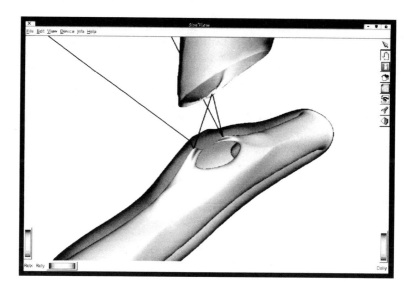

Figure 3. A close up still image of the geometry around the suture penetrating the vessel wall. The adventitia (the exterior of the vessel) is partly removed by choosing low opacity parameters whereas the endothelium/intima (the interior layer of the vessel) is displayed with more details.

4. Discussion

Physical models made of synthetic material or from animal preparations have been implemented in many surgical training programs [10-11]. Although, physical models expose realism in regard to tissue behavior, we believe that digital training simulators with proper haptic devices will be more eligible as a training aid in the future, especially due to its assortment of educational features as:

- Individual digital proctors can serve as an integrated part of the simulator based on skills and ambitions of the students. The (virtual) individual proctor can provide relevant training scenarios as well as report progress and comparative information.
- The quality and effectiveness of carrying out a simulated procedure can be recorded, and the data can form valuable feedback by analyzing the instrument trajectories and visualizing the results e.g. simulating an angiographic sequence after a coronary bypass.
- The clinical diversity experienced in real life due to differences in anatomy, different pathological processes and stages, requires a large and flexible model basis that is probably only possible with a digital trainer.
- Several digital trainers might be connected in a network that renders an effective way to maintain and update the systems. Furthermore, a database that includes recordings from the training sessions might provide valuable statistical information.

- New medical technologies like surgical robots also demand innovation in design of new instruments and visualization systems. Production, testing and distribution of such prototypes are expensive which might exclude good ideas to be tried out. However, by introducing a virtual model in a digital simulator important feedback might be provided from the users to the designers before physical prototyping and testing – virtual "beta-testing".

- Video database, 3D-anatomical atlas, multimedia presentations and videoconferences from "live" procedures may run on the same digital platform as the digital simulators, and thereby enhance the quality and extend the content of training sessions.

- The same technologies applied in surgical simulators might be utilized in surgical planning, as a tool in developing new clinical procedures and in the future it might serve as an enabling technology for autonomous robotic systems.

- The purchase expense of a physical model based training system is most likely to be lower than it is for a digital system, but the total cost of ownership with much use may be higher.

- Training with a digital simulator is a novel approach with versatile pedagogic potentials that might motivate physicians to improve their skills and better assess new techniques.

A variety of programs and systems are today available in surgical training. Some training centers can also provide digital training methods. One digital training tool currently applied, is the simulator MIST (Virtual Presence, London, UK) that is designed for training two-handed laparascopic procedures by creating a virtual environment representing tasks not similar to a real clinical situation, but rather part-tasks constructed for training coordination and instrument manipulation [12]. The employment of the MIST is based on the idea that many of the part-tasks that constitute a clinical procedure can be learned without working on realistic tissue and suture models. This concept has been shown to improve the learning curve in laparoscopic procedures [13-14].

Our objective in developing an anastomosis simulator for robotic assisted Endoscopic Coronary Artery Bypass Grafting (Endo-CABG) is to focus on the most critical part of the procedure and produce a virtual environment that in addition to instrument coordination also reflects the anatomy and tissue mechanics similar to clinical situations. By including other features possible with digital simulators we believe that in the future the number of animal trails can be reduced, and more important that the overall clinical performance can be significantly improved.

The technology applied in the simulator, is a geometry format that describes the organs as continues, non-discrete, surfaces in a very compact and efficient way. This representation and its corresponding data structure also entail utilization of the technology in situations when, e.g. endoluminal implants and artificial valves are virtually placed in soft tissue and analyzed and evaluated by simulation. This utilization of the geometrical format is very appropriate since all the derived vectors as gradients would be continues in contradiction to situations with discrete polygon-based models.

The geometry format also provides an enabling technology when simulations are carried out through a network with limited bandwidth and critical time delays. Especially, when it comes to handling of soft tissue dynamics, as in tele-surgery where time delays are very critical. However, the time delays in remote control can partly be bypassed by working on virtual models reflecting the reality where the models are constantly being updated by the obtainable information. Implementation of such a hybrid control design would require efficient dynamical models as in simulators.

References

[1] S. L. Dawson and J. A. Kaufman. The imperative for medical simulation. Proceedings of the IEEE. 86(3):479-83, 1998

[2] P. J. Gorman, A. H. Meier, and T. M. Krummel. Simulation and virtual reality in surgical education: Real or unreal? Archives of Surgery. 134:1203-8, 1999

[3] R. M. Satava and S. B. Jones. Current and future applications of virtual reality for medicine. Proceedings of the IEEE. 86(3):484-9, 1998

[4] G. Székely, C. Brechbühler, R. Hutter, A. Rhomberg, N.Ironmonger and P. Schmid, Modelling of Soft Tissue Deformation for Laparoscopic Surgery Simulation, First International Conference on Medical Image Computing and Computer-Assisted Intervention MICCAI'98, 1998

[5] E. Fosse, F. Laerum, JS Rotnes The Interventional Centre-31 months experience with a department merging surgical and image-guided intervention. Minimally Invasive Therapy and Allied Technologies. 8 (5) : 361-369, 1999

[6] Computer Motion, Inc., 130-B Cremona Drive, Goleta, CA, USA, http://www.computermotion.com/

[7] M. Bro-Nielsen. Finite element modeling in surgery simulation. Proceedings of the IEEE. 86(3):490-503, 1998

[8] S. Cotin, H. Delingette, and N. Ayache. Real-time elastic deformations of soft tissues for surgery simulation. IEEE Transactions On Visualization and Computer Graphics, 5(1):62-73, 1999

[9] U. Kühnapfel, H.K. Çakmak and H. Maaß. 3D Modeling for Endoscopic Surgery. In: Proc. IEEE Symposium on Simulation, Delft , NL, Oct. 13, 1999. 22-32, 1999

[10] Rex De L. Stanbridge, David O'Regan, Ashok Cherian and R.Ramanan, Use of a Pulsatile Beating Heart Model for Training Surgeons in Beating Heart Surgery, Department of Cardiothoracic Surgery, St Mary's Hospital, London W2 1NY UK. Presented at the Second Annual Meeting of the International Society for Minimally Invasive Cardiac Surgery, Palais dés Congres, Paris, France, May 21-22, 1999 http://www.hsforum.com/vol2/issue4/1999-8488.html

[11] The Chamberlain Group, MA, USA http://www.thecgroup.com/

[12] Virtual Presence Limited, The Canvas House, London, SE1 2NL, UK http://www.vrweb.com/WEB/DEV/MEDICAL.HTM#MIST

[13] A. Chaudhry, C. Sutton, J. Wood, R. Stone and R. McCloy, Learning rate for laparoscopic surgical skills on MIST VR, a virtual reality simulator: quality of human-computer interface, Annals of the Royal College of Surgeons of England. 81(4):281-6, 1999

[14] A.G. Gallagher, N. McClure. J. McGuigan. I. Crothers and J. Browning, Virtual reality training in laparoscopic surgery: a preliminary assessment of minimally invasive surgical trainer virtual reality (MIST VR), Endoscopy. 31(4):310-3, 1999

Medicine Meets Virtual Reality 2001
J.D. Westwood et al. (Eds.)
IOS Press, 2001

A NEW PORTABLE EQUIPMENT FOR DETECTION OF PSYCHOPHYSICAL CONDITIONS

A. Rovetta (*), A. Cucè (**), D. Platania (**),C. Solenghi (*)

(*) Politecnico di Milano, Dipartimento di Meccanica
Piazza Leonardo da Vinci, 32 20133 Milano (MI)
E-Mail: alberto.rovetta@polimi.it
Fax: +39-02-70638377
(**) STMicroelectronics, Soft Computing Operation Group
Via Bramante, 65 26013 Crema (CR)
E-Mail: Tonino.Cuce@st.com
Fax: +39-0373-282040

Keywords: virtual reality, biorobotics, Parkinson disease

Abstract

This paper deals with the Disease Detector (DDX) that is a virtual reality control system for detection of Parkinson disease.
The control system consists of a small board with an internal fuzzy micro controller capable of acquiring, through the joystick, the well known three basic parameters (reaction, speed and force) in order to detect the state of health and perform them by fuzzy rules. The resulting output can be visualized through a display or transmitted by a communication interface.

1. Introduction

This paper deals with the Disease Detector (DDX), a new portable equipment with detection of response time and psychophysical conditions in normal and exceptional environments also with virtual reality measurements with a fuzzy-based control system. It may be adopted for earth and space applications, because of its portability, in order to measure all the reactions in front of external effects. The external effects require 1) the response to sounds, 2) a soft touch of a button, 3) by pronouncing a word, 4) the touch of the finger in front of a virtual reality drawing of the finger itself, and the equipment is able to measure the reaction time of the person.
On the other hand, the development of internet and satellite communications makes remote health diagnosis very useful and interesting. It could be possible to check individual states of health whilst they are leading their normal lives.

2. Tools

DDX (Disease Detector) is an experimental bioengineer system for the acquisition and the restitution of some data about human finger movement. It has been originally applied for the analysis of neural disturbs with quantitative evaluation of both the response times and the dynamics action of the subject. Now, it is applied in the clinical activity, daily for the diagnostic of progressing of pathology of the Parkinson disease.

The system obtains such goal using the following protocols:

- Fast Movement: starting from a fixed point of initial reference, the person must use the index finger to touch as fast as possible the target which measures the impressed force; in parallel, other parameters are measured, as the angular position, the speed of finger and the time of reaction.

- Movement with Virtual control: the person looks at a virtual image on a graphical display of his own finger and when he touches real target, then the virtual one changes color indicating that it has been caught up and this is the end of the test.

3. Purpose

Through DDX it is possible to point out some characteristics about the extension of the index finger of one hand with the target to find and to estimate the kinematics characteristics, the control of the movement and the impressed force.

The system is composed by:

- a skeleton: mounted on a support structure to acquire the finger position of the patient who puts his hand in a glove in vertical position.

- variable rotational resistors: sited in correspondence of the phalanx are able to retrieve finger movements.

- surface active electrodes: these send a signal to the electromiograph through a double channel probe.

The other parameters are acquired from the button and these are: reaction time (defined as the delay time from acoustic signal of buzzer to the starting of pressure), speed (calculated from the starting point to the end point of button race) and force (by using a strain gage). So the mechanics of button was the following one.

4. Methods

In figure we introduce the block diagram which describes, from the functional point of view, the structure of the new proposed system DDX.

The block (1) is the press button. This is the input patient interface and its function is to capture indirectly three basic information for diagnosis: the response time, the speed and the pressure of the fingertip. Effectively, it captures the start time of button pressure, the end time and the force impressed by using a strain gage.

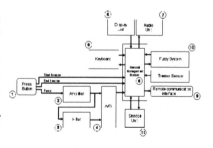

The analog force signal is first amplified in block (2), after it is filtered by block (3) and then converted in a 8-bit digital form by block (4). All these three information are collected from block (6) which is the heart of the system and directs the informations flow among peripherals. Blocks (5,8) represents the medical operator interface to give commands and to read outputs. The block (6) manages all informations and stores them in block (11) if it is necessary. Tremor is also caught up by a very cheap switch accelerometer that we call "Tremor Sensor".

The block (10) performs fuzzy rules on acquired data and return diagnosis results that will be output on display (5). The audio unit, composed by a simple buzzer, is used to synchronize the patient actions in relation to the kind of test.

5. Results

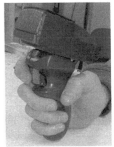

The target is the realisation of a portable, user-friendly machine, like a mobile phone, with more efficient diagnostic results in order to gain advantages compared to existing detection systems. The ability to hold the joystick with a single hand is the fundamental aspect of this system. A person's state of health may be tested daily.

In order to avoid putting patients off, the color scheme has been altered accordingly.

6. Conclusions

In this paper, we have described an innovative system for Parkinson disease detection. Present systems of detection are very reliable but not portable.

The solution proposed, by using virtual reality, takes the advantage of portability without losing in efficiency and in diagnosis efficiency.

It is also provided the ability of transferring diagnosis through a remote communication interface in order to monitor daily the state of health of a patient.

The system is an intelligent-machine based on soft computing techniques and so, its efficiency can be improved considering more example for membership function calibration or, moreover, improving the response correctness by using a self learning technique.

References

[1] A. Rovetta, F. Lorini, M. Canina, A New Project for Rehabilitation and Psychomotor Disease Analysis with Virtual Reality Support, IOS Press , (1998) Medicine Meets Virtual Reality .

[2] A. Antonini, A Rovetta., R. Fariello, M. Barichella, F. Lorini M. Canina, G. Pezzoli, A novel device in the evaluation of motor impairement in Parkinson Disease, Fifth International Congress of Parkinson's Disease and Movement Disorders, New York, October 10-14, 1998

[3] J. C. Eccles, How the Self controls its Brain, 1994

[4] J.P. Changeux, L'homme neuronal, Paris, 1983

[5] H. Lopes Da Silva, Spatio-temporal analysis of brain signals, Workshop: "Detection and Multimodal Analisys of Brain weak Signals to Study Brain Function Desease", Politecnico di Milano, 29 November 1997

Medicine Meets Virtual Reality 2001
J.D. Westwood et al. (Eds.)
IOS Press, 2001

3D Visualization and Stereographic Techniques for Medical Research and Education

Martin Rydmark, MD, Ph.D., Torben Kling-Petersen, Ph.D.,
Ragnar Pascher and Fiona Philip

Mednet (The Computer Laboratory of the Medical Faculty),
Göteborg University, Box 417, SE 405 30 GÖTEBORG (SWEDEN)
E: martin.rydmark@mednet.gu.se , URL: http://www.mednet.gu.se

Abstract. While computers have been able to work with true 3D models for a long time, the same does not apply to the users in common. Over the years, a number of 3D visualization techniques have been developed to enable a scientist or a student, to see not only a flat representation of an object, but also an approximation of its Z-axis. In addition to the traditional flat image representation of a 3D object, at least four established methodologies exist:

Stereo pairs. Using image analysis tools or 3D software, a set of images can be made, each representing the left and the right eye view of an object. Placed next to each other and viewed through a separator, the three dimensionality of an object can be perceived. While this is usually done on still images, tests at Mednet have shown this to work with interactively animated models as well. However, this technique requires some training and experience.

Pseudo3D, such as VRML or QuickTime VR, where the interactive manipulation of a 3D model lets the user achieve a sense of the model's true proportions. While this technique works reasonably well, it is not a "true" stereographic visualization technique.

Red/Green separation, i.e. "the traditional 3D image" where a red and a green representation of a model is superimposed at an angle corresponding to the viewing angle of the eyes and by using a similar set of eyeglasses, a person can create a mental 3D image. The end result does produce a sense of 3D but the effect is difficult to maintain.

Alternating left/right eye systems. These systems (typified by the StereoGraphics CrystalEyes® system) let the computer display a "left eye" image followed by a "right eye" image while simultaneously triggering the eyepiece to alternatively make one eye "blind". When run at 60 Hz or higher, the brain will fuse the left/right images together and the user will effectively see a 3D object. Depending on configurations, the alternating systems run at between 50 and 60 Hz, thereby creating a flickering effect, which is strenuous for prolonged use.

However, all of the above have one or more drawbacks such as high costs, poor quality and localized use.

A fifth system, recently released by Barco Systems, modifies the CrystalEyes system by projecting two superimposed images, using polarized light, with the wave plane of the left image at right angle to that of the right image. By using polarized glasses, each eye will see the appropriate image and true stereographic vision is achieved. While the system requires very expensive hardware, it solves some of the more important problems mentioned above, such as the capacity to use higher frame rates and the ability to display images to a large audience.

Mednet has instigated a research project which uses reconstructed models from the central nervous system (human brain and basal ganglia, cortex, dendrites and dendritic spines) and peripheral nervous system (nodes of Ranvier and axoplasmic areas). The aim is to modify the models to fit the different visualization techniques mentioned above and compare a group of users perceived degree of 3D for each technique.

1. Introduction

During the last decade 3D-modelling has emerged from the specialized laboratories equipped with high-end computers, now easily accomplished with competent PCs and Macs. Over the years, a number of 3D visualization techniques have been developed to enable a scientist or a student to see not only a still and flat representation of an object, but also an approximation of its depth. At least four established methodologies exist:

Interactive 3D models displayed in 2D, where the movement produces the necessary depth cue, are probably the most common. Examples of this technique are web based VRML, QuickTime 3D, Cult 3D and desktop applications such as TGS 3-SpaceAssistant. We usually refer to these techniques as "Pseudo3D".

Early attempts within the scientific community to display 3D objects using 2D techniques eventually resulted in the generation of two semi-identical images usually 5-10 degrees apart, generally referred to as "stereopairs". This technique was adopted, especially within areas such as organic chemistry and morphology, where the need to see a molecule or similar in 3D is very important. This approach requires at most, a set of plastic binoculars although many experienced users quickly accomplish this without any paraphernalia.

The approach taken by the movie industry to accomplish 3D visualization, as part of a motion picture, is to overlay two images (one tinted red and one tinted green). Issuing the audience with red/green spectacles allows each eye to see the "correct angles image", which produces a 3D image in the mind of the viewer. While inexpensive, this technique unfortunately destroys most, if not all, of the color in the image. The red/green separation technique is also very difficult to endure for a long period of time.

A further development, of the above mentioned techniques, is still dependant on supplying each eye with an image with the correct angle of viewing. Modern computers with fast graphics cards do this by displaying alternating images for the left and right eye, usually with a frequency of 60 Hz or more. Synchronized to these shifts is a set of specialized glasses where an LCD screen is made transparent in the same alternating pattern as the screen. As the frequency is faster than the human visual system, the brain will fuse these images into a coherent 3D image. At lower frequencies the flickering is strenuous for prolonged use. This technique is however, by far, the most expensive and not all software can use these systems.

Taken together, all of the above methods have one or more drawbacks such as high costs, poor quality and localized use.

A fifth system, recently released by Barco Systems, modifies the CrystalEyes system by projecting two superimposed images, using polarized light, with the wave plane of the left image at right angle to that of the right image. By using polarized glasses, each eye will see the appropriate image and true stereographic vision is achieved. While the system requires very expensive hardware, it solves some of the more important problems mentioned above, such as the capacity to use higher frame rates, the use of relevant color and texture and the ability to display images to a large audience. At Mednet, Göteborg University, we do not have this Barco Systems facility.

Mednet has instigated a research project, where we use 3D reconstructions of cellular components, cells, tissues and organs from our research, in web-distribution and 3D visualization. By modifying the 3D models to fit the different visualization techniques, mentioned above, we will compare how a group of users perceive the degree of 3D, for each technique. This preliminary, very restricted study, is aimed at obtaining guidelines from a few selected test persons, for a more extended experiment on web-distributed 3D and VR (see Mednet«s home page for previous achievements: http://www.mednet.gu.se).

2. Material and methods

2.1. Neurobiological preparative work

Two objects were selected for display, one node and one dendritic spine. In both cases cat nervous tissue specimens were prepared for electron microscopy. Consecutive ultra thin sections (each about 50-100 nm thick) series were examined and sections covering a specimen thickness of some hundred micrometers were photographed. Images were realigned according to in-house produced routines [1]. The Ranvier«s node was from a nerve fiber of a spinal root; here the Schwann cell cytoplasm (the outer covering of the nerve fiber) was rendered with both its inner and outer outlining, giving the rough topology of a hollow fluted tube, constricted in the mid-part. The dendritic spine was from a neuron in hippocampus and had the topology of a branched tree, with an outer surface. In Figures 1 and 2 stereopairs of the two objects are shown.

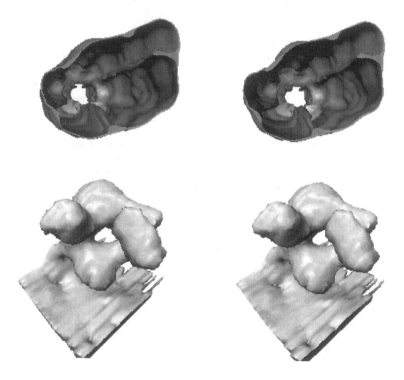

Figures 1 and 2. 3D renderings of a Ranvier s node (top) and a dendritic spine (bottom) displayed as stereopairs.

2.2. 3D-modelling

The models used in this work were created using Mednet's SGI cluster and in-house software according to techniques reported earlier [2, 3].

2.3. PC-visualization

Testing (see below) was done on an Intergraph ZX-10 workstation [www.intergraph.com] (2 x 833 MHz Pentium PC with 512 Mb RAM and a WildCat 4110 graphics card [www.intense3d.com]). The following equipment was used: for red/green separation one pair of standard red/green plastic glasses was used, for the stereopairs we used a Reflecting Stereoscope (VCH Verlagsgesellschaft, Weinheim, Germany), and the stereoscopic visualization by alternating left/right eyeglasses was accomplished using CrystalEyes CE-2 glasses [www.stereographics.com].

Visualization and generation of the various stereographic displays was done in 3-SpaceAssistant (TGS Software). Optimization of the stereo separation was done individually for each test, according to the individual test person's preferences.

2.4. Test persons

The following seven test persons were selected: one male and one female medical student at a level prior to the course in neurobiology, one male Ph.D. in zoology, one male Ph.D. in biomedicine and expert in computer science and VR (co-author Kling-Petersen), one male MD/Ph.D./Associate Professor with long time experience in 3D reconstruction, neurobiology and teaching (author Rydmark), and one male and one female professor in neurobiology.

2.5. Test and Questions

The 3D objects were presented individually for the test persons in a sequence - "pseudo 3D", "stereo pairs", "red/green separated", "crystal eyes" – first as still objects, then rotated, zoomed, etc. The following questions and possible answers followed each display situation:

1) The still object is perceived as 3D - immediately, after a few seconds, after >30 sec, never.
2) The 3D nature of the object is easier to perceive when you rotate it - (The following answering alternatives are valid for questions 2-6. – "correct", "fairly", "hardly", "no")
3) Zooming improves the perception of 3D.
4) When you are told "What the object depicts", the 3D perception is improved.
5) Color and texture are of great importance for the perception of the object.
6) A large size of the object is of great importance for the perception.

The answers were interpreted and registered as scores with 4 for the first alternative, to 1 for the last. A spreadsheet covering the objects, visualization techniques, manipulations, test persons and questions were examined for visual clues of similarities and correlation.

At the end of each individual test, each test person was asked to express pros and cons for computer based 3D, especially in comparison to magazines and books, and any other general comments.

3. Results

There was no obvious expression of differentiated 3D perception neither between the two objects (the node and the spine), nor between gender of the test persons, or the estimation of the various visualization techniques and the manipulations of the objects. However, there was a student to professional difference in the appreciation of what the object was depicting; students required (asked for) information about the object.

On this background average values of scores, rounded to one significant digit, were computed (See Table 1).

Table 1. 3D perception	Answers　　(4: yes to 1: no)				
Questions	pseudo 3D	stereo	red/green	crystal	all
1　perceived as 3D quickly?	3	4	4	4	3
2　rotating -> improved 3D?	4	4	3	4	4
3　zooming -> improved 3D?	4	3	3	3	3
4　naming -> improved 3D?	2	2	2	2	2
5　color -> improved 3D?	3	3	4	3	3
6　big size -> improved 3D?	4	3	3	3	3
		NB. Values are rounded to one significant digit			

The overall perception of 3D was quickly accomplished for all visualization techniques, although somewhat faster for the "true" 3D (N.B. Time for adjustment of the equipment was required.). The possibility to rotate and to zoom the objects was appreciated; as were color and texture and a large rendering of the object. In the case of color and texture a certain ambiguity in the answers was detected, namely, when testing "red/green" the test persons focused on the necessity to have familiar colors and texture. Further, the appreciation of a large rendering of the object was most stressed in the "pseudo 3D" situation.

Among free comments the following was noted: The male student found rotation and zooming increased the perception in all techniques and stated that the size of the object was not critical when using "crystal eyes". Further he expressed a wish for a good name indication technique of object sub-details. The female student stated that it is a great advantage to use computer assisted 3D in regard to comprehending connectivity among objects. On the other hand, books and magazines are more convenient to carry around and are more common. In conclusion, she applauded the developmental efforts for computer based visualization. The male Ph.D. zoologist's sole comment was that "pseudo 3D" was to be preferred, as one does not have to keep track of all the special equipment. The male professor said that the nature of the material is key if computer assisted 3D is to be advantageous. Further, he initially found "stereo pairs" best, but gradually "crystal eyes" improved with use. The female professor commented that computer assisted 3D could be advantageous in selected cases. "The author and the co-author" prefer to give their comments in the "Discussion" part of this work.

4. Discussion

This is not an investigation with any statistical value. The material is selected; as are the test persons. The questions clearly have a steering tendency in their semantics. On the other hand, the aims were to obtain guidelines, or rather support, for experiences or presumptions gained by the authors Rydmark, Kling-Petersen and Pascher during 10-15 years of computer assisted 3D reconstruction and education in biomedicine.

Our research profile at Mednet contains a strong component of getting research results quickly and widely distributed among research colleagues and students. Today, that means web distribution. Currently, few individuals in laboratories or universities (or home) have more than competent PCs and Macs, giving access to "pseudo 3D", and at best "stereopairs". This small survey supports the idea that "pseudo 3D" and "stereopairs" (most individuals quickly learn to fuse "stereopairs" without special equipment) could be sufficient, after a little training, given that the objects are possible to interact with, i.e. rotate, zoom, name, and have a large size.

Still the "true" 3D is advantageous in respect to quality of perception and independence of size, color/texture and interaction.

5. References

[1] Rydmark M, Jansson T, Berthold CH, Gustavsson T (1992) Computer assisted realignment of light micrograph images from consecutive section series of cat cerebral cortex. J. Microsc. 165, 29-47

[2] Kling-Petersen T, Pascher R, Rydmark M (1999) Virtual Reality on the web: the potential of different methodologies and visualization techniques for scientific research and medical education. Stud Health Tech Inf, 62, 181-186

[3] Kling-Petersen T, Rydmark M (2000). Modeling And Modification Of Medical 3D Objects. The benefit of using a haptic modeling tool. Stud Health Tech Inf, 70, 162-167.

Medicine Meets Virtual Reality 2001
J.D. Westwood et al. (Eds.)
IOS Press, 2001

Decision Support System for Medical Triage

Sarmad Sadeghi, M.D., Afsaneh Barzi, M.D., Neda Zarrin-Khameh, M.D.
7227 Fannin St. suite #200, Houston TX 77030

Abstract

The paper explains the application of an artificial intelligence tool for the purpose of medical decision-making. The first product of this application is a triage engine, available on the Internet, to help laypersons make a decision about the urgency of their situation by providing tailored and accurate information. The expansion of this tool can lead to diagnostic tools for professionals or for educational purposes.

1. Introduction

This is a new attempt at using Bayesian Networks for the purpose of medical decision-making[6]. Out of different approaches to medical decision-making, such as, decision trees and neural networks, a Bayesian network approach probably has the strongest rationale of all. Our tool addresses triage, a simple medical decision-making problem[7].

2. Background/Problem

Triage is one simple medical decision-making problem that has been recognized as easily manageable outside clinical facilities. As a result, several attempts have been made at making triage advice available to end users through books, software, and nurses' call centers. The decision-making scheme in almost all of the above-mentioned approaches is simple decision trees. However, this approach has a number of shortcomings, including the inability to accommodate missing or incomplete information resulting in failure to reach a decision, as well as the geometric increase in maintenance time as the number of decision nodes increases. Most significantly, decision trees fail to appropriately handle uncertainty. Consequences of these shortcomings include referral of too many patients to urgent care settings, unnecessarily, or conversely, missing patients who require urgent care. Bayesian networks follow the closest path to the way medical decisions are, or better yet, should be, made[9].

3. Methods and Tools

By using Bayesian network technology and influence diagrams, uncertainty is effectively handled. For making a decision under uncertainty a utility-based approach could be used[1-4,8]. Both of these elements, Bayesian networks and utility, are provided in Hugin software. We use an iterative approach to modeling a medical domain starting by a chief complaint and collecting information necessary for correctly triaging the case. All necessary probabilities and utilities are elicited from practicing doctors through carefully designed interviews and questionnaires[5]. After this process, networks will undergo a sophisticated quality assurance process and all foreseeable errors will be fixed.

As the purpose of triage tool is helping patients make a decision, the evidence that are available to this system are subjective, such as, associated symptoms with the chief complaint, chronological appearance of the symptoms and severity of the symptoms. There are diagnoses that are inseparable based on these subjective data. We have put them under one category, umbrella diagnosis, if the utility for their disposition is the same. An example is spontaneous bacterial peritonitis and peritonitis because of a perforated bowl, both of these diagnoses need urgent care, and therefore, could fall in the same category of peritonitis.

The questions asked for each chief complaint are the components of the domain knowledge. These components may be conditionally dependent on one another, e.g. the interpretation of certain symptoms may vary with age. The dependencies among the components and probabilities are extracted from the literature or the domain experts, in our case medical specialists. This step is called knowledge elicitation.

In the run time a user answers a series of questions and receives a recommendation and up to three differential diagnoses, which are the most probable cause of the user's complaint. For triage purposes we have four decisions, *call 911*, *have someone drive you to the ER*, *make an appointment with your physician within 24 to 48 hours*, and *observe your symptoms at home*.

The utility values used for making a decision based on posterior probabilities for diagnoses must also be elicited from experts. Within each chief complaint we need the utility of each decisions for each differential diagnosis. The appropriate utility values are elicited from doctor interviews. This process involves multiple questionnaires each presenting a clinical situation under certain assumptions. Based on the answers provided by doctors, the appropriate utility value for each of the decisions will be calculated.

Considering the number of combinations in the system and impracticality of a manual QA process to verify all combinations, the QA is structured to cover the most common presentations of each diagnosis. This could mean that uncommon presentations might not be diagnosed correctly. However, since the primary purpose of this tool is to provide the appropriate disposition rather than diagnosis, the effects of possible misdiagnosis of the uncommon presentation of a diagnosis will be negligible.

The testing process starts with running cases from the board review books on the system and comparing the results with expected diagnoses. In case of any discrepancies, the reason will be investigated and appropriate changes will be made. The next step of testing is running the cases that practicing physicians confront in their practice.

After reaching the expected level of confidence in the models they will be implemented on a website allowing a user to log on, choose a chief complaint, answer a series of questions and receive appropriate advice and up to three possible diagnoses.

4. Results

Preliminary clinical reviews, including extensive case studies, show that, in most instances, the diagnosis provided by the system is accurate, and, in almost all cases the decision made by the system is appropriate for the medical condition presented to the system.

Many of the problems with nurses' call centers that perform the triage task such as irreproducibility, interpersonal, and intra personal changes in the decisions made for a patient are due to differences in experience, personality and psychological conditions of the person in charge of triage. This system provides a reproducible result that can be logged verified.

5. Conclusion

We conclude that the use of Bayesian networks for simple medical decisions, such as triage, is an efficient way of performing triage in emergency rooms and brings consistency and reproducibility of results and reduces human or systematic errors. This is helpful in creating a standard for triaging patients. There is also hope that adding objective evidence and expanding on the network design could help build a more powerful diagnostic tool.

References

1 Baron, J. Why expected utility theory is normative, but not prescriptive [editorial; comment]. Med Decis Making 1996; 16(1):7-9.

2 Cohen, B. J. Is expected utility theory normative for medical decision making? [see comments]. Med Decis Making 1996; 16(1):1-6.

3 Cohen, B. J. Reply: Utilitarianism, Risk Aversion, and Expected Utility. Med Decis Making 1996; 16(1):14.

4 Cohen, B. J. Do the expected utility axioms hide flaws? [letter; comment]. Med Decis Making 1997; 17(4):498-499.

5 Druzdzel, M. J., van der Gaag, L. C. Elicitation of Probabilities for Belief Networks: Combining Qualitative and Quantitative Information.Proceedings of the Conference on Uncertainty in Artificial Intelligence: Morgan Kaufmann, San Francisco, CA., 1995.

6 Jensen, F. V. An Introduction to Bayesian Networks. Springer-Verlag New York, Inc., 1996.

7 Lurie, J. D., Sox, H. C. Principles of medical decision making. Spine 1999; 24(5):493-498.

8 Nease, R. F., Jr. Do violations of the axioms of expected utility theory threaten decision analysis? [see comments]. Med Decis Making 1996; 16(4):399-403.

9 Pearl, J. Probabilistic Reasoning in Intelligent Systems. Morgan Kaufmann, San Mateo, CA., 1988.

Medicine Meets Virtual Reality 2001
J.D. Westwood et al. (Eds.)
IOS Press, 2001

Comparison of Tracking Techniques for Intraoperative Presentation of Medical Data using a See-Through Head-Mounted Display

Tobias Salb, Oliver Burgert, Tilo Gockel, Björn Giesler and Rüdiger Dillmann

Industrial Applications of Informatics and Microsystems (IAIM)
Building 07.21, Department for Computer Science
Universität Karlsruhe (TH), 76128 Karlsruhe, Germany
Tel.: ++49 721 608 7126, Fax: ++49 721 608 8270
Email: salb@ira.uka.de, WWW: http://wwwiaim.ira.uka.de/users/salb/

Tracking of a see-through head-mounted display is a necessary precondition for proper overlay of virtual data and real scenes within the display. In our contribution ,the intention and technique for Intraoperative Presentation will be presented. Focus will be the tracking of the display device. We will illustrate and compare three different optical tracking approaches and the results achieved by using them.

1 Introduction and purpose of the work

Nowadays many tools for preoperative planning and simulation of surgical interventions are available in the clinical environment, while the surgical procedure itself still lacks the computer based assistance. At the Institute for Industrial Applications of Informatics and Microsystems (IAIM) at Universität Karlsruhe (TH), Germany, we are working on a solution for closing this gap using augmented reality. A technique called Intraoperative Presentation has been developed in order to superimpose virtual computer-generated information with a real patient using a see-through head-mounted display [2].

The purpose of our development is to visualise results from preoperative work, like planning and simulation information, radiological data, risk regions, target areas or any other important data within the see-through glasses. Clinical tests have been done with the display to ensure proper functionality and to receive considerations for the design of the visualisation software [1]. The concept of Intraoperative Presentation has been compared to other solutions [3] and was described in detail on the SPIE 2000 conference [2].

In this paper our focus is on the tracking of the see-through head-mounted display. Precise real-time tracking is necessary for achieving sufficient results in data presentation. Three different optical tracking algorithms have been implemented at our institute. Methods and results are being presented below.

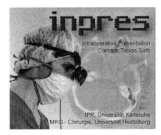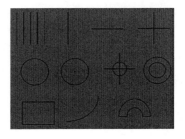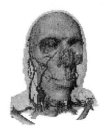

Figure 1: Start GUI for Intraoperative Presentation, data for clinical trials of the display, virtual information that shall be visualised within the glasses (from the left to the right)

2 Methods

Intraoperative Presentation of image data causes hard accuracy requirements. It is challenging to track the see-through glasses with sufficient precision in order to transform the image data correctly and to supply the surgeon with an optimal superimposition of virtual and real data.

The first tracking method we call a "standard machine vision approach" using two Pulnix monochrome CCD cameras. Light emitting diodes are mounted on top of the display as artificial landmarks. The cameras are fixed in the operation room for tracking the display. For the tracking software, the Matrox Imaging Library has been used as a basis. Besides this standard setup, two miniature cameras will be mounted on both sides of the display in order to enhance precision of the tracking.

The second tracking system is the commercial optical navigation system "Polaris". The system, manufactured by NDI, is distributed by the Surgical Navigation Network (SNN). Results of the SNN tracking software have been combined with our visualisation system. Moreover, special rigid bodies with passive markers have been designed for proper tracking results.

The last tracking method we are realising is an innovative tracking approach using a "parabolic mirror" which has been used in mobile robotics before. Artificial landmarks are distributed all over the operation room. Images are being taken using a single CCD camera attached on top of the head-mounted display. A parabolic mirror which is coated on the outside is mounted on the camera. This setup enables us to take a 360 degree image of an operation room. Using this type of images we search for the landmarks in order to do dynamic localisation and navigation of the display. The approach is still under development and will be presented in a separate paper in detail.

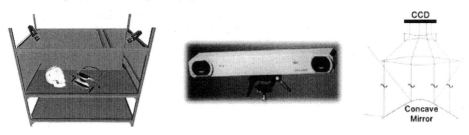

Figure 2: The different optical tracking approaches: Standard camera-based setup, NDI Polaris system and parabolic mirror approach (from the left to the right)

3 Results

All tracking setups show sufficient time behaviour. While the Polaris system has been developed for real-time usage, the two self-made approaches had to be tuned properly. Fast PCs are being used in order to ensure real-time tracking. Because of the single camera within the setup, the parabolic mirror approach shows a better time performance.

First clinical trials have been done for testing accuracy. After registration, the particular tracking bodies of the different approaches have been placed in measured positions and orientations. Then the results of the respective tracking software have been analysed with regard to the measured data.

The SNN Polaris tracking has been able to reach a sub-millimetre accuracy in translation and a sub-degree accuracy in rotation. This high accuracy has been proposed by the company before. Our self-made camera-based approach has been worse in the test, with an accuracy of about 2-3 millimetres and about 2 degrees. The parabolic mirror approach has shown a good rotational behaviour in first trials while translation behaviour is worst.

No	Setup type	Translation accuracy	Rotation accuracy
1	Standard camera-based	=< 3mm	=< 2,5 degrees
2	SNN Polaris	< 0,3 mm	< 1 degree
3	Parabolic mirror	=< 5 mm	=< 1,5 degrees

Figure 3: Accuracy test results

4 Conclusion

For use in Intraoperative Presentation we have developed and compared three optical tracking systems. Best behaviour has been shown by an enhanced setup, based on the commercially available Polaris system. Much worse in translation but comparable in rotational behaviour are our self-made methods, using a parabolic mirror or a standard camera-based approach. Results are nevertheless satisfying and visualisation of data will be realised soon using the different tracking systems.

References

[1] Brief, J., Hassfeld, S., Salb, T., Burgert, O., Münchenberg, J., Pernozzoli, A., Grabowski, H., Redlich, T., Raczkowsky, J., Krempien, R., Kotrikova, B., Wörn, H., Dillmann, R., Mühling, J. and Ziegler, C.: Clinical evaluation of a see-through display for Intraoperative Presentation of planning data. Proceedings of conference: Israeli Symposium on Computer-Integrated Surgery, Medical Robotics and Medical Imaging (ISRACAS), Haifa, May 2000.

[2] Salb, T., Brief, J., Burgert, O., Hassfeld, S. and Dillmann, R.: Intraoperative presentation of surgical planning and simulation results using a stereoscopic see-through head-mounted display. Proceedings of conference: Stereoscopic Displays and Applications, Part of Photonics West (SPIE), San Jose, CA, January 2000.

[3] Salb, T., Brief, J., Burgert, O., Hassfeld, S., Mühling, J. and Dillmann, R.: Towards augmented reality in medicine - Overview and approach. Proceedings of workshop: Computer Aided Surgery (CAS), Erlangen, October 1999.

Medicine Meets Virtual Reality 2001
J.D. Westwood et al. (Eds.)
IOS Press, 2001

A New Concept for Intraoperative Matching of 3D Ultrasound and CT

Oliver Schorr, Heinz Wörn Ph.D.

University of Karlsruhe (TH), Institute for Process Control and Robotics
Kaiserstraße 12, 76128 Karlsruhe, Germany, e_mail: schorr@ira.uka.de

Matching of ultrasound images with CT or MRI scans is an awkward and unsatisfactory task when using conventional methods. Wide ranging differences in modality of ultrasound and CT/MRI require new techniques to be explored for successful alignment. Ultrasound images characteristically show comparable high noise ratio due to scattering inside the region of interest and the surrounding area. Additionally, shadowing and tissue dependent echo response time produce geometric artifacts. These image distortions are sophisticated to recover. Though image quality and geometric relationship are poor, ultrasound images show the potential for fast, low-cost, non-invasive and flexible image acquisition, predestinated for intraoperative application. The fusion of intraoperative ultrasound and preoperatively acquired CT/MRI images provides both, geometric invariance and flexible fast image acquisition, merging in a powerful tool for augmented three dimensional reality.

In this paper we describe a completely new concept for alignment with abstaining from direct rigid or elastic matching of ultrasound to CT/MRI. Instead of placing those images in direct relationship, our approach involves a simulation of ultrasound wave behavior in order to predict B-mode images.

1. Introduction

In a wide range of applications the operating surgeon needs to have information about the patient's condition pre- and intraoperatively provided by imaging systems. In order to determine changes between both images and to simplify the geometric relation of the images to one another, alignment methods need to be used which correlate both images.

Methods for monomodal or bimodal alignment of CT or MR images have been well developed, resulting in algorithms for rigid or elastic matching based on landmarks [4][5] or gray value distributions [3][6]. These methods have been proven to be accurate enough for the resolution provided by CT or MR imaging systems. Especially the alignment by maximization of mutual information is an effective procedure which produces highly accurate alignments without the need of identifying natural or artificial corresponding points in images.

Unfortunately, the intraoperative usage of both systems, MR and CT has essential disadvantages. In the need of CT, an intraoperative CT scanner must be available, surgeons and the additional personal as well as the patient are exposed to radiation and the patient has to be fixed in order to precisely determine a position inside the human body. In contrast to CT, MRI scanners are less invasive but significantly more expensive in purchase and operation and the duration of image acquisition is comparably high. Additionally, fixing the patient still remains the problem.

In order to overcome these drawbacks whenever MR or CT scanning is not absolutely indicated, surgeons want to revert to intraoperative imaging by ultrasound. Ultrasound shows the potential for fast, low-cost, non-invasive and flexible image acquisition, predestinated for intraoperative application. Therefore, investigations and experiments were done in order to determine in which way intraoperative ultrasound can be aligned with preoperative images from CT or MR scanners.

The outcome showed that methods used for bimodal matching of CT with MR images or v.v. are not suitable for the application to ultrasound images. Reasons are the significant disadvantages in image quality of ultrasound images. Scattering produces high noise ratio inside the scanned region. Physical effects due to the properties of acoustical waves like shadowing and tissue dependent response time contribute their degradation of image quality. Especially image distortions resulting in geometric inaccurate representations make it a difficult task to align ultrasound images with highly accurate and geometric invariant images produced by CT scanners.

Currently, different research groups are working on modified mutual information algorithms in order to overcome these shortcomings [8]. Other research groups are trying to solve the problem with modification of the image itself by elimination of artifacts.

The concept that we present in this paper tries a completely different way by processing from bottom up. It consists of four steps: (1) preoperative acquisition of 3D data sets with highly geometrically invariant techniques like CT or MRI, (2) estimation and approximation of density, attenuation and scattering based on gray value distributions of those scans, (3) simulation of B-mode ultrasound images referring to the parameters determined in the step before, (4) matching of the acquired ultrasound images and the images simulated in the preceding step. The outcome of this matching is a transformation showing the relation between simulated and measured images.

We do not place ultrasound image and CT/MR image in direct relationship. Instead, we use the preoperatively acquired CT/MR image as input in order to determine ultrasound specific properties of the region scanned later by ultrasound transducers. The aim of our simulation is to produce reasonable images or volumes corresponding to real ultrasound images and to calculate a transformation describing essential geometric distortions from CT/MRI to ultrasound images. We are investigating a new method for B-mode ultrasound simulation which relates accuracy and runtime. The emphasis is not put on realistic ultrasound images, nor do we try to find another representation for tissue properties. Our goal is a fast calculation of the most relevant structures and properties of the regarded volume highlighting ultrasound specific geometric distortions.

The main idea of our new approach is to combine the transformations received in the previous steps of simulation and matching (steps three and four). The inverse concatenation of both transformations leads to a complete description of the transformation from real ultrasound to CT/MRI providing an accurate matching of high quality. The usage of the simulator bypasses ultrasound specific geometric distortions and allows us a description of the matching result from bottom up. Of course additional computation time will be necessary, but should be weighed up against significant accuracy improvement.

Our concept for augmented reality will be used to intraoperatively visualize CT/MR image and ultrasound image three dimensional in correct correlation to one another. It enables the surgeon to compare the intraoperative and preoperative conditions of the patient. The advantages of our concept are obvious: fast and flexible intraoperative image acquisition with combination of accurate and high resolution provided by preoperatively taken CT/MR data. Image details which can not be visualized with ultrasound, can be faded in throughout CT/MR image.

2. Methods

2.1.   System overview

Our concept consists of a process flow with four absolutely necessary steps and one optional step. CT/MRI data and ultrasound data are entering the workflow in different steps. Figure 1 shows the processing queue.

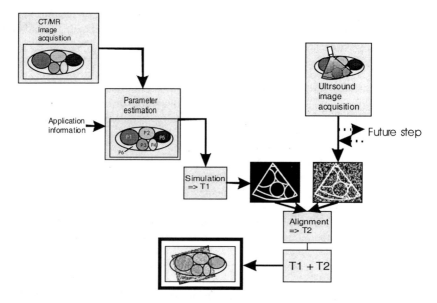

Figure 1: Overall system processing queue. The queue has two different entry points for input data (CT/MR images or ultrasound images) and four steps. A fifth step is planned to preprocess ultrasound images before entering the queue.

The first step is a preoperative step and involves the acquisition of a 3D dataset from CT or MR scanners. The resolution of these images needs to fulfill the surgeons accuracy requirements and has to be at least as high as the resolution of ultrasound images. It is important that the images contain the whole volume of interest including the surface on which the ultrasound probe will be put on intraoperatively. Otherwise, the ultrasound simulation can fail according to missing tissue property estimations at the entry point of the acoustic waves in the patient's body.

The next step tries to estimate ultrasound specific properties of the tissue scanned in the preceding step. The estimation is based on two different input data: the gray value distribution included in CT/MR data and additional information about the clinical application our proposed system is applied to. For instance, we can separate neurosurgical interventions from abdominal ones and include this additional information in order to map gray values in CT/MR data to ultrasound properties. This mapping process can be performed preoperatively as well.

Step three is the first step which is performed intraoperatively and includes our simulation process. The simulation is done based on the parameters calculated and estimated in step two and the position of the ultrasound probe during three dimensional intraoperative image acquisition. Referring to the probe's position, our simulator produces images which show characteristic ultrasound image drawbacks. These distortions and artifacts are measured during simulation so that they are recoverable.

The proceeding step aligns the simulated and the real acquired ultrasound image by usage of modified conventional registration algorithms. Currently we are working on a modified mutual information algorithm in order to abstain from the usage of landmarks.

In the last and conclusive step we concatenate the transformation calculated in the preceding step and the measured distortions and artifact influences measured in step three. This results in a complete description of the transformation from ultrasound image to CT/MR or vice versa which enables us to superimpose CT/MR data and ultrasound data for intraoperative assistance of the surgeon.

2.2. Estimation of ultrasound specific tissue properties

The behavior of ultrasound waves with respect to human tissue has already been described in several publications before [1][2]. Referring to these, important properties influencing ultrasound B-mode images are velocity, mass density and attenuation. Whenever ultrasound images are to be simulated, these parameters will have to be taken into account. However, the study of these parameters shows that there is no proper formulation of the relation between specific tissue and these parameters. This statement can be drawn from table 1 showing the parameters of some human tissues.

Table 1: Typical values for velocity, mass density and attenuation in some human tissues [2]

Tissue	c (m/sec)	ρ (g/cm³)	attenuation (dB/MHz cm)
Fat	1470	0,97	0,5
Muscle	1586	1,04	2
Liver	1540	1,055	0,7
Brain	1530	1,02	1
Bone	3600	1,7	4 – 90
Water	1492	0,9982	0,002

Even though it does not appear clearly, the variance of the values shown in table 1 depends on the tissue and is always a mean value. Whereas the calculation of a mean value was possible in the cases for fat, muscle, liver and brain the variance of attenuation in case of bone is that high that a description by mean value is senseless. Therefore, a value needs to be chosen best describing the behavior of ultrasound waves in bones.

The idea of our estimation concept is to describe the mentioned ultrasound parameters mainly by the incoming CT or MR image. Consequently, we formulate a relation mapping gray values of the incoming image to ultrasound parameters. The main problems of this task are that (1) we get one parameter as input and need to estimate three parameters and (2) there is no direct dependency between gray value and these parameters. Hence, mapping is a difficult process and we are trying to support our mapping method by context sensitivity. This means as second input we are supplying information about the application our system is used for. Whether we are scanning brain, liver or leg i.e. influences the mapping from gray values to ultrasound parameters.

2.3.   Localization and ultrasound image acquisition

Our current ultrasound acquisition system is a commercial 2D array scanner with linear and convex transducer probes. In order to gain 3D datasets, the probe's position is tracked during hand performed motion and the acquired images are post processed to a 3D volume. The advantage of this method compared to 3D matrix ultrasound scanners is that we can apply our system to more medical applications because of its small size and its easy use. This is very useful when the probe is put on curved surfaces. Moreover, shading effects can be removed by changing the probes orientation.

Since we are working with a tracking device, the localization of the ultrasound probe is already provided. Unfortunately, the position we get for the probe is relative to the tracking device. The acquired images just have to be put in the right correlation to each other. But in our case, we need to put patient and ultrasound in an absolute relationship in order to do the correct simulation. However, we are also investigating in methods to overcome that issue described in section 2.5 below.

2.4.   Ultrasound simulation

Various tools and programs are available for the simulation of ultrasound behavior and B-mode images [1][9][10]. However, in most cases they lack from speed of execution which makes them unsuitable for the intraoperative application. Typical numbers, depending on the complexity of the simulation method of course, can be found in [1] and vary from hours until days just to produce a 2D B-mode image. As our needs are 3D volumes which have to be calculated as fast as possible in order to fulfill the intraoperative needs, a less complex simulation method is currently under exploration.

We abstain from detailed description of all physical effects and focus on the most relevant ones dominating the image. Physical effects mostly taken into account are reflection, refraction, diffraction, doppler effect, interference, attenuation and noise[1]. The manner and how much these effects influence each calculation also depends on the applied method. Studying the literature one can find methods based on finite element method [11], finite difference method [1], spatial impulse response [10]. In order to overcome time consumption, our approach is mostly based on reflection and attenuation. We are not describing ultrasound waves, but acoustic intensities propagated through the volume. Accordingly, we are not able to take into account effects like interference. Moreover, our method treats the scanned region on a per ray basis. The substantiation of this approach is based on the fact that in some scanning systems each transducer element of an ultrasound probe is responsible for a certain section within the scanned volume.

Although we apply strong restrictions to our simulation method, we are able to describe image distortions very well allowing their recovery. In a pre-simulative step our method randomly selects arbitrary coordinates within the incoming CT or MR data. During simulation, for each reflection we check whether it appears at any of the preselected points. If so, the coordinates of that point and the time when the reflected ray reaches the transducer element again are stored for later retrieval. This enables us to get a relation between elapsed time and coordinates. Hence, we can exactly determine where any of the preselected points producing pixel values greater than zero in the ultrasound data can be found in the incoming CT or MR data. Our image warping method interpolates the information about all preselected points resulting in a transformation describing affine and elastic local and global distortions from CT/MR to ultrasound. A standard method based on radial base-functions is used to warp the images.

2.5. Registration and Alignment

Our ultrasound simulation process is based on the information where the ultrasound transducer is located. This is necessary, because image distortions depend on the orientation and position of the transducer relative to the scanned tissue. Consequently, we register the ultrasound data relative to the incoming CT/MR data. This can be done by using fiducials which can be identified by ultrasound as well as CT or MRI. We want to stress that we do not use the information about the transducers location in order to align ultrasound data with CT/MR data. The information is solely used for finding the entry point of the ultrasound waves in the human body. We are also developing a new registration method which manages registration without fiducial markers based on a combined back-loop mechanism involving simulation and registration.

The outcome of our simulation process are synthetic ultrasound data. This dataset needs to be aligned with the measured one in order to complete our process queue and to superimpose both. We are using an algorithm introduced by Viola [3] for alignment. As this algorithm is based on mutual information we can align both images without any additional information like corresponding points. Currently, we are modifying the algorithm in order to better fulfill our needs for the alignment of synthetic and real ultrasound data.

2.6. Transformation concatenation

In our concept the correct superimposition of intraoperative ultrasound image and preoperative CT/MR image is done by the concatenation of two transformations:

- image warping transformation describing image distortions during ultrasound simulation based on the incoming CT/MR data and
- affine or elastic transformation describing the path from synthesized to measured ultrasound data.

A conventional concatenation of both transformations is sufficient in our case. Nevertheless, it must be remembered that the resulting transformation of our concept is local and has to be applied in such a way. We are not able to describe the transformation from CT/MR to ultrasound by global transformations.

3. Discussion and Conclusion

We present a new concept to relinquish direct matching of CT/MRI and ultrasound. Instead, a simulation based on CT/MRI scans is preformed calculating geometric distortions during ultrasound image acquisition of the same volume. By watching this process we can determine an inverse transformation from simulated images back to CT/MRI scan. Common techniques for matching the simulated ultrasound data and acquired data are used in the next step.

We hope that our concept is generic enough to be applicable to any intraoperative setting. Even if our concept is not implemented yet, we expect our concept to describe geometric distortions more accurate.

Future improvement will be done by preprocessing the ultrasound image acquired by the ultrasound scanner in regard to scattering and other blur and noise artifacts. Another approach for the future will be to use elastic instead of rigid matching when minimizing mutual information previously introduced by Hata et al [6].

References

[1]   T. Rohlfing, *Simulierte Ultraschallbildgebung und in der medizinischen Diagnostik auftretende Arte-fakte*, Master Thesis, Karlsruhe, Germany, 1998
[2]   H. Morneburg (Hrsg.), *Bildgebende Systeme für die medizinische Diagnostik*, Erlangen, Publicis MCD Verlag, Germany, 1995
[3]   P. A. Viola, *Alignment by Maximization of Mutual Information*, Cambridge, USA, MIT Technical Report No. 1548, 1995
[4]   K. S. Arun, T. S. Huang, and S.D. Blostein, *Least-Squares Fitting of Two 3D Point Sets*, IEEE Transactions on PAMI, vol. 9 no. 5, pp. 698-700, 1987
[5]   A. Bürkle, *Elastische Deformation Anatomischer Modelle*, Master Thesis, Karlsruhe, Germany, 1998
[6]   N. Hata, T. Dohi, S. Warfield, W. Wells III, R. Kikinis, F. A. Jolesz, *Multimodality Deformable Registration of Pre- and Intraoperative Images for MRI-Guided Brain Surgery*, In Proceedings of Medical Image Computing and Computer Assisted Intervention (MICCAI), Boston, USA, 1998
[7]   J. M. Blackall, D. Rueckert, C.R. Maurer Jr., G. P. Penney, D. L. G. Hill, D. J. Hawkes, *An Image Registration Approach to Automated Calibration for Freehand 3D Ultrasound*, In Proceedings of Medical Image Computing and Computer Assisted Intervention (MICCAI), Pittsburgh, USA, 2000
[8]   A. Roche, X. Pennec, M. Rudolph, D. P. Auer, G. Malandain, S. Ourselin, L. M. Auer, N. Ayache, *Generalized Correlation Ratio for Rigid Registration of 3D Ultrasound with MR Images*, In Proceedings of Medical Image Computing and Computer Assisted Intervention (MICCAI), Pittsburgh, USA, 2000
[9]   S. Holm, *Simulation of Acoustic Fields from Medical Ultrasound Transducers of Arbitrary Shape*, Noridic Symposium in Physical Acoustics, Ustaoset, Norway, 1995
[10] J. A. Jensen, *Simulating Arbitrary-Geometry Ultrasound Transducers Using Triangles*, IEEE International Ultrasonic Symposium, San Antonio, Texas, USA, 1996
[11] W. Cao, *Design Simulation of Composite Transducers*, Whitaker Ctr. for Med. Ultrasonic Transducer Eng., PA, USA , 1997

Medicine Meets Virtual Reality 2001
J.D. Westwood et al. (Eds.)
IOS Press, 2001

Human Perception of Haptic Information in Minimal Access Surgery Tools for Use in Simulation

A. Seehusen, P.N. Brett, A. Harrison

University of Bristol, Department of Mechanical Engineering
Queen's Building, University Walk
Bristol, England BS8 1TR

Abstract. This paper describes research on human perception of haptic information in minimal access surgery (MAS) instruments, for use in a MAS simulator. Understanding the thresholds of human perception is important in determining which haptic information must be provided for realistic feedback and which information can be ignored without compromising the immersive quality of the simulator. Initially this research has determined the limits of perception for non-continuous change of force amplitude and frequency in a scissors-grasping position.

1. Introduction

Haptic force feedback systems have become an important part of surgical simulation. Many early computer surgical simulators did not address the issue of haptics because it was argued that haptic feedback was not important and that a training surgeon could learn a lot by manipulating real instruments and watching the tissue interaction on a video screen. These first attempts, however, were found to lack a certain amount of reality or immersion into the virtual environment. It was decided that immersion did not hinge solely on the visual realism of the system, but rather on a user's feeling of presence in a virtual environment [1]. Since haptic feedback plays an important role in tissue-tool interactions, which account for a large percentage of surgical simulation, haptic feedback is key to the immersive quality of a surgical simulator. Most surgical simulators in recent years have reflected this by including haptic feedback systems.

When designing haptic force feedback systems for MAS simulators it is important to consider the limitations of human perception. Understanding the limitations for human perception will allow simulator force feedback systems to be optimised, preventing the simulation of excessive haptic information that a surgeon cannot feel. An understanding of human perception will also ensure the inclusion of important haptic information and the quality of a simulator's haptics.

Haptic perception incorporates and relates local tactile stimuli to the larger kinaesthetic spatial awareness of the body and involves the exchange of tactile information between the body and the outside world [2,3]. Haptic perception is composed of several haptic cues, or characteristics that contribute to the overall sensation of touch. To understand how to mimic haptic perception these haptic cues must be identified. The most important haptic cues are frequency, amplitude and phase. For each haptic cue there is a limit of human perception which is linked to a frequency above which the cue becomes of decreasing importance to the overall haptic sensation. This idea is illustrated in figure 1. Understanding perception limits will provide guidelines for the design of a simulator with an optimised force feedback system.

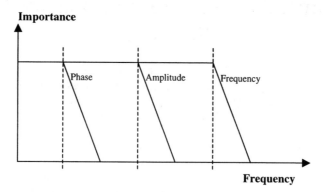

Figure 1: Cut-off Frequencies for Important Haptic Cues

Presently, there is no instrument manipulation or scissors-grasping specific haptic sensing information available. However, data existing for single fingertip stimulation will be useful in determining the range of frequencies that can be expected. The range of vibration perception appears to lie from 2 Hz-400 Hz, but higher frequencies (1kHz-10kHz) cannot be ruled out as important. The ability to discriminate one signal from another drops after 300Hz and the minimal detectable amplitude of movement is 5-10 μm [4-9]. Similar types of information will be determined in this research. To begin with, we have chosen to look at the ability of humans to perceive non-continuous changes in force amplitude and frequency.

2. Methods

Though a MAS tool has several degrees of freedom in which these tests could be performed, the degree of freedom used for haptic testing does not change the ability of a human to perceive haptic cues. Therefore, the handle-action degree of freedom was used because this is where the greatest precision of tool movement is found.

The testing rig was composed of a MAS tool cut in the middle with the scissor action control mechanism connected to a linear actuator (Linear Drives, Ltd Thrust Tube 2504) as shown in figure 2. A PC controlled the linear actuator's movement and force. Initially, there were two experiments testing 10 subjects of different gender, age and occupation.

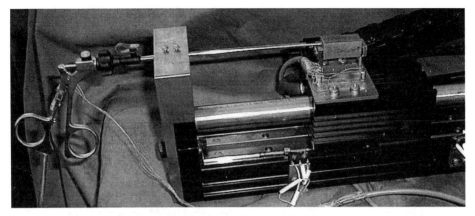

Figure 2: Human Perception Test Rig

The experiments investigated human ability to perceive non- continuous changes in force amplitude and frequency. Non-continuous changes were used so the accuracy requirements of force amplitude and frequency reproduction in simulation could be determined. These step change perception tests were conducted first because they were easy and quick to perform and they gave results that will be useful in determining subsequent experiments.

For each test, equally spaced sets of 2-second sinusoidal pulses were imposed. Examples for each test are shown in figures 3 and 4.

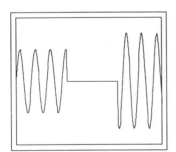 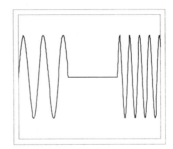

Figures 3&4: Sinusoidal Pulses for Change in Force Amplitude and Frequency Test

In the examination of the force amplitude a constant frequency of 4Hz was used because initial experimentation showed test subjects could follow this frequency with ease. The force amplitude step changes ranged from 1N to 5N representing a large scope of possible changes. The overall force amplitude range was chosen from 15-35N using the forces of a MAS tool (10-20N) during manipulation and the lower limits of the linear actuator (15N) [10]. In the investigation of frequency a constant force amplitude of 30N was provided representing the upper end of forces used in the amplitude tests and a force amplitude that was easily followed. The frequency steps examined were 2Hz, 4Hz and 6Hz, a range determined using initial experimentation. For each test the force amplitude or frequency either increased or decreased by the specified step, or else remained the same. The test subject held the handle of the MAS tool lightly and was asked to compare the force amplitude or frequency of a pulse to the previous pulse. The perceived response for each pulse was noted.

3. Results

Force Amplitude Test

The amplitude tests give the expected result. The smaller the overall force amplitude the more accurate a step change of force amplitude must be to be perceived. The results are summarised in table 1. The detectable step is determined to be the point where less than 80% of a test subject's answers are correct. Table 1 suggests suitable guidelines for reproducing force amplitude in surgical simulation. The table also recommends that small force amplitude changes at high force amplitudes do not need to be accurate, or to exist at all. Larger force amplitude changes however need to be more accurate to maintain immersion in the simulation.

Range (N)	Minimum Step	% of Total Amplitude
15-25	3.5	17.5
25-35	4.5	15.0

Table 1: Force Amplitude Step Limits of Perception

Frequency Test

The limits of perception for a step change in frequency can be summarised by table 2. The frequency results occur as expected: the greater the frequency change the higher the overall frequency can be before the change is no longer detectable. The point where test subjects could not accurately perceive changes in frequency (about 80% correct responses) defines the limit of perception. Table 2 suggests suitable guidelines for accuracy in frequency reproduction. It also recommends that if simulating a small frequency change at a high frequency, the change does not need to be accurate or, if the frequency is high enough, it can be left out altogether.

Step Frequency (Hz)	Limit of Perception (Hz)	% of Total Frequency
2	15	13.3
4	34	11.8
6	48	12.5

Table 2: Frequency Limits of Change Perception

4. Conclusions

The perception of non-continuous changes in a MAS tool for both force amplitude and frequency are dependent upon the percentage of the overall signal that the changes make up. Therefore, the accuracy of the force amplitude or frequency in a simulation only needs to be accurate to the specified percentage. For force amplitude the accuracy needs to be about 15%-17.5% of the force amplitude being simulated. When simulating the frequency of MAS tools the accuracy needs be about 12%-13% of the overall frequency.

These results also suggest that force amplitude and frequency changes do not need to be particularly accurate. For force amplitude changes below the 15% mark can probably be ignored altogether, while changes in the 17.5%-15% range should probably exist, but do not need to be entirely accurate. However, changes above 17.5% of the overall signal should be accurate. The same idea applies for step changes in frequency. Step changes for frequency do not need to be accurate up to about 12%. Above 12% a change in step is more readily detectable and will need to be more accurately reproduced.

5. Further Testing

These tests are only the initial tests in the unravelling of the human perception of the haptic information that is simulated in MAS. Further testing will look at the overall ability of humans to perceive force amplitude and frequency. It will also look at perception of phase and the ability to detect movement. Once these tests are complete a simple simulator will be used to compare human perception of unfiltered haptic information to filtered haptic information. The filters will be determined by the guidelines set out by the previously mentioned testing. This testing will allow the guidelines to be tested and fine tuned and will help to optimise the design of future simulators.

6. Acknowledgements

A very special thanks to Jenny Guy and Simon Wheat for their help in the set-up and running of this research.

References

[1] W. Barfield and C. Hendrix, Factors Affecting Presence and Performance in Virtual Environments. In: K. Morgan et al. (eds.), Interactive Technology and the New Paradigm for Healthcare. IOS Press, Amsterdam, 1995, pp. 21-28.

[2] M.H. Lee and H.R. Nicholls, Tactile Sensing For Mechatronics-A State of the Art Survey, Mechatronics 9 (1999) 1-31.

[3] V. Hayward and O.R. Astley, Performance Measures for Haptic Interfaces. In: G. Giralt et al. (eds.), Robotics Research: The 7th International Symposium. Springer Verlang, New York, 1996, pp. 1-11.

[4] T.L. Brooks, Telerobotic Response Requirements, IEEE International Conference on Systems, Man, and Cybernetics (1990) 113-120.

[5] G. Burdea and J. Zhuang, Dextrous Telerobotics with Force Feedback - An Overview. Part 1: Human Factors, Robotica 9 (1991) 171-178.

[6] R.E. Ellis et al., Design and Evaluation of a High - Performance Haptic Interface, Robotica 14 (1996) 321-327.

[7] R.H. La Motte and V.B. Mountcastle, Capacity of Humans and Monkeys to Discriminate Between Vibratory Stimuli of Different Frequency and Amplitude: A Correlation Between Neural Events and Psychophysical Measurements, Journal of Neurophysiology 38 (1975) 539-559.

[8] U. Lindblom and B. Lindstrom, Tactile Thresholds of Normal and Blind Subjects on Stimulation of Finger Pads with Short Mechanical Pulses of Variable Amplitude. In: Y. Zottlerman (ed.), Sensory Function of the Skin in Primates (with Special Reference to Man). Pergamon Press, Oxford, 1976, pp. 105-111.

[9] V.B. Mountcastle *et al.*, Detection Thresholds for Stimuli in Humans and Monkeys: Comparison With Threshold Events in Mechanoreceptive Afferent Nerve Fibers Innervation the Monkey Hand, *Journal of Neurophysiology* **35** (1972) 122-136.

[10] V. Gupta *et al.*, Forces in Surgical Tools: Comparison Between Laparoscopic and Surgical Forceps, *Proceedings of the 1996 18th Annual International Conference of the IEEE Engineering in Medicine and Biology Society* **1**(1996) 223-225.

Medicine Meets Virtual Reality 2001
J.D. Westwood et al. (Eds.)
IOS Press, 2001

Design and Construction of a Computer-Based Logical System for Medical Diagnosis

Hisham M. Sherif *, M.D., Sarmad Sadeghi, M.D., Greg Mogel, M.D.
Research Associate, askRed.com, 7227 Fannin Street, Houston, Texas 77030, USA

1. Introduction

Over the past two decades, research teams have been engaged in the use of computers and Artificial Intelligence systems to perform several diverse tasks in the health care field. In particular, researchers have worked to reproduce the process by which clinicians examine patients' presenting data to reach a diagnosis. Some of these attempts date back to 1977.[1,2,5]

Efforts in this field have dramatically increased in the last decade, as increasingly powerful computer systems were being developed, and especially with the advent of the Internet, the World Wide Web and the explosive growth in information resources and databases.

One of the main research objectives in most of these endeavors has been to develop a fairly precise and reproducible tool that would help improve clinicians' diagnostic accuracy, be an educational tool to develop and perfect these diagnostic skills, and be another ancillary tool in outcome predictions and quality assurance in different aspects of health care practice.[7]

Most of these endeavors have involved the design and construction of a computer-based Logical Algorithm specifically designed to undertake a single task, such as a scoring system for acute appendicitis or a decision-support tool evaluating a particular condition presenting in the emergency department.[3,13]

Most researchers have used a traditional approach -- the team essentially develops a computer analog of the familiar decision tree or algorithm that is used by clinicians in office, clinic and hospital settings. A frequently cited remark in this context is that one component of the diagnostic process relies significantly on the clinician's experience or "clinical sense," and that it would be extremely difficult to "program intuition."

These research endeavors have met with variable degrees of success. Factors involved or implicated in these results include: inadequate data categorization, inadequate identification of all the variables involved, inadequate data input or an inherent limitation of the system itself; e.g., the limitations imposed by the nature of the software used.[4,5,6]

2. Research Objectives

We established several objectives that had to be met when designing, constructing and implementing a computer-based logical medical diagnostic system. These objectives are: simplicity, flexibility, adaptability, expandability, standardization, upgrading, logic, integration and interface, and implementation.[8,15]

Simplicity

The system design and structure has to be as simple and uncomplicated as possible, using the simplest possible software and requiring the least possible hardware.

Flexibility

The system must be able to adequately perform a range of different tasks, and must not be designed to fit or be limited to a unique one.

Adaptability

The system should be able to maintain the same level of performance in different or diverse environments, including contextual variations (e.g., clinical versus laboratory application, interactive applications versus quality assurance, etc.) This should require minimal, if any, adjustments or changes to the basic system configuration.

Expandability

The system should be designed, constructed and implemented to be able to perform in an extended range of applications, or in different parallel applications of the original task (e.g., extended range of diagnostic application).

Standardization

The system must be constructed in a systematized, standardized way, thus rendering it readily and easily reproducible.

Upgrading

The system must have room for growth; it should also allow for constant and regular upgrading and improvement. This should be with reference to the continual changes in health care knowledge and data.

Logic

The logical system or Artificial Intelligence medium used should allow for fuzzy reasoning and logic, thereby being able to accept and to handle a wide range of variability in the data used, as well as being receptive to different applications.

Integration and Interface

The system should be able to interface with, be integrated with and be compatible with other existing knowledge bases and information databases.

Implementation

The system usage should be as friendly and easy to learn and implement as possible, and not require special knowledge or training.

3. System Configuration

The system is designed to examine and analyze the relevant data about a certain defined condition, presentation, problem or situation, to make a diagnosis of the possible causes and to plot solution choices.

Applying this to health care, the system will be required to examine the relevant data about a symptom, sign and/or a presentation, make a diagnosis and present the treatment options applicable. The system consists of the following components: target task, data pool, possible answers, system architecture, and diagnosis.

Target Task

The Target Task is the first step to be defined in the system. It is the problem that the system will endeavor to solve. In our present context of online medical diagnosis, this task will represent a symptom, a symptom cluster, a sign, a presentation or a condition.

Data Pool

The Data Pool represents all the available or obtainable information that pertains to the Target Task. In our context, this will include information such as epidemiological data about disease prevalence and incidence, and information about the clinical picture of the condition being examined, e.g., associated symptoms and signs, clinical course, etc.

Possible Answers

Upon examining and analyzing the given sets of information from the previously discussed components, the system will provide a list of possible explanations or answers to the Target Task. In other words, the system will describe the list of possible causes of the problem. This list of possible answers should relate well to and represent the trends, patterns and logical relationships between the data subsets.

System Architecture

System Architecture is the actual computer software configuration that will analyze and correlate the data provided to reach the required conclusion. The choice of the most suitable medium should take into consideration several factors: The logical system used should work fast, handling data from multiple sources, working in a non-linear fashion. It should handle the data in a low-dimensional plot, using fuzzy logic pathways, and also offer a significant margin of flexibility in architecture with ease of learning and use.[9]

Diagnostic Approach

Diagnosis is the main process that the system will perform. It consists of correlating all the available data, examining and analyzing the laws, trends, patterns and logical relationships that exist among the different data subsets and also against the list of possible answers, to decide upon the best explanation for the Task at hand.[10,11,14]

The Diagnostic Approach is the thinking process that is used to arrive at the one or two best diagnoses that will explain the symptom or condition being examined.

Defining this reasoning process has been at the very heart of developing every medical diagnostic system designed. There are three approaches that have been commonly employed to achieve this:

<u>Possibilistic Approach:</u> Approach in which the system examines ALL the existing possible answers for the presenting condition.

<u>Probabilistic Approach</u>: A widely used approach in which the system focuses only on the answers that are more likely to happen. It is, in effect, a short list of the ones that the first approach will describe.

<u>Prognostic Approach</u>: A more practical approach. It mainly examines first those answers that have a serious or grave impact on the condition (e.g., emergency conditions, conditions with serious or life-threatening complications).

Each of the three approaches has its merits as well as its shortcomings. To have a comprehensive, fast and practical diagnostic system, we have found that using a combined approach yields the best results.

At first all the possible diagnoses are listed and examined, then the more common or likely conditions are brought into focus, while giving special consideration to the life-threatening, emergent and serious conditions.

4. System Interaction and Correlation

Here we discuss the basic concepts, guidelines and relationships that govern the way each component of the system will interact with the other components.

These considerations include the differentiation, organization, categorization and representation of the data subsets or groups; defining the directions, pathways and patterns of data processing flow; and determining the governing factors that will direct and influence the flow of data between those different subsets. The basic concepts in this regard include identification of the determinants, modifiers and associated data variables, and assigning the probability values.[12]

Identification of the Determinants

The data subset of determinants describes the data values that will remain constant and not change with regard to the task, application or usage. Examples of such data include percentage of people in certain age groups, percentage of high-risk groups within a specific population, etc.

Identification of the Modifiers

The data subset of modifiers includes those data values that are in direct relation to, are affected by and are changing with regard to the main task. Examples of such data include the onset of pain, the level of fever, the physical characteristics of a rash, etc.

Identification of the Associated Data Variables

The data subset of variables includes those data values that are also related to the main task, but they may or may not change in accordance to the main task at any given point in time. By definition, this data subset is the most variable, and it is also one area where the diagnostic system will display considerable flexibility. Examples of this kind of data include presence of nausea or vomiting with abdominal pain, the presence of different types of cough with fever, a history of alcohol use in headache, etc.

Assigning the Probability Values

The logical system works by correlating the relative probability of the data subsets, and from this interaction of probability determination, the logical conclusion is drawn in the form of the solution. Data subsets can have either a base probability value (commonly with reference to the general population being examined) or a dependent probability value (determined in relation to the other data subsets).

Determining the Data Flow

This includes the logical relationships and pathways which the system will use to correlate the different probability values of different data subsets. The system will recognize data subsets according to their influence and/or dependability on other data subsets, i.e.:

- Data subsets that influence all the other subsets
- Data subsets influencing only a specific number of other subsets
- Data subsets being under the influence of (dependent on) other subsets. This dependency can be a sequential relationship (one present following the other) or a conditional relationship (one present only if the other is)

Developing a Hierarchy

This is the concept of assigning a different priority order to each of the data subsets as they are being examined, correlated or output. This concept's greatest impact will be on the order of the solutions presented after the information is processed.

5. Concluding Remarks

Dr. Denton A. Cooley, who stands in the pantheon of the gods of cardiac surgery, once said that he could train a monkey to perform heart surgery. This remark, we presume, reflects how important it is to develop a well-structured and standardized system to handle any given task, with the least requirements of knowledge or training.

In our own experience in designing, building and implementing a logical medical diagnostic system, we have found out that a well-detailed, structured and standardized system can be used to handle different diagnostic tasks in different environments while requiring minimal adjustment of its internal configuration. It will also require the least operator adjustment, effort and time.[6]

We believe that Artificial Intelligence systems are quite capable of performing diagnostic tasks in the medical field, if they are designed, built and implemented with a well-structured reasoning framework.

We are looking forward to increased involvement of Artificial Intelligence systems in various aspects of health care management, which we can only envision as beneficial to the health care community, and to the general public.

References

1. Rogers SK; Ruck DW; Kabrisky M; Artificial Neural Networks for early detection and diagnosis of cancer: Cancer Letters 1994,77 (2-3):79-83, Mar 15.
2. Taleit E; Reibnegger G; Artificial Neural Networks in laboratory medicine and medical outcome prediction: Clin Chem Lab Med 37(9):845-853,1999.
3. Ercal F; Chawla A; Stoecker WV; Neural Network diagnosis of malignant melanoma from color images:IEEE Transaction on Biomed Engineering,41(9):837-45,Sep 1994.
4. Stempczy~nska J; Kacki E; Problems of knowledge acquisition automation in medical expert systems: Medinfo, 8 Pt 1(-HD-): 857-60,1995.
5. Long W; Medical diagnosis using a probabilistic causal network; Applied Artificial Intelligence,3:367-383,1989.
6. Wellwood J; Johannessen S; Spiegelhalter DJ; How does computer-aided diagnosis improve the management of abdominal pain? : AnnR Coll Surg Engl, 74(1):40-6,1992 Jan.
7. de Dombal FT; Dallos V; McAdam WA; Can computer aided teaching packages improve clinical care in patients with acute abdominal pain?: BMJ,302(6791):1495-7,1991,Jun 22.
8. Henry SB; Borchelt D; Schreiner JG; Musen MA; A computer-based approach to quality improvement for telephone triage in a community AIDS clinic: Nurs Adm Q, 18(2):65-73,1994,Winter.
9. Moreno HR; Plant RT; A prototype decision support system for differential diagnosis of psychotic and organic mental disorders: Med Decis Making, 13(1):43-8,1993,Jan-Mar.
10. Wang S; el Ayeb B; Echav'e V; Preiss B; An intelligent interactive simulator of clinical reasoning in general surgery: Proc Annu Symp Comput Appl Med Care, -HD-(-HD-):419-23,1993.
11. Wilson DH; et al; Diagnosis of acute abdominal pain in the accident and emergency department: Br J Surg, 64(4): 250-4,1977,Apr.
12. de Dombal FT; The OMGE acute abdominal pain survey. Progress report,1986: Scand J Gastroenterol Suppl,144(-HD-):35-42,1988.
13. Ohmann C; et al; Clinical benefit of a diagnostic score for appendicitis: JAMA,134(9),Sept 1999.
14. Richardson WS; et al; Users' Guide to the Medical Literature: XV. How to use an article about disease probability for differential diagnosis: JAMA, 281(13),Apr 7, 1999.
15. Whalley LJ; Ethical issues in the application of virtual reality to medicine: Comput Biol Med, 25(2):107-14,Mar,1995.

Medicine Meets Virtual Reality 2001
J.D. Westwood et al. (Eds.)
IOS Press, 2001

Surgical Trainee Assessment using a VE Knee Arthroscopy Training System (VE-KATS): Experimental Results

K.P.Sherman[1], J.W.Ward[2], D.P.M.Wills[2], V.J.Sherman[3], A.M.M.A.Mohsen[1]

1. Orthopaedic Department, Hull and East Yorkshire Hospitals NHS Trust, Hull, UK
2. Department of Computer Science, University of Hull, Cottingham Road, Hull, UK
3. University of Cambridge, UK

Abstract. Previous work has described the development of a Virtual Environment Knee Arthroscopy Training System (VE-KATS): a collaborative project between the Orthopaedic Department, Hull and East Yorkshire Hospitals NHS Trust, Hull, U.K., and the Department of Computer Science, University of Hull, U.K. This work describes the initial results obtained by Orthopaedic Surgical Trainees using VE-KATS. The results showed that differences between individual trainees could be measured using the scoring system incorporated within VE-KATS. There was a weak correlation with the seniority of the surgical trainees.

1 Background

There is a perceived need for improved training of higher surgical trainees for arthroscopy. Virtual environment simulators offer the potential for improved training in such techniques, whilst avoiding risk to patients [1,2]. Such simulators must provide evaluation of performance to have teaching effectiveness. We have incorporated an objective scoring system into a knee arthroscopy simulator. The scoring system evaluates time to task and the percentage of each anatomical structure visualized using the virtual arthroscope. The work described here was undertaken to evaluate the scoring system.

2 Method and Materials

The current version of VE-KATS [3] takes the physical form of a limb "shell" with an outer skin made of foam rubber. This outer skin is formed from the same foam material as that used for artificial limbs and is supplied as a contoured cylinder. The skin has been found to give realistic deformation and conformation. Portals placed in this foam give a realistic feel to the physical instruments and subjectively behave in a similar mechanical fashion to portals placed through skin, subcutaneous tissue and fascia. Inside the skin is a polypropylene hard liner for the thigh and calf, with multi-axial hinges joining the two components together. The physical model of the thigh, knee and leg can thus be flexed and extended, and the model can also be rotated at the thigh component. The position of the lower leg part of the limb can be monitored using one of the sensors of a Polhemus Fastrak electromagnetic tracking system.

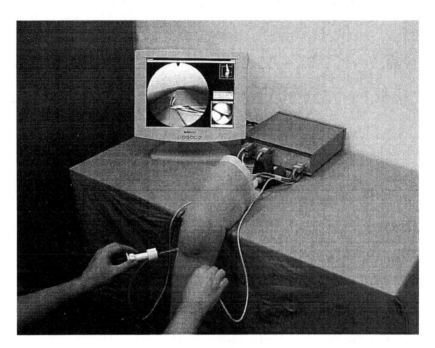

Figure 1 Current version of VE-KATS

The physical model arthroscope is made from hard plastic and allows independent rotation of the camera around the long axis of the arthroscope. The probe is also modeled in hard plastic. The position of the arthroscope and probe are both monitored with a Polhemus Fastrak™ electromagnetic tracker. The physical shape of the arthroscope analogue has been designed to match closely that of contemporary video-arthroscopes. The camera on the arthroscope can be rotated independently to allow maximization of the effective field of view without changing the orientation of the picture on the monitor, i.e. the arthroscope can be rotated to sweep the field of view around the knee whilst holding the camera in one position. The independent rotation of the arthroscope camera is tracked using an encoder, which is able to measure 360° continuous rotation. This component is contained within the physical model. The arrows in Figure 2 indicate the rotation point.

The software is hosted on a PC with graphics accelerator card, (a Pentium II 300MHz PC with Fire GL 1000 Graphics accelerator card). The use of this computer allows the system to be made portable. The current PC-based system allows refresh rates of 40Hz with scoring operational. The software has been developed using C++ and OpenGL.

In addition to the simulated arthroscopic view, a window can be opened to show an anatomical overview of the position of the arthroscope and probe to allow the beginner to locate the position of the instruments when they cannot be located through the arthroscopic view. A further window can be opened on screen to display a video-clip showing a real arthroscopic procedure. In the current version the angled fields of view can be reproduced, views of 0°, 30° or 70° can be selected. Previous work has demonstrated optical distortion produced by the use of wide-angled lenses in arthroscopes [4]. This distortion is simulated in real time within VE-KATS.

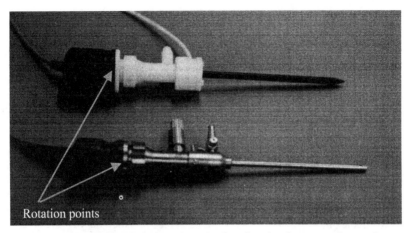

Rotation points

Figure 2 VE-KATS Arthroscope (top) and real arthroscope (bottom)

The current model uses a linear tetrahedral Finite Element Method (FEM) for modeling the deformable tissues [5]. The Voxel Intersection method is used for detecting collision with non-deformable tissues as this allows calculations to take place at a rate several orders faster than the polygon intersection method used for the deformable tissues [2].

The system incorporates objective scoring of performance. Evaluation of performance is based on a validated scoring system [6,7]. The ICI scripting language [8] has been used for the scoring system incorporated within VE-KATS. The system allows performance to be assessed on several independent criteria. The area being viewed can be calculated at any time, allowing a measure to be made of the area of any specific structure that has been visualized. The area that has been probed can be calculated in a similar way. The format of a training session can take the form of a tutorial. The system has the capability for separate subtasks to be demonstrated on the screen using a pre-recorded clip. The trainee then commences the subtask evaluation/practice using a footswitch. The subtask is then scored. At the completion of a training session a total score can be produced. This scoring allows the trainee to self-assess his/her progression in learning the appropriate practical skills and also allows a supervising trainer to evaluate the stage of development the trainee has reached.

Once the separate subtasks have been mastered the trainee can then proceed to perform an entire diagnostic arthroscopy. In its current form the score is given in a numeric % form, with a breakdown into the percentage of each individual structure which has been visualized. A minimum time of visualization is required to avoid cursory scanning or accidental scans over the surface of a structure without proper intentional visualization.

The individual movements of the virtual instruments' analogues are recorded and the entire procedure can then be played back to allow the trainee to review his/her performance. As the subsequent playback is a reconstruction based on the recording of the individual movements themselves it is possible to re-apply the scoring using subsequent modifications to the scoring system (such as different minimum visualization registration times). As an example the results using minimum visualization registration times of 2 seconds, 3 seconds and 4 seconds could be compared.

Forty-three Orthopaedic higher surgical trainees attending their annual appraisal were asked to complete a standardized diagnostic arthroscopy using VE-KATS. Each trainee was presented with an explanatory sheet explaining the criteria used for scoring.

Time was then allowed for the trainee to become familiarized with the system. Once the trainee was satisfied that he or she was ready to commence they were asked to press the footswitch and then complete a diagnostic arthroscopy, visualizing key specified anatomical structures. The structures could be visualized in any order. On completion of the procedure they were asked to press the footswitch again. The scores obtained for each trainee were formatted into a report, which detailed the percentage of each key structure which had been visualized, together with the time taken to complete the test. Each trainee also completed a questionnaire evaluation of VE-KATS.

3 Results

Twenty-nine of the trainees had previously used a plastic knee model. These trainees evaluated the usefulness of VE-KATS in its current form as being very close to that of currently available physical knee models (ratings of 6.67 and 6.86 out of 10 respectively).

Differences in performance between individual trainees could be identified. The scores for the percentage of each anatomical structure visualized were averaged to obtain a mean score. A composite score was calculated for each trainee by dividing the mean score for visualization by the time taken to complete the procedure. The time-to-completion, mean scores and composite scores for the trainees were plotted against their year group on the training scheme (Figure 3).

The results were analysed using SPSS. When the scores were aggregated for each year group Pearson Correlation Coefficients (r) of 0.4 (p < 0.21), 0.57 (p < 0.11) and 0.73 (p < 0.05) were obtained for time to completion, mean score and composite scores respectively. However, when the composite score for each individual trainee was plotted against their year on the training scheme the scatter plot demonstrated a wide variation in performance within each year group and the Pearson Correlation Coefficient did not reach the 0.05 level of significance (r = 0.24, p < 0.16). Regression ANOVA showed poor linearity (sum of squares regression 0.51, residuals 8.68, mean square regression 0.51, residuals 0.51, F = 2.06) (Figure 4).

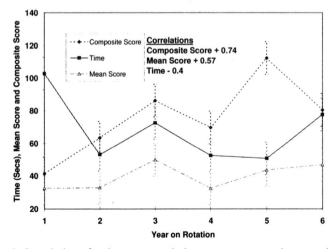

Figure 3 Correlations for time-to-completion, mean score and composite score v seniority of trainee

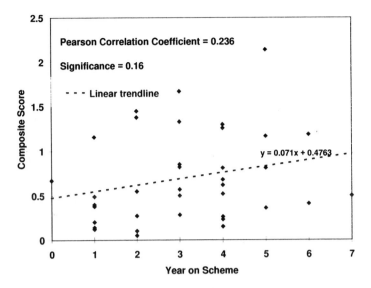

Figure 4 Correlation of composite score v seniority of trainee

4 Conclusions

In its present form the scoring system incorporated within VE-KATS has been shown to identify differences in performance between individual trainees. There is, however, only a poor correlation between the seniority of the trainees and the scores obtained. There are a number of possible explanations for this observation. Surgeons may employ a number of techniques to achieve efficient navigation of instruments within the joint cavity. Such techniques include the use of visual, haptic and kinesthetic cues. An example of haptic navigation cues would include touching the side of the instrument against rigid structures within the joint. It is suggested that more experienced surgeons may rely less on visual cues and more on haptic and kinesthetic feedback. This will be the subject of further research.

It is concluded that VE-KATS has concurrent validity. The potential educational value was rated highly by surgical trainees. Future development should concentrate on the introduction of haptic feedback [9,10] and improving the sophistication of the scoring system (including evaluation of the proportion of specific structures probed).

References

[1] D. P. M. Wills, I. P. Logan, R. D. Macredie, K. P. Sherman, A. M. M. A. Mohsen, Human Factors Issues in the Design of an Arthroscopic Simulator, *Proc. IEEE Conference "Virtual Reality - User Issues.* Cheltenham UK, March 1996 pp. 9/1-9/4.

[2] I. P. Logan, D. P. M. Wills, N. J. Avis, A. M. M. A. Mohsen, K. P. Sherman, *Simulation in* Virtual Environment Knee Arthroscopy Training System, *Synthetic Environments '96, Simulation Series* **28 (4)** (1996) pp. 11-16.

[3] K. P. Sherman, J. Ward, D. P. M. Wills, A. M. M. A. Mohsen, A Portable Virtual Environment Knee Arthroscopy Training System with Objective Scoring. In: J. D. Westwood, H. M. Hoffman, R. A. Robb, D. Stredney (Eds), Studies in Health Technology and Informatics, 62, IOS Press Ohmsha, Amsterdam, 1999, p. 335.

[4] A. M. M. A. Mohsen, J. Ward, D. P. M. Wills, K. P. Sherman, Improved Optical Distortion Simulation for a Virtual Environment Knee Arthroscopy Training System, *Proc. SICOT 99 Sydney* 18–23 April 1999, p. 600.

[5] I. P. Logan, J. Ward, D. P. M. Wills, K. P. Sherman, Arthroscopic training in a virtual environment: Is it a reality?, *Proc MEDTEC '97 Medical Technology Conference and Exposition,* Tysons Corner VA, 1997.

[6] D. Bartram, M. Crawshaw, A. Geake, K. P. Sherman, Prediction of Performance in Arthroscopic Surgery, *Proc. British Psychological Society Occupational Psychology Conference,* Jan 1999, pp. 110-114.

[7] A. Geake, D. Bartram, M. Crawshaw, K. P. Sherman, The Development of an Objective Scoring System for Arthroscopic Surgery, *Proc. British Psychological Society Occupational Psychology Conference,* Jan 1999, pp. 110–114.

[8] ICI Scripting Language http://www.zeta.org.au/~atrn/ici

[9] J. Ward, D. P. M. Wills, K. P. Sherman, A. M. M. A. Mohsen, "The Development of an Arthroscopic Surgical Simulator with Haptic Feedback" in: *Future Generation Computer Systems,* **550** (1998) pp. 1–9.

[10] J. Ward, K. P. Sherman, D. P. M. Wills, A. M. M. A. Mohsen, M. Crawshaw, The Acquisition of Force Feedback Data For a Virtual Environment Knee Arthroscopy Training System, *Proc. Industrial & Business Simulation Symposium 1999 Advanced Simulation Technologies Conference,* San Diego, April 1999, pp. 87–92.

Medicine Meets Virtual Reality 2001
J.D. Westwood et al. (Eds.)
IOS Press, 2001

Haptic palpation of Head and Neck cancer patients – Implications for education and telemedicine

Joacim Stalfors MD[1], Torben Kling-Petersen PhD[2],
Martin Rydmark MD, PhD[2] and Thomas Westin MD, PhD[1]
[1]*Dept. of Otolaryngology, Head and Neck surgery, Sahlgrens University Hospital*
[2]*MEDNET. Göteborg University, Göteborg, Sweden*

Abstract. Malignancy in the head and neck area is a disease that often gives high morbidity in functions like speech, eating, breathing and cosmetics. To ensure a treatment of high clinical standard these patients are presented for a multidisciplinary tumor-team at Sahlgren University hospital. The team usually involves ENT-surgeons (Ear, Nose and Throat), oncologists, radiologists, pathologists, plastic surgeon, general surgeon and oral surgeons. The aim of the presentation is to classificate the tumor and suggests a treatment. The patients presented are from the whole western region of Sweden, and therefore some patients have to travel long distances. To minimize travel telemedicine was introduced 1998 with success [1]. One concern, when presenting a patient with telemedicine, has been the lack of possibility to palpate the tumor and the tissue surrounding it.

To address this problem a 3D model of the tumor visualizes the region and possibly allows haptic palpation. Based on a series of high resolution CT/MR scans, a model of the region around the patients tumor is created. Haptic properties are added to the skin and subcutaneous structures (including the tumor) of the model. Initially, the haptic tuning is done by an examining physician, but in the final telemedical application, the aim is to develop a sensory device for this purpose (e.g. a position sensitive glove, such as Virtual Technologies, Inc. CyberGlove [2] and a graded system for setting firmness of the tissue). The model with its haptic properties can then be examined visually and haptically, the latter using a haptic device such as the SensAble PHANToM [3].

The present system uses a 3D model in VRML format based on reconstructed structures in the ROI (which includes the jawbones, the vertebra, the throat, major muscles and the skin) from high resolution CT. Haptic properties are added using MAGMA 2.5 (ReachIn Technologies AB, Sweden) [4]. Haptic force feedback is provided using a PHANToM Desktop (SensAble Technologies Inc) [3]. Visual feedback can be either monoscopic or stereoscopic (StereoGraphic CrystalEyes) [5].

The system will be used for concept testing and for evaluating possible limitations and/or the need for a modified examination protocol. Once a reliable set of parameters has been generated (using both professionals and medical students at various levels), the remote components will be added.

[1] Telemedicine in regional tumor conference on ear, throat and neck diseases
    Rapport from SPRI, http://www.lf.se/telemedicin
[2] http://www.vertex.com
[3] http://www.sensable.com
[4] http://www.reachin.se
[5] http://www.stereographics.com

1. Introduction

Patients with head and neck cancer are very seriously ill and will often die from their disease. The treatment offered is dependent on several factors such as age, general condition, histology and localization of the tumor. The disease and the treatment will often affect important functions such as eating, breathing speech and cosmetics. Palpation of the tumor in relation to normal tissues can sometimes be of crucial value when the surgeon decides on whether or not to operate and also to assess the extent of the surgery necessary.

In the western part of Sweden all patients with a cancer in the head and neck area are presented to a multidisciplinary tumor-conference at Sahlgrens University hospital. The conference usually involves ENT-surgeons (Ear, Nose and Throat), oncologists, radiologists, pathologists, plastic, general and oral surgeons. The purpose of this conference is to classificate the tumor and suggests a treatment. Many patients presented at this conference have to travel more than 150 miles. To minimize travel telemedicine was introduced in 1998 and its effects studied [1,2]. Telemedicine is now used as an integrated tool during the tumor-conference. However, palpation still cannot be offered by means of telemedicine and therefore some cases need to be seen face-to-face by the surgeon for palpation. This has especially been found to be on patients with tumors in the hypopharynx, mesopharynx and thyroid gland [2].

Since the lack of palpation is a limitation during a telemedicine conference this project was initiated. First step is to provide an interactive 3D image that the participants at the conference can use for further understanding of the tumors localization. Furthermore, if haptic sensations can be integrated into this image, understanding of anatomical relations over a distance can be more comprehendible.

2. Materials and Methods

2.1 Present model

For concept testing purposes, a simplified model is used. Based on a series of high resolution CT/MR scans from a patient, 35 slices (3 mm apart) are selected from the neck and face region. Discrimination of important structures is done by hand and includes the jawbones, skin, muscles, larynx, spinal column and a tumor. The segmented areas are triangulated and modeled using in-house software (for description see [3, 4]). Once the discrete model is complete, the file is converted into VRML97 (VRML 2.0) format for further manipulation in Magma® (ReachIn Technologies AB, Sweden).

Magma® is a programming API/environment allowing interactive manipulation of a 3D model using a haptic interface. In the present model, we use a PHANToM® from SensAble Technologies Inc. Using Magma® (version 2.5), we assigned dynamic and tactile properties to the different part of the model. In principle, bone is set to exhibit a very stiff structure while skin is set to exhibit low friction and high elasticity. Muscles, tumor etc are given properties in-between according to the recommendation of a trained medical practitioner.

Once the model is given its properties, single point palpation is performed to assess the degree of realism and determine the feasibility of the project. The results are described below.

2.2 Hardware

In addition to the equipment mentioned above, the model is created using the Medical Faculty Computer laboratory's SGI cluster. Haptic interface programming is done using an Intergraph Zx-10 workstation (2x 833 MHz Pentium PC with 512 Mb RAM and a WildCat 4110 graphicscard). According to user preferences [4] monoscopic or stereoscopic visualization can be accomplished using a standard CrystalEyes CE-2 setup (Stereographics Inc) [www.stereographics.com].

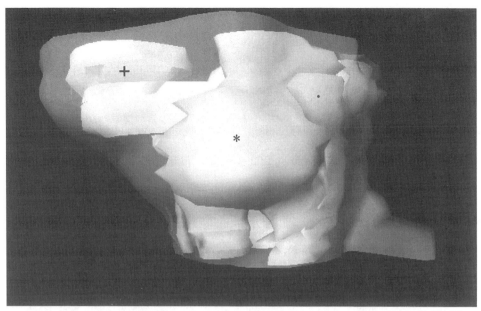

Figure 1. Semi transparent view of the simplified model (seen from lower left). The tumor(*) can be seen covering most of the left cheek around the jawbone (+). Posterior to the tumor the sternoclaidomastoid muscle (O) can be seen.

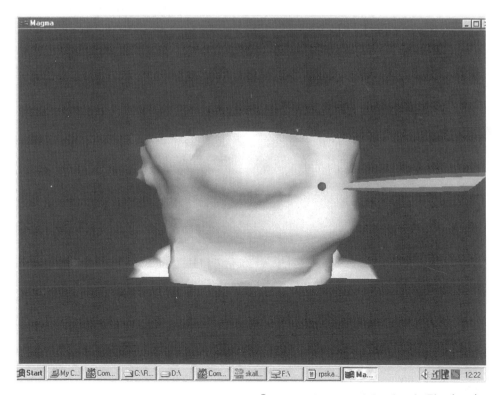

Figure 2. The model displayed in Magma° viewed from straight-ahead. The haptic interface (i.e. a PHANToM Desktop°) is visualized as a ball and a grip.

3. Results and discussion

The simplified model produced for the concept testing in the present work contained, in addition to the tumor, important landmarks such as the jawbone, the larynx, muscle groups and skin (see fig 1). Once the model has been transferred to Magma®, the view is locked to a forward view angle and the skin is made non-transparent.

Palpation, usually done with two hands and several fingers is reduced to a single point. However, the contact of this point with the reconstructed model produces propriosensory feedback and haptic resistance not unlike normal palpation. While some of the internal structures are difficult to palpate, this is due to the limitations of Magma. Better support for multiple interaction layers and object to object collision detection will solve this problem. While Magma displays some limitations, the built in support for PythonScript, new algorithms for tissue deformation as well as future support for multiple PHANToMs, will make Magma a very versatile VR environment.

The difficulty of accurate sensing of deeper structures led us to allowing penetration of the skin with the haptic userinterface. This allowed us to palpate inner structures without the interference of skin, muscles and fatty tissue. While this needs to be explored further, we believe that it may end up being a major improvement to traditional palpation, giving the examining physician more detailed information as to the medical state of the patient.

Future developments. Once an acceptable set of parameters has been established, the telemedical phase will be implemented. Using a generic model of a head (neck-throat region), patient specific data will be added. For the telemedical application, a CyberGlove (Virtual Technologies, Inc.) will be used by the examining physician (at a selected rural hospital) to palpate the patient and using a keypad, appropriate parameters for texture and dynamic properties is set for both specific landmarks as well as possible pathological findings. Once the examinations are done, the data is downloaded to the main hospital.

Based on the downloaded data, the generic model is modified and a specialist can perform an examination of the patient specific model at his leisure. Data obtained using the above mentioned approach as well as data generated from CT scans, can be used as a training tool for medical students, thereby providing patient relevant training models.

In summary, the present pilot study clearly indicates that this is a valid approach to enhanced medical examinations. While the telemedical angle has yet to be explored, we feel that most of the technical problems highlighted by the present study, will be possible to solve and the addition of remote model generation will open up new ways of diagnosis as well as new tools to educate future specialists.

4. References

[1] Telemedicine in regional tumor conferences on ear, throat and neck diseases Rapport from SPRI, http://www.lf.se/telemedicin
[2] A Tele-oncology simulation indicates good accuracy compared to face to face consultations during a head and neck cancer conference. Stalfors J et al. In manuscript.
[3] Kling-Petersen T, Pascher R, Rydmark M (1999) Virtual Reality on the web: the potential of different methodologies and visualization techniques for scientific research and medical education. Stud Health Tech Inf, 62, 181-186
[4] Kling-Petersen T, Rydmark M (2000). Modeling And Modification Of Medical 3D Objects. The benefit of using a haptic modeling tool. Stud Health Tech Inf, 70, 162-167.
[5] Rydmark M, Kling-Petersen T, Pascher R and Philip F. (2001). 3D Visualization and Stereographic Techniques for Medical Research and Education. This publication.

Medicine Meets Virtual Reality 2001
J.D. Westwood et al. (Eds.)
IOS Press, 2001

Implementing a Virtual Reality Paradigm in Human Anatomy/Physiology College Curricula

Helen St. Aubin, Ph.D.
Central Arizona College
Superstition Mountain Campus, Apache Junction, AZ 85222
E-mail: hstaubin@msn.com

Abstract

Modes of instruction in the college course called Human Anatomy/Physiology are changing. Due to ethical concerns and the ever-increasing source of new physiological data, there is a need for enhancements to assist the instructor and student. The computer science of virtual reality (VR) provides a method to electronically educate, train, prototype, test and evaluate new enhancements to the college curricula. This study detailed the modeling and simulation of a skeletal human hand with degrees of freedom of movement, which provided the students with a physiological representation of some of the movements of the hand. The primary objectives of the study were to assess the use of the VR simulation by college students and to assess the potential learning outcomes of students in their use of the VR simulation. The simulation was implemented into classes of Human Anatomy/Physiology as an adjunct enhancement for the students' use. The expectation centered on the constructivist theory that students develop an analytic outlook to the various articulations of the human skeleton. Positive results were shown based on the answers to the questionnaire, summary and post-test taken by the students, after their use of the VR simulation. The results supported the constructivist theory that critical thinking took place. The results showed that the virtual reality simulation enhanced the learning ability of the students. The recommendations of the study include future experimentation to be done on increasing the number of VR simulations, incorporating the VR simulations into undergraduate courses, testing the outcomes, and following the progression of students into graduate programs that are using VR simulations. Faculty and administration are advised to consider implementing the paradigm of VR simulations in undergraduate courses of Human Anatomy/Physiology.

1 Introduction

The virtual reality simulation environment is a major change in the paradigm of medical education, and the motivation of the student to utilize a virtual reality simulation for education may prove to be a cost savings. Considerations are in the planning stages for virtual reality simulations in the science courses in the undergraduate programs in colleges and universities. Students planning a career in most medical fields are required to take an under-graduate course called Human Anatomy/Physiology, which is a foundational course for advanced topics that place emphasis on problem solving, and it is necessary to help students to develop necessary synthetic, analytic, and diagnostic thinking skills. Past teaching practices in the course would rely heavily on the students memorizing large amounts of data without the cognitive ability to reason the need for all the data and how it applies to the human body.

Changes in the college curricula are being researched, developed and implemented, but new paradigms need to be researched to enhance the present methods of instruction. These paradigms, that may include virtual reality simulations, will enable students to continue into the medical school environment with an introductory background in virtual reality applications in the study of human anatomy/physiology. Further, instead of testing factual recall on textbook memorization, the inference functions built into the symbolic virtual reality model make it possible to develop assessment measures that can evaluate whether the student is applying some productive reasoning strategies in problem solving. This constructivist type of exercise can provide a better foundation for the assessment of diagnostic reasoning and a very different modality of instruction and testing. With the challenges of attracting more students into the college environment, new innovative methods are being pursued.

2 Goals

The goals of this research were the modeling, simulation and implementation of a virtual reality simulation of the human skeletal hand with some degrees of freedom movement in the fingers and thumb. The VR simulation was used as an enhancement in the science lab in the study of Human Anatomy/Physiology (one of the courses taught by the author). The goals of the study were, also, to assess the use of the VR simulation by college students, and to assess the potential learning outcomes of students in their use of the VR simulation.

3 Methods

The author created the model (using a software program called MultiGen Creator 2.1 [1]), developed the simulation (using a software program called EON Studio 2.5 [2]) and implemented the virtual reality simulation (using EON Viewer [2]) in three college classes of Human Anatomy/Physiology. The VR simulation was a non-immersive stereoscopic screen display and it was placed on desktop personal computers in college lab environments. The students used the keyboard and mouse for the manipulation of the VR simulation. The decision to develop a non-immersive VR simulation was based solely on cost to the college. The two colleges, in this study, have computers available but do not have the funds for any peripheral devices that would be necessary for an immersive VR simulation.

The movements of the hand were limited in order to reduce the size of the file, so that it could be placed on a 3¼ floppy (2HD) disk for transportability to the various colleges. Also reducing the size of the file will enable future experimentation with the use of the file via the Internet for web-based college distance learning classes. In addition to the VR simulation the author created a booklet of reference material, a questionnaire and post-test of semantic differential scale and Likert scale type questions and a summary evaluation to be used by the students.

4 Results

The virtual reality simulation of the human skeletal hand provided the students with a physiological representation of some of the movements of the hand. At present, in classes, students have no representation of the skeletal hand movement; all they have is the text material describing in short detail the physiological movements of the hand. The cadaver that is now available in some of the college labs, that basically has replaced cat dissection (due to ethical reasons and cost), is already dissected (by a professional) and the students view the cadaver as the instructor does a "show and tell". The plastic skeleton models available to students in the lab also have rigid hands that are held in place by wires, thus permitting no finger and thumb movement.

The students viewed the VR simulation by using the mouse. They were able to move the VR simulation of the skeletal hand, using the mouse, by rotating it left to right, right to left, and basically moving the hand wherever in the screen (using the x, y, and z axis). By clicking with the mouse, on the phalanges of the fingers and the thumb, the students could see the various movements of the fingers and the thumb. They saw flexion and extension movements of the hand. At the time abduction and adduction of the fingers and thumb were not included because of the amount of computer memory and speed necessary for real-time simulation. Also, the special action of the thumb called opposition was not available, as opposition uses the motion of the metacarpal bone. No movement of the metacarpals was available in the VR simulation.

A questionnaire, summary evaluation and post-test were given the students after they were finished using the VR simulation and the results and comments were all positive. The questionnaires and post-tests with Likert-type and semantic differential type variables were analyzed using frequency distributions. To date there are very few evaluations of the use of VR simulations in the classroom, especially in the undergraduate college level.

5 Conclusions

The goal of the creation and implementation of the VR simulation of the human skeletal hand with some degrees of freedom movement in the fingers and thumb was achieved. The implementation of the VR simulation took place in three labs of Human Anatomy/Physiology in on-site classes. The VR simulation was developed to show that it was a teaching skill that was relevant to the real task performance, and although it was not totally realistic, a virtual reality simulation needs only to be realistic enough so that the students who use the VR simulation feel they have learned something or done something they could not ordinarily learn or do.

Despite the software, hardware, and other problems, the author observed very positive attitudes exhibited by all the students when they used the VR simulation. The experience was new, the students were interested, some were excited, some were amazed, and some were taken back when they saw the fingers and the thumb move in the VR simulation. From the student answers on the questionnaire, it was concluded that the VR simulation enhanced the student learning of hand movement and gave them better understanding of the movement of the fingers and thumb. The results indicated that students want to see other VR simulations of the human joints, want to see other science courses using VR simulations, prefer to use a VR simulation to just reading the information in the textbook, enjoy using the VR simulation, and were encouraged to think more about the movements of the hand and the other joints of the body. It was a first-of-a-kind experience.

Observing the students was a positive experience, and seeing the positive results of the questionnaire, summary and post-test were encouraging for the new technology of VR simulation. Introducing a new paradigm of instruction into a class has problems, but the advantages can outweigh the disadvantages. The learning experience gained by the students was the priority and that priority was met and exceeded the author's expectations.

Constructivist theories assert that students learn by taking in information from their environment and constructing their own meaning from the experience. The use of the VR simulation of the hand enhanced this constructivist concept when the curriculum role of the instructor changed to facilitator and more control was turned over to the students. Finally, for an effective curriculum for the course of Human Anatomy/Physiology, better cooperation, understanding, communication, and compromise need to take place among the faculty and administration. Also needed is a consensus on the use of computer-based enhancements for the course.

An effective curriculum must integrate a problem-solving and decision-making experience. Unfortunately, faculty resistance is one of the most commonly cited reasons for the lack of widespread implementation of new technologies, such as virtual reality simulations. Instructional methods are changing in the 21st century, and it is imperative for instructors to keep up with change to assist the students to further their educational goals and be interested in learning.

References

[1] MultiGen Creator 2.1. (1998). Software program and User Guide. CA: MultiGen-Paradigm Inc. (available at http://www.multigen.com/

[2] EON Studio 2.5. (1999). Software program and user Guide. CA:EON Reality, Inc. (available at http://www.eonreality.com/

Medicine Meets Virtual Reality 2001
J.D. Westwood et al. (Eds.)
IOS Press, 2001

Collaborated surgical works (Surgical planning) in virtual space with tactile sensation between Japan and Germany

Naoki SUZUKI [a], Asaki HATTORI [a], Shigeyuki SUZUKI [b], Kazuki SUMIYAMA [c],
Susumu KOBAYASHI [c], Yoji YAMAZAKI [c], Yoshitaka ADACHI [d]

[a] Institute for High Dimensional Medical Imaging, Jikei Univ. School of Med.,
4-11-1 Izumihoncho, Komae-shi, Tokyo, 201-8601, Japan
[b] Graduate School of Science & Engineering, Waseda Univ.
[c] Dept. of Surgery, Jikei Univ. School of Med.
[d] Suzuki Motor Corp., R&D Center

Abstract. Surgeons in Japan and Germany applied tele-virtual surgery and a force feedback device during a hepatectomy simulation. Using this system, surgeons in each country were able to perform various surgical maneuvers upon the same patient. They palpated abdominal skin made electrical scalpel incisions and widened the incision line by using surgical tools in virtual space. While surgeons performed a virtual operation. the force feedback device conveyed tactile sensations. In each location. the force feedback devices and two graphic workstations of equal capability were employed. As each workstation communicated only event signals through an ISDN (64Kb) line. it was possible to obtain real time tele-virtual surgery without a large capacity communication infrastructure.

1. Preface

Three dimensional images reconstructed from MRI or CT images are currently used in various applications. The application of virtual reality (VR) techniques to 3D images has a large potential to provide future medical treatments through tele-diagnosis and tele-medicine[1-4].

In this paper, we report the results of a tele-virtual surgery experiment between Japan and Germany. Apparatus at both sites were connected by an ISDN line and equipped with a VR surgery system which had a force feedback function. Using this system, surgeons in each location shared identical tactile sensations.

2. Surgical simulation system

Surgical simulation systems have useful applications in the medical field. Such systems allow a user to repeatedly perform virtual surgery until a suitable procedure is established. They are especially useful for educational medical training.

Taking into consideration the needs of the medical field, we have been developing a virtual surgical simulation system upon the following requirements:

1) The system should enable the user to design and determine surgical procedures based on 3D model reconstructed from the patient's data.

2) By using force feedback device, the system must transmit authentic tactile sensations to the user during organ manipulations.

In our system, the surgeon (user) is able to perform various surgical maneuvers with suitable surgical tools as interactive actions in a virtual space[5,6]. This system allows the surgeon to

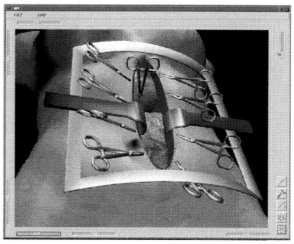

Fig.1 An application of surgical simulation used in this experiment

make a scalpel incision, widen the incision line and secure it with forceps (Fig. 1). All surgical procedures on a 3D object in a virtual space proceed in real-time. Also 3D human structures are reconstructed from 3D patient data that give such anatomical characteristics as vascularity. Numerical parameters such as location, depth, direction to the targeted organ and excised tissue volumes are measurable with quantitative accuracy.

The basic system is function displays various viewpoints, scales and angles. It can also alter the transparency of an organ's multiple layers. Rendering by wire frames is also possible. In addition, each organ model is shaded by light sources set within the system space and separated by easily distinguishable colors. In order to determine possible incision points, these models are texture mapped by using images of the patient's skin and extracted organ texture.

3. Force feedback device

Recently, we have developed a haptic device which allows the user to experience tactile sensations. We also have been developing a force feedback device which possesses 16 degrees-of-freedom (DOF) for manual interactions with virtual environments. The features of the device manufactured for our virtual surgery system can be summarized as follows.

1) The force feedback system is composed of two types of manipulators: a force control

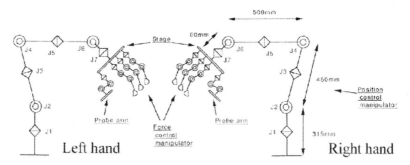

Fig.2 A block diagram of the force feedback device

manipulator and a motion control manipulator.

2) Three force control manipulators are attached to the end of the motion control manipulator.

3) Both ends of each force control manipulator are attached to the thumb, forefinger, and middle finger of the operator.

4) The force control manipulator has a joint structure with minimal inertia and less friction.

5) The motion control manipulator has mechanical stiffness.

Fig.2 shows the block diagram of the force feedback device. Both the right and left force feedback devices have the same internal structure and functions. The force feedback device for the right hand is a mirror image of the left one. On both hands, the force control manipulator producing haptic sensation is attached to the thumbs, forefingers and middle fingers of the right and left hands respectively. Fig.3 illustrates how the user's fingers are attached to the manipulators. Fig.4 shows a user and the devices attached to both hands. These devices communicate data (finger location etc.) with the surgical simulation system through a LAN. When an interaction occurs between the user's fingers and a 3D object in a virtual space, a force parameter of tactile sensations calculated by the sur-

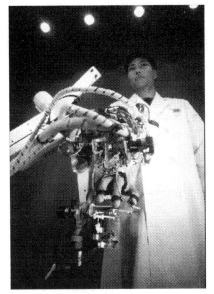

Fig.3 Force feedback device attached to fingers of the right hand

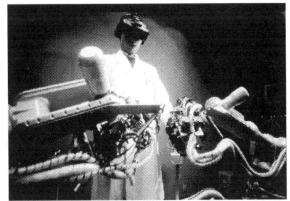

Fig.4 A demonstration of the force feedback devices for the right and left hands

gical simulation system, is transferred to these devices. This allows the user to experience tactile sensations in each finger. Fig.5 shows the linkage between the device and the real time image. The user's hand is perceived as a 3D image in order to identify its location as it comes in contact with the liver surface. When the liver surface was compressed on the image the user's finger experienced tactile sensations.

4. Tele-surgical simulation system

In this experiment, we used a 1ch ISDN line (64Kb/s), because we intended to utilize tele-virtual surgery without a large capacity communication infrastructure. However, it was diffi-

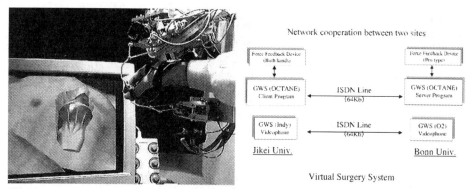

Fig.5 An experiment to touch a liver surface with the   Fig.6 System outline of tele-virtual surgery system
3D image manipulator

cult to transfer images of simulation results to each location in real-time. Therefore, we installed a simulation program and the patient's 3D modeling into each system. The MRI images produced 3D data of the skin surface, liver, liver vessels, liver tumor and colon. The system transmitted and received only event signals related to the simulation. The event signal included force feedback device location data, the application's GUI event (buttons, sliders etc.) and the calculated force of the force feedback device. The size of data per event is about 200 bytes. In this way, both sites were able to observe an identical simulation result in real-time.

The system's outline is shown in Fig.6. Participants at each location employed two graphic workstations (Japan site: Octane, Indy, German site: Octane, O2. All workstations are SGI inc. products) for the surgical simulation and teleconference. The workstations were connected by an ISDN line via an ISDN router. Each workstation had a force feedback device. In Japan, the force feedback was a glove type device attached to both hands, while a pen type device was used in Germany. These devices conveyed tactile sensations to the surgeons during the virtual surgical operation.

For communicating between each site, we used a teleconference application InPerson (SGI inc.) and video image and audio functioning at 300x200 pixels. This application's video frame was about 0.5 frame/sec.

When using network communication as in this experiment, we have to consider the data transfer delay. As this system doesn't manage event time, the delay causes a different results between two sites. We measured the delay between Japan and Germany by using UNIX command ping. The ping command result was 300ms (round-trip time). At this speed, the user didn't need to wait for the processing completion However, if both users in each site had interacted with a 3D object simultaneously, each site's simulation result would have been different. Therefore, each user conducted their procedures in turns.

5. Results

A simulated hepatectomy was chosen for the experiment. The scene of the experiment at the both sites is shown in Fig.7. Surgeons in each location palpated the patient's abdominal skin (Fig.8a) and discussed an incision position while observing the tumor location and vascularity of the liver. While doing so they changed the transparency of the skin and liver surface. In Germany, surgeons made an incision on the skin surface (Fig.8b) while a Japanese

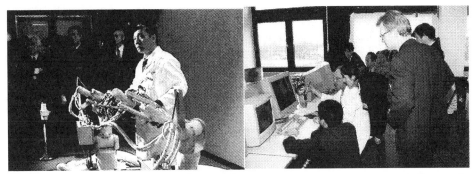

a. Japanese site   b. German site

Fig.7 Scene of the experiment at both sites

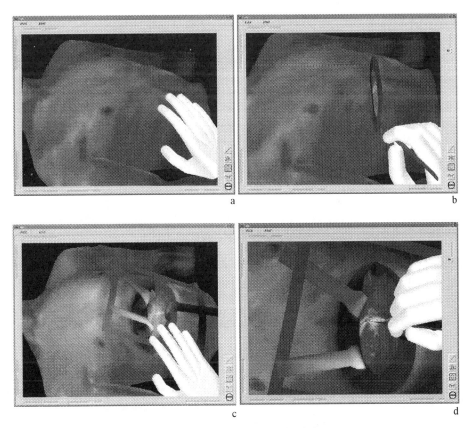

a

b

c

d

Fig.8 Images of a hepatectomy simulation

surgeon widened the incision line using a surgical tool. After widening, they palpated the exposed liver and deliberated upon an incision to the liver (Fig.8c). Finally, a German surgeon made an incision to the liver to complete the hepatectomy (Fig.8d).

In this system, the display's frame rate was 6-7 frame/sec. However, considering the surgeons action during the surgical simulation, the frame rate was acceptable for the simulation. Both surgeons evaluated this system and the experiment, but had no negative comment on the frame rate. The Japanese surgeon commented that he felt in close proximity the German surgeon and didn't sense any delay in the operation. The German surgeon observed that he could discuss surgery procedures in detail with the Japanese surgeon in order to find a solution to the surgical problem.

6. Discussion

We conducted an experiment in which two surgeons simulated virtual surgery while sharing identical tactile sensations over a long distance. It was possible to obtain real-time tele-virtual surgery without a large capacity communication infrastructure.

However, this system has a limitation. Both sites operated on a 3D object in turn, due to time delays when communicating event signals. The delay cause different results between two sites. Therefore, we need to evaluate the effects of time delay on the surgical simulation and develop a system which enable users to manipulate a 3D object simultaneously. If possible, the revised system will be the basis of an enhanced tele-surgery system.

The drawbacks of the force feedback function were caused by a 3D model structure. This model's elasticity is configured only on the surface, and can't take into account the organ's internal structure. To counter this problem, we are developing another 3D model called the "Sphere filled model". This model is reconstructed as a surface model filled with small element spheres with which a force acting on the internal structure can be calculated. By applying this model, tactile sensations will improve.

References

[1]   Suzuki. N. Takatsu. A. Kita. K. Tanaka. T. Inaba. R. Fukui. K: Development of a 3D image simulation system for organ and soft tissue operations.: Abstract of the World Congress on Medical Physics and Biomedical Engineering 1994: 39a: 609.

[2]   Robb RA. Hanson DP: The ANALYZE software system for visualization and analysis in surgery simulation. In: Computer Integrated Surgery. Eds. Steve Lavalle. Russ Taylor. Greg Burdea and Ralph Mosges. MIT Press. 1995. pp.175-190.

[3]   Robb RA. Cameron B: Virtual Reality Assisted Surgery Program. In: Interactive Technology and the New Paradigm for Healthcare. Eds.. R. Satava. et al.. Vol. 18. 1995. pp.309-321

[4]   Kikinis R. Langham Gleason P. Jolesz FA: Surgical planning using computer-assisted three-dimensional reconstructions. In: Computer Integrated Surgery. Eds. Russel Taylor. Stephane Lavallee. Grigore Burdea. and Ralph Mosges. MIT Press. 1995. pp.147-154.

[5]   N. Suzuki. A. Hattori. A. Takatsu: "Medical virtual reality system for surgical planning and surgical support". J. comput. Aided Surg.. 54-59. 1(2). 1995.

[6]   N. Suzuki. A. Hattori. S. Kai. T. Ezumi. A. Takatsu: "Surgical planning system for soft tissues using virtual reality". MMVR5. Eds: K.S. Morgan et al.. pp.159-163. IOS Press. 1997.

Medicine Meets Virtual Reality 2001
J.D. Westwood et al. (Eds.)
IOS Press, 2001

Web-based Educational Tool
for Cleft Lip Repair using XVL

Daigo Tanaka[1], Masahiro Kobayashi[1], Hiroaki Chiyokura[2],
Tatsuo Nakajima[1], Toyomi Fujino[3]
Department of Plastic and Reconstructive Surgery, Keio University[1]
Faculty of Environmental Information, Keio University[2]
International Medical Information Center[3]
Shinano-machi 35, Shinjuku, Tokyo, JAPAN, 160-8582

Abstract. Recent web-based technologies have brought a variety of new
possibilities to the field of medical information. Nevertheless, transferring 3D
patient models through usual low-band-width networks is difficult because of the
large size of data file. XVL (eXtensive VRML with Lattice), a new framework for
3D Data representation with high quality surface shape, has solved this problem. In
cooperation with Lattice Technology Inc., we have created XVL-formatted patient
3D models. The XVL model takes less than 100 kilobytes, whereas the same quality
model in Virtual Reality Modeling Language(VRML) format requires more than 5
megabytes. Because of the many advantages of XVL, we have created a 3D web-
based educational tool for repair of cleft lip -- plastic surgery for congenital defects
of the lips that requires complex incisions and reconstruction. Our system can
interact with the model and 3D visualization of the incision lines, displacement of
skin flaps, and suturing. Our educational tool for cleft lip repair has demonstrated
that the XVL model and its web-based application can open up new possibilities for
3D medical information systems. We are currently refining the XVL model and
developing XVL-based applications to simulate the actual surgery on the World
Wide Web.

1. Introduction

Rapid evolution of 3D Computer Graphics (CG) such as volume rendering has given us
precise 3D pictures of the human body. More recently, the expansion of the internet has
enabled us to transfer 3D medical images to any place in the world. Hendin et al.[1] have
developed a system to display volume rendered images on a web browser. This system is
very acceptable to surgeons because volume rendering is already a practical method for
diagnosis. John et al. [2, 3] have created a virtual training system for surgery making use of
Virtual Reality Modeling Language (VRML) technology. In addition to viewing patient
models, one can also simulate operational procedures such as ventricular catheterization by
manipulating virtual surgical instruments. This promises to make surgical expertise more
widely accessible through out the world. However, one problem that prevented these web-
based systems from being used practically is that 3D medical information files are very
large, and take a long time to transfer across low-bandwidth networks.

Looking at the fields of 3D Computer Aided Design (CAD) and CG industry, we can
find similar problems and solutions. One excellent technology is Lattice Modeling, created
by *Lattice Technology Inc.* While VRML expresses model shapes in polygonal mesh,
Lattice modeling expresses them in high quality surface. This feature enables the model
surface to be very smooth. Saved in a file format called eXtensive Vrml with Lattice (XVL),
the Lattice Model can be transferred through the internet and can also be viewed on the

Microsoft Internet Explorer^{TM} (IE) browser software. XVL files are very small compared to VRML files. In cooperation with *Lattice Technology Inc.*, we have developed a system that can convert polygonal mesh to a Lattice Model, and then save in the XVL format. The method is very suitable for medical data and is very practical because it can reduce data size without omitting model details.

In this paper, we evaluated this new method by developing a 3D educational tool for Cleft lip repair surgery. Cleft lip is a congenital lip defect the repair of which requires a complex surgical procedure. Surgeons have to understand the 3D structure of the patient's lip, and the surgical procedure is like a 3D puzzle of the skin flap. Currently, teaching materials include surgery textbooks that are expressed in 2D illustrations or photographs, VTRs, or silicon models of patients. None of these educational tools can show the 3D structure of lips and the surgical procedure in animations. Using XVL, our new textbook can show on-demand angle images of cleft lip, and the suture of skin flaps in 3D animation. It is a very practical tool for trainees because the contents of the textbook come in a few seconds through the internet from the server. In addition, trainees can communicate with each other and view synchronized images with XVL's multiuser function. This feature facilitates distant learning and teleconferencing in the clinic.

In section 2, we show an overview of our web-based educational tool for cleft lip repair using XVL. Section 3 presents the modeling method from Computed Tomography (CT) data and briefly describes how XVL reduces data size. Section 4 introduces the procedure of making a 3D textbook of cleft lip repair integrating XVL, Hyper Text Markup Language (HTML), and JavaScript. Section 5 describes some evaluation of XVL, and the textbook showing some snapshots in comparison to current textbooks. We conclude this paper in section 6 with future studies.

2. System Overview

Figure 1 shows the system architecture. The server has 3D cleft lip models, and descriptions that are written in HTML. Upon request, it sends models and descriptions through the internet. The textbook is browsed by IE with *XVL player*^{TM} which is plug-in software for viewing Lattice models. JavaScript codes are also embedded in the HTML coding. This provides some user interface, and mediates user input into the XVL player. Thus, the textbook can display animations like suture of skin flaps interactively.

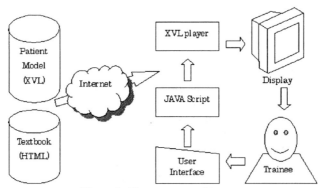

Figure 1. The system architecture

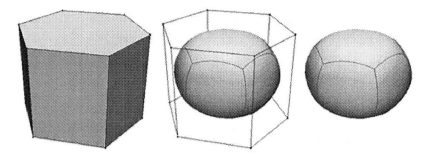

Figure 2. Lattice mesh and Lattice surface conversion.

3. 3D Modeling and Data reduction

The cleft lip models are made constructed from CT data of an actual patient. 3D models are obtained by extracting skin contours from CT images, doing surface reconstruction, reducing data with XVL, and then adjusting models manually for textbook use.

Modeling from CT image data

The CT data was acquired with the cooperation of a patient and parents. The patient was 1 month-old female baby. The CT data set was 100 slices of 512 x 512 images. The distance between adjacent slices was 1.5 mm. We extracted the lip contours by thresholding CT images. We extracted the cleft palate shape by hand tracing because it cannot be separated from other tissues by CT values. Hand tracing is also done when we omitted the lower lip shape to make the model can be conserved from inside the mouth. The contouring process is done with our original system, and surface reconstruction is executed with NUAGES[4]. The 3D model output from NUAGES is in STL format polygonal mesh model, and the average file size is 5 MB.

Data reduction by XVL

We adopted XVL to reduce the size of the files without omitting details. XVL gives high quality surface data using the Lattice Model. The Lattice Model consists of a Lattice surface and Lattice mesh. The Lattice surface is free-form surface data [6] represented by Gregory patches [7]. The Lattice mesh is a simple polygonal mesh which has connectivity data (vertices, edges, faces). Because the Lattice surface and mesh have one-to-one correspondence, the high quality Lattice surface data can easily be converted to a simple and compact Lattice mesh. Figure 2 shows the conversion of two data representations.

We have developed a system to convert STL to XVL. To obtain a precise XVL model, the free-form Lattice surface has to fit the polygonal mesh. To achieve this, we extended the surface fitting method proposed by Takeuchi et al.[8]. In their method, the mesh is simplified based on the Quadric Error Metrics (QEM) technique [9]. We extended this method as follows: At the mesh simplification scheme, we used the points on the Lattice surface as evaluators of QEM and constructed a Lattice mesh that controls the free-form surface. As noted in [6], a vertex L_0 of the Lattice mesh is mapped one-to-one to a vertex P_0 of a Lattice surface. P_0 is represented by L_0 and its neighbors as follows:

$$P_0 = (1 - w_0)L_0 + w_0 \; \Sigma \; k_j l_j ...(1)$$

where w_0 denotes a weight needed for rounding operations.

As shown in [10], at each edge collapse operation, the evaluation function Q^f for calculating an optimized position of v is:

$$Q^v(v) = \Sigma\ area(f)Q^f(v) \ ....(2)$$

$$Q^f(v) = (n^Tv + d)^2 = v^TAv + b^Tv + c\ ....(3)$$

n denotes the normal vector of a face f and d is a scalar. A is a symmetric 3 x 3 matrix, b is a vector and c is a scalar.

As Q^v is a quadratic function, a minimum value is found by simply solving a linear Equation delta Q = 0. We apply P_0 to Equation (2), that is to solve delta $Q^v(P_0)$ = 0. By this extended simplification, a Lattice mesh is constructed.

Manual adjustment of the model

Patient models that are automatically generated do not have enough anatomical features to be used in the field of plastic surgery. This is because CT data does not give information like boundary lines between red lip and white lip. In plastic surgery, this information becomes an important landmark when making the incision line on the tissue. So we edited the Lattice mesh manually to make the edges on the XVL model match the anatomical landmarks. Figure 3 shows two Lattice mesh that represents before and after the editing process.

After changing the edge directions, we colored on each region of the model such as skin, red lip, and white lip.

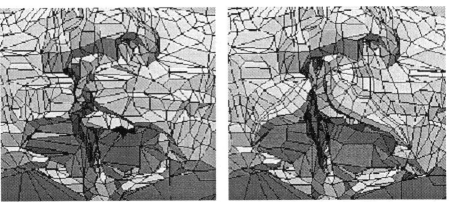

Figure 3. Editing the model to enhance anatomical landmarks

4. Integrating data into a textbook

Embedding the 3D model in HTML

XVL can be embedded in HTML. Once embedded, we can examine the model changing the viewpoint, angle, and scale by mouse dragging. To make the textbook interactive, we also embed buttons on HTML documents using JavaScript. When the user submits a request by clicking the button, JavaScript sends the requests to the XVL player. Using this feature, we can make interactive animations including local dformation of the skin flaps. Even after the deformation the models are still smooth in shape because the XVL animation is based on free-form deformation.

Multi user function

XVL has multi-user function. It reflects the operations of one user to multiple other users. Using this function in the textbook takes the greatest advantage of the internet. enabling distance education and teleconferencing.

5. Evaluation

Data transfer

As an example, we viewed the textbook on a client PC (PentiumII 366MHz, 192 MB RAM) with IE (version 5). The textbook data was downloaded from the server through a low-bandwidth (ISDN, 64K) network. The files of the models created for this textbook were 60 kilobytes each, and were transferred to client computer within a few seconds. After downloading, the XVL player automatically started up in IE window and took a few more seconds to convert the Lattice mesh data to Lattice surface. The rendering performance is totally depended on the specifications of the PC although one can select appropriate rendering quality from several choices provided by the XVL player. The file size and model transferring time are clearly suitable for low cost PCs and a low-bandwidth network, making this system appropriate for distance educations.

The textbook

Clinical conferences are held in our plastic surgery department twice a week. Conferences are held for pre-operational planning and post-operational review, and they are a time for the training of young surgeons. We evaluated this textbook at clinical conferences. Figure 4 shows a snapshot of our textbook that illustrates showing some animations for skin flap movement.

Studying cleft lip repair surgery is a very difficult task, even if the trainees have many chances to see the actual surgery. Good textbooks are therefore required. Figure 5 shows typical illustrations of cleft lip repair surgery. The left one shows the incision design, and the right one explains the sutures of the skin flap. It is very difficult to understand these procedures with 2D illustrations, and figure 6 shows how much more effective 3D illustrations are for understanding.

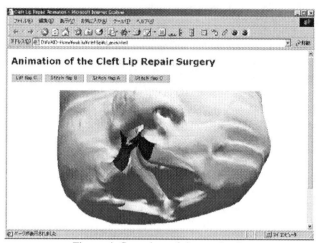

Figure 4. Snapshot of the textbook

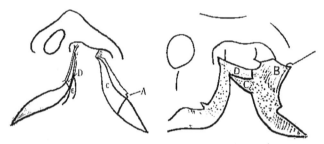

Figure 5. Typical illustrations for cleft lip repair

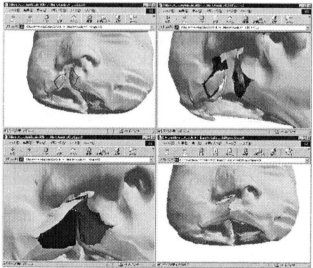

Figure 6. Several scenes of the surgery:
The incision design (top left), lifting a skin flap (top right),
suture of two parts of the lip (bottom left), completion of the surgery (bottom right).

6. Conclusions and Future studies

In this paper, we have proposed a new method to transfer 3D medical data through the internet, and applied this to a textbook of cleft lip repair surgery. Using XVL technology, the textbook clearly illustrates the complex surgical procedures, and is suitable for browsing through a low-bandwidth network.

We anticipate the development of more complex systems, for example surgical simulation, using the XVL framework. Currently we are working to represent the soft tissue deformation after the lip muscle suture.

We are also gathering feedback from surgeons about our textbook. The textbook can be browsed on the World Wide Web,

http://www.prs.med.keio.ac.jp/

using Lattice Technology's XVL.

Acknowledgements

The authors would like to thank Akira Wakita and Takamichi Hayashi from Chiyokura laboratory, Keio University for the discussions and help with the software development.

This research has been done as a part of the Center Of Excellence (COE) project of Keio University funded by the Ministry of International Trade and Industry, Japan.

References

[1] Hendin, O., et al., "Medical volume rendering on the WWW using JAVA and VRML", *Medicine Meets Virtual Reality 1998* (1998), IOS Press, pp.34-40.
[2] John, N. W. et al., "Surgical Simulators Using the WWW", *Medicine Meets Virtual Reality 2000* (2000), IOS Press, pp.146-152.
[3] John, N. W. et al., "A VRML simulator for ventricular catheterisation", *Eurographics UK*(1999).
[4] Geiger, B., "Three-dimensional modeling of human and its application to diagnosis and surgical planning", *Tech. Rep. 2105*, Institut National de Recherche en Informatique et Antomatique, (1993), France.
[6] Wakita, A., "XVL:A Compact And Qualified 3D Representation With Lattice Mesh and Surface for the Internet", *Web3D Consortium Proceedings* (1999), ACM Press, New York, pp209-216
[7] Chiyokura, H., et al., "Design of solids with free-from surfaces", *SIGGRAPH '83 Proceedings* (1983), ACM Press, New York, pp.289-298
[8] Takeuchi, S., et al. "Subdivision surface fitting with QEM-based mesh simplification and reconstruction of approximated B-spline surfaces", *Pacific Graphics 2000* (2000), pp.202-212
[9] Garland, M et al. "Surface simplification using quadric error metrics", *SIGGRAPH '97 Proceedings* (1997), ACM Press, New York, pp.209-216

Medicine Meets Virtual Reality 2001
J.D. Westwood et al. (Eds.)
IOS Press, 2001

Keeping Sharp:
Internet CE Update and Experience

T. Bradley Tanner, M.D., Mary P. Metcalf, Ph.D., and Meghan B. Coulehan
Clinical Tools, Inc., 431 W. Franklin St. #30, Chapel Hill, NC 27516

Abstract. The Internet as a distance-learning tool is evolving rapidly. Most Internet-based Continuing Education (CE) experiences follow a standard didactic approach as demonstrated by lectures, slide presentations, written journals, videotape, and audiotape; however, some Internet-based educators are exploring the full interactive, problem-solving potential of Internet technology. With support from NIMH we are reviewing the state of the art in Internet-based CE and developing CE courses targeted toward primary care providers that aim to alter clinical skills related to depression treatment.

1. Background

There were over 736,000 physicians (M.D.s and D.O.s) in 1996 [1], almost all requiring Continuing Education (CE) each year. There are many strategies used to educate physicians via CE, including seminars, printed material, office based training, lectures, and videotapes [2-7]. The majority of existing medical CE is conference/lecture based. Unfortunately, the value of conference based CE is not supported by the literature. A 1995 review of the literature revealed, "Relatively short (1 day or less) formal CME events such as conferences generally effected no change; six [of six] interventions demonstrated negative or inconclusive effects" [8]. Other standard approaches to CE have also shown marginal results. Davis's review of the literature revealed that, "Educational materials (e.g., printed monographs or audiovisual programs) demonstrated a positive effect in four interventions, but failed to demonstrate an effect in seven instances" [8]. Conference/lecture-based CE is also clearly inconvenient and expensive.

Continuing Education provided via the Internet has grown rapidly and become common and inexpensive. Potential benefits of Internet CE offerings include easy access, low expense, support for previewing, support for multiple media, easy updating, and an ability to create interactive clinical cases. These benefits create a high potential for enthusiasm for Internet-based continuing education when compared with competing Continuing Education learning formats, such as conferences, lectures, written materials, or audio/video materials. However, it is not clear if current examples of Internet-based CE utilize the potential of the Internet.

2. Methods

We are completing a thorough review of existing Internet-CE to fully evaluate online providers of CE on multiple parameters. A database is being developed that includes site name and URL, supporting agency/funding source/type of agency, number of courses offered and usage, course areas covered/topic covered/format, CE credits available and cost per credit, target audience, usability features (e.g., registration requirements, free previewing, payment options, and ability to obtain instant credit), and adherence to quality and privacy standards.

We are also developing a novel interactive CE experience to teach primary care physicians how to detect, diagnose, and treat depression. The first phase of this project designed, implemented, and evaluated an Internet based Continuing Medical Education course entitled *"Mental Health in Primary Care: A Patient with Tiredness."* This course is available at *www.vlh.com* or *www.healthcme.com*. The goals of the course are to teach primary care physicians (or any interested physician) how to recognize Major Depression as defined in the DSM-IV and begin treatment. Issues surrounding suicide are also addressed. The course is designed to affect improved knowledge, attitude, depression clinical skills, self-efficacy, and awareness of resources. It is one in a series of Internet-based courses we are developing that will emphasize learning via a case-based approach. In addition, these courses will include unique features possible with web-based courses, including support for user control and feedback, discussion and communication, an accompanying news/resource area, patient education materials, and links to other information resources.

We completed a comprehensive literature search on depression diagnosis and treatment. Focusing on the identified issues, we worked with our consultants to establish both the necessary educational content and the appropriate approach in presenting this content. In addition, input from physicians was gathered. We also investigated design issues, such as page length (and need for scrolling), amount of graphics, and navigation.

The software was demonstrated to two different professional focus groups comprised of resident physicians at the University of Pittsburgh. All focus group participants completed a demographics form, pre and post attitude survey, and pre and post knowledge test. All forms were completed online. They all viewed the *"Mental Health in Primary Care: A Patient with Tiredness"* CME course. The first focus group (n=19) provided input on and assessed the value of the course via a structured intervention. The purpose of this focus group was to evaluate and refine the course and the knowledge assessment instrument. They answered knowledge questions and an attitude survey concerning treatment of depression, mental health related CME, and Internet based CME. Following this group, both the course and the knowledge test were revised and a second focus group (n=16) was conducted. A simple pre–post knowledge test was given to all participants. No control group was involved.

We also subjected the course to a "real world evaluation" after it gained approval for Category I CME credit by making it live on the Virtual Lecture Hall (VLH). Satisfaction results from the first 287 users of the course on VLH are summarized below.

3. Results

Our initial feedback in developing the course was that a simple "clinical case" based approach was superior in terms of user interest and ease of creating the course. We also found that "didactic" information could be inserted into the course with minimal difficulty and without harming the flow of the course. Such information is crucial to learning, but can be detrimental in an environment where the user can easily quit learning with a click of a mouse.

The course had a dramatic effect on the attitude of residents in our second focus group towards both Internet-based CME and mental health focused CME. Prior to the course experience almost all users reported that they were not interested in either Internet-based CME or mental health CME. After taking the course, 94% were interested in taking more

Internet based CME, and 92% were interested in more mental health oriented CME. The course also had an effect on knowledge. Of the 48% of users who failed the knowledge pretest (<70%, the usual standard), 67% of those passed the knowledge test after viewing the course. We feel that these results argue strongly for the success of our course as a method of educating physicians in primary care about depression and related mental health topics.

Physicians taking our depression course online at the Virtual Lecture Hall were very positive. Self-report measures of satisfaction all scored over 4 on a 1 to 5 scale. The question of how well learning objectives were met received an average score of 4.14 on a 5-point scale. Users rated the relevance of the information in the course to their clinical practice as an average of 4.24 on a 5-point scale. The program was rated overall as a 4.10 on a 5-point scale.

The Virtual Lecture Hall also provides a means for users to provide public comments. Comments on the course have been overwhelmingly positive. Users have commented on the course's relevance to their daily practices, the conciseness of the course, and the ease of use of the interface. When users have offered suggestions for improving the course, we have altered the course when possible.

4. Conclusions

Existing CE very rarely capitalizes on the ability of the Internet to provide an easy to use, timely, interactive, and challenging experience. There is tremendous potential to provide an Interactive clinical experience via the Internet via clinical case-based scenarios, yet this potential is mostly unmet. Physicians respond favorably to this method of learning. Future studies will evaluate if such learning leads to improved performance and changes in self-perception of clinical skill.

This project is supported by a grant from the National Institute of Mental Health, Grant #R43 MH57604-01A1.

References

[1] American Medical Association. AMA Enterprise Information Base. October 1996. *http://www.ama-assn.org/physdata/physnow/physnow.htm* (March 29, 2000). 1999.
[2] Basen-Engquist K, O'Hara-Tompkins N, Lovato CY, Lewis MJ, Parcel GS, Gingiss P. The Effect of Two Types of Teacher Training on Smart Choices: A Tobacco Prevention Curriculum. Journal of School Health 1994; 64:334-339.
[3] Carney PA, Dietrich AJ, Freeman DH, Mott LA. A Standardized-Patient Assessment of a Continuing Medical Education Program to Improve Physicians' Cancer-Control Clinical Skills. Acad. Med. 1995; 70:52-58.
[4] Kristeller J, and Ockene J. Tobacco Curriculum for Medical Students, Residents, and Practicing Physicians. *Indiana Medicine*, Vol. 89 (2), p.199-204. 1996.
[5] Montner P, Bennett G, Brown C. An Evaluation of a Smoking Cessation Training Program for Medical Residents in an Inner-city Hospital. *Journal of the National Medical Association* 1994, 86:671-675.
[6] Williams PT, Eckert G, Epstein A, Mourad L, Helmick F. In-Office Cancer-Screening Education of Primary Care Physicians. J Cancer Educ. 1994; 9:90-95.
[7] Wood GJ, Cecchini JJ, Nathason N, Hiroschige K. Office-Base Training in Tobacco Cessation for Dental Professionals. *JADA* 1997; 128:216-224.
[8] Davis, David A. MD; Thomson, Mary Ann BHSc; Oxman, Andrew D. MD; Haynes R. Brian, PhD MD Changing Physician Performance: A Systematic Review of the Effect of Continuing Medical Education Strategies, Volume 274(9), 6 September 1995, pp 700-705.

Medicine Meets Virtual Reality 2001
J.D. Westwood et al. (Eds.)
IOS Press, 2001

Using Virtual Reality to teach special populations how to cope in crisis: The case of a virtual earthquake

Ioannis Tarnanas MSc.
Dr. George C. Manos, PhD. Professor
Aristotle University of Thessaloniki
ioannist@psy.auth.gr
1st Emm. Papa,
55236 Thessaloniki, Greece
Tel+30-31344831
Fax+30-31344548

Abstract. The unique characteristics of special populations such as pre-school children and Down syndrome kids in crisis and their distorted self-image were never studied before, because of the difficulty of crisis reproduction. This study proposes a VR setting that tries to model some special population's behaviour in the time of crises and offers them a training scenario. The sample population consisted of 30 pre-school children and 20 children with Down syndrome. The VR setting involved a high-speed PC, a VPL EyePhone 1, a MR toolkit, a vibrations plate, a motion capture system and other sensors. The system measured and modelled the typical behaviour of these special populations in a Virtual Earthquake scenario with sight and sound and calculated a VR anthropomorphic model that reproduced their behaviour and emotional state. Afterwards one group received an emotionally enhanced VR self-image as feedback for their training, one group received a plain VR self-image and another group received verbal instructions. The findings strongly suggest that the training was a lot more biased by the emotionally enhanced VR self-image than the other approaches. These findings could highlight the special role of the self-image to therapy and training and the interesting role of imagination to emotions, motives and learning. Further studies could be done with various scenarios in order to measure the best-biased behaviour and establish the most natural and affective VR model. This presentation is going to highlight the main findings and some theories behind them.

1. Introduction

Crisis situations are not very common for special populations. In fact special populations, especially at the case of pre-school children and children with Down syndrome, are highly protected and come at little or no risk without the presence of a trained personnel. Yet these crises, whenever they arrive, even at the presence of the trained personnel, do not leave their psychodynamics unharmed [1].

Psychoanalytic theory hypothesizes that all of mental life exists on two levels: within the realm of conscious-ness, and also within a less accessible realm that Freud labeled the unconscious. Some psychic or emotional symptoms that these special populations can show in crisis arise from aspects of mental life that were at least in part unconscious [2].

These special populations show yet another difficulty. Due to their "egocentric" and distorted self-image, psychodynamic psychotherapy and cognitive-behavioural therapy must be applied with caution so that we do not create more problems than we intended to solve [3]. Therefore a clinical investigation of how these special populations cope in crisis is "critical", especially in countries, where crisis situations, such as earthquakes, are not so rare.

In Psychotherapy, the virtual cyberspace offers a series of powerful and valid applications for diagnosis and treatment. The qualities that make VR software reliable and particularly useful in the practice of assessment and rehabilitation of certain psychopathological dysfunctions emerge with extreme clarity from the specialist literature [4], [5]. Virtual reality technology takes its place as an experience that is able to reduce the gap existing between imagination and reality.

The feeling of "actual presence" is perhaps the peculiar characteristic of this tool [5], [6] and is made possible both by the realistic reproduction of the cybernetic environments and by the involvement of all the sensorimotor channels during interaction. A virtual earthquake would immerse the user in a crisis situation, where his psychological responses and behaviour would be monitored *"in vivo"*.

The prevalent elements in cognitive-behavioural therapies are that of exposing the subject to the stimuli that produce the dysfunction and of generating responses that are antagonistic to the maladaptive ones [7]. A virtual earthquake facilitates both of these processes of treatment. Using a VR earthquake scenario we were able to monitor the maladaptive behaviour of the pre-school and Down syndrome children. Afterwards we developed an innovative implementation of a virtual PCT (panic control treatment [8]) in order to train the children how to cope in crisis.

The purpose of the current study was to examine and model the behaviour of pre-school and Down syndrome children inside a virtual earthquake scenario and uses a virtual variation of the panic control treatment in order to "teach" these children how to cope in crisis.

2. The Virtual Environment design and implementation

The VR earthquake scenario was developed using a custom virtual reality system at the Aristotles University of Thessalonica, Department of Polytechnics. The system was a Pentium III based immersive VR system (700Mhz, 128Mb RAM, graphic engine: Matrox G400 Dual Head, 32Mb WRam) including an HMD subsystem (VPL EyePhone 1), a two-button joystick-type motion input device and some EEG sensors.

The VPL EyePhone 1 head mounted provided the visual display. The HMD displays 800 lines of 255 pixels to each eye and uses LCD technology (two active matrix 7" color LCDs). An InterSense InterTrax 30 tracker provided head tracking. The tracker can sense azimuth, elevation and roll with a sensitivity of 360 degrees per second. The response latency is 38ms+/-2ms. Due to the possible "impetuosity" of the virtual earthquake scenario we did not use a stereoscopic display and accepted the possible trade-off in realism.

The data glove-type motion input device is very common in virtual environments for its capability of sensing many degrees of freedom simultaneously. To provide a easy way of moving in the virtual scenario, sitting on top of the vibrating plate, we used an infrared two-button joystick-type input device: pressing the upper button the operator moves forward, pressing the lower button the operator moves backwards. The direction of the movement is given by the rotation of operator's head.

The virtual earthquake is an interactive (see Figure 1) virtual environment developed using the MR toolkit. The main attraction is the interior of a school classroom within a typical Greek elementary school. The possible variations include a kindergarten, a high school and a special children academic institution. The therapist constantly monitors the session using the panic control treatment techniques implemented in a VR AVATAR that is calculated in real-time, modelling the emotional and behavioural responses of the children. In particular the therapist can define the length of the virtual experience, its end and the instructions that the AVATAR is going to propose according to the phase of the session.

3. The Clinical Protocol

All the subjects were assessed at pre treatment, upon completion of the clinical trial and after a 1-month, 3-month and 6-month follow-up period. The following psychometric tests will be administered at each assessment point:

1. **BDI** - Beck Depression Inventory (Beck, Ward, Mendelson, Mock & Erbaugh, 1961) [9]; contains 21 items which address behavioural, physical, cognitive, and affective components of depression. Each item has four choices that are scored from 0 to 3 in terms of severity.

2. **STAI** - State-Trait Anxiety Inventory (Spielberger, Gorsuch, Lushene, Vagg & Jacobs, 1983) [10]; measures a person's situational (or state) anxiety, as well as the amount of anxiety a person generally feels most of the time (trait). The two scales contain 20 items each, which may be scored 1 (not at all) to 4 (very much so). Trait anxiety has a reliability of .81 and state of .40, with internal consistency of between .83 and .92.

3. **FQ** - Fear Questionnaire (Marks & Mathews, 1979) [11]; the questionnaire consists of a subscale of agoraphobia, which has five items and is limited to the evaluation of motor behaviour.

During the assessment were also used:
- Objective measurements (EEG monitoring)

- Subjective Units of Distress (SUDs) during exposure to virtual environments. In particular SUDs will be taken at baseline, after 10 minutes and after 20 minutes. (scale is from 0 = no anxiety to 100 = maximum anxiety)

4. The Procedure

The subjects were split into a group that received an interactive VR approach (VR earthquake treatment), a group that took an alternative edition of the VR earthquake and a verbal instructions group (control group). The VR earthquake treatment was usually delivered in 12 weekly sessions, individually to pre-school and Down syndrome children. The VR earthquake approach included 3 introductory and 9 treatment session. In early sessions, children are taught about the nature and function of fear and its nervous system substrates. At these sessions the fear response is presented as a normal and generally protective state that enhances our ability to survive and compete in life. The Panic attacks inside the VR environment are conceptualised as inappropriate fear reactions arising from spurious but otherwise normal activation of the body's fight-or-flight nervous system. In addition to normalizing and demystifying panic attacks, the educational component of PCT provides children with a model of anxiety that emphasizes the interaction between the mind and body and provides a rationale and framework for the skills to be taught during treatment. Due to the sensitivity surrounding the exposure of special children into risk conditions, we constantly monitored the procedure with a digital camera and some EEG sensors.

The general treatment strategy used at the later sessions was panic control treatment (PCT). The general goal of PCT is to foster within children the ability to identify and correct maladaptive thoughts and behaviours that initiate, sustain, or exacerbate anxiety and panic attacks. In service of that goal, the VR earthquake treatment combines education, cognitive interventions, relaxation and controlled breathing procedures, and exposure techniques. The innovative aspect of our current approach is that the above treatment was given using an anthropomorphic VR model (AVATAR), calculated in real-time by the emotional and behavioural responses of the children, which lived and interacted at the same environment with the children as their friend. That way we applied the PCT using the same principles as with biofeedback, but with minimum physical intervention. We chose this approach because we hypothesized based on psychological data [12], [13], that it would be easier to enter the world and the "egocentric" perception of these populations if we "disguise" ourselves as their digital ego. As a consequence the therapist had full control at the cognitive schemas of the children inside the VR environment by interacting with their computerized self-image.

Using this computerized VR self-image, a three-component model was used, in which the dimensions of anxiety were grouped into physical, cognitive, and behavioural categories. The physical component includes bodily changes (e.g., neurological, hormonal, cardiovascular) and their associated emotional outcome that was represented at the computerized self-image. The cognitive component consists of the rational and irrational thoughts, images, and impulses that accompany anxiety or fear (e.g., thoughts of dying, images of losing control, impulses to run). These thoughts were treated at various sessions using the computerized self-image according to the PCT in order to gain an objective self-awareness and expectation that their thinking is distorted. Finally, the behavioural component contains the things people do when they are anxious or afraid (e.g., pacing, leaving or avoiding a situation, carrying a safety object). Most important, these three components were described as interacting with each other at the "body" of the computerized self-image.

Having laid this foundation, the VR earthquake scenario then teaches children skills for controlling each of the three components of anxiety. The whole approach constituted a VR role-playing scenario, where children were essentially mimicking their "ideal self". We did not include a more systematic situational exposure component in PCT because we wanted to focus initially on the experience of panic attacks, rather than on avoidance behaviour, since this had not been done previously. An optional agoraphobia supplement was developed later, for use with children who have significant situational avoidance.

The alternative version of the VR earthquake scenario did not follow the PCT approach. The experience that the children had with this version was a VR environment where they "lived" along with an exact replica of their selves that behaved exactly as they behaved. We chose this scenario in order to test the efficacy of the computerized self-image alone. One of the fundamental parameters in assessing the effectiveness of therapies is the ratio existing between the "cost" of administration of the therapeutic procedure and the resulting "benefits". By cost it is meant the expenditure not only in terms of money and time, but also in terms of emotional involvement by the person to whom the therapy is directed. The benefits regard the effectiveness of the treatment, i.e., the achievement of the target set, in the shortest time possible.

5. Results – Discussion - Conclusion

We found that 87% of the children in the VR earthquake PCT group were panic free by the end of treatment, compared with 50% in the non-PCT condition and 33% in the control group. A 3-months follow-up of PCT completers found that gains were maintained. At post treatment, 85% of PCT-treated children were panic free, versus 30% in a waitlist condition. We evaluated cognitive interventions alone as treatment, and the results were varied, with effect sizes ranging from –0.95 to 1.10 (mean ES = 0.18). The results of the questionnaires pre and post the treatment showed a statistically significant difference at the frequency of the negative responses (F(df=1)=8,024,p<0,05).

The pre-school and Down syndrome children were left by the experience of the VR earthquake not only unharmed but also improved in terms of negative thoughts. They were able to control their digital self in ways that were only possible for adults by biofeedback treatments. Despite their distorted self-image they were able to mimic their "ideal self-image". The results of the post treatment and the follow up suggest that the memories that the children acquired were not blunted.

The possibilities offered in this framework by virtual technology are numerous and all extremely advantageous. The administrations at the model of the computerized self-image, guided by the therapist, in VR of scenes that favour the induction of relaxation response have shown extremely positive results. This is primarily due to the intrinsic effects of the VR tool. The feeling of actual presence offered by the realistic reproduction of cybernetic environments and by the involvement of all the sensorimotor channels enables the subject undergoing treatment to live the virtual experience in a more vivid and realistic manner than he could through his own imagination.

Several psychologists have already emphasized the significance of mental images and of imagination at psychotherapy and phobias [6], [14]. Yet the significance of mental images in large-scale physical crisis was never tried before. This study demonstrated that with serious and careful experimentation even the more sensitive populations, such as the pre-school and Down syndrome children could enjoy the numerous advantages offered by immersive VR and by technological development. This innovative tool produces a change with respect to the traditional relationship between client and therapist. The new configuration of this relationship is based on the awareness of being more skilled in the difficult operations of recovery of past experiences, through the memory, and of foreseeing of future experiences, through the imagination.

VR-assisted therapy offers a strong impulse to the development of new possibilities of prevention and care of psychological health. Though this study was not intended to alter the cognitive abilities of the Down syndrome children under consideration, it seems like the subjects undergoing treatment perceived the advantage of being able to re-create and use a real experiential world inside the VR earthquake scenario by mimicking their "ideal self image". More studies are required in order to investigate in detail the possible impact of this kind of role-playing scenarios on the cognitive abilities of this population.

References

[1] Leonard HL, Rapoport JL: Anxiety disorders in childhood and adolescence, in American Psychiatric Press Review of Psychiatry, vol 8, edited by Tasman A, Hales RE, Frances AJ. Washington, DC, American Psychiatric Press, 1989, pp 162–179
[2] Breuer J, Freud S: Studies on hysteria (1895), in The Standard Edition of the Complete Psychological Works of Sigmund Freud, vol 2, translated and edited by Strachey J. London, Hogarth Press, 1959, pp 1–183 Press, 1959, pp 77–174
[3] Roy-Byrne PP, Geraci M, Uhde TW: Life events and the onset of panic disorder. Am J Psychiatry 1986; 143:1424–1427 in children of parents with panic disorder and agoraphobia.
[4] Riva G (1997). Virtual reality as assessment tool in psychology. In: Riva G, ed., *Virtual reality in neuro-psycho-physiology: Cognitive, clinical and methodological issues in assessment and rehabilitation.* Amsterdam: IOS Press, 95-112.
[5] Riva G, Galimberti C. (1997) The psychology of cyberspace: a socio-cognitive framework to computer mediated communication. *New Ideas in Psychology*;15:141-158.

[6] Vincelli F., Molinari E., (1998). Virtual reality and imaginative techniques in Clinical Psychology. In Riva G., Wiederhold B.K., Molinari E. (Eds.) *Virtual environments in Clinical Psychology and Neuroscience.* IOS Press Amsterdam.

[7] Rothbaum BO, Hodges L, Kooper R. (1997) Virtual reality exposure therapy. *J Psychother Pract Res*;6:219-226.

[8] Craske MG, Meadows E, Barlow DH: Therapist's Guide for the "Mastery of Your Anxiety and Panic II" and "Agoraphobia Sup-plement." Albany, NY, Graywind, 1994

[9] Beck A.T., Ward C.H., Mendelson M., Mock J. & Erbaugh J. (1961) An inventory for measuring depression. *Archives of General Psychiatry, 4, 561-571.*

[10] Spielberger C.D., Gorsuch R.L., Lushene R., Vagg P.R. & Jacobs G.A. (1983) *Manual for the Stait.Trait Anxiety Inventory.* Palo Alto,CA, Consulting Psychology Press.

[11] Marks I.M. & Mathews A.M. (1979) Brief standard self-rating for phobic patients. *Behavior Research and Therapy, 17, 263-267.*

[12] Greenspan S. & Benderly B. (1998). The Growth of the Mind. Perseus Books; ISBN: 0738200263.

[13] Shapiro T: The concept of unconscious fantasy. J Clin Psychoanal 1992; 1:517–524 19.

[14] Vincelli F. (1999). From imagination to virtual reality: the future of Clinical Psychology. *CyberPsychology & Behavior. 2; 3; 241-248.*

Figure 1. *Virtual Earthquake View*

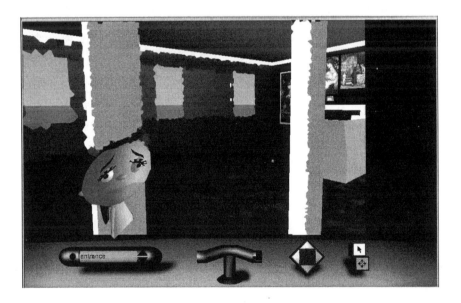

Medicine Meets Virtual Reality 2001
J.D. Westwood et al. (Eds.)
IOS Press, 2001

3–D Simulation of Craniofacial Surgical Procedures

Matthias Teschner

Telecommunications Laboratory
University Erlangen, Germany
teschner@LNT.de

Sabine Girod

National Biocomputation Center
Stanford University, USA
sgirod@biocomp.stanford.edu

Bernd Girod

Information Systems Laboratory
Stanford University, USA
girod@ee.stanford.edu

Abstract

An integrated system for simulating craniofacial surgical procedures is presented. The system computes nonlinear soft–tissue deformation due to bone realignment. It is capable of simulating bone cutting and bone realignment with integrated interactive collision detection. Furthermore, soft–tissue deformation and cutting due to surgical instruments can be visualized. The system has been tested with several individual patient data sets.

Simulation processes are based on a 3–D model of a patient's preoperative bone structure of the skull derived from a computer tomography scan and on a 3–D, photorealistic model of the patient's preoperative appearance obtained by a laser range scanner.

The multi–layer soft–tissue model is represented by nonlinear springs. Very fast and robust prediction of nonlinear soft–tissue deformation is computed by optimizing a nonlinear cost function.

1 Introduction

The simulation of surgical procedures and the prediction of their outcome are especially useful in craniofacial surgery. Craniofacial surgery is aimed at the restoration of the skeletal anatomy of the head and at the improvement of the patient's aesthetics. Simulation techniques can be used to support osteotomy planning and to predict the patient's postoperative appearance.

The idea of estimating soft–tissue deformation due to bone realignment was formulated by Vannier in 1983 [20]. In 1992, further approaches to surgery simulation were introduced by Kikinis [12, 1], followed by Delingette in 1994 [5, 6], Bohner in 1996 [2], Koch in 1996 [13], and Bro-Nielsen in 1998 [3]. These approaches use deformable volumes, mass–spring models, or finite elements to predict soft–tissue changes.

In [14], a framework for facial surgery simulation is presented. This approach is based on a photorealistic surface scan of a patient's face and a CT scan of a patient's skull, which is the same approach for photorealistic prediction of soft–tissue deformation already proposed by Keeve [10]. In [14], a finite–element system is employed for tissue modeling. The model is restricted to linear elasticity. Bone cutting and realigning without collision detection can be performed and restricted soft–tissue deformation can be computed. Simulation results for several real patient data sets are presented. Computation of soft–tissue deformation takes approximately half an hour on an high–end graphic workstation.

In [4] a system for computing soft–tissue deformation with integrated collision detection for deformable models is introduced. A finite–element approach is used that models nonlinear strain–stress relationship of soft–tissue. However, differentiated elasto–mechanical properties of soft tissue are not considered. Soft–tissue deformation can be computed in real–time, but the simulation requires several hours of preprocessing time for each configuration of soft–tissue properties. Soft–tissue cutting can not be simulated.

A virtual environment for surgical planning and analysis (VESPA) has been developed at the National Biocomputation Center, Stanford University Medical Center [16]. The objective of this project is to provide visualization and interaction between the surgeon and patient data sets consisting of various modalities. The developed surgical planning station allows to simulate surgical procedures regarding the patient's bone structure. However, soft–tissue deformation cannot be predicted.

A finite–element approach to soft–tissue simulation using tetrahedral grids is proposed by Zachow [21]. Bone cutting, bone realigning and and soft–tissue deformation can be simulated. Results are presented using real patient data sets. Due to the complexity of the soft–tissue deformation approach, computational time is about 5min on high–end graphics workstation.

The authors have investigated methods for surgery simulation based on 3–D computer models since 1993 [8, 11, 17, 18, 19]. In this paper, a realistic soft–tissue model with nonlinear elasto–mechanical properties and a very fast and robust technique for direct computation of global soft–tissue deformation are proposed. They are part of an integrated craniofacial surgery simulation system which has been tested with a variety of real patient data sets. The system is capable of simulating craniofacial surgical procedures. Furthermore, it consists of components for simulating bone cutting and bone realignment with integrated interactive collision detection and avoidance.

The paper is organized as follows. Sec. 2 describes the simulation of bone cutting and bone realignment. Sec. 3 introduces the soft–tissue model and the approach to direct computation of soft–tissue deformation.

2 Manipulation of the Bone Structure

The simulation of bone cutting is essential in the craniofacial surgery planning process. The introduced system employs a cutting tool which is proposed in [10, 11]. This tool uses a rectangle as cutting plane. In its initial state this rectangle is part of the $Z = 0$ plane. The cutting plane can be translated and rotated arbitrarily. The transformation of the cutting plane is described by matrix **M**. A cut is performed by applying the inverse transformation $\mathbf{M}^{-1}$ to the object and retriangulating all triangles that intersect the $Z = 0$ plane in the area of the cutting plane.

The main purpose of the cutting tool is to separate bone structures in order to realign them independently. Therefore, a post–processing step is performed to estimate separated triangle structures and to reorganize the data structure of the bone model accordingly.

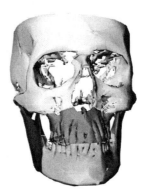

Figure 1: Skull with resected ramus and ascending branches of the lower jaw, and upper jaw.

Fig. 1 shows a typical preparation of a bone model that is used for dysgnathia correction planning. The cutting instrument is usually used to resect the ramus and ascending branches of the lower jaw and to extract the upper jaw. This allows to realign these structures separately in the surgical planning process.

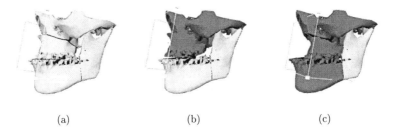

(a)   (b)   (c)

Figure 2: Realignment of the upper jaw. Dark bone structures indicate collisions. Interactive realignment with integrated collision detection is provided by the system.

The process of craniofacial surgery simulation requires a simulation of the transformation of bone structures. In combination with the bone cutting tool this enables the realistic simulation of any osteotomy of facial and skull bones.

In order to provide the simulation system with interactive collision detection, the software library RAPID [9] is integrated. RAPID has shown to be very robust. It enables interactive collision detection and avoidance for bone models with up to 50000 triangles.

As the collision detection test depends on the geometry of the bone models, it is not possible to specify a maximal computation time. However, collision tests are always performed faster than 0.05s on an SGI O2, R10000. Fig. 2 shows an image sequence of upper jaw movement. Dark parts indicate collisions. The user can decide, whether collisions are indicated or avoided.

3 Direct Computation of Soft–Tissue Deformation

The introduced approach to soft–tissue deformation is based on a mass–spring model. Soft tissue is discretized into mass points **p** which are linked by nonlinear springs. The force–deformation relationship of these springs is given as

$$F = k \left(\frac{x}{L}\right)^n \tag{1}$$

with F denoting the magnitude of force, k denoting the spring constant, x denoting the magnitude of deformation, and L denoting the initial spring length.

Experiments for estimating the relationship between applied force and deformation for living tissue are rare. However, measurements of stress–strain relationships for a resting papillary muscle of a rabbit are presented in [7]. In order to approximate this relation, k is set to 10^4N and n is set to 5.

The introduced approach for estimating soft–tissue deformation optimizes a nonlinear cost function which describes internal forces of the soft–tissue model. Instead of simulating the dynamic model behavior by numerical integration of positions and velocities of mass points through time, the proposed method directly determines a stable equilibrium of the system.

The force at soft–tissue point $\mathbf{p_i} \in \mathbb{R}^3$ due to all forces caused by springs connected to this node is referred to as force $\mathbf{F_i}$:

$$\mathbf{F_i} = \sum_{j|j \in S_i} k_j \left(\frac{\left|\mathbf{p_j^2} - \mathbf{p_j^1}\right| - L_j}{L_j}\right)^n \frac{\mathbf{p_j^2} - \mathbf{p_j^1}}{\left|\mathbf{p_j^2} - \mathbf{p_j^1}\right|} \tag{2}$$

with S_i denoting the set of all adjacent springs connected to $\mathbf{p_i}$. $\mathbf{p_j^1}$ and $\mathbf{p_j^2}$ are end–points of spring j. End–point $\mathbf{p_j^1}$ of spring j corresponds to $\mathbf{p_i}$.

The set P_{free} represents all points **p** which are considered in the deformation process. Function $f_{force}(P_{free})$ describes the sum of all magnitudes of forces at soft–tissue points:

$$f_{force}(P_{free}) = \sum_{i|\mathbf{p_i} \in P_{free}} |\mathbf{F_i}|. \tag{3}$$

This function is parametrized by all positions of free soft–tissue points $\mathbf{p_i} \in P_{free}$. Points at the edge of the model are not considered in the deformation process to avoid global transformation. Furthermore, soft–tissue points which represent attachments to the underlying bone structure are not considered.

In the initial state of the deformation process the soft–tissue model is in a stable equilibrium: $f_{force}(P_{free}) = 0$. The realignment of bone structures causes forces at soft–tissue points which leads to $f_{force}(P_{free}) > 0$. A multidimensional conjugate gradient method is applied in order to solve $P'_{free} = \text{argmin}\, f_{force}\,(P_{free})$ with P'_{free} denoting a set of displaced soft–tissue points.

Minimizing $f_{force}\,(P_{free})$ corresponds to varying the positions of free soft–tissue points in order to neutralize forces $\mathbf{F_i}$ at all free soft–tissue points $\mathbf{p_i}$. The minimum corresponds to a stable equilibrium of the model with the bone structure realigned. In this case forces at all free soft–tissue points are zero.

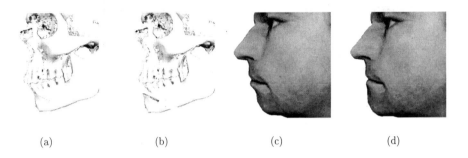

      (a)   (b)   (c)   (d)

Figure 3: Original bone structure (a), simulated realignment of the chin (b), and corresponding face models (c) and (d), respectively.

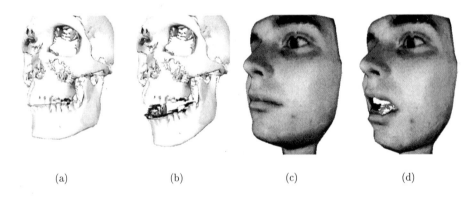

      (a)   (b)   (c)   (d)

Figure 4: Simulated physiological lower jaw movement. Bone models (a), (b) and corresponding face models (c), (d), respectively.

Fig. 3 shows a simulated realignment of a chin. In this case, the soft–tissue model consists of 1838 points and 11763 springs. Computing the soft–tissue deformation took 3.6s on an SGI Octane, MIPS R12000, 300 MHz. Fig. 4 illustrates a simulated physiological lower jaw movement. The model consists of 1472 points and 9726 springs. The deformation process required 7.9s.

Fig. 5 exemplifies a simulated soft–tissue cut. Fig. 5(a) shows a synthetic soft–tissue model. Fig. 5(b) illustrates deformation due to a surgical instrument. A soft–tissue cut is initiated in case of large external forces at free soft–tissue points. This is shown in Fig. 5(c).

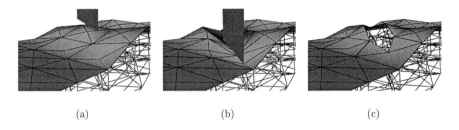

(a)   (b)   (c)

Figure 5: Simulated deforming (b) and cutting (c) due to a surgical instrument.

4 Conclusion

In this paper, a system for craniofacial surgery simulation has been presented. It can be used to simulate bone cutting, bone realignment, nonlinear soft–tissue deformation and soft–tissue cutting. A new, very efficient and robust approach to nonlinear soft–tissue deformation has been introduced, which can be used to simulate soft–tissue deformation due to bone realignment and due to surgical instruments. The approach takes into account the nonlinear stress–strain relationship of soft tissue.

Ongoing work focusses on the integration of muscles in order to simulate the patient's postoperative facial expressions. Furthermore, it is intended to perform clinical studies to estimate appropriate parameters for the introduced soft–tissue model. Postoperative surface scans, which are registered with the preoperative surface scan, will be used to compare the simulated soft–tissue deformation and the actual surgical result.

References

[1] D. Altobelli, R. Kikinis, J. Mulliken, H. Cline, W. Lorensen, F. Jolesz. "Computer-Assisted Three-Dimensional Planning in Craniofacial Surgery", *Journal of Oral and Maxillofacial Surgery Suppl.*, Vol. 92, 1993.

[2] P. Bohner, P. Pokrandt, S. Hassfeld. "Simultaneous Planning and Execution in Cranio-Maxillo-Facial Surgery", *MMVR4 '96*, San Diego, CA, USA, 1996.

[3] M. Bro-Nielsen. "Finite Element Modeling in Surgery Simulation", *Proceedings of the IEEE: Special Issue on Virtual & Augmented Reality in Medicine*, 86(3):524–530, March 1998.

[4] S. Cotin, H. Delingette, N. Ayache. "Real-Time Elastic Deformations of Soft Tissues for Surgery Simulation", *IEEE Trans. on Visualization and Computer Graphics*, 5(1):62, 1999.

[5] H. Delingette, G. Subsol, S. Cotin, J. Pignon. "A Craniofacial Surgery Simulation Testbed", *INRIA, Rapport de Recherche, Nr. 2199*, Sophia-Antipolis, 1994.

[6]   H. Delingette. "Toward Realistic Soft-Tissue Modeling in Medical Simulation", *Proc. of the IEEE: Special Issue on Virtual & Augmented Reality in Medicine*, 86(3):524–530, 1998.

[7]   Y. C. Fung, *"Biomechanics - Mechanical Properties of Living Tissues,"* ISBN 0–387–97947–6 (New York), ISBN 3–540–97947–6 (Berlin), Springer, Berlin, New York, 1993.

[8]   S. Girod, E. Keeve, B. Girod. "Soft Tissue Prediction in Orthognatic Surgery by 3D CT and 3D Laser Scanning", Journal of Oral and Maxillofacial Surgery Suppl., Vol. 51, 1993.

[9]   S. Gottschalk, M. C. Lin, D. Manocha, "OBBTree: A Hierarchical Structure for Rapid Interference Detection," *Proc. SIGGRAPH'96, Computer Graphics*, ACM, New York, NY, USA, pp. 171–180, August 1996.

[10] E. Keeve, S. Girod, P. Pfeifle, B. Girod. "Anatomy–Based Facial Tissue Modeling Using the Finite Element Method", In *Proc. IEEE Visualization*, San Francisco, CA, USA, 1996.

[11] E. Keeve, S. Girod, R. Kikinis, B. Girod. "Deformable Modeling of Facial Tissue for Craniofacial Surgery Simulation", *Computer Aided Surgery*, 3(5):228–238, 1998.

[12] R. Kikinis, H. Cline, D. Altobelli, M. Halle, W. Lorensen, F. Jolesz. "Interactive Visualization and Manipulation of 3D Reconstructions for the Planning of Surgical Procedures", In *Proceedings of Visualization in Biomedical Computing VBC '92*, pages 559–563, 1992.

[13] R. M. Koch, M. H. Gross, D. F. Bueren, G. Frankhauser, Y. Parish, F. R. Carls. "Simulating Facial Surgery Using Finite Element Models", *SIGGRAPH '96, ACM Computer Graphics*, 30, August 1996.

[14] R. M. Koch, S. H. M. Roth, M. H. Gross, A. P. Zimmermann, H. F. Sailer, "A Framework for Facial Surgery Simulation," *ETH Zurich, CS Technical Report #326, Institute of Scientific Computing*, June 18, 1999.

[15] W. E. Lorensen, H. E. Cline. "Marching Cubes: A High Resolution 3D Surface Construction Algorithm", *SIGGRAPH '87, ACM Computer Graphics*, 21(4):163–169, 1987.

[16] K. Montgomery, M. Stephanides, S. Schendel, M. Ross. "Virtual Surgical Tools for Planning Craniofacial Surgery", *Medicine Meets Virtual Reality*, 1999.

[17] J. Richolt, M. Teschner, P. Everett, M. B. Millis, R. Kikinis. "Impingement Simulation of the Hip in SCFE Using 3D Models", *Computer Aided Surgery*, 4(3):144–151, 1999.

[18] M. Teschner, S. Girod, B. Girod. "Optimization Approaches for Soft-Tissue Prediction in Craniofacial Surgery Simulation", *Proc. MICCAI'99*, pp. 1183–1190, Cambridge, England, September 1999.

[19] M. Teschner, S. Girod, B. Girod. "Surgical Planning", In *Principles of 3D Image Analysis and Synthesis*, Girod, Greiner, Niemann (ed.), Kluwer Academic Publishers, Boston, 2000.

[20] M. W. Vannier, J. L. Marsh, J. O. Warren. "Three Dimensional Computer Graphics for Craniofacial Surgical Planning and Evaluation", *SIGGRAPH '83, ACM Computer Graphics*, 17(3):263–273, 1983.

[21] S. Zachow, E. Gladiline, H.–C. Hege, P. Deuflhard , "Finite–Element Simulation of Soft–Tissue Deformation," *Proc. CARS'00*, San Francisco, USA, pp. 23–28, June , 2000.

Medicine Meets Virtual Reality 2001
J.D. Westwood et al. (Eds.)
IOS Press, 2001

A Medical Platform for Simulation of Surgical Procedures

Lennart Thurfjell[1, 2], Anna Lundin[1], John McLaughlin[1]

[1]*Reachin AB, Stockholm, Sweden*
[2]*Centre for Image Analysis, Uppsala University, Uppsala, Sweden*

Abstract: Surgery simulation is a promising technique for training of surgical procedures. The overall goal for any surgical simulator is to allow for efficient training of the skills required and to improve learning by giving the user proper feedback. This goal is easier achieved if the training is performed in a realistic environment. Therefore functionality such as soft tissue deformation, tearing and cutting, penetration of soft tissue etc. is necessary. Furthermore, a realistic simulator must provide haptic feedback so that all senses match, that is, there should be a correspondence between what you see and what you feel with your hands. In this paper we describe a medical platform that provides all this functionality. It is based on the ReachIn Magma API, which has been extended for surgery simulation. We describe the development of the platform and illustrate the use of it for the development of two different types of surgical simulators, both of which represents work in progress.

1. Introduction

Surgery simulation is becoming an increasingly important tool for training surgical procedures. In laparoscopic surgery, a video camera and surgical tools are inserted through small incisions and the surgeon performs the surgery guided by an indirect view of the site of operation. Today's surgery is usually performed using a monoscopic system and the working conditions are very different from those during open surgery with a major difficulty lying in the hand-eye coordination. Furthermore, the manipulative freedom is restricted due to the geometrical constraints posed by the control of the instruments through the trocar hull. Therefore, training is especially important and many of today's simulators have been developed for training of minimal invasive techniques [1, 2, 3]. Other areas where training is important include various lifesaving surgical procedures such as those taught in the Advanced Trauma Life Support (ATLS) course from the American College of Surgeons. Every surgeon should be confident in performing these procedures but this is rarely the case because training in real life is impossible due to the nature of the procedures.

We are developing a laparoscopic cholesystectomy simulator and a simulator for training the airway management part of the ATLS course. However, the focus in this paper is not on these applications but on the development of the *medical platform* on which we base our surgical simulators. The medical platform in turn is built on the Magma API from ReachIn [4]. Magma is an API for combined graphics and haptics rendering using the same scene-graph. It is hardware independent and can be used with various display systems and haptic devices.

2. Methods

2.1   The Magma API

The Magma API was developed as the first truly hapto-visual scene-graph API. Prior to Magma there existed just one commercial haptics API – GHOST [5] and several commercial graphics APIs such as OpenInventor, Cosmo3D, Direct3D, etc. The main problem with these was that they specialised in either graphics or haptics. Therefore in order to develop commercial hapto-visual applications there were essentially four options:

1. Extend a graphics API to add haptics rendering.
2. Extend a haptics API to add graphics rendering.
3. Integrate the use of a graphics and a haptics API, providing a unifying API layer.
4. Develop a hapto-visual API "from the ground up" which is designed for multi-sensory rendering.

The problem with the first two options is that the API in question was not general enough to allow for extension to a completely different mode of rendering. In each case, crucial design decisions had been made that skew the API towards a particular mode (graphics or haptics). The problems also affect option 3. When developing software according to option 3, one finds that a significant portion of the code and effort is targeted at synchronising the objects that are represented in both the graphics and haptics APIs. This, together with the redundancy of representation, makes option 3 unappealing.

Therefore option 4 was settled upon. The basis for this hapto-visual API is OpenGL on the graphics side and a low-level device driver on the haptics side. This driver simply communicates force/torque vectors to the device and reads back position/orientation information from the device. This vector-based interface is simple enough that it can easily be substituted for different drivers and haptics devices.

The scene-graph structure

The Magma scene-graph is modelled after the VRML specification [6]. This open standard provides an excellent recognizable framework to start with. While some aspects of the specification that are tailored towards web browsers have been ignored – the vast majority of the specification is relevant to multi-sensory rendering.

The nodes in the VRML standard have been expanded upon to allow for specification of haptics behaviour, dynamic motion and configuration of a stereoscopic display.

Use of scripting

C++ is an excellent language for defining efficient node functionality, however it is a very poor language for constructing and configuring scene-graphs. While using VRML to define the C++ class hierarchy and node structure of the API, it seemed obvious to provide a VRML parser and loader in order to quickly configure and specify Magma scene-graphs. The creators of VRML intended scripts to be useful for distributing content on the Internet; in Magma we use VRML as a development environment. Magma also provides a Python [7] scripting environment for defining application functionality and behaviour. Python is a free byte-code compiled object-oriented scripting language.

The VRML and Python components allow the developer to work in an environment free of recompilation. This produces a qualitative change in the test/implement development cycle.

Developing with Magma

We may describe the development domains of Magma as follows.

- *C++ development* – this domain is ideal for creating scene-graph nodes. These may contain performance-critical routines defining haptics functionality. Nodes created in C++ provide an interface so that they may be instantiated from VRML or Python.

- *VRML scripting* – this domain is ideal for constructing a scene-graph, specifying geometry data, and visual and haptic appearance. No recompilation is required.

- *Python scripting* – this domain is extremely useful for rapid prototyping and also for full-scale application development. This language is byte-code compiled (similar to Java) and provides many high-level interfaces to services such as networking, string manipulation, etc.

- *Content production* – this involves the preparation of geometry, visual images and images used for haptics rendering (such as bumpmaps, etc). In this case mostly third-party tools such as Photoshop and various CAD tools are used.

2.2 Extensions of Magma for surgery simulation

As described above, Magma can be used for a wide range of applications. However, for surgical simulation, a number of features that are not part of Magma are required. This includes functionality for:

- Deformation of organs as a result of interaction with surgical tools.
- Communication between objects for modelling how neighbouring organs interact, for example, when one of the organs is moved as a result of a force supplied from one of the surgical tools.
- Tearing and cutting of tissue.
- Punctuation and penetration of soft tissue.
- Modelling of different surgical tools and other devices such as tubes and catheters.

We are implementing the above-mentioned features in what we call a medical platform, which can be viewed as a layer on top of Magma.

Different organs have different elasticity properties and it is important that the behavior of the real organ is simulated in a realistic way. The behavior of a specific organ is modelled through a number of parameters including surface friction parameters and parameters for modelling the amount and the range of deformation as well as the forces sensed when the surgical tool is pushed against the organ (Fig. 1). The parameters for each organ must be set individually, which requires the knowledge of an expert. To accomplish this we have developed a graphical interface where the user can interactively change the parameters for a selected organ.

The above-mentioned features constitute what we call *simulation blocks.* These are the basic building blocks of a simulator and are independent of the application. The simulation blocks are then combined into *skill modules.* A skill module is a basic entity that describes a specific skill such as setting a clip, making an incision, connecting two tubes of different diameters etc.

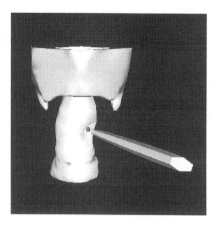 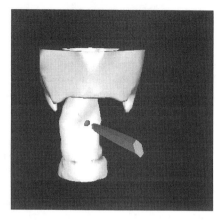

Figure 1. The figure shows the deformation of an object when the stylus is pushed against the surface. The parameter that controls the range of deformation was changed from a narrow range (left image) to a slightly wider range (right image).

2.3 Development strategy

The Magma API and the medical platform provide the basis for our development of different surgical simulators. However, it should be emphasized that it is not enough to build a realistic simulator. It is vital that we identify in detail 1) the surgery skills required, 2) how to train these skills, and 3) how to assess them. In fact, realism is not by itself a goal. It is rather a means to build an environment where the necessary surgery skills can be trained.

We use the Universal Modelling Language (UML) for modelling the surgical procedures. We describe the procedures using UML's activity diagrams and activity specification. We then take on a "use case"-centric approach in the development process. A use case is a way to describe how an actor interacts with the system and we employ use cases to describe the different lessons available in the simulator. This strategy provides us with a structured approach for communicating with medical experts. Once we have reached consensus with the medical expertise on the correctness of the domain model and on which use cases to include in the simulator, the rest of the development process follows a relatively standard approach for object oriented software development.

3. Application examples

In this section we will illustrate the use of the medical platform on two applications. Both projects represent works in progress.

3.1   Airway management in acute trauma situations

The course in Advanced Trauma Life Support (ATLS) from the American College of Surgeons (ACS) teaches the student strategies for management of trauma patients [8]. The course teaches a number of life saving procedures for keeping a free airway, control of ventilation and circulation and managing shock. The surgical procedures involved includes crico thyroidotomy, tube thoracostomy, pericardiocentesis and periotenal lavage. These procedures are today trained using anesthetized animals or cadavers. There are several ethical and practical problems with this; animals do not present the correct anatomy and cadavers are difficult to obtain and there are post mortem changes to the tissue properties. Furthermore, there is no feedback given to the student about the quality and precision of the task performed. These limitations may be overcome if the procedures are trained instead in a simulated environment. The first virtual reality based training system for a procedure in ATLS, a system for performing pericardiocentesis, was recently presented by Kaufmann et al. [9].

We are addressing the airway management component of the ATLS course. When a patient has a blocked airway, the practicing doctor must rapidly find the cause and take the right decision. It is generally a step-by-step procedure that should be performed where choices between different possible actions are made. If none of the non-invasive actions such as chin lift, insertion of a nasal tube, intubation, etc. helps a surgical cricothyroidotomy must be performed. If so, a cut through the cricothyroid membrane is made and a tube is inserted into the trachea. The purpose of the simulator is to train both the decision making and the skills required for performing the surgical intervention.

The challenge in the context of this paper is to develop the functionality for palpation where the student use his/her finger to identify the location of the cricothyroid membrane, for cutting through the skin, fat and the membrane, and for inserting the tube into the trachea. All this functionality has been developed based on the medical platform described above.

3.2   Laparoscopic Cholesystectomy

As our first laparoscopic application, we have chosen cholecystectomy which is an application where the gallbladder is removed. The simulator will address training of the entire procedure from start to stop, but due to our modular approach, with a number of independent skill modules, it will also be possible to train basic skills. A first prototype has

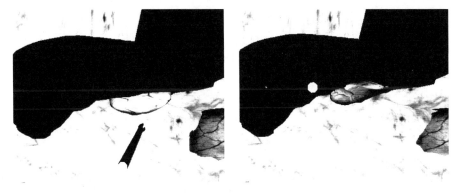

Figure 2. The figure shows a model of the liver, the gallbladder and surrounding fat. The left image shows the model in the resting state while the right image shows the model when the user grabs the gallbladder with a tool and pulls out and upwards.

been built for testing that the soft tissue deformation is sufficiently realistic (Fig. 2).

4. Discussion

We have developed a medical platform that includes functionality that can be shared among a wide range of surgery simulation applications. Our results show that, by having this platform and the underlying Magma API as the base, new applications can be developed very efficiently. The model we use for soft tissue simulation, including organ deformation, punctuation, palpation etc. is realistic and efficient. However, it should be pointed out that we use a surface representation for our models. This works well for our current applications since the cutting involved is more of a separation of one object from another (e.g., when freeing the gall bladder from surrounding tissue) or making an incision in an object. Modelling of more complex cutting, for example, removal of a liver segment will require the use of a volumetric model and a more elaborate soft tissue simulation such as previously reported in [1, 3, 10].

The development of the laparoscopic and airway management applications represents work in progress, but our results so far allow us to conclude that the described platform is suitable for a wide range of applications in surgery simulation. The applications we are working with are quite different in the sense that the laparoscopic cholesystectomy application uses a standard 2D display for an indirect view of the site of operation while the airway management simulator requires a co-located hand-eye environment. For this we use the ReachIn Display, a stereoscopic workspace using the Phantom haptic device from SensAble Technologies.

Although we have not addressed validation in this paper, it is important to emphasize that a surgical simulator is not useful until it has been validated. It is also important that a complex simulator such as our cholesystectomy application is validated first module-by-module and then as a whole. This work is currently underway and will be carried out in multi-center studies in collaboration with our clinical partners.

References

[1] S. Cotin, H. Delingette, J.-M. Clement, V. Tassetti, J. Marescaux, and N. Ayache. Volumetric deformable models for simulation of laparoscopic surgery. In *Proceedings of the International Symposium on Computer and Communication Systems for Image Guided Diagnosis and Therapy, Computer Assisted Radiology (CAR'96)*, volume 1124 of *International Congress Series*. Elsevier, June 1996.,

[2] Jambon AC, Qerley D, Dubois P, Chaillou C, Meseure P, Karpf S, Geron C. SPIC Pedagogical simulator for gynecologic laparoscopy. In Westwood et al. (Eds), Medicine Meets Virtual reality, IOS Press, 2000; pp. 139-145.

[3] Székely G, Brechbühler C, Hutter R, Rhomberg A, Ironmonger N, Schmid P, Modelling of soft tissue deformation for laparoscopic surgery simulation, Medical Image Analysis, In press.

[4] magma.reachin.se , www.reachin.se

[5] www.sensable.com

[6] www.web3d.org

[7] www.python.org

[8] American College of Surgeons Committee on Trauma, Advanced Trauma Life Support for Doctors, 6th edition, Chicago, IL (1997).

[9] Kaufmann C, Zakaluzny S, Liu A, First steps in eliminating animals and cadavers in advanced trauma life support. .In MICCAI'2000, October 2000, vol. 1935 of Lecture Notes in Computer Science, pp. 618-623, Springer.

[10] Moor A, Kanade T, Modifying soft tissue models: progressive cutting with minimal new element creation. In MICCAI'2000, October 2000, vol. 1935 of Lecture Notes in Computer Science, pp. 598-607, Springer.

Medicine Meets Virtual Reality 2001
J.D. Westwood et al. (Eds.)
IOS Press, 2001

Clinical Validation of Computer Assisted Pelvic Surgery using Ultrasound. A percutaneous safe Technique with low Radiation Exposure

Tonetti J, MD; Carrat L, PhD; Blendea S, MD;
Troccaz J, PhD; Merloz Ph, MD; Lavallee S, PhD; Chirossel J-P, MD.
Orthopaedic and Trauma department
Hospital Michallon – BP 217 – F 38043 Grenoble France.
Phone (33)476 76 55 32   Fax (33)476 76 52 18   jerome.tonetti@imag.fr

Abstract. This study presents early results of the clinical experience of computer assisted surgery (CAS) applied to percutaneous iliosacral screwing. The results of these 10 first cases (4 patients) are compared to an historical series of 51 cases (30 patients). The CAS technique shows better screw placement without outside bone screw and a very low radiation exposure.

1. Introduction

Letournel did the first publication of an iliosacral screwing technique, in 1978 [1]. This procedure involved 6 to 25 % of wound complications[2]. Matta and Saucedo, in 1989, introduced the fluoroscopic operative control [3]. To be less invasive, several authors proposed percutaneous techniques; under fluoroscopy [Matta et Saucedo [3], Simonian et al. [4], Shuler et al. [2], Remiger et al. [5], Routt et al. [6] or under CT-scan [Ebraheim et al. [7], Starr AJ et al [8]]. Fluoroscopic technique is delicate. The screw placement must be strictly inside the bone, because of the neurologic trunk's neighborhood: lumbosacral trunk and S1 root [Templeman et al. [9]]. The tip of the screw takes an anchorage in the strong S1 body. Two screws are placed into the S1 body, through the iliosacral joint, using a narrow corridor of 22 mm by 11 mm (mean values) [Tonetti et al. [10]]. The procedure done under CT scan causes a lot of irradiation for the patient and staff and requires CT in the operative room or surgery in the CT room.

Recently, computer assisted surgery was proposed. Khaler et al. [11] use a registration based with prior implanted pins and markers on the iliac crest. Others authors use virtual fluoroscopy navigation (Gruetzner et al. [12]), but the major drawback is that it doesn't offer real 3D information.

One other CT-based navigation is proposed, using for the first time an ultrasound-based registration [Tonetti et al. [13]]. This technique is the subject of the present paper. Clinical results being documented and compared to previous series of patients who underwent traditional fluoroscopic percutaneous surgery.

2. Surgical procedures

2.1 Fluoroscopic procedure

The patient was installed in supine position, which allowed the external reduction. To approach the optimal trajectory a canulated screw ancillary was used (7 mm screw diameter - Mathys inc - Etupe, France). The trajectory was checked directly on the screen during repetitive Inlet, Outlet, AP and lateral view [15].

2.2 Computer assisted surgery (CAS) procedure

Preoperative CT-scan segmentation and surgical planning. A CT-scan acquisition of nearly 50 images with a 3mm slice thickness was performed with a spiral CT GE Hispeed Advantage (General Electric - Buc, France). The examination field was included the whole sacrum. A semi-automatic segmentation of the bone was performed in order to obtain a 3 Dimensional CT model of the pelvis. Using an interactive interface that allowed the computation of arbitrary planes, the surgeon was defined on CT model the optimal screw trajectories.

Operative ultrasound acquisition and registration. The patient was installed in prone position. At the beginning of the operative time, all the reduction maneuvers were done like with fluoroscopic procedure. A 6D optical localizer (Polaris, NDI – Toronto, Canada) was used. It was located the position and orientation of wireless customized rigid-bodies equipped with reflective markers (TIMC laboratory). Rigid-bodies were fixed on surgical tools.

- A standard ultrasound probe of 7,5 MHz frequency with an examination field of 2 cm width and 5 cm depth (Hitachi EUB-405 - Tokyo, japan).

- A linear tool used for registration validity checking and drilling trajectory approach (TIMC laboratory).

- A standard surgical power drill (landos Landanger - Chaumont, France).

- A linear tool guide used during drilling and screwing (TIMC laboratory).

A reference rigid-body was firmly fixed on the sacrum. It was defined the intraoperative reference coordinate system, that was used during the whole surgery. Using the ultrasound probe, nearly 30 ultrasound images of the soft tissue and sacrum interface were stored [14]. Then, a manual segmentation procedure was enabled the surgeon to build curves of 2D points that was corresponded to the bone surface. These curves were converted in 3D clouds, referenced in the intra-operative coordinate system. The cloud of points was registered with the preoperative CT scan model of the sacrum using a surface-based registration algorithm (TIMC laboratory). As a result, the preoperative CT scan defined screw trajectories were known in the intraoperative coordinate system.

The passive drilling guidance. During each step of the guidance, real-time tool tracking and re-sliced images showing the tool position in the CT scan images were displayed on the computer screen. An important step were the registration validation, witch were consisted in verified if the displayed image really were corresponded to the specific anatomical elements, palpated with the linear tool. Then, screwing was done using the calibrated tools. A final X-ray control was done, using inlet, outlet, AP and lateral views.

3. Patient population

3.1 Fluoroscopic group

They were 30 patients, 23 males and 7 females. The average age of 34.7 years, ranging from 17 to 60. All the patients had a recent traumatic lesion of the iliosacral joint or of the sacral ala. The Tile classification [16] was used. The B1 lesion was found in 3 cases, C1 in 17 cases, C2 in 4 cases, C3 in 5 cases. One patient presents an isolated fracture of the sacrum. The average ISS was 30.8 (maximum score 75) range from 5 to 75. 51 screws were implanted. The preoperative examination found 8 neurologic lesions of the lumbosacral trunk or of the S1 root, 13 patients without any lesion. For 9 patients, the clinical preoperative examination were impossible because of early general anesthesia (severe multiple trauma).

3.2 Computer assisted surgery (CAS) group

From February 2000 to April 2000, this new technique was used in 4 patients, 1 male and 3 females. The average age was 48.5 years, ranging from 34 to 71. Two (2) patients had an. unilateral recent traumatic lesion of the sacral ala with a vertical instability, C type according to Tile classification. The injury severity scores (ISS) were 9, respectively 47. One other patient needed a circular fusion of the pelvic ring, because of tumor reconstruction, with bilateral iliosacral arthrodesis.The last patient presented a delayed union of an iliosacral disruption and needed a deferred iliosacral arthrodesis. 10 screws were implanted with CAS. The preoperative neurological examinations did not found any deficit at the lower limbs.

4. Method of evaluation

During surgery, the duration (minutes), voltage (Kvolt), intensity (mA) of the irradiation were stored. The patients underwent rigorous postoperative neurological evaluation of the lower body, including the territory of the superior gluteus nerve.

A post-operative CT scan was performed for each patient. The position of the screws was checked in the transversal plane. "A" was the distance from the screw to the anterior cortex of the sacrum, "B" - the distance from the screw to the spinal canal or to the S1 foramen. There was established a security score in function of "A" and "B" values such as: If A or B equal 0, security score is 0% because one anatomical limit is reached. If A = B, security score is 100% because the screw is accurately centered. The score was not calculated for negative values.

No statistic comparison tests were done, because of the small Number of patients in the CAS group.

5. Results

5.1 Fuoroscopic procedure

Fifthty one screws (51) were placed with fluoroscopic procedure. The average length of the screws was 85,5 mm, ranging from 65 to 110 mm. The mean operating time was 25 minutes for one screw and 40 minutes for 2 screws. The average of irradiation time by patients was 1.03 minutes ranging from 0.1 to 3.1. The average of irradiation time by screw was 0.6 minutes. The voltage and intensity of the irradiation exposure was measured for 16 patients, showing an average voltage of 74.9 Kvolt by patient (64 to 110) and an average intensity of 3.6 mA by patient (2.1 to 7.1). The postoperative CT scans control data found 12 misplaced screws (23%). The average score were calculated only for inside bone trajectories (n=39) and was 63%. Postoperative neurological evaluation found 11 patients without any deficit. One patient died in the resuscitation unit, so the evaluation was not possible. 18 patients had neurological lesions. 8 lesions were known preoperatively and 10 lesions were unknown. 7 of those lesions can be explained by outside bone trajectories (13%) - see table.

5.2 Computer assisted surgery procedure.

Ten (10) screws were implanted. The average length was 76 mm, ranging from 70 to 85 mm. The mean operating time was 50 minutes for one screw and 60 minutes for 2 screws. The average of irradiation time by patients was 0.35 minutes ranging from 0.1 to 0.5. The average voltage was 78 Kvolt by patient (68 to 89) and the average intensity was 3.1 mA by patient (3.1 to 3.2). All the screws were well placed. The average score was 62%. No postoperative neurological lesion was found - see table.

Table: Comparative results between

Fluoroscopic group and Computer assisted surgery group (CAS)

	FLUOROSCOPY	CAS
n patients	30	4
n screws	51	10
mean irradiation time / patient (min)	1.03 (3.1 - 0.1)	0.35 (0.1-0.5)
mean irradiation time / screws (min)	0.6	0.14
mean voltage / patient (Kvolt)	74.9 (64 to 110)	78 (68 to 89)
mean intensity / patient (mA)	3.6 (2.1 to 7.1)	3.1 (3.1 to 3.2)
Score of placement	63% (n=39)	62% (n=10)
Outside bone trajectories	12 (23%)	0 (0%°
Neurological lesion due to the screw	7 (13%)	0 (0%)

6. Discussion

Despite of the insufficient statistical analysis, the tendencies are clear.

With the traditional fluoroscopic procedure all the outside bone trajectories occur for the first 15 patients, a good training being necessary. With the CAS procedure, no outside bone trajectories was found. It was a new technique for the authors, but no learning curve is observed. This technique looks safe for the surgical students. Nevertheless, the score of placement is the same in the both groups for the inside bone screws. The explanation is that the choice of the entry point decides if the trajectory will be inside or outside the bone. For a good entry point, the drill slips easy between the cortical bone of the sacral ala. In consequence, no postoperative neurological lesion is found in the CAS group. The aim of the percutaneous fluoroscopic procedure is to be less invasive than the open surgery, but as shown in this study, the results are not always so good. We mean that an augmented reality tool is necessary to perform a routine percutaneous surgery.

The second advantage of the CAS technique is the decrease of the irradiation time. Fluoroscopic views are required only at the end of the procedure, to verify the screw placement.

Other CT-based navigation is also safe, but require the introduction of fiducial markers into the bones, prior building the preoperative model. The patient must have two anesthesias: first to insert pins and second do perform the screwing. When the surgical team use external fixator for reduce the pelvic ring displacement, this technique is interesting. In our trauma center, we use traction for vertical instability and pelvic clamp for reduces the transversal displacement, in the emergency room. No anesthesia is necessary. Thus, new anesthesia for implant the fiducial is for us too much invasive.

The virtual fluoroscopy is full of promise: no CT registration, faster technique. Early results presented by Gruetzner et al. [13] shows an average operative time of 50 to 105 minutes with a very large irradiation exposure of 1.83 to 4.33 minutes. Two different papers shown outside bone screws: Gruetzner et al. [13] and Stöckle et al. [18] found respectively 2 wrong trajectories for 12 screws and 9 wrong trajectories for 60 screws. This technique actually is not decisive in comparison of Routt's advice [19].

The major drawback of the ultrasound-based registration is the ultrasound images segmentation. In this study, the segmentation is done manually, being very delicate and need a well trained engineer in the surgical room. This step is time consuming and increase the operative time. The registration is delicate too. Manual approach of the registration is sometime necessary. Research is currently performed to develop an automatic segmentation and registration of ultrasound acquisition.

7. Conclusion

The percutaneous screwing of the posterior lesion of the pelvic ring fractures is a delicate procedure, requiring a well-trained surgeon. Some tools of augmented reality are necessary. The ultrasound-based registration with CT guidance is a very low radiation dose method. The CAS procedure is safe and accurate in clinical use. This tool aids the inexperienced surgeon for realize new interventions without learning curve and iatrogenic lesions.

References

[1] E Letournel, Pelvic fractures, *Injury* 10 (1978) 145-148.

[2] TE Shuler, DC Boone, GS Gruen, AB Peitzman, Percutaneous iliosacral screw fixation: early treatment for unstable posterior pelvic ring disruptions, *J trauma* 38 (1995) 453-458.

[3] JM Matta and T Saucedo, Internal fixation of pelvic ring fracture, *Clin Orthop Rel Res* 242 (1989) 83-97.

[4] PT Simonian, C Jr Routt, RM Harrington, AF Tencer, Internal fixation for the transforaminal sacral fracture, *Clin orthop Rel Res* 323 (1996) 202-209.

[5] A Remiger and P Engelhardt, [Percutaneous iliosacral screw fixation of vertical unstable pelvic ring fractures], *Swiss Surg* 6 (1996) 259-263.

[6] ML Jr Routt, PJ Kregor, PT Simonian, KA Mayo, Early results of percutaneous iliosacral screws placed with the patient in the supine position, *J Orthop Trauma* 3 (1995) 207-214.

[7] NA Ebraheim, JJ Russin, RJ Coombs, WT Jackson, B Holiday, Percutaneous Computer-Tomography Stabilization of Pelvic Fractures: Preliminary Report. *J Orthop Trauma* 1 (1987) 197-204.

[8] AJ Starr et Al, Percutaneous Fixation of the Columns of the Acetabulum : A new Technique, *J Orthop Trauma* 1 (1998) 51-58.

[9] D Templeman, A Schmidt, J Freese, I Weisman, Proximity of Iliosacral Screws to Neurovascular Structures after Internal Fixation, *Clin Orthop Rel Res* 329 (1996) 194-198.

[10] J Tonetti, O Cloppet, M Clerc, L Pittet, J Troccaz, P Merloz, J-P Chirossel, [Optimal Placement of the Iliosacral Screws: 3D Computer Tomography Simulation], *Rev Chir Orthop* 86 (2000) 360-369.

[11] DM Khaler, K Mallik, Computer Guided Percutaneous Iliosacral Screw Fixation of posterior Pelvic Ring Disruption compared to Conventional Technique, Syllabus of CAOS USA 2000, Pittsburgh pn June 15-17 (2000) pp 185-187.

[12] PA Gruetzner, B Vock, F Holz, A Wentzensen, Virtual Fluoroscopy in acute Treatment of Pelvic Ring Disruptions, Syllabus of CAOS USA 2000, Pittsburgh pn June 15-17 (2000) pp 197.

[13] J Tonetti, L Carrat, S Lavallee, L Pittet, P Cinquin, P Merloz, J-P Chirossel, Percutaneous Iliosacral Screw Placement using Image Guided Techniques, *Clin Orthop Rel Res* 354 (1998) 103-110.

[14] C Barbe, J Troccaz, B Mazier, S Lavallee, Using 2.5d Echography in Computer Assisted Spine Surgery, Engineering in Medicine and Biology Society Proceedings, San Diego, Institute Of Electrical And Electronics Engineers Inc (1993) pp 160-161.

[15] ML Jr Routt; PT Simonian; SG Agnew; FA Mann, Radiographic Recognition of the Sacral Alar Slope for Optimal Placement of Iliosacral Screws: A Cadaveric and Clinical Study, *J Orthop Trauma* 3 (1996) 171-177.

[16] M Tile, Fractures of the Pelvis and Acetabulum. Williams And Wilkins, Baltimore 1984.

[17] U Stöckle, B König, R Hofstetter, LP Nolte, NP Haas, Virtual Fluoroscopy : Safe Zones for Pelvic Screw Fixations, Syllabus of CAOS USA 2000. Pittsburgh Pn June 15-17 (2000) pp 199.

[18] ML Jr Routt, PT Simonian, WJ Mills, Iliosacral Screw Fixation: Early Complications of the Percutaneous Technique. *J Orthop Trauma* 8 (1997) 584-589.

Medicine Meets Virtual Reality 2001
J.D. Westwood et al. (Eds.)
IOS Press, 2001

The Interaction of Spatial Ability and Motor Learning in the Transfer of Training From a Simulator to a Real Task

Michael R. Tracey, MS and Corinna E. Lathan, Ph.D.

The Catholic University of America, Dept. of Biomedical Engineering
Washington, DC 22206
and
AnthroTronix, Inc.
387 Technology Drive, College Park, MD 20742
email: mike@anthrotronix.com

Abstract: Virtual Reality (VR) based simulators have been used as a training tool in many settings, although very few studies examine transfer of training from simulators to a real world task, particularly for manipulation tasks. Simulators could play a key role as an enabling technology for manipulation tasks related to teleoperation, and medical procedure training. We investigated the relationship between motor tasks and participants' spatial abilities. This relationship was further examined with respect to learning in a simulator and to transfer of training from the simulator to the real world on a pick-and-place task. Spatial abilities were characterized using a battery of recognition and manipulation figural tests. Subjects with lower spatial abilities demonstrated significant positive transfer from a simulator based training task to a similar real world robotic operation task. Subjects with higher spatial skills did not respond as positively from training in a simulated environment.

1. Introduction

Computer-simulated environments are part of an emerging set of human interface technologies, with a multitude of applications. Although applications span entertainment, medicine, data manipulation, aviation, and rehabilitation, questions concerning appropriate applications and tasks for computer-simulated environments still need to be addressed before this technology can make a significant impact in these areas [1, 2].

This paper will focus on issues pertinent to perceptual-motor skill learning. This refers to the learning of motor skills such as flying, surgical training, or assembly / building tasks. Although complex motor tasks, such as flying and surgery, may have a lot in common in terms of the appropriate use of simulators for training, very little performance data exists to quantify transfer of training from the virtual environment into the real world [3].

The learning of specific motor skills is an integral component of the learning process in simulated environments. The skills learned in the controlled environment are then transferable to real-world situations. For example, the medical community is looking at Virtual Reality (VR) based simulators as a tool for continued medical education and even as an accreditation tool for medical students. Prototypes of VR systems to train surgeons in surgical procedures have also been developed [4-6].

A key aspect of learning in simulators is the effective use of spatial information, such as navigation through an environment, or determination of the best trajectory for manipulating objects in a pick and place task. Navigation in VR is been addressed by many researchers and is summarized by Stuart [7]. Cromby [8] demonstrated transfer of training from a navigation task to the real world by studying subjects with severe learning disabilities. Operators trained to complete a shopping task in a virtual environment had positive transfer to a real environment. Experiments concerning the transfer of training of manipulation tasks from VR have conflicting results [9, 10].

The degree of spatial ability (SpA) required to accomplish tasks can vary. For example, pilots perform better than non-pilots on some visual-spatial tasks such as mental rotation of objects [11]. This paper will characterize some aspects of participants' spatial abilities and explore the relationship of their spatial ability to the transfer of training from a simulator to the real world, on a manipulation perceptual-motor task.

2.   Methods and Tools

2.1   Spatial Ability Testing

SpA is defined as the ability to reason about visual scenes. It is a basic dimension of human intelligence, and it is comprised of a domain of abilities rather than a single skill. Pellegrino reports one classification [12] using three factors to categorize SpA: spatial relations, spatial visualization, and spatial orientation. However, after 70 years of psychometric research, the number of distinct spatial processing factors that exist and how best to characterize each one is not conventionally defined.

Complex spatial tests have been correlated with performance on figural tests (paper and pencil tests), which have led to hundreds of off the shelf paper and pencil tests of SpA. Eliot [13] classified figural spatial tests as having two divisions based on Kelley [14], recognition and manipulation. Recognition involves "sensing and retention of visual forms," and manipulation involves "the mental manipulation of shapes."

The recognition tests used in this experiment were the Gestalt Completion Test and Stumpf's Spatial Memory Test. The Gestalt Completion Test requires subjects to recognize an incomplete picture, and thus impose meaning upon ambiguous stimuli. The Stumpf Spatial Memory Test has two parts. First the subject memorizes figures and then in the second part must recall the same figures after an interval.

The manipulation tests used were a Paper Folding Test and Stumpf's Cube Perspectives Test. The Paper Folding Test draws upon figural memory and demands both sequential and cumulative reasoning. The Stumpf Cube Perspectives Test is part of a pre-medical school screening battery used in Germany and has been administered to several thousand subjects. It requires the subject to make positional judgments about an object displayed 3-Dimensionally in 2-Dimensions.

The SpA tests were given in a random order to 42 volunteer subjects. The distribution of SpA scores is presented in Figure 1. The score was calculated as the number of successful design answers divided by the total number of designs. The scores for each test were averaged to calculate a total composite score for each participant.

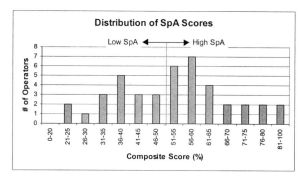

Figure 1: SpA Score Distribution.

2.2   Task Development

Real and simulated environments were created to test and train operators. The task required operators perform a pick and place task using an articulated robot arm with a touch pendant input device. The dependent variables are performance on the spatial tests and the time to task completion. The number of errors committed was also recorded.

The real-world environment used a SCORBOT ER V robot arm (Serial No. 141360; Tel Aviv, Israel) with an ER V Tech Pendant (Serial No. 170960; Tel Aviv, Israel) to perform a pick and place task. One wooden block, with a hook in the top to assist grasping with the robot arm was placed on brick towers. Figure 2 shows the robot experiment set up. To limit the use of stereoscopic cues, a flat screen was placed between the operator and the robot. Although the operator still had some 3-D perspective, the screen limited the operator to one seating position.

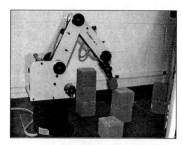

Figure 2: Real-world pick and place task using a robot arm.

The simulator environment was designed to emulate the real task as closely as possible using Transom Jack 2.0 (Transom Technologies, Inc., Ann Arbor, MI) on a Windows NT 4.0 Workstation. An AccelGraphics 3D 8-MB video card was used with a VX1100 monitor. Monitor resolution was 1280 x 1024 with a pixel depth of 16.

The fidelity of the task interface was the focus of the simulator design. The use of an IntelliKeys keyboard (IntelliTools, Inc., Novato, CA, Serial No. T7956) permitted the design and implementation of an input device that identically matched a real world robot input keypad. However, the use of the IntelliKeys keyboard prohibited the use of several advanced displays, which would have provided a greater level of immersion. Head mounted displays with stereoscopic vision and sound systems present the operator with a more realistic 3-D perspective, but the operator would not have been able to use the input tablet.

A Tcl/Tk interface file was created to manipulate the end effector of simulated robot in the Transom Jack environment. Keystroke commands directed the end effector of the robot to move in Cartesian space, and grab or release an object. The speed of movements was altered to match the default speed of the real robot as closely as possible. Figure 3 shows the simulator input device (left) and real robot touch pendent (right).

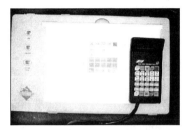

Figure 3: Input devices for the simulator and the real task.

Simple geometric objects (blocks and towers) were created in Transom Jack and saved as part of the environment. The towers and blocks used in the simulator environment were of identical relative dimensions to those used in the real world task. The operator would move one virtual block from a starting position to the top of one of three towers. A collision detection routine was implemented to alert the operator to intersection of the robot with a tower and contact of the block with the top of the tower. Figure 4 presents a photo of the screen and display used in the simulator.

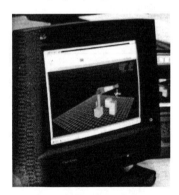

Figure 4: Simulator Screen

2.3   Subjects

Twenty-two volunteer subjects were taken from the subject pool (5 male and 17 female) and divided into two classifications, high and low SpA. Those with scores greater than the average were considered to have "higher" spatial ability and those with less had "lower" spatial ability. The groups will be referred to as "High" and "Low" although it should be stated that these are relative terms applied only in our subject pool and this particular set of tests. Each group was then split into a robot (control) training group and a simulator (experimental) training group, resulting in four groups, "Experimental High", "Experimental Low", "Control High", and "Control Low".

The experimental groups trained in the simulator and then performed a similar testing task using the real robot. The control groups performed the same testing task and results between groups (experimental and control) and with groups (high and low SpA) were compared. Performance was measured as time to complete task and number of errors. A Simple Factorial ANOVA analysis was used (SPSS Release 10.0.5) on all data. Significance levels were tested at $p<0.05$. Post-hoc analysis of pairwise comparisons was made using a Least Significant Difference test.

The subjects were all students or employees of The Catholic University of America with ages ranging from 18-47. All subjects were pre-screened to ensure they did not have experience with the particular robot used in this experiment and attempts were made to randomize age, gender, academic major and degree of technical comfort. All subjects signed IRB approved consent forms and were paid $20 for completing the experiment.

2.4   Procedure

Roughly half of the experimental high group and half of the experimental low group were randomly selected to train in the simulator. Each subject was seated before the monitor with the IntelliKeys keyboard directly in front of him or her. The directions of the coordinate axis were described and the subjects were given up to two minutes to familiarize themselves with the simulator and input method. Three training exercises were performed. The maximum allowed time to complete the task was 6 minutes.

Similar to the simulator training, each control subject was allowed up to two minutes to familiarize themselves with the robot and pendent. Three training exercises were performed. The directions of the Cartesian coordinates were given to the subject. The robot was configured in Cartesian space mode where inputs affect the XYZ position of the end effector. The robot-testing task was identical to the training task. The simulator-trained group was given up to two minutes to experiment with the real robot.

3.   Results

A significant difference in time to complete task was found ($p<0.05$) between SpA groups, with superior performance among high SpA operators. No similar significance was found for errors. A significant difference in performance between experimental and control groups is seen in the low SpA group. The experimental group performed significantly better ($p<0.05$) than the control group and demonstrated an average 14.95% transfer from the VE to the real world. Training transfer was calculated as:

$$Transfer = \frac{Performance_{Control} - Performance_{Experimental}}{Performance_{Control} + Performance_{Experimental}}$$

The experimental high SpA group did not demonstrate any significant improvement in performance.

Power law of practice calculations predict that the high SpA (experimental and control) and low SpA (control) operators leveled off in performance by the fifth trial [15]. Note the time to complete task was significantly better for the high SpA groups than the low SpA control group. The low SpA experimental group is predicated to improve performance to a level significantly better (p<0.05) than the low SpA control group and should equal performance of the high SpA groups within six trials.

The order in which the tests were taken had no effect upon how any individual scored. Also, the sample size was not large enough to test effects of gender, age, and major, however a few observations were made. There were only four men in the subject pool and all three with technical backgrounds scored in the high range. Also, the subjects who scored higher on the spatial ability tests tended to be students studying science and engineering-related fields. Three of the experimental group subjects did not understand Cartesian X-Y-Z coordinates.

The average time to complete each trial is presented in figure 5, separated by high SpA and low SpA. The standard deviation of time measurements for the low SpA group ranged from 9.2 to 5.7 seconds (experimental) and 15.2 to 3.4 seconds (control). The standard deviation of time measurements for the high SpA group was 13.4 to 8.4 seconds (experimental) and 10.1 to 4.0 seconds (control).

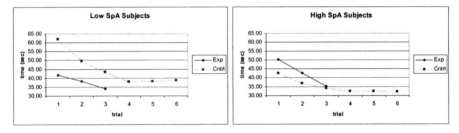

Figure 5: Time to Complete Task

The number of tower strikes was intermittent across all subjects and was not significantly different across any factor. Many subjects had no tower strikes and those that did, reduced the number of tower strikes to zero by the end on the training series.

4.   Conclusions

Simulations serve as an effective manipulation task training tool and provide the most benefit to operators with lower SpA. We have found that for our perceptual-motor task, VR is an effective training tool for operators with lower SpA. Training in a simulator did not have significant benefit to higher SpA operators but did not seem to hinder overall performance. This suggests that a simulator is an effective training tool.

Future experiments will further examine the ability of spatial testing to predict performance on spatial-motor manipulation tasks in virtual reality and subsequent transfer of training. Recognition and manipulation figural tests seemed to be an effective means of assessing subject spatial ability. Future test batteries should include other performance spatial tests to determine the utility of such tests.

An important factor that potentially limits the predictive validity of spatial ability tests is the fact that all conventional tests are restricted to judgments about static spatial displays. In contrast, many real world activities that presumably tap visual spatial reasoning involve objects moving in space (Pellegrino 1991). One potential solution is to use movie or computer-based spatial ability testing, which may be a more appropriate way to test computer-based tasks. Computer-based testing would also provide instantaneous feedback on spatial ability and could be used to customize a VR training task as a function of the individual's score.

Acknowledgments

This research was supported in part by the Dept. of Army, US Army Medical Research Acquisition Activity, MCMR, Assistive Technology and Neuroscience Research Center (ATNRC), grant # DAMD 17-00-1-0056.

References

[1]   Durlach, N.I. and A.S. Mavor, eds. *Virtual Reality: Scientific and Technological Challenges.* . 1995, National Academy Press: Washington, DC.

[2]   Stanney, K.M., R.R. Mourant, and R.S. Kennedy, *Human Factors Issues in Virtual Environments: A Review of the Literature.* Presence: Teleoperators and Virtual Environments, 1998. **7**(4): p. 327-351.

[3]   Pausch, R., T. Crea, et al., *A literature survey for virtual environments: Military flight simulator visual systems and simulator sickness.* Presence, 1992. **1**(3): p. 344-363.

[4]   Delp, S.L., *et al.*, *Surgical Simulation: An Emerging Technology for Training in Emergency Medicine.* Presence, 1997. **6**(2): p. 147-159.

[5]   Lathan, C.E., K. Cleary, and R. Greco. *Development and evaluation of a spine biopsy simulator.* in *Medicine Meets Virtual Reality.* 1998: IOS Press, Amsterdam.

[6]   Lathan, C. and K. Cleary. *Performance feedback in a spine biopsy simulator.* in *Proceedings of Surgical-Assist Systems.* 1998. San Hose, CA: SPIE.

[7]   Stuart, R., *The Design of Virtual Environments.* 1996, New York.: McGraw-Hill.

[8]   Cromby, J.J. and P.J. Standen, et al. *Successful transfer to the real world of skills practiced in virtual environment by students with severe learning difficulties.* in *Proc. 1 Euro. Conf. Disability, Virtual Reality & Assoc. Tech.* 1996. Maidenhead, UK.

[9]   Kozak, J.J., *et al.*, *Transfer of training from virtual reality.* Ergonomics, 1993. **36**(7): p. 777-784.

[10]   Kenyon, R. and M. Afenya, *Training in virtual and real environments.* Annals of Biomedical Engineering, 1995. **23**: p. 445-455.

[11]   Dror, I.E., S.M. Kosslyn, and W.L. Waag, *Visual-Spatial Abilities of Pilots.* Journal of Applied Psychology, 1993. **78**(5): p. 763-773.

[12]   Pellegrino, J., W. and E. Hunt, B., *Cognitive Models for Understanding and Assessing Spatial Abilities.*, in *Intelligence: Reconceptualization and Measurement*, H. Row, A.., Editor. 1991, Lawrence Erlbaum Associates: New Jersey. p. 203-225.

[13]   Eliot, J., *Models of Psychological Space: Psychometric, Developmental, and Experimental Approaches.* 1987, New York: Springer-Verlag.

[14]   Kelley, T.L., *Crossroads in the mind of man: A study of differentiable mental abilities.* 1928, Stanford: Stanford University Press.

[15]   Proctor, R.W. and A. Dutta, *Skill Acquisition and Human Performance.* 1995, London: Sage Publications.

528

Medicine Meets Virtual Reality 2001
J.D. Westwood et al. (Eds.)
IOS Press, 2001

An Enabling System for Echocardiography Providing Adaptive Support Through Behavioral Analysis

Sabine TROCHIM, Michael WEIDENBACH, Stefan PIEPER, Christoph WICK, Thomas
BERLAGE
GMD German National Research Center for Information Technology
Institute for Applied Information Technology
Schloss Birlinghoven,D-53754 St. Augustin,'Germany
{trochim\stefan.pieper\wick\berlage@gmd.de
University of Cologne, Cologne, Germany
weidenbach@mmkmail.gmd.de

Abstract. Echocardiography requires the integrated application of a broad spectrum of cognitive and practical skills, e.g. diagnostic knowledge (symbolic), image interpretation (visual perception) and handling of the ultrasound probe (sensorimotor). This complex expertise is acquired through extensive practical training guided by a skilled cardiologist that is often incompatible with clinical reality.

Especially for beginners, the most critical point during an echocardiographic examination is the steering of the ultrasound probe to navigate between different cardiological standard planes (sensorimotor skill) without loosing orientation. These transitions or "standard trajectories" can roughly be described by specific movement patterns.

We propose an enabling system based on an Augmented Reality simulator for two-dimensional echocardiography imitating this apprenticeship [1]-[3]. During a simulated ultrasound examination the system monitors the activities of the trainee and analyzes the motion pattern of the ultrasound probe. The simulator reacts by mapping the motion patterns onto cognitive orientation demands and providing adaptive feedback in the form of context sensitive help (animations). It partly takes the role of the critical teacher.

1. Introduction

During the last few years the number of simulation-based medical training systems has been steadily growing in order to deal with the lack of practical training. Most of them are surgical simulators like, e.g. [4] and [5].

But also imaging techniques like ultrasound need extensive practical training. Echocardiography, for example, requires the integrated application of *cognitive skills* (diagnostic knowledge), *visual perception* (image interpretation) and *sensorimotor skills* (steering of the ultrasound probe). Figure 1 shows the involved cognitive modes. This integral expertise can only be acquired within the application context. However, sufficient practical training guided by a skilled cardiologist is incompatible with clinical reality. That is why we need a training system imitating this cognitive apprenticeship approach ([6]).

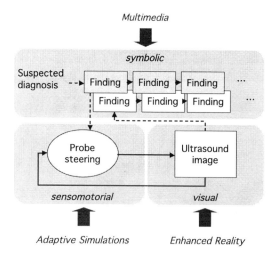

Figure 1: Cognitive modes

One possible solution is the combination of the real world and a virtual simulation environment to build an *Augmented Reality* scenario where the real situation is explained by the mental model of an expert (see Fig. 2) [1], [2]. The simulator enables the learner to slice a three-dimensional ultrasound data set similar to a real echocardiographic examination using a dummy ultrasound probe and a human torso model. A reference scene provides continuous visual feedback using a virtual heart model, which indicates the current orientation of the slice plane in relation to the patient's heart. The training method is mainly based on *self-assessment* using visual feedback.

In this paper we add intelligent tutoring/training capabilities analyzing the sensorimotor system interactions in order to provide adaptive feedback in the form of context sensitive help animations. The main ideas are the inference of semantic concepts describing the current ultrasound plane and the transducer head movements (e.g. correct behavior or indications of orientation misconceptions). Methods used are *fuzzy rules* and stochastic *hidden Markov models*.

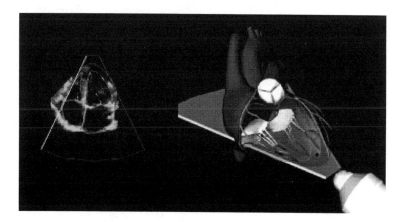

Figure 2: Augmented Reality Simulator

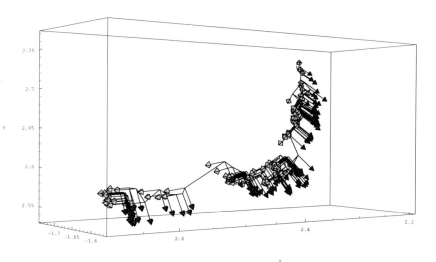

Figure 3: Trajectory for parasternal long axis -> parasternal short axis

2. Methods

All sensorimotor interactions with the system, i.e. every position and orientation of the ultrasound probe are logged and analyzed using fuzzy rules and hidden Markov models. Ota, Loftin et al. have used fuzzy rules for performance assessment in VR surgical simulators [7]. Hidden Markov models have been utilized for the same task by Rosen et al. [8]. The inferred semantic concepts can then be used to provide adaptive help.

2.1 Characteristics of transducer head trajectories

Echocardiography relies on well-defined *standard planes*. These standard planes are echocardiographic views, which guarantee that all relevant structures are seen and measurements are made comparable. Especially for beginners, the most critical point during an echocardiographic examination is the steering of the ultrasound probe to navigate between different cardiological standard planes (sensorimotor skill) without loosing orientation. These transitions or "standard trajectories" can roughly be described by specific movement patterns.

The sensorimotor data consist of a sequence of tuples containing a translation vector and a vector-angle pair. These tuples describe the current orientation of the ultrasound plane. Transitions between standard planes, e.g. *parasternal long axis* to *parasternal short axis* involve typical movement patterns (here e.g. *clockwise rotation of about 90 degrees*. Figure 3 shows an example trajectory, where the arrows represent the direction and normal vectors respectively.

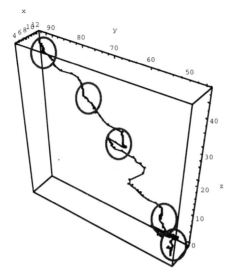

**Figure 4: Tilting of the transducer head in the course of time.
Clusters in the vicinity of standard planes**

2.2 Inference of standard planes by fuzzy rules

Standard positions can be recognized by smaller distances between successive trajectory points (c.f. Fig. 4) and by angle movements near zero. This information is useful for segmentation (start and end of a transition) of a trajectory.

Moreover a fuzzy cluster analysis of the ultrasound plane normal vectors can be used for describing standard positions. The algorithm is a variation of the fuzzy c-means algorithm (see e.g. [9]) using an angle-based distance measure [10]. The resulting cluster prototypes are used to derive fuzzy rules for recognition of standard planes.

Transitions can be checked by rules comparing the angle sums (tilting parallel to the plane, tilting orthogonal to the plane and rotating around the direction axis) with the values of a prototype transition. Moreover fuzzy concepts describing the *straightness* of movements can be formulated. Low straightness or strong shaking may indicate disorientation.

2.3 Fuzzy cluster analysis of Euler angles and hidden Markov models

A fuzzy cluster analysis of the Euler angles between successive time stamps has been used to analyze motion patterns of three different standard trajectories including six standard planes. We have shown that specific movement patterns like, e.g. *"slight rotation counter-clockwise"*, *"strong tilting forward"*, can be identified.

The cluster prototypes serve to determine the number of states and the initial shapes of hidden Markov models (HMMs) [11] describing transitions between standard positions. Using HMMs intended transitions can be detected before they are completed and interruptions of a transition followed indicate possible cognitive orientation demands. Fig. 5 shows a hidden Markov model for the transition *parasternal short axis Aorta* to *parasternal short axis Mitral valve*. The normal movement pattern consists only of tilting forward. But slight deviations like repetitions of part trajectories are tolerated.

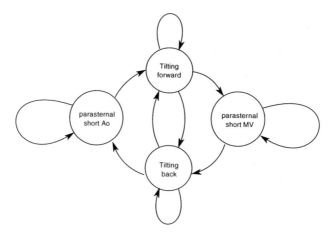

Figure 5: HMM for transition para-short Ao to para-short MV

In addition to models describing normal trajectories, *disorientation models* can be conceived, which describe uncontrolled movements occurring when the learner has lost spatial orientation. Fig. 6 shows a possible disorientation model for *"fanning"*.

These concepts are then used to build rules like the following, which diagnoses possible causes in case of disorientation.

IF *fanning* **AND** *Position (para_s_Ao)*
    THEN *possible misconception (Transition Ao->MV unknown)*

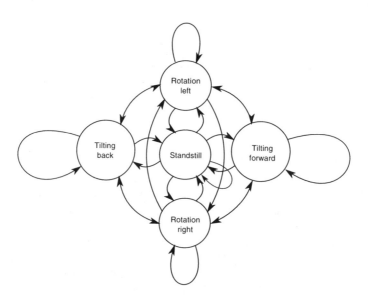

Figure 6: HMM for disorientation

3. Results and further work

Fuzzy rules and hidden Markov models describing standard planes and the transitions between them have been used to analyze sensorimotor behavior. Using the inferred concepts (standard positions, transitions and disorientation), adaptive feedback can be provided. For example, if the matching degree of the recognized standard plane is not sufficient, the following system reactions are possible:

♦ multimedia tutoring modules explaining the standard plane with the characteristic structures

♦ animations showing the difference of the current and the optimal plane

♦ showing the normal trajectory to this position, if there are detected movement errors

4. Conclusions

A medical training system supporting the acquisition of complex integrated medical expertise as it is achieved in clinical practice has to provide situated learning. This is only possible in a realistic learning environment, which can react according to the learner's behavior.

The inferred orientation demands can be used for providing adaptive feedback similar to hints an experienced cardiologist would give, in the sense that the situation "talks back" to the learner.

References

[1]   Berlage, T., T. Fox, G. Grunst, and K.J. Quast. *Supporting Ultrasound Diagnosis Using An Animated 3D Model of the Heart.* in *IEEE Multimedia Systems.* 1996. Hiroshima, Japan.

[2]   Weidenbach, M., C. Wick, S. Pieper, K.J. Quast, T. Fox, G. Grunst, and D.A. Redel, *Augmented Reality Simulator for Training in Two-Dimensional Echocardiography.* Computers in Biomedical Research, 2000. **33**(1): p. 11-22.

[3]   Wick, C., M. Weidenbach, S. Pieper, T. Fox, and T. Berlage. *An Echocardiographic Teleconsultation Environment Using a Virtual Heart Model for Visual Guidance.* in *Medicine Meets Virtual Reality 2000.* 2000: IOS Press.

[4]   Billinghurst, M. and e. al. *The Expert Surgical Assistant: An Intelligent Virtual Environment with Multimodal Input.* in *Medicine Meets Virtual Reality '95.* 1995.

[5]   Voss, G., U. Bockholt, J.L. Los Arcos, W. Müller, P. Oppelt, and J. Stähler. *LAHYSTOTRAIN Intelligent Training System for Laparoscopy and Hysteroscopy.* in *Medicine Meets Virtual Reality 2000.* 2000. Newport Beach, CA: IOS Press.

[6]   Collins, A., J.S. Brown, and S.E. Newman, *Cognitive apprenticeship: Teaching the crafts of reading, writing, and mathematics,* in *Knowing, Learning, and Instruction,* L.B. Resnick, Editor. 1989, Erlbaum: Hillsdale, NJ. p. 453-494.

[7]   Ota, D., B. Loftin, T. Saito, R. Lea, and J. Keller, *Virtual Reality in Surgical Education,* http://www.vetl.uh.edu/surgery/vrse.html. 2000.

[8]   Rosen, J., C. Richards, B. Hannaford, and M. Sinanan. *Hidden Markov Models of Minimally Invasive Surgery.* in *Medicine Meets Virtual Reality 2000.* 2000: IOS Press.

[9]   Bedzek, J.C., *Pattern Recognition with Fuzzy Objective Function Algorithms.* 1981, New York: Plenum Press.

[10]   Klawonn, F. and A. Keller. *Fuzzy clustering based on modified distance measures.* in *IDA'99.* 1999: Springer-Verlag.

[11]   Rabiner, L. and B.-H. Juang, *Fundamentals of Speech Recognition.* 1993, Englewood Cliffs, N.J.: Prentice Hall.

Medicine Meets Virtual Reality 2001
J.D. Westwood et al. (Eds.)
IOS Press, 2001

The development of an evaluation framework for the quantitative assessment of computer-assisted surgery and augmented reality accuracy performance

Warren J Viant

Department of Computer Science, University of Hull, Hull, UK

Abstract. The paper describes a framework for the quantitative assessment of errors within a computer assisted surgical system. The framework diagrammatically describes the registration process and simulates the error propagation chain based on the assumption that errors can be described through the use of a normal distribution model. The projection error associated with a fluoroscopic image intensifier is given as an example.

1 Introduction

Prototype Computer Assisted Surgery (CAS) systems integrated with virtual environment technology are becoming more prevalent within the operating theatre. Cost and performance benefits are well publicised for their use within research hospitals, but not in the wider medical community.

The measurement of performance, especially when linked to patient risk, is sensitive. The primary method for assessing system performance is through a series of cadaveric or clinical trials. The complexity of CAS systems, in particular the real-time and multi-sensor aspects, necessitate a large trial size to achieve reliable performance figures. An objective method to quantitatively assess performance during development and before the commencement of trials would be beneficial.

A typical test procedure for a CAS system, in this case CAOSS developed at the University of Hull [3], proceeds as follows. A series of plastic bone trials are conducted in the laboratory with results qualified with a Co-ordinate Measurement Machine (CMM). Electrical, mechanical, electromagnetic compatible and biocompatible risks are assessed, and steps taken to reduce either their potential severity or occurrence. The plastic bone trials are re-conducted in a theatre environment, where conditions are as realistic as possible. Medical Device Agency (or Federal Drug Administration), Hospital and ethical approval for a series of clinical trials are sought. At this stage the system is considered "safe" except for the remaining question of accuracy of implant placement within the patient's anatomy. As CAOSS is essentially a passive system, where the surgeon maintains complete control, a series of dry trials can then proceed. A dry trial is where the position and orientation of the implant is intra-operatively planned, but not actually implemented.

Pilot trials can then take place on patients. After the valuable feedback from the pilot trials, the series of clinical trials can proceed.

This lengthy test procedure, whilst ensuring patient safety, leaves the assessment of accuracy to near the end of the product's development lifecycle. A requirement therefore exists for an effective method to quantitatively assess CAS performance during the development lifecycle and before the commencement of clinical trials.

The problem is that CAS systems are complex real-time systems that typically integrate: one or more imaging modalities; one or more 3D position tracking systems; one or more physical instruments; and four or more independent coordinate systems. All of these require registration and contribute to system accuracy. One distinguishing feature of a CAS system that makes it rather unique is the limited scope for visual feedback to correct for errors. This is mainly due to the fact that the desired implant position is within an anatomic region that is not visible without the aid of an imaging modality.

The proposal is to develop an evaluation framework to characterise the accuracy within a complex real-time system. The framework diagrammatically describes the registration process and simulates the error propagation chain, based on the principle that errors can be described through the use of a statistical model.

Lea [1] introduces a diagrammatic notation (Lea diagram), for describing registration strategies. The notation uses a graph-theoretic framework to visually describe the registration connectivity between system components. Lea states that although this diagrammatic technique provides a good representation of the registration problem it does not provide any indication of the system accuracy.

2   Method

The evaluation framework [2] takes the main components of the Lea diagram [1], namely the node and the link, representing key features within the registration strategy and expands and augments them with a normal distribution error model supported by a set of computer simulations. The normal distribution error model provides accuracy information for each link within the evaluation framework. This information enables an understanding of the error propagation and resultant accuracy of a CAS system.

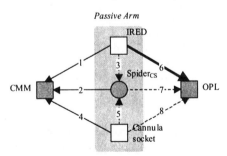

Figure 1. An evaluation framework of a Passive Arm

Figure 1 illustrates an evaluation framework of a Passive Arm, a typical CAS subsystem. The Passive Arm includes three components represented by nodes on the diagram: IRED, an array of infrared diodes; Cannula socket, a tube for the support of a surgical cannula; and a Spider, a local co-ordinate system. Two measurement devices are also represented: Co-ordinate Measurement Machine (CMM), to calibrate the Passive Arm;

and Optical Position Localiser (OPL), to provide real-time tracking of the IRED array on the Passive Arm and hence the position of the surgical cannula.

The aim of the evaluation framework is to quantitatively analyse the performance of a CAS system or sub-system. The system or sub-system is decomposed into a series of patterns, which are represented on an augmented Lea diagram. Each pattern has an associated computer simulation, which predicts component accuracy. An iterative cycle propagates errors across the system or sub-system providing both a total system error and visualisation of error propagation.

2.1 Nodes

The Lea diagram introduced the concept of a node to represent key features within the registration strategy. Nodes that exist on the same physical superstructure are represented in the original Lea diagram as a *motion group,* presented as a rounded box. Nodes within a motion group are constrained to maintain a constant spatial relationship with all other nodes in the group. The evaluation framework extends the node concept to include:

- *Abstract node* (circle): Abstract concept or non-physical features e.g. the surgical plan.
- *Co-ordinate system node* (shaded circle): A refinement of the abstract node, an arbitrary location in space defined by a co-ordinate frame.
- *Physical node* (square): Physical feature involved in the registration strategy e.g. IREDs.
- *Measurement node* (shaded square): A refinement of the physical node representing the class of physical objects that are capable of measurement e.g. CMM or OPL.

2.2 Links

The original Lea diagram introduced links to connect nodes. Lea states "Links represent the act of measurement which establishes a known spatial relationship between the objects represented by the two nodes" [1]. The link does not represent the actual spatial relationship, as two objects may be spatially related even though a link has not established the fact.

To capture the dynamic aspects of registration Lea introduced the concept of an *event* and the *induced link.* When objects move relative to one another, measurements (links) that were previously valid become invalid. An event is used to tag all the links that simultaneously become invalid. The induced link represents a spatial relationship between two nodes that is derived from an indirect connection of links via a common third node. The induced link can only be derived if the indirect connection of links to the third node is tagged with the same event, or all three nodes belong to the same motion group. The induced link is considered persistence and is presented as a dotted line.

The temporal aspects of links can also be represented in the original Lea diagram with the *transient* or *sustained link.* The transient link represents a discrete measurement operation between two nodes, presented as a thin solid line e.g. link between the CMM and cannula socket node. The sustained link represents a continuous measurement operation between two nodes, presented as a thick solid line e.g. link between the OPL and IRED nodes.

It is within the link structures that the distinction between the original and augmented Lea diagrams becomes evident. The augmented Lea diagram makes a stronger distinction between types of link. The types of link are associated to a specific normal distribution simulation. The following list of link types is not exclusive but is extendible, dependant on the nature of the registration strategy being evaluated. Currently the link types include:

- *Measurement*: Represents the process of measuring between two nodes.
- *Transformation*: Represents the process of transforming from one node to a second node.
- *Registration*: Represents the process of registering one co-ordinate system with a second, by means of a common set of reference points, whose position is known in each coordinate system.
- *Reconstruction*: Represents the process of reconstructing a link given other external data. This link is different from the previous three, in that it is both application specific and requires external data.

The original Lea diagram represents the link as a straight line, of varying consistencies, joining two nodes. This representation is maintained along with representation of transient, sustained and induced links. Link properties in the augmented Lea diagram are mapped to rows in an associated table.

Links in the augmented Lea diagram are directional, with an arrow indicating the sense. Traversal of the link in the direction of the arrow is a forward traversal and against the arrow is an inverse traversal.

2.3 Process

The basic registration problem illustrated in Figure 1 contains: a measurement node, the CMM; a physical node, the IRED array; and a co-ordinate system node, the Spider local co-ordinate system. The local co-ordinate system on the Spider is based around a set of physical features, which in this case can be measured by the CMM. Both the IRED array and the Spider co-ordinate system belong to the same motion group, represented by the rounded box, and hence have a fixed spatial relationship. The simulator, using accuracy measurements for the Spider co-ordinate system feature, calculates the error propagation along link 2. A co-ordinate system has one set of normal distribution error models per measurement link connected to the node. Each error model is relative to the node at the other end of the associated measurement link.

The normal distribution error model provides accuracy information for each link within the augmented Lea diagram. This information enables an understanding of the error propagation and resultant accuracy of a CAS system. Once the augmented Lea diagram is completed, the normal distribution error models are generated in a two-stage process. A normal distribution error model is created for each measurement link. The values for the statistical model are derived from manufacture's equipment specifications, through experimentation or through simulation. An iterative error propagation cycle ensures that all remaining induced links are modelled. The sequence of this iteration follows the order of the event tags in the augmented Lea diagram.

Error model connectivity extends the basic connectivity detailed by Lea [1]: Error propagation requires that there exists a connected sub graph for the purpose of fulfilling basic, control and sustained connectivity such that all links contain an error propagation model.

2.4 Framework templates

Similarities exist within the evaluation frameworks for related CAS systems. The proposal is to exploit any similarities with the use of design templates, analogous to class patterns in object oriented software design.

The template approach is based on the premise that an evaluation framework for a CAS system contains a number of recurring patterns within the node and link structure. Identification of these patterns permits a logical decomposition of the problem into a number of sub-problems. Each sub-problem can be mapped directly onto an existing error model template. This process both decreases the time required to develop a framework and reduces the possibility of introducing errors during model creation. The templates detailed in this paper are sufficient to describe the general registration problem and more specific x-ray registration problems. If a sub-problem does not map directly to an existing template, then a new specialised template can be created e.g. x-ray source reconstruction.

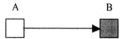

Figure 2. A link between a physical node (A) and a measurement node (B)

In Figure 2, node A is connected to node B via a link directed towards B. This link establishes the spatial relationship between nodes A and B. Mathematically this relationship is defined as:

$$B = RA + t$$

Where R is a 3x3 rotation matrix and t a translation vector defining the transformation between the co-ordinate system local to A and the co-ordinate system inherent to B. Links between a co-ordinate system node and a non co-ordinate system node are directed towards the former. Links between two co-ordinate system nodes are unconstrained.

Templates have been developed for both generic and application specific problems. Each template is associated with one of the basic link types:

- *Measurement*: error propagation template
- *Transformation*: error and co-ordinate system transformation templates
- *Registration*: registration template
- *Reconstruction*: x-ray projection, x-ray source reconstruction, x-ray target reconstruction and other application specific templates.

The templates provide the flow of control for the evaluation framework simulation. The templates are derived from a direct mapping of the nodes and links, following system decomposition. The static and dynamic behaviour of the simulation are determined by a set of states associated with each link and node. Many of these states will be initially undefined. Upon successful completion of the simulation all states should be fully defined.

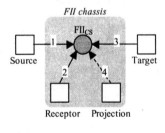
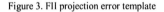

Figure 3. FII projection error template

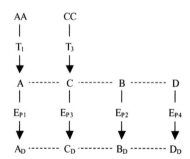

Figure 4 Simulation FII projection error

2.5   FII projection error template

The FII projection error template is given as one example of an application specific template, with attached normal distribution modelling simulation.

The FII projection error template (Figure 3) represents the process by which the projection error during FII image generation can be determined, given the positional accuracy of the x-ray source, receptor and target. The process is represented on the augmented Lea diagram as a reconstruction link (link 4) between the FII co-ordinate system and the projection.

The simulation of the FII projection error template is described in the following algorithm, and illustrated in Figure 4. The FII projection error is given in variable E_{P4}.

AA, perfect geometry of the source in its local co-ordinate system.

T_1, transformation that maps the source's local co-ordinate system onto the FII's co-ordinate system.

E_{P1}, accuracy with which the position of the source is known relative to the FII's co-ordinate system.

A, geometry of AA, transformed error free by T_1 to the FII's co-ordinate system.

A_D, geometry of A when perturbed by positional accuracy E_{P1}.

B, perfect geometry of the receptor plane.

E_{P2}, accuracy with which the position of the receptor is known.

B_D, geometry of B when perturbed by positional accuracy E_{P2}.

CC, perfect geometry of the target in its local co-ordinate system.

T_3, transformation that maps the target's local co-ordinate system onto the FII's co-ordinate system.

E_{P3}, accuracy with which the position of the target is known relative to the FII's co-ordinate system.

C, geometry of CC, transformed error free by T_3 to the FII's co-ordinate system.

C_D, geometry of C when perturbed by positional accuracy E_{P3}.

D, geometry of the intersection of the line A to C with the plane B.

D_D, geometry of the intersection of the line A_D to C_D with the plane B_D.

E_{P4}, accuracy of which the position of projection D is known, obtained through comparison of D and D_D.

3   Validation of the framework

Experimentation has shown that the process of registration is sufficiently complex to require a large sample size for a reliable result to be obtained from the normal distribution error model. Consequently the framework has been validated with a set of small controlled experiments, where the emphasis is placed on large sample sizes rather than complexity.

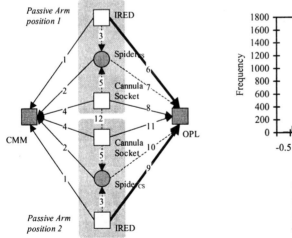

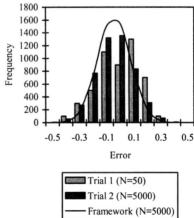

Figure 5. An augmented LEA diagram of a Passive Arm calibration experiment

Figure 6. Results of validation experiment described in Figure 5.

Figure 5 illustrates one of the validation experiments. A passive arm was first calibrated with a CMM. The arm was then moved so as to place a fixed rod in the cannula socket, in such as way as to constrain the movement of the arm to travel along the rod or rotate about the rod. The OPL was used to determine the location of the passive arm in many positions about the rod (i.e. N=5000). The error measurement is represented on the augmented Lea diagrams by link 12. The results from the evaluation framework and experimentation are compiled in Figure 6.

4 Discussion

The evaluation framework provides a valuable tool for the development of CAS systems. In particular:

- Testing of new components within a simulated CAS system, e.g. registration algorithms.
- Examination of error propagation through a CAS system.
- Confidence testing for a completed CAS system.

Although primarily developed for the evaluation of CAS systems, the framework is adaptable to accuracy measurement of any complex multi-sensor system. Any virtual or augmented reality application, were accuracy is a key issue, can utilise the framework.

Quantitative assessment of the two significant types of registration strategy for image-guided surgery, based on a C-arm image intensifier, has been performed using the evaluation framework.

5 References

[1] Lea JT, Santos-Munne JJ, Peshkin MA, Diagramming Registration Connectivity and Structure, MMVR3, San Diego, Jan 1995.

[2] Viant WJ, An evaluation framework to support accuracy analysis of computer assisted surgery systems, SCSC 2000, Vancouver, July 16-21 2000

[3] Viant WJ, Bielby MS, Chawda MN, Phillips R, Mohsen AMMA and Sherman KP, Computer-Assisted Compression Hip Screw Placement, CAOS5, Davos, 17-19 February 2000.

Medicine Meets Virtual Reality 2001
J.D. Westwood et al. (Eds.)
IOS Press, 2001

541

3D registration through pseudo x-ray image generation

Warren J Viant and Frederic Barnel

Department of Computer Science, University of Hull, Hull, UK

Abstract. Registration of a pre operative plan with the intra operative position of the patient is still a largely unsolved problem. Current techniques generally require fiducials, either artificial or anatomic, to achieve the registration solution. Invariably these fiducials require implantation and/or direct digitisation. The technique described in this paper requires no digitisation or implantation of fiducials, but instead relies on the shape and form of the anatomy through a fully automated image comparison process. A pseudo image, generated from a virtual image intensifier's view of a CT dataset, is intra operatively compared with a real x-ray image. The principle is to align the virtual with the real image intensifier. The technique is an extension to the work undertaken by Domergue [1] and based on original ideas by Weese [4].

1 Introduction

The registration of a pre-operative plan with an intra-operative patient is problematic. Within Computer Assisted Surgery a plan can be derived from information extracted from pre-operative datasets. Many registration techniques have been previously investigated including digitisation of anatomical features, fiducial markers and image matching, all aiming to register the patient to the dataset.

The approach detailed in this abstract is an extension to the work undertaken by Domergue [1], based on original ideas by Weese [4].

2 Method

The approach is based on the principle of image comparison. A pseudo x-ray image [2] is generated from a CT dataset absorber, by a virtual image intensifier (II) using ray-tracing techniques. The pseudo x-ray image is intra-operatively compared to a real fluoroscopic II image to determine a similarity measure. The position and orientation of the virtual II is then refined in light of the similarity measure. A registration solution is achieved when the position and orientation of the virtual II is located in a similar position, relative to the patient, as the real fluoroscopic II.

A correlation between techniques used in algebraic cone-beam reconstruction for CT datasets [3] with this registration approach has resulted in a comparative study between a basic ray-tracing technique [1] and a ray-driven splatting technique. The latter has been found to be advantageous in the perspective cone-beam situation. By using an interpolation kernel, added to the ray-driven splatting, artefact generation within the rendered image can be reduced. This research has also investigated the issue of real x-ray image resolution and CT dataset resolution on the accuracy and speed of the final registration solution.

The original work of Domergue [1] used a simulated annealing based global optimisation technique to ensure both a rapid convergence and a near optimal refinement of the virtual II's position and orientation. Within this paper the simulated annealing has been replaced in favour of enhanced simplex global optimisation.

The comparison of a real x-ray image with a pseudo x-ray image can be unreliable. The approach used here increases the robustness and accuracy of the comparison by the inclusion of additional artefacts into the pseudo image i.e. image distortion, image noise, contrast variation and image blurring [1].

Domergue matched pseudo x-ray images with a single real x-ray image to obtain a registration solution. Subsequent experimental evidence has identified errors that can be considerably reduced with an additional real x-ray image. The principle is to take two real x-ray images from orthogonal viewing directions and simultaneously match the pair of real images to pairs of pseudo x-ray images to determine the registration solution.

3 Results

Domergue [1] performed controlled tests on calibrated geometric objects at known positions and orientations, to determine registration accuracy. The further development of the registration strategy to utilise CT-datasets, has enable the replacement of the geometric objects within the tests. A controlled environment is achieved by substituting a high-resolution pseudo x-ray image (with added noise) for the real x-ray image, hereafter referred to as the real x-ray image.

The ray-tracing technique for image generation proved superior to the ray-driven splatting technique in quality of pseudo x-ray image. The ray-driven splatting was significantly faster, but the performance differential diminished when a perspective rather than orthogonal image was generated. The study concluded that a ray-tracing rather than ray-driven splatting technique is currently more compatible with this registration strategy. Work is continuing on improving the ray-driven splatting, as its performance potential is seen as significant.

Down scaling the resolution of the CT dataset and real x-ray image by a factor of two, matched predictions that the performance of image generation would increase twofold and fourfold respectively. Down scaling the resolution of both CT and x-ray image by a factor of two or four did not significantly affect the accuracy of the registration solution.

A precondition of the image comparison function is that the images are of equal size. If the pseudo image is generated at a lower resolution than the real x-ray image, to increase performance, then post processing is required to shrink the real x-ray image to the dimensions of the pseudo x-ray image. The post processing, in this case a mean filter, resulted in the reduction in accuracy of the registration solution. This presents a problem for the optimisation of the registration strategy. Performance increases when the resolution of the CT-dataset or pseudo x-ray image is decreased, but the resultant size discrepancy between the pseudo and real x-ray images causes a corresponding degradation in registration solution accuracy.

The similarity value returned by the image comparison function provided a useful measure of the reliability of the registration solution. Analysis indicated that a primary cause of poor registration accuracy was the initial state of the simplex. With a priori knowledge a registration solution with a large final similarity value was discarded and the simplex reinitialised. This approach reduced the standard deviation of registration solution error.

The expansion of the registration strategy to two rather than one real x-ray image resulted in a significant increase in registration accuracy, particularly in the direction normal to the first x-ray image. The only disadvantage of the use of two x-rays was the increase in radiation exposure to the patient.

The registration algorithm has demonstrated that the registration accuracy previously obtained on a geometric dataset is comparable to that from a CT dataset.

4   Discussion

The advantage of this particular registration strategy over alternative approaches is that it is both non-invasive and non-user intensive. Furthermore, the approach does not require the segmentation of either the CT dataset or x-ray image, thus eliminating a further source of inaccuracy.

The research has identified a number of areas that require further investigation. An increase in the quality of ray-driven splatting images would make viable their inclusion in the registration strategy with the obvious performance improvement. On the basis of the improvement achieved by using two rather than one image, the effect of further increasing the quantity of real x-ray images has to be considered.

5   References

[1] Domergue G, Viant WJ. 3D Registration through Pseudo X-ray Image Generation, MMVR-8, Los Angeles, Jan 2000.

[2] Gouzinis H, Viant WJ. Simulation of the X-ray Image Generation Process, Virtual Reality & 3D Modelling Symposium, ASTC'99, SCS, ISBN 1-56555-167-2, 1999.

[3] Mueller K. Fast and accurate three dimensional reconstruction from cone-beam projection data using algebraic methods, PhD thesis, Ohio State University, 1998.

[4] Weese J, Buzug TM, Lorenz C and Fassnacht C. An approach to 2D/3D registration of a vertebra in 2D X-ray fluoroscopies with 3D CT images, CVRMed-MRCAS'97, Lectures notes in Computer Science, Springer, ISBN 3-540-62734-0, 1997.

544

Medicine Meets Virtual Reality 2001
J.D. Westwood et al. (Eds.)
IOS Press, 2001

A VR-Based Multicomponent Treatment For Panic Disorders With Agoraphobia

F. VINCELLI [1-2], Y.H. CHOI [3], E. MOLINARI [2], B.K. WIEDERHOLD [4], G. RIVA [1-2]

[1]Laboratorio Sperimentale di Psicologia, ATN-P Lab, Istituto Auxologico Italiano, Verbania, Italy
[2]Department of Psychology, Università Cattolica, Milan, Italy
[3]Seoul Paik Hospital, Inje University, Seoul, South Korea
[4]Center for Advanced Multimedia Psychotherapy, CSPP Research and Service Foundation, San Diego, California

Abstract: Agoraphobia consists of a group of fears of public places such as going outside, using public transportation and being in public places, which cause serious interference in daily life.

Many studies demonstrated the effectiveness of a multicomponent cognitive-behavioral treatment strategy for panic disorder with agoraphobia. The traditional protocol involves a mixture of cognitive and behavioral techniques which are intended to help patients identify and modify their dysfunctional anxiety-related thoughts, beliefs and behavior. Emphasis is placed on reversing the maintaining factors identified in the cognitive and behavioral patterns.

We use Virtual Reality (VR) to support Panic Disorder treatment. The preliminary treatment protocol for Panic Disorder and Agoraphobia, named Experiential-Cognitive Therapy (ECT), was developed at the Applied Technology for Neuro-Psychology Lab of Istituto Auxologico Italiano, Verbania, Italy, in cooperation with the Psychology Department of the Catholic University of Milan, Italy. The actual version included the efforts of researchers from the Center for Advanced Multimedia Psychotherapy, California School of Professional Psychology, San Diego (CA), USA, and from the Seoul Paik Hospital, Inje University, Seoul, Korea.

The goal of ECT is to decondition fear reactions, to modify misinterpretational cognition related to panic symptoms and to reduce anxiety symptoms. The characteristics of the approach will be presented through the description of the clinical protocol.

1. Introduction

A review of epidemiological studies suggests that in different geographic, cultural and racial groups approximately 5% of the population will have agoraphobia and 3.5% will have panic disorder at some time in their life [1].

Within the Diagnostic and Statistical Manual of Mental Disorders (DSM-IV) framework, the essential feature of panic disorder (PD) is the occurrence of panic attacks. A panic attack is a sudden onset period of intense fear or discomfort associated with a cluster of physical and cognitive symptoms, which occurs unexpectedly and recurrently, such as pervasive apprehension about panic attacks, persistent worry about future attacks, worry about the perceived physical, social or mental consequences of attacks, or major changes in behavior in response to attacks. The disorder is often associated with circumscribed phobic disorders such as specific phobias, social phobias, and especially with agoraphobia [2,3]. Indeed, avoidance of public places in order to reduce fear or panic becomes the main cause of incapacity in patients, who, in more serious cases, are confined to their homes [4,5].

Evidence collected over the past 20 years has consistently shown the effectiveness of a multicomponent cognitive-behavioral strategy in the treatment of panic disorder with agoraphobia. The treatment package includes exposure to the feared situation, interoceptive exposure, cognitive restructuring, breathing retraining, and applied relaxation. On an average the duration of the protocol is twelve-fifteen sessions. The protocol involves a mixture of cognitive and behavioral techniques which are intended to help patients identify and modify their dysfunctional anxiety-related thoughts, beliefs and behavior. Emphasis is placed on reversing the maintaining factors identified in the cognitive and behavioral patterns [10,11,12,13,14].

2. Traditional versus Virtual Reality Therapy

One of the fundamental parameters in assessing the effectiveness of therapies is the ratio existing between the "cost" of administration of the therapeutic procedure and the resulting "benefits" [15].. By cost it is meant the expenditure not only in terms of money and time, but also in terms of emotional involvement by the person to whom the therapy is directed. The benefits regard the effectiveness of the treatment, i.e., the achievement of the target set, in the shortest time possible. Exposure therapy traditionally is carried out "in imagination" or "*in vivo*". In the first case, the subject is trained to produce the anxiety-provoking stimuli through mental images; in the second case, the subject actually experiences these stimuli in semi-structured situations. Both of these methods present advantages and limitations as regards the cost-benefit ratio. In the first case, the prevalent difficulty is represented by teaching the subject to produce the images that regard experiences associated with anxiety: the majority of failures linked to this therapy are those subjects who present particular difficulties in visualizing scenes of real life. The cost of the application, however, is minimal, because the therapy is administered in the physician's office, thus avoiding situations that might be embarrassing for the patient and safeguarding his privacy. In the second case, the difficulty lies in structuring, in reality, experiences regarding the hierarchically ordered anxiety-provoking stimuli, with the result that the cost in terms of time, money and emotions is high. At the same time, the advantage of contending with real contexts increases the likelihood of effectiveness of the "*in vivo*" procedure [16,17,18].

Using VR software, it is possible to re-create, together with the subject undergoing treatment, a hierarchy of situations corresponding to reality, which he may experience in an authentic way thanks to the involvement of all his sensorimotor channels[27]. The realistic reproduction of virtual environments enables the interacting individual to immerse himself in a dimension of real presence. This makes it possible to limit the costs as compared to traditional procedures of treatment, as pointed out above, and to consolidate the effectiveness of the treatment thanks to the possibility of re-creating a "three-dimensional world" within the walls of the clinical office [18].

Table 1 summarizes the main clinical applications of Virtual Reality, taken from international scientific literature. Through the analysis of these investigations of VRT (Virtual Reality Therapy) some conclusions, which are common to various scientific studies, can be drawn as to the effectiveness of virtual experience.

First of all, individuals subjected to virtual environments have experienced the feeling of being present like real experience even when the virtual environment did not faithfully match the real world situations. This statement was confirmed by the evidence that the reactions and emotions originating from virtual experience were equal to those experienced by subjects involved in real experience. Another rather frequent conclusion in the analyzed studies concerns the fact that the concentration on a task shown by subjects engaged in virtual experience significantly increases if compared to the control groups treated "in vivo". In addition, perception and behaviour connected with real world can be changed thanks to experience into virtual experience. This last datum confirms that it is possible to extend the results obtained by "in vitro" treatments, which make use of VR, to "in vivo" situations too.

3. The Experiential-Cognitive Therapy Protocol

At the beginning the Experiential-Cognitive Therapy (ECT) protocol for Panic Disorder and Agoraphobia was developed at the Applied Technology for Neuro-Psychology Lab of Istituto Auxologico Italiano, Verbania, Italy, in cooperation with the Psychology Department of the Catholic University of Milan, Italy [19]. The actual version included the efforts of researchers from the Center for Advanced Multimedia Psychotherapy, California School of Professional Psychology, San Diego (CA), USA, and from the Seoul Paik Hospital, Inje University, Seoul, Korea [20]. The goal of ECT is to decondition fear reactions, to modify misinterpretational cognition related to panic symptoms and to reduce anxiety symptoms. This is possible in an average of seven sessions of treatment plus an assessment phase and booster sessions, through the integration of Virtual Experience and traditional techniques of CBT. We decided to employ the techniques included in the cognitive-behavioral approach because they showed high levels of efficacy. Through virtual environments we can gradually expose the patient to feared situation: virtual reality consent to re-create in our clinical office a real experiential world. The patient faces the feared stimuli in a context that is nearer to reality than imagination.

Hodges L.F., Bolter J., Mynatt E., Ribarsky W., Van Teylingen R.	1993	Acrophobia
Lamson R.	1994	Acrophobia
Rothbaum B.O., Hodges L.F., Kooper R., Opdyke D., Williford J.S., North M.	1995	Acrophobia
North M.M., North S.M., & Coble J.R.	1995	Agoraphobia
Rothbaum B.O., Hodges L., Watson B.A., Kessler G.D., Opdyke D.	1996	Fear of flying
Strickland D., Mesibov G.B., Hogan K.	1996	Autism
North M.M., North S.M., Coble J.R.	1997	Fear of flying
Hirose M., Kijima R., Shirakawa K., Nihei K.	1997	Autism
North M.M., North S.M., Coble J.R.	1997	Social phobia
Botella, C., Baños, R. M., Perpiña, C., Villa, H., Alcañiz, M., Rey, A.	1998	Claustrophobia
Bullinger A.H., Hoessler A., Mueller-Spahn F.	1998	Claustrophobia
Riva G., Bacchetta M., Baruffi M., Rinaldi S., Molinari E.	1998	Eating disorder
Alcañiz, M., Perpiña, C., Baños, R., Lozano, J.A., Montesa, J., Botella, C., Garcia, A.	1999, 2000	Body image disturbances
Riva G., Bacchetta M., Baruffi M., Rinaldi S., Vincelli F., Molinari E.	1999, 2000	Eating disorder Body image disturbances
Vincelli F., Choi Y.H., Molinari E., Wiederhold B., Riva G.	2000	Panic Disorder Agoraphobia

Table 1: The main clinical applications of Virtual Reality published on peer-reviewed journals

For ECT we developed the Virtual Environments for Panic Disorders - VEPD - virtual reality system. VEPD is a 4-zone virtual environment developed using the Superscape VRT 5.6 toolkit. The four zones reproduce different potentially fearful situations - an elevator, a supermarket, a subway ride, and large square. In each zone the characteristics of the anxiety-related experience are defined by the therapist through a set-up menu. In particular the therapist can define the length of the virtual experience, its end and the number of virtual subjects (from none to a crowd) to be included in the zone.

Zone 1: In this zone, an elevator in which the subject has to enter, the subject becomes acquainted with the appropriate control device, the head mounted display and the recognition of collisions.

Zone 2: this zone show a supermarket in which the patient can go for shopping. The subject can pick up objects and pay for them at the cash-register.

Zone 3: this zone reproduces a subway ride. The subject is located in the train which moves between different stations.

Zone 4: the last zone is a large square in which are located a medieval church, different buildings, and a pub.

Subjects. Subjects will be consecutive patients seeking treatment who met will DSM IV criteria for panic disorders and agoraphobia for a minimum of 6 months as determined by an independent clinician on clinical interview. Individuals will be excluded if they were acutely suicidal, medically ill or pregnant, had abused alcohol or drugs within the last year or had evidence of cardiac conduction disease. Before starting the trial, the nature of the treatment will be explained to the patients and their written informed consent will obtained

3.1   Assessment

Subjects will be assessed by independent assessment clinicians who will not involved in the direct clinical care of any subject. They will be MA-level chartered psychologists or PhD-level chartered psychotherapist. For the clinical interview they will use a semi-structured interview with the aim of identifying relevant DSM IV diagnostic criteria in the subjects. All the subject will be assessed at pre treatment, upon completion of the clinical trial and after a 1-month, 3-month, 6-month, 12-month and 24-month follow-up period. The following psychometric tests will be administered at each assessment point:
1. **BDI-II** - Beck Depression Inventory [21];
2. **STAI** - State-Trait Anxiety Inventory [22];
3. **ACQ** - Agoraphobic Cognitions Questionnaire [23];
4. **FQ** - Fear Questionnaire [24];
During the assessment will be also used:
-   Subjective measurements (self reports, diaries)
-   Subjective Units of Distress (SUDs) during exposure to virtual environments. In particular SUDs will be taken at baseline, after 10 minutes and after 20 minutes.

3.2   Treatment

The first goal of session 1 is to discuss with our patient the etiologic model of Panic Disorder and Agoraphobia and to describe the program of Experiential-Cognitive Therapy. The description is necessary to obtain an active role of the patient in the therapy.

Then we introduce our patient to Virtual Reality through the use of head mounted display and joystick. The innovative principle of ECT is to integrate cognitive and behavioral techniques with the experiential possibilities offered by Virtual Reality. Then the next step of the first session is to structure the Graded Exposure procedure to virtual environments.

The second step is to show the patient the role of avoidance as the main source of agoraphobic and panic behaviors. The therapist underlines the importance of regular exposure to feared situation and structures with his patient a self-exposure schedule. In vivo graded self-exposure as homeworks, initially with the co-therapist (when it is possible), is very important to empower the efficacy of the therapy. This step can be more easily approached by graded exposure to virtual reality and produce important advantages for the patient: reducing the number of sessions, reducing dependency on the therapist and helping to maintain therapeutic achievements.

Before to pursue graded exposure work we teach Breathing Retraining and Relaxation. A consistent percentage of panickers describe hyperventilatory symptoms as being very similar to their panic attack symptoms. This observation had stimulated the idea that hyperventilation may play an important causal role in panic attacks. In this conception panic attacks are viewed as stress-induced respiratory changes that provoke fear because they are perceived as frightful and augment fear elicited by other panic stimuli.

The goal of this step is to teach the patient a technique to control panic symptoms during exposure therapy in Virtual Reality and during self-exposure.

Each session starts with the review of the homeworks, to verify the difficulties that have emerged during self-exposure and to reinforce the patient for the tasks that have been carried out. After the graded exposure procedure, session three is based on Cognitive Restructuring. In panic disorder cognitive treatment focuses upon correcting misappraisals of bodily sensations as threatening. The cognitive strategies reduce attentional vigilance for symptoms of arousal, level of chronic arousal, and anticipation of the recurrence of panic.

Session 1
- Description of the etiologic model according cognitive-behavioral approach
- Programmation of Cognitive-Experiential Treatment
- Introduction to Virtual Environments.
- Graded exposure to virtual environments

Session 2
- Breathing retraining and Relaxation
- Graded exposure to virtual environments
- Introduction and scheduling of in vivo Self-Exposure
- Homework: in vivo Self-Exposure with co-therapist

Session 3
- Homework's Review
- Graded exposure to virtual environments
- Cognitive Restructuring
- Homework: in vivo Self-Exposure with co-therapist

Session 4
- Homework's Review
- Graded exposure to virtual environments using relaxation
- Cognitive Restructuring
- Homework: in vivo Self-Exposure with co-therapist

Session 5
- Homework's Review
- Interoceptive Exposure
- Graded exposure to virtual environments using relaxation
- Homework: in vivo Self-Exposure

Session 6
- Homework's Review
- Cognitive Restructuring
- Graded exposure to virtual environments using relaxation

Session 7
- Homework's Review
- Cognitive Restructuring
- Prevention Relapse
- Booster sessions schedule

Booster sessions
- Follow-up after 1 month, 3 months and 6 months
- Review and Reinforcement of patient's tasks
- Management and Prevention of future relapse

Table 2: The Experiential-Cognitive Therapy Protocol for the treatment of Panic Disorder with Agoraphobia (Vincelli & Riva, 2000)

Cognitive treatment starts by reviewing with the patient a recent panic attack and identifying the main negative thoughts associated with the panic sensations. Once patient and therapist agree that the panic attacks involve an interaction between bodily sensations and negative thoughts about the sensations, a variety of procedures are used to help patients challenge their misinterpretations of the symptoms.

A lot of patients interpret the unexpected nature of their panic attacks as an indication that they are suffering from some physical abnormality. In these cases information and psycho-education about the nature of anxiety can be helpful, especially if it is tailored to patients' idiosyncratic concerns. One of prevalent types of errors in cognitions is *overestimation*. The panickers are inclined to jumping to negative conclusions and treating negative events as probable when in fact they are unlikely to occur. Another type of cognitive error is misinterpreting events as *catastrophic*. Decatastrophizing means to realize that the occurrences are not as "catastrophic" as stated, which is achieved by considering how negative events are managed versus how "bad" they are. This is best done in a socratic style so that clients examine the content of their statements and reach alternatives. The cognitive strategies are conducted in conjunction with behavioral technique of graded exposure in virtual reality. The schedule of session four is the same of session three. The first part is dedicated to graded exposure. The second part is dedicated to the careful inquiry of cognitive distorsions and their modification.

The key feature of session five is Interoceptive Exposure [6,9]. The theoretical basis for interoceptive exposure is one of fear extinction, given the conceptualization of panic attacks as "conditioned" alarm reactions to particular bodily cues. Since according to the cognitive model panic disorder is considered as a *"phobia of internal bodily cues"*, the purpose is to modify associations between specific bodily sensations and panic reactions. This technique can be used also during the exposure to the virtual environments. After the induction of panic-like sensations the patient uses Breathing retraining and Relaxation to control symptoms. After cognitive restructuring, prevention relapse is an important step of the last session. In this session we have to schedule the homeworks of self-exposure, the Booster sessions and to reinforce the patient for the tasks that have been carried out and for the future tasks.

The number of booster sessions can be scheduled according to the results of our patients. In our experience three sessions after 1, 3 and 6 months is an appropriate number for supporting the results of the therapy. The objective of booster sessions is to verify the difficulties that have emerged and to reinforce the patient for the tasks that have been carried out. During this phase it is possible to repeat some steps of the therapeutic techniques to improve or to stabilize the results of treatment [19,20].

4. Conclusion

The feeling of actual presence offered by the realistic reproduction of cybernetic environments and by the involvement of all the sensorimotor channels, enables the subject undergoing treatment to live the virtual experience in a more vivid and realistic manner than he could through his own imagination. VR constitutes a highly flexible tool which makes it possible to programme an enormous variety of procedures of intervention on psychological distress. The possibility of structuring a large amount of controlled stimuli and, at the same time, of monitoring the possible responses generated by the user of the programme offers a considerable increase in the likelihood of therapeutic effectiveness, as compared to traditional procedures. Great care must be however taken when operating since this instrument too is characterized by a number of limits and undesired side effects which must be kept under control. These limits are relevant both to technical factors and to factors connected with the peculiarity of the research within the field of mental health. The former are mainly caused by the costs and by the technological complexity required for setting up virtual environments.

Acknowledgment

The present work was partially supported by the Commission of the European Communities (CEC), specifically by the IST programme through the VEPSY UPDATED (IST-2000-25323) research project (http://www.psicologia.net).

References

[1] H.U. Wittchen & C.A. Essau, The epidemiology of Panic Attacks, Panic Disorder and Agoraphobia, in *Panic Disorder and Agoraphobia*, J.R. Walker, G.R. Norton & C.A. Ross, Eds. Pacific Grove: Brooks/Cole Publishing Company, 1991, pp. 103-149.

[2] APA (1994). *Diagnostic and statistical manual of mental disorders*, 4th edition (DSM-IV). Washington, DC: American Psychiatric Press.

[3] Goisman, R. M., Warshaw, M. G., Peterson, L. G., Rogers, M. P., Cuneo, P, Hunt, M. F., Tomlin-Albanese, J. M., Kazim, A., Gollan, J. K., Epstein-Kaye, T., Reich, J. H., & Keller, M. B. (1994). Panic, agoraphobia, and panic disorder with agoraphobia: Data from a multicenter anxiety disorders study. *Journal of Nervous and Mental Disease, 182(2)*, 72-79.

[4] Barlow, D. H., & Mavissakalian, M. (1981). Directions in the assessment and treatment of phobia: The next decade. In M. Mavissakallan & D. H. Barlow (Eds.), *Phobia:Psychological and pharmacological treatment*. New York: Gullford Press.

[5] Chambless, D. L., & Goldstein, A. J. (1983). *Agoraphobia: Multiple perspectives on theory and treatment*. New York. Wiley.

[6] Barlow, D. H. (1988). *Anxiety and its disorders: Tbe nature and treatment of anxiety and panic*. New York: Guilford Press.

[7] Telch, M. J., Lucas, J. A., & Nelson, P. (1989). Nonclinical panic in college students: An investigation of prevalence and symptomatology. *Journal of Abnormal Psychology, 98, 300-306*.

[8] Barlow, D. H., & Craske, M. G. (1994). *Mastery of your anxiety and panic II*. San Antonio, TX: Harcourt Brace & Co.

[9] Clark, D. M., Salkovskis, P., Gelder, M., Koehler, C., Martin, M., Anastasiades, P., Hackmann, A., Middleton, H., & Jeavons, A. (1988). Tests of a cognitive theory of panic. In I. Hand & H. Wittchen (Eds.), *Panic and phobias II*. Berlin: Springer-Verlag.

[10] R.M. Rapee & D.H. Barlow, The cognitive-behavioral treatment of panic attacks and agoraphobic avoidance, in *Panic Disorder and Agoraphobia*, J.R. Walker, G.R. Norton & C.A. Ross, Eds. Pacific Grove: Brooks/Cole Publishing Company, 1991, pp. 103-149.

[11] Clark, D., Salkovskis, P., & Chalkley, A. (1985). Respiratory control as a treatment for panic attacks. *Journal of Behavior Therapy and Experimental Psychiatry, 16*, 23-30.

[12] Clark, D. M., Salkovskis, P., Hackmann, A., Middleton, H., Anastasiades, P., & Gelder, M. (1994). A comparison of cognitive therapy, applied relaxation, and imipramine in the treatment of panic disorder. *British Journal of Clinical Psychology, 164*, 759-769.

[13] Gitlin, B., Martin, M., Shear, K., Frances, A., Ball, G., & Josephson, S. (1985). Behavior therapy for panic disorder. *Journal of Nervous and Mental Disease, 173*, 742-743.

[14] Shear, M. K., Ball, G., Fitzpatrick, M., Josephson, S., Klosko, J., & Francis, A. (1991). Cognitive-behavioral therapy for panic: An open study. *Journal of Nervous and Mental Disease, 179*, 467-471.

[15] Vincelli F. (1999). From imagination to virtual reality: the future of Clinical Psychology. *CyberPsychology & Behavior. 2; 3; 241-248*.

[16] Rothbaum BO, Hodges L, Kooper R. (1997) Virtual reality exposure therapy. *J Psychother Pract Res;6:219-226*.

[17] Riva G, Galimberti C. (1997) The psychology of cyberspace: a socio-cognitive framework to computer mediated communication. *New Ideas in Psychology*;15:141-158.

[18] Vincelli F., Molinari E., (1998). Virtual reality and imaginative techniques in Clinical Psychology. In Riva G., Wiederhold B.K., Molinari E. (Eds.) *Virtual environments in Clinical Psychology and Neuroscience*. IOS Press Amsterdam.

[19] Vincelli F., Riva G. (2000) Experiential Cognitive Therapy for the treatment of panic disorders with agoraphobia. *MMVR 2000, Medicine Meets Virtual Reality Conference*. January 27-30.

[20] Vincelli F., Choi Y.H., Molinari E., Wiederhold B., Riva G. (2000). Experiential Cognitive Therapy for Treatment of Panic Disorder with Agoraphobia: definition of a clinical protocol. *CyberPsychology & Behavior. 3; 3; 375-385*.

[21] Beck A.T., Ward C.H., Mendelson M., Mock J. & Erbaugh J. (1961) An inventory for measuring depression. *Archives of General Psychiatry, 4, 561-571*.

[22] Spielberger C.D., Gorsuch R.L., Lushene R., Vagg P.R. & Jacobs G.A. (1983) *Manual for the Stait.Trait Anxiety Inventory*. Palo Alto,CA, Consulting Psychology Press.

[23] Chambless D.L., Caputo G.S., BrightP. & GallagherR. (1984) Assessment of fear of fear on agoraphobics. The Bodily Sensation Questionnaire and the Agoraphobic Cognitions Questionnaire. *Journal of Consulting and Clinical Psychology, 52, 1090-1097*.

[24] Marks I.M. & Mathews A.M. (1979) Brief standard self-rating for phobic patients. *Behavior Research and Therapy, 17, 263-267*.

Medicine Meets Virtual Reality 2001
J.D. Westwood et al. (Eds.)
IOS Press, 2001

Virtual Reality as Clinical Tool: Immersion and Three-Dimensionality in the Relationship between Patient and Therapist

Francesco VINCELLI [1-3], Enrico MOLINARI [1-3], Giuseppe RIVA [2-3]

[1] Laboratorio Sperimentale di Psicologia, Istituto Auxologico Italiano, Verbania, Italy

[2] Applied Technology for Neuro-Psychology Lab., Istituto Auxologico Italiano, Verbania, Italy

[3] Department of Psychology, Catholic University, Milan, Italy

Abstract: VR represents the maximum level of evolution in interaction between man and computer systems. In Clinical Psychology, the virtual cyberspace offers a series of powerful and valid applications for diagnosis and therapy.

The qualities that make VR software reliable and particularly useful in the practice of assessment and rehabilitation of certain psychopathological dysfunctions emerge with extreme clarity from the specialist literature. VR constitutes a three-dimensional interface that puts the interacting subject in a condition of active exchange with a world re-created via the computer. The possibility of not limiting the paradigm of interaction in a unidirectional sense represents the strong point of the new technology: man is not simply an external observer of pictures or one who passively experiences the reality created by the computer, but on the contrary may actively modify the three-dimensional world in which he is acting, in a condition of complete sensorial immersion. The nature of this exchange means that the subject feels actually present in this new context. The feeling of "actual presence" is perhaps the peculiar characteristic of this tool and is made possible both by the realistic reproduction of the cybernetic environments and by the involvement of all the sensorimotor channels during interaction.

In this paper we focus on the characteristics of the new configuration in the relationship between patient and therapist.

1. Introduction

Virtual Reality (VR) is usually defined with reference to some technological instruments: computers, head mounted displays and sensors (trackers) for recording the movements of head and limbs. However this definition does not adequately emphasize the usefulness of this tool within a psychosocial context. Beyond common sense, which considers virtual experience a sort of cybernetic game, the scientific community is increasingly giving its agreement on the use of virtual technologies for the simulation of reality in medicine and psychology [1, 2].

"… If you only could see me in those moments, doctor, what I am now telling you would be clearer. I totally lose control, I get the impression that my body has become detached from my mind. That's why it's so difficult to describe what is actually happening to me…" This type of statement is often made by patients during a typical clinical examination. The evaluation of this discomfort and of how it reveals itself is made on the basis of a reconstruction of reality as perceived by the subject requiring the treatment. In the therapist-patient relationship, it is sometimes difficult to clearly outline the mental representation as well as the symptomatology appearing at the time of the discomfort occurrence. But should it be possible, through direct observation, to see how the patient reacts to pathogenic stimuli, we would have a larger amount of useful information available to set up the therapeutic action.

In clinical practice, observation and in-vivo treatment are usually uncommon procedures because of the number of problems they involve. First of all, the cost of the treatment, both in terms of time and money, is rather high. Furthermore, in order to guarantee validity and effectiveness, direct observation must submit to the ecological criterion – it must assure the respect of the environment – so that the observer's presence does not affect the behavioral real sequences. The compliance with this rule makes on-the-spot observation rather complex although still being a useful and sensitive instrument. On the basis of these observations and of the results obtained by experimental methods, we believe that the use of VR in clinical practice can allow to overcome these limits, partially at least, thus reducing the gap between the "in vitro" and the "in vivo" methods of treatment [3, 4].

2. The patient-therapist dialogue

The research aimed at increasing psychotherapy effectiveness is quite active and its priority target is to find the application limits of the different treatments. Specialized literature clearly reports that virtual experience makes it possible to overcome some of these limits with regard to an ever increasing amount of different types of psychopathological disorders.

To better explain the advantages offered by this technology, let us examine, for instance, the so-called "Graded Exposure". One of the essential components of cognitive-behavioural therapies is the exposure of the subject to the stimuli causing his disorder. Virtual reality allows to make this stage of the treatment easier. VR software makes it possible to re-create, together with the subject under treatment, a hierarchy of reality-matching situations, which the subject will experience in a real way thanks to the involvement of all sensory and motor channels. The realistic reproduction of virtual environments enables the interacting individual to immerse himself in a condition of real presence.

Another factor which plays a major role in the psychotherapeutic treatments connected with the different schools of psychology is the elicitation of antagonist responses rather than of maladjusted ones. The development of the ability to induce a condition of psychophysical relaxation is one of the goals aimed at by any psychotherapist anxious to limit the negative effects involved by psychophysiological arousal. In all cases in which dysfunctional thoughts and maladjusted behavior are combined with the manifestation of the disorder through the hyperactivation of the psychophysiological parameters, some training to control one's own psychosomatic responses in a more adaptive way becomes essential.

But the effectiveness of this technique largely depends on the ability shown by the subject for whom the therapy has been designed, to produce the images which are generally suggested by the therapist. The more these images will become vivid and realistic in the subject's fancy the more it will be easy to obtain a relaxation response [5].

The opportunities offered by virtual technology in this field are manifold and quite favorable. The guided administration by the VR therapist of scenes helping to induce a relaxation response has been fairly successful [6, 7]. This is mainly due to the intrinsic effects of the VR instrument. The feeling of being really present as provided by the realistic representation of the cybernetic environments and by the involvement of all sensory and motor channels enables the subject under treatment to live the virtual experience more vividly and realistically than he would do through his own imagination [4].

Virtual Reality is a highly flexible instrument allowing to program manifold ways of managing psychological troubles. The opportunity to structure a large number of controlled stimuli and at the same time to monitor any response aroused by the program user allows to increase the chance of therapeutic success as compared to traditional procedures. The potential offered by this technology mainly comes from the central role played in psychotherapy by imagination and by memory [8]. The limits of these two factors, which are essential in the life of all of us, are either absolute or connected with individual potentials.

Thanks to virtual experience some of these limits can be overcome. Re-created world can sometimes be more vivid and real than the world that a large number of subjects can describe through their own imagination and through their own memory.

This innovative instrument brings about a change in comparison with the traditional relationship between patient and therapist [9]. The new pattern of this relationship is based of the awareness of being more capable to manage in the difficult operation of recovering past experience and of predicting future experience. The therapist who knows and is aware that he can make use of and derive benefit from this effective instrument in his own therapeutic practice feels more efficient and capable to act in a more incisive way on the course of the disorder suffered by his patient [8]. At the same time, the subject under treatment perceives the advantage of being able to re-create and make use of a real experimental world within the walls of his own therapist's surgery.

3. Conclusion

Virtual Reality Assisted Therapy gives therefore a substantial impulse to the development of new opportunities for the prevention and treatment of psychological health. On the other hand, research-connected factors deal with the difficult cooperation between the community of experts concerned with Virtual Reality and the community of experts who establish the official standards for mental health investigations.

Quite often the results achieved by VR are not taken into consideration by experts who carry out their researching activity within some particular nosological environments, since this method of study is not included in the guidelines of traditional research. Although their attitude is rather common in our culture, being consistent with the difficulties shown by each of us in accepting innovations and differences, this limit can be overcome only through the establishment of specific standards to be applied to the guidelines for Virtual Reality research.

Acknowledgment

The present work was supported by the Commission of the European Communities (CEC), specifically by the IST programme through the VEPSY UPDATED (IST-2000-25323) research project (http://www.psicologia.net).

References

[1] F. Vincelli, From imagination to virtual reality: the future of clinical psychology, *CyberPsychology & Behavior*, vol. 2, pp. 241-248, 1999.

[2] G. Riva and L. Gamberini, Virtual Reality in Telemedicine, *Telemedicine Journal*, vol. 6, pp. 325-338, 2000.

[3] C. Botella, C. Perpina, R. M. Banos, and A. Garcia-Palacios, Virtual reality: a new clinical setting lab, *Studies in Health Technology and Informatics*, vol. 58, pp. 73-81, 1998.

[4] F. Vincelli and E. Molinari, Virtual reality and imaginative techniques in clinical psychology, in *Virtual environments in clinical psychology and neuroscience: Methods and techniques in advanced patient-therapist interaction*, G. Riva, B. Wiederhold, and E. Molinari, Eds. Amsterdam: IOS Press, 1998, pp. 67-72.

[5] F. Vincelli, Y. H. Choi, E. Molinari, B. K. Wiederhold, and G. Riva, Experiential cognitive therapy for the treatment of panic disorders with agoraphobia: Definition of a clinical protocol, *CyberPsychology & Behavior*, vol. 3, pp. 375-386, 2000.

[6] G. Riva, M. Bacchetta, M. Baruffi, S. Rinaldi, and E. Molinari, Virtual reality based experiential cognitive treatment of anorexia nervosa, *Journal of Behavioral Therapy and Experimental Psychiatry*, vol. 30, pp. 221-230, 1999.

[7] G. Riva, M. Bacchetta, M. Baruffi, S. Rinaldi, F. Vincelli, and E. Molinari, Virtual reality based Experiential Cognitive Treatment of obesity and binge-eating disorders, *Clinical Psychology and Psychotherapy*, vol. 7, pp. in press, 2000.

[8] F. Vincelli and G. Riva, Virtual reality as a new imaginative tool in psychotherapy, *Studies in Health Technology and Informatics*, vol. 70, pp. 356-358, 2000.

[9] G. Riva, Design of clinically oriented virtual environments: A communicative approach, *CyberPsychology & Behavior*, vol. 3, pp. 351-358, 2000.

Medicine Meets Virtual Reality 2001
J.D. Westwood et al. (Eds.)
IOS Press, 2001

THE VIBE OF THE BURNING AGENTS: SIMULATION AND MODELING OF BURNS AND THEIR TREATMENT USING AGENT-BASED PROGRAMMING, VIRTUAL REALITY, AND HUMAN PATIENT SIMULATION

D.K.J.E. von Lubitz[a], H. Van Dyke Parunak[b], H. Levine[a], K-P. Beier[a], J. Freer[a], Tim Pletcher[a], J. Sauter[b], D. Treloar[a], Eric Wolf[a]; Medical Readiness Trainer (MRT), University of Michigan, Ann Arbor, MI[a] and ERIM, Ann Arbor, MI[b], USA

"SAPERE AUDE"
Horace, Ars Poetica

Animal models in biomedicine

Accordingly to the Concise Oxford Dictionary of English (1982), a model is a "representation in three dimensions of existing or proposed structure, etc. esp. on a smaller scale (working model); simplified description of system etc. to assist calculations and predictions". Webster's New Riverside University Dictionary of English (1988) expands the concept and adds "2. A preliminary pattern serving as the plan from which an item not yet constructed will be produced. 3. A tentative description of a theory or system that accounts for all of its known properties.

Seen in their most restrictive context, none of the definitions fit what is collectively described as "models" of injury. None of the current models work on a smaller scale since pathologies of rat and human appear to be very similar. A cell in the cell culture exposed to anoxic conditions or mechanical damage can hardly be viewed as a "plan" for future construction of the processes involved in, e.g., traumatic brain injury. And, despite the massive accumulation of new data, we are still very far from a "tentative description that accounts for all known properties" of most, if not all, forms of injurious processes that affect living organisms.

The linguistic definitions of a "model" apply only when used in the context of human pathologies that a trauma team confronts following a major car accident. It is also in this context that a debate on the utility of the currently used models of injury is conducted. The best example of this situation are studies of stroke where "validity of rodent brain-ischemia models is self-evident" (14). Yet, while experimental therapies are quite effective, there is practically no demonstrable effect of these studies on clinical outcomes (9, 20). Moreover, the art of modeling pathological processes in the brain did not progress much during the past 10 years. The currently used tools in injury research are still the same and are based on cell and cell culture methods, isolated tissue (e.g., brain or heart slices), and surgical/pharmacological manipulation of animals to produce conditions similar to those observed clinically. It is the range of the analytical tools and techniques that now assist in the discovery, analysis, and understanding of the processes evoked by our modeling efforts that has changed and it is these new analytical methods that helped to discover phenomena whose existence, until quite recently, was entirely unsuspected. Yet, in similarity to with all experimental approaches to human disease, majority of these methods have demonstrable limitations (5, 8,17). Interpretation of the results is also quite difficult, and often involves translation of phenomena characterized by the high spatial and temporal complexity of the constituent events into linear patterns of cause and effect that are inadequate to represent biological interactions. Implementation of computer-based models may assist in circumventing this critical problem.

Computer-based models of normal and pathological cell/tissue interactions

Despite highly promising results of the initial work, computational models and simulation have not yet gained the popularity they deserve (21, 29. Several reasons may explain the reluctance in accepting the blend of very advanced computing, simulation, visualization, and information technologies in the studies of stroke and brain injury. First of all, the level of the required knowledge is seemingly daunting – maximum utilization of the techniques that are becoming rapidly available and approach "off the shelf" level exceeds current technical abilities of many among biomedical investigators. "Communication gap" that still separates the computer and medical scientists prevents meaningful exchange of ideas (3). The underlying mistrust within the biomedical spheres that meaningful simulation-based models of systems as complex as the brain can be ever attained (2) also ads to the reluctance with which computer-based simulation finds acceptance. Finally, the costs of simulation using the most widely accepted object-based approach may be very high, and the equipment needs exceed the capacity of the majority of biomedical research centers (11, 16). Even at the laboratories equipped with the necessary hardware, the practical execution of a simulation session may require very creative approaches in order to provide the necessary materiel support (16)!

The difficulties notwithstanding, substantial results have been already obtained in simulation/modeling of cytotoxic and vascular events in ischemia (19), pathogenic mechanisms in stroke (15), calcium-related physiology (6), blood flow dynamics (28), and spreading depression in focal cerebral ischemia (30). Very importantly, computational models of cognitive deficits following brain damage that are currently developed (7, 22) and will provide a natural extension of the model-based studies of cerebral pathology. The creation of the GENESIS simulator-based database (part of the Human Brain Project; see 2) and several other neural simulation programs (10) indicates that the field of simulation rapidly gains strength as an important research tool.

Contemporary approaches to computer based modeling of cell/tissue interactions

Formal models of complex physiological and metabolic processes are conventionally created using coupled differential equations (1, 4, 12, 13, 18, 23). While this approach is appropriate for monolithic systems, it has serious shortcomings for systems with many interacting components such as brain. In the latter systems, the monolithic models quickly become cumbersome to construct, debug, and maintain. Furthermore, small differences in parameter values in different components of a system (represented by a single "lumped" parameter in a monolithic model) may lead to divergent trajectories of system components due to the nonlinearity of the underlying dynamics.

Current approaches to tissue/organ modeling are based either on the concepts of linear relations and dependencies that result in very inaccurate "toy" models used in high-school education (31). More sophisticated approaches are based on object-based programming suitable for modeling complex systems providing these are adequately described by differential equations. The best example of the latter is the model of Purkinje cell (11). However, in the ultracomplex systems (e.g., brain) in particular, variations within the "assumed constants" (lumped constants) will be particularly pronounced, especially when pathological environments are modeled. As the direct result of the cumulative effect of such progressively increasing deviation from reality the model will perform either inaccurately or even erroneously.

The New Wave: agent-based modeling of injury

Agent-based modeling (ABM) represents a new and powerful alternative to the dilemma of simulation and modeling of complex biomedical events, where each entity in the system is represented by a separate computational process. While experience in implementing both classes of models (object-based vs. agent-based) has led to a deep understanding of the relative strengths and weaknesses of these alternative modeling methods (25, 26), agent-based approaches have never been tested in biomedical applications. Yet, the advent of agent-based modeling may represent the most exciting avenue for simulation and modeling of complex biological systems both under normal and pathological conditions encountered in humans

In agent-based modeling, each agent is represented by its own independent computational element that, apart of its characteristics (code and persistent state), is also endowed with a "will", i.e., the ability to sample the environment and respond to it in an appropriate manner. Moreover, there is no scale to the agent: a receptor subunit may be an agent as much a treating physician. Thus, a very large number of agents can represent a multidimensional system in which spatial and temporal determinants play as important role as the functional characteristics of the involved elements as, for example, in the penumbra zone of a focally injured brain or periphery of a severe burn. Agent based modeling offers the additional advantages of integration with the visual rendition of the physiological processes either in a fully immersive (CAVE) or semi-immersive virtual reality (e.g., ImmersaDesk) systems (31), and of creating interactive environments that are essential for experimentation, testing hypotheses, etc. Thus, agent-based models that operate visual interfaces capable of responding to interactive manipulation represent a substantial leap in the ability of an investigator to observe a very large number of processes taking place within a cell while standing within its virtual cytoplasm, manipulate individual subsystems of that cell (e.g., turn off metabolic pathways, activate receptors or enzymes, control expression of intracellular messengers, etc.), and observe the cumulative effect of these interactions.

VIBE (Virtual Interactive Burn Environment) – the first step

VIBE (Virtual Interactive Burn Environment) represents the first attempt at a practical implementation of agent-based modeling directed at biomedical problems. The goal of VIBE project initiated recently through collaboration of University of Michigan and ERIM is to provide a sophisticated training and research tool assisting in dealing with the complex issues of the treatment of burns (32)

Physiological response to thermal injury (and the potential danger) depends on the extent rather than the intensity of the burn, and the physiological processes involved in burns interact in complex ways. There are four kinds of dynamics involved in burn pathologies (Table 1) and the agent-based model "driving" the Virtual Burn Mode will support all four classes of dynamics.

The distinction between "slow" and "fast" (Table 1) is relative to the time scale of interventions in the ER. Fast dynamics are virtually instantaneous in comparison with ER activities, and agents that participate in them can communicate instantaneously by messages even if they are remote from one another. Slow dynamics evolve concurrently with medical interventions, and agents that participate in them must propagate their influences step-wise over space.

It is straightforward to assign an individual agent to each localized system in Fig. 1. Dynamics in the distributed systems are represented by a one-dimensional (for circulatory and nervous pathways) or two-dimensional (for tissue) structure of agents. Although the current work with distributed dynamics performed at ERIM uses a regular hexagonal grid (27), in the burn model, it may prove advantageous to use an irregular tiling of the patient based on the polygonization underlying the visual display. Thus, while the burned patient is presented visually in three dimensions, the major dynamics occur within the dermis, a two-dimensional covering over the body. Thus the initial phase of the functional model will consist of a two-dimensional structure

Table 1: Four classes of dynamics in burn pathologies. The systems listed are examples, not an exhaustive list.

	Localized	Distributed
Slow	Kidney Heart	Skin Circulatory system
Fast	Brain	Nervous system

representing the dermis, and supporting pathological processes involving first and second degree burns. A subsequent phase will implement a parallel two-dimensional structure representing processes in the subdermal tissues, coupled to the dermal layer, thus accounting for dynamics into the third dimension

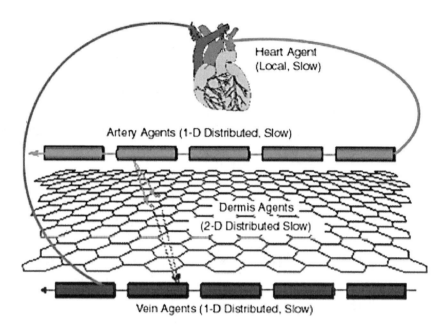

Figure 1. Interactions of various agent dynamics. VIBE combines localized and distributed agents, with both slow and fast dynamics.

The coupling between local and global dynamics occurs is by means of anatomical pathways (e.g., nerve bundles, veins and arteries) that join global agents with selected local agents, corresponding to the anatomical distribution of these features. For example, Figure 1 shows a partial schematic of agent interactions to account for the diffusion of fluid that eventually leads to tissue edema. Each agent (polygon) in the model of dermis aggregates the interactions of capillaries, cells, and inter-cellular spaces within its region, and takes on the average pressure at its center. Several approaches are available to model the interactions within an agent, including rule-based programming, Petri nets, neural nets, and systems dynamics models.

Modeling fluid diffusion between polygons using methods is inspired by finite-element analysis. Thus, each polygon exchanges with its neighbors proportional to their shared boundaries, the pressure differential between them, and the distance between their centers of gravity. Veins and arteries interact directly with the polygons through which they run, and generate pressure differentials that drive the diffusion between intermediate tissues.

Nerve pathways are similarly adjacent to selected polygons. However, they differ in two ways from the circulatory pathways. First, they constitute a one-way path to the brain; the return path is mediated via the circulatory system. Second, because nerves are "fast," propagation along a nerve is not modeled although the distributed nature of the nerves is. Thus, injury mediated signal interruption, e.g., if the nerve is cut, can be represented. However, as long the pathway is intact, propagation of the signal from an offended site to the brain is considered to be instantaneous.

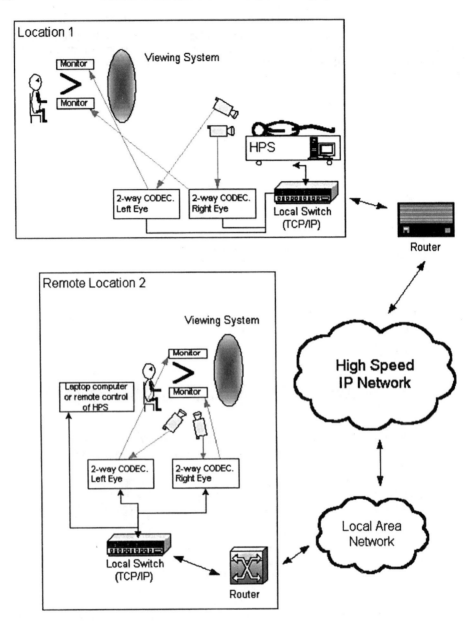

Figure 2. Schematic diagram of Advanced Distributing Learning system capable of providing training at ultra-long distances. CAVE, ImmersaDesk, Ethereal Technologies, Inc. "MIRROR", and other devices can be used the interactive components of the viewing/training environments.

The resulting model includes three classes of techniques indicated in Figure 1 that schematically depicts an agent-based model. Interactions among distributed slow agents, whether one-dimensional (circulatory system) or two-dimensional (dermis) will draw on techniques from finite element modeling. The internal dynamics of individual agents will draw on a tool kit that includes system dynamics models.

The fact that agent-based models are computer-based permits their eventual placement in the "e-world", as public-owned Web based tools available to any investigator anywhere on the globe. Thus, providing appropriate standards are developed (as, for example an extension of the already existing KQML or FIPA), the existing models can be continuously enriched with the latest discoveries, and the accuracy of their performance can be continuously monitored and tested. and their practical use as rapid hypothesis-testing tools will increase the speed of research. Moreover, the inherent plasticity of agent based modeling allows fusion of models with training simulation either in virtual reality alone or using Human Patient Simulators integrated with virtual environments. Basic concepts of distributed training using Human Patient Simulators remotely operated from the distance of 3000 miles have been recently explored (Fig. 2, see ref.32).

Dimidium facti cui coepit habet: sapere aude

The complexities of the suggested simulation and modeling effort cannot be underestimated. Neither can be its scientific and, ultimately, economic importance. Major injury, such as burns, brain or open trauma, etc. are still the leading causes of morbidity and mortality and is associated with an enormous economic burden. The "economy of injury" is encumbered even further by the rapidly raising costs of new drug development that combines with the increasing restrictions on the experimental use of animals already felt in Europe and soon to arrive in the USA as well. The cumulative impact of the last two factors may have catastrophic repercussions on the effective development of new drugs, and advanced simulation and modeling will become the only viable alternatives. The urgency of rapid introduction of simulation and modeling tools into routine medical practice is also stressed by the need to maintain adequate readiness of medical personnel. It is a particularly daunting task in the context of rural and remote regions and where advanced computer-based simulation tools appear to provide a realistic solution to the dilemma of dwindling skills, limited access to training, and their most dangerous consequence: the less-than-adequate treatment of major injury (Fig.2, see also ref.32).

References

1. Bauer RD, Busse R, 1978, The Arterial System: Dynamics, Control Theory & Regulation. Springer-Verlag (Berlin)
2. Beeman D, Bower JM, De Schutter E, Efthimiadis E,N, Goddard N, Leigh N, 1997, The GENESIS simu based neuronal database. In Neuroinformatics: An Overview od the Human Brain Project, Koslow SH, Huerta MF (Eds.), Lawrence Erlbaum Associates (Mahwah, NJ), 57 – 81
3. Bower JM, Koch C, 1992, Experimentalists and modelers: can we just get along? Trends Neurosci. 15, 458 – 461
4. Cardiovascular System Dynamics Society. 2000, Cardiovascular System Dynamics Society Home page., vol. 2000, 2000. Http://www.hopkinscme.org/CSDS/main.html.
5. Choi DW, 1990, Limitations of in vitro ischemia. Prog. Clin. Biol. Res. 361, 291 – 9
6. Coomber C, 1998, Current theories of neuronal information processing. Comput. Chem. 22, 251 – 63
7. Christiansen C, Abreu B, Ottenbacher K, Huffman K, Masel B, Culpepper R, 1998, Task performance in virtual environments used for cognitive rehabilitation after traumatic brain injury. Arch. Phys. Med. Rehabil. 79, 888 – 92
8. De Graba TJ, Pettigrew LC, 2000, Why do neuroprotective drugs work in animals but not humans. Neurol. Clin. 18, 475 – 493

9. De Keyser J, Sulter G, Luiten PG, 1999, Clinical trials with neuroprotective drugs in acute ischemic stroke: are we doing the right thing. Trends Neurosci. 22, 535 – 40

10. De Schutter E, 1993, Neural Simulation Software Demonstration.
    http://www.bbf.uia.ac.be/publications/pub014/TNB_pub14_abst.shtml

11. Eichler West RM, De Schutter E, Wilcox GL, 1999, Using evolutionary algorithms to search for control parameters in nonlinear partial differential equation.
    http://science-rainessance.org/rogene/Papers/IMA/IMA_chapter.html

12. Fell DA, 1997, Systems Properties of Metabolic Networks. In Proceedings of International Conference on Complex Systems (Perseus), 163-178

13. Ghista DN, Patil MK, Oliver C, Woo DM. 1971, Development in Vivo Simulation and Medical Utility of a Control System Model for the Mechanics of the Human Left Ventricle. In Proceedings of Summer Computer Simulation Conf., Simulation Councils, Inc.

14. Ginsberg MD, 1996, The validity of rodent brain-ischemia models is self-evident. Arch. Neurol. 54, 350

15. Goodall S, Reggia JA, Chen Y, Ruppin E, Whitney C, 1997, A computational model of acute focal lesions, Stroke 28, 101 – 9

16. Howell FW, Dhyrfjeld-Johnsen J, Maex B, Goddard N, De Schutter E, 1999, A large scale model of the cerebellar cortex using PGENESIS, Elsevier preprint, in press

17. Hunter AJ, Green AR, Cross AJ, 1995, Animal models of acute ischemic stroke: can they predict clinically successful neuroprotective drugs? Trends Pharmacol. Sci. 16, 123 – 8

18. Hyndman BW. 1987, The Eighth International Conference of the Cardiovascular System Dynamics Society: A Special Issue of the Journal Automedica. (Gordon & Breach)

19. Kocher M, Treuer H, Voges J, Hoevels M, Sturm V Muller RP, 2000, Computer simulation of cytotoxic and vascular effects of radiosurgery in solid and necrotic brain. Radiother. Oncol 54, 149 – 5

20. Lanier WL, 1999, The prevention and treatment of cerebral ischemia. Can J. Anesth. 46(5 Pt2):R46 – 56

21. Lansner A, Liljenstrom H, 1994, Computer models of the brain – how far can they take us. J. Theor. Biol. 171, 61 – 73

22. Mayall K, 1998, Methodology and validity in the construction of computational models of cognitive deficits following brain damage. Artif. Intell. Med. 13, 13 – 35

23. Mojtahedzadeh MT, Kazemeynee M, Azizkhan H, 1992, Renal Stone Model. In Proceedings of Proceedings of the 1992 International System dynamics. Conference of the System Dynamics Society, The System Dynamics Society, 445 – 454

24. MRT, 2000, Immersive virtual reality platform for medical education: introduction to Medical Readiness Trainer. In, Medicine Meets Virtual Reality 2000: Envisioning Healing: Interactive Technology and the Patient Practitioner Dialogue, IOS Press (Amsterdam), 207 – 213

25. Parunak HVD, Savit R, Riolo RL, 1998 Agent-Based Modeling vs. Equation-Based Modeling: A Case Study and Users' Guide. In Proceedings of Workshop on Multi-agent systems and Agent-based Simulation (MABS'98), Springer, 1998, 10 –25

26. Parunak, HVD, 1998, The DASCh Experience: How to Model a Supply Chain. In Proceedings of Second International Conference on Complex Systems

27. Parunak HVD, Brueckner S, Sauter J, Matthews R, 2000, Distinguishing Environmental and Agent Dynamics: A Case Study in Abstraction and Alternative Modeling Technologies. In Proceedings of Engineering Societies in the Agents' World (ESAW'00), 2000.

28. Piechnik, S, Czosnyka M, Smielewski P, Pickard JD, 1998, Indices for decreased bloood flow control – a modeling study. Acta Neurochir. Suppl. 71, 269 -71

29. Reggia JA, Ruppin E, Brandt RS, 1997, Computer modeling: a new approach to the investigation of disease. MD Comput. 14, 160

30. Revett K, Ruppin E, Goodall S, reggia JA, 1998, Spreading depression in focal ischemia: a computational study. J. Cereb. Blood Flow Metab. 18, 998 – 1007

31. Van der Valk J, Dewhurst D, Hughes I, et al., 1999, Alternatives to the use of animals in higher education. ATLA, 27:39 – 52, 1999.

32. von Lubitz, D.K.J.E., Beier, K.-P., Freer, J., Levine, H., Van Dyke Parunak, H., Sauter, J., Treloar, D., Wolf, E., 2001, IMERSME in VIBES, Proceedings ITEC 2001, Lille, in press

Medicine Meets Virtual Reality 2001
J.D. Westwood et al. (Eds.)
IOS Press, 2001

ICAPS
An Integrative Computer-Assisted Planning System for Pedicle Screw Insertion

Gerrit VOSS, Dipl.-Inform., Alex BISLER, Dipl.-Inform., Uli BOCKHOLT, Dipl.-Math.,
Wolfgang K. MÜLLER-WITTIG, Albert SCHÄFFER MD
Fraunhofer-Institut für Graphische Datenverarbeitung (Fraunhofer-IGD)
Department Visualization & Virtual Reality
Rundeturmstraße 6, D-64283 Darmstadt, Germany
Phone: +49-6151-155277, Fax: +49-6151-155196
E-mail: {vossg\bisler\bockholt\muellerw}@igd.fhg.de
URL: http://www.igd.fhg.de/www/igd-a4

Robot Assisted Surgery (RAS) Systems win more and more recognition in the field of orthopaedics. Especially in Hip Surgery RAS has proved to be suited for application in medical routine. Often Robot Assisted Surgery Systems consist of a planning- and an interoperative component. According to specifications done with the planning software the tools are driven. Benefits of the robot assisted surgery should be higher precision and a better surgical outcome. In the co-operation project of several Fraunhofer Institutes "RoMed" (Robots and Manipulators for Medical Application) an exemplary application of robot aided spine surgery is developed [1]. The planning software used in this context is proposed in this article.

1. Tools & Methods

Based on experiences with the planing system for computer assisted Total Knee Replacement [2] the Fraunhofer–IGD is developing the ICAPS system, where the surgeon should be supported in preparation of pedicle screw insertion. The basic module provides a graphical user interface where based on patient's tomography scans the appropriate position and size of the pedicle screw can be defined (c.f. Figure 1). This planning process starts with loading and checking of the tomography scans. The surgeon navigates through three orthogonal views of the tomography data and marks the pedicle. The next step is to define the insertion direction of the screw in the sagittal and frontal quadrant. The transversal plane is adjusted to this direction. Now the correct diameter and length can be measured in the transversal quadrant and the appropriate implant can be loaded from the implant database. The surgeon is able to validate his planning results using the virtual x-ray option, where the tomography data including the implants is accumulated along virtual x-rays.

This basis module of the ICAPS system can be enhanced by a biomechanic extension, where Finite Element Methods are applied to foster a better insight into the patient specific case. To achieve this, the three dimensional representations of the vertebrae and the intervertebral disks have to be discretized with numerical grids. To define the boundary conditions of the FEM simulation a biomechanical model is established taking patient specific parameters like height, weight and abdomen perimeter into account[2]. Afterwards commercial FEM software packages are applied for the solution of the calculations.

To offer the surgeon a tailored visualization of the simulation a hybrid rendering system is developed based on the volume slicing technique[3]. This system overlays the patients tomography data with the reconstructed surface models and the simulation results (c.f. Figure 2). This gives the surgeon the possibility to analyse and to verify the Finite Element simulation.

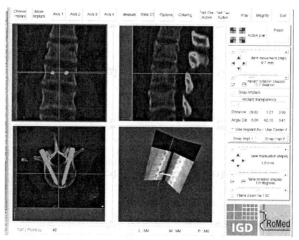

Figure 1: Graphical User Interface of the ICAPS Planning System

2. Results

Using the basic module of ICAPS the surgeon is able to precisely specify the intervention by selecting the appropriate implant components and the optimal placement of the implants within the patient specific data set. The system produces the preoperative plan to be used by the surgical robot system.

The FEM component offers interesting possibilities for additional support, but it is still in the development phase. Particular an evaluation method verifying the simulation results has to be established.

3. Conclusions

This planning system for computer-assisted pedicle screw insertion demonstrates that based on patient specific image data and a catalogue of implants the use of highly interactive 3-D visualization techniques is well suited to enhance accuracy of transpedicular screw placement.

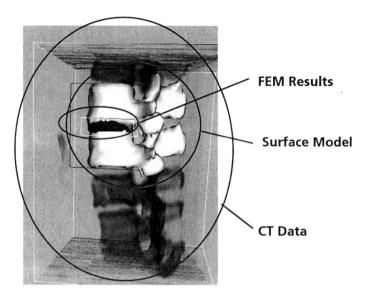

FEM Results

Surface Model

CT Data

Figure 2: Hybrid Rendering System

Acknowledgements

We thank Prof. Dr. h.c. Dr.-Ing. José L. Encarnação for providing the environment in which this work was possible. We also thank all our colleagues and students at our laboratory, especially Berit Klahsen, Mario Becker, and Siegfried Bauer, without their work we would not have been able to achieve the results presented herein.

References

[1]   Müller W. http://www.igd.fhg.de/igd-a4/projects/medicine/RoMed.html
[2]   Müller W., Bockholt U., Voss, G., Lahmer A., Börner M., Planning System for Computer Assisted Total Knee Replacement, Proceedings of Medicine Meets Virtual Reality, pp. 214-219, Imperial Beach CA, 2000
[3]   Ghista, D.N., Subbaraj, S., Mazumdar, J., Rezaian, S.M.: The Biomechanics of Back Pain, in: IEEE Engineering in Medicine and Biology Volume 5 Issue 6, pp. 36-41, 1998
[4]   Robert Grzeszczuk R, Henn C, Yagel R, *Advanced Geometric Techniques for Ray Casting Volumes*, SIGGRAPH 1998

564

Medicine Meets Virtual Reality 2001
J.D. Westwood et al. (Eds.)
IOS Press, 2001

Psychometric Properties of the *driVR*™: A Virtual Reality Driving Assessment

Jaye Wald[1] and Lili Liu[2]

Ph.D. Cand., Department of Educational and Counseling Psychology, and Special Education, University of British Columbia, Vancouver, B.C., Canada, jwald@interchange.ubc.ca[1]
Associate Professor, Department of Occupational Therapy, University of Alberta, Edmonton, Alberta, Canada, lili.liu@ualberta.ca[2]

Abstract. This study provides data on the psychometric properties of the *driVR*™, a virtual reality assessment used to assess driving in persons with brain injury. Several *driVR*™ measures were compared to other established indicators of driving performance. Many concurrent validity coefficients over r = 0.3 were identified between *driVR*™ measures of lane tracking with on-road, Trail Making Test, and the Driver Performance Test II scores. The results provide further evidence to support the concurrent validity of the *driVR*™. Continued research addressing other aspects of validity and reliability is recommended.

1. Introduction

The residual effects of brain injury can interfere with the ability to safely drive an automobile. As a result, health care and rehabilitation specialists are often required to make decisions about the driving fitness of individuals who have sustained a brain injury. These decisions are often based on results from a combination of measures that assess physical, visual, neuropsychological, and behavioral functioning, as well as their integration via road and simulator testing. However, many measures designed to assess driving competency have limited validity and reliability data.

One virtual reality driving simulator, the *driVR™*, has undergone considerable empirical research. A normative study [1] included 148 non-head injured participants across eight age categories. A discriminative validity study [1] identified *driVR*™ variables that could distinguish between virtual driving performance in brain-injured and uninjured persons. The *driVR*™ can detect age-related changes in virtual driving performance, and appears suitable for the older adult population [2]. A pilot study found initial evidence to support the *driVR*™'s concurrent validity [3].

2. Purpose

Our objective was to provide further data on the psychometric properties of the *driVR*™, with a larger sample of persons with brain injury by obtaining concurrent validity coefficients between *driVR*™ scores with on road, visual-attention/perceptual, and driving video test results.

3. Method

Sample. The sample (n = 35) was drawn from a database of clients who received a driving evaluation at Community Therapists Inc., Vancouver, British Columbia. The selection criteria for the sample included completion of the *driVR™* assessment, and to control for age effects, those over 60 years of age were excluded. The sample's mean age was 37.8 years (SD = 11.4) and ranged from 20 to 59 years old. Driving experience of this sample ranged from zero to 41 years, with a mean of 18.1 years (SD = 12.4). Twenty-five held a valid driver's license. The mean year of brain injury was 1994 and ranged from 1964 to 1999.

The Driving Evaluation. The evaluation consisted of a standardized assessment administered by an occupational therapist. Visual attention/perceptual tests included the Trail Making Test (Part A and B) and the Baylor Adult Visual Perceptual Test. Driving video tests consisted of the Driver Performance Test II and Driver Risk Index II, which respectively examined, driver knowledge and risk taking behavior. The road test was conducted by a certified driving instructor from Young Drivers of Canada, accompanied by the occupational therapist. Road testing included two standardized routes that involved residential and business areas of Vancouver. Scores were based on the standards of the Motor Vehicle Branch of British Columbia, which included Number of Demerits and Number of Fails for test routes one and two.

The driVR™. The *driVR™* simulator was developed by Imago Systems Inc. [4]. The system consists of a Pentium computer with 3D graphics software, which handles the interfacing with controls, image generation, and data management of test results. Driver controls include a steering wheel, gas, and brake pedals. The head mounted display and head tracker unit provides visual and auditory input. The *driVR™* route includes a practice route and standardized test routes. The test course consists of a series of sequential scenarios, which are described in [1]. For this study, as described in Table 1, selection of scenarios included those which were found to be statistically significant, or approached statistical significance, in discriminating brain injured from non-brain injured individuals [1].

Table 1. Description of *driVR™* Scenarios and Scores.

Scenario	Description	Score
Follow Traffic Event	Following a pace car; lane tracking measure	distance from pace car, # times crossing center and shoulder lines
Shop Road	Driving by parked cars on side of road; lane tracking measure	distance from center line, # times crossing center and shoulder lines
Opposite Road	Driving with oncoming vehicles; lane tracking measure	distance from center line, # times crossing center and shoulder lines
Driveway Choice Event	Parking in a driveway	pass/fail
Avoid Traffic Event	Avoiding a car backing up	pass/fail
Stop Signs Missed	Stopping at stop signs	# of incomplete stops

4. Results

Table 2 presents the concurrent validity coefficients (r = 0.3 and greater) between *driVR™* measures of lane tracking (Follow Traffic Event, Shop Road, and Opposite Road) with on-road, driver video, and visual attention/perceptual tests. Correlations between the other *driVR™* variables and other driving measures were consistently below r = 0.3.

Table 2. Concurrent Validity Coefficients Between Lane Tracking *driVR™* Measures with On-Road, Driver Video, and Visual Attention/Perceptual Tests.

	Follow Traffic			Shop Road			Opposite Road		
	Distance from lead car	# times cross center line	# times cross shoulder line	Distance from center line	# times cross center line	# times cross shoulder line	Distance from center line	# times cross center line	# times cross shoulder line
Road Test 1									
# Demerits	.3	.7	.8	.3	.6	.5	.3	.7	.6
# Fails		.5	.4	.3	.3	.3	.4	.5	.9
Road Test 2									
# Demerits							.3	.3	.3
# Fails		.3		.3		.6	.3	.3	.6
Driver Performance		-.5	-.3		-.4	-.3	-.3	-.5	-.5
Driver Risk	.3								
Trails Part A		.4	.5	.4	.5		.6	.4	.7
Part B			.4	.4	.5	.5		.3	.6
Baylor	-.3							-.6	-.5

5. Conclusions

Results of this study further support the concurrent validity of the *driVR™*, particularly lane tracking measures with road test, Trail Making Test, and Driver Performance Test scores. These moderate to strong correlations suggest that they could be measuring similar driving skills, such as visual attention and visual processing speed. Lower correlations between some measures (e.g., Driver Risk Index and *driVR™* lane tracking measures) indicate that these tests may be measuring different abilities or constructs. Limitations of this study included uncontrolled mediating or moderating variables (e.g., age-related effects, driving experience), unknown reliability and validity of the on-road test, and restricted range for some variables. Future research with larger samples should replicate these findings and continue addressing other aspects of the *driVR™*'s validity and reliability.

6. Acknowledgments

The Insurance Corporation of British Columbia provided funding for this research project.

References

[1] L. Liu,, M. Miyazaki, & B. Watson, Norms and validity of the "DriVR" - a virtual reality driving assessment for persons with head injury, Cyberpsychology and Behavior 2 (1999) 53-67.
[2] L. Liu, B., Watson, & M. Miyazaki, VR for the elderly: Quantitative and qualitative differences in performance with a driving simulator, *Cyberpsychology and Behavior 2* (1999) 567-576.
[3] J. Wald, L., Liu, & S. Reil, Concurrent validity of a virtual reality driving assessment for persons with brain injury, Cyberpsychology and Behavior 3 (2000), 643-654.
[4] Imago Systems Inc., *driVR user guide.* Author, Vancouver, 1996.

Medicine Meets Virtual Reality 2001
J.D. Westwood et al. (Eds.)
IOS Press, 2001

A Prototype Haptic Suturing Simulator

Roger W. Webster PhD[1], Dean I. Zimmerman[1], Betty J. Mohler[1],
Michael G. Melkonian MD[2] Randy S. Haluck MD[2]

[1]*Department of Computer Science, School of Science and Mathematics*
Millersville University of Pennsylvania, Millersville, PA 17551
[2]*Department of Surgery, Penn State College of Medicine*
The Pennsylvania State University, MC H070, PO Box 850, Hershey, PA 17033

Abstract. A new haptic simulation designed to teach basic suturing for simple wound closure is described. Needle holders are attached to the haptic device as the graphics of the needle holders, needle, sutures and virtual skin are displayed and updated in real time. The simulator incorporates several interesting components such as real-time modeling of deformable skin, tissue and suture material and real-time recording of state of activity during the task using a finite state model.

1. Background/Problem

Simple wound closure by suturing is a fundamental procedure utilized by a number of types of healthcare providers worldwide. Poor techniques can result in sub-optimal outcomes in terms of healing, infection, and cosmetics. Using a haptic suturing simulator, students can practice the virtual procedure at any time to potentially improve their technique.

Researchers and developers have attempted to solve the problems that arise in the development of a generalized anatomical force feedback surgical simulator, however, a complete system is still unavailable [1-4]. By limiting their training application, i.e. bronchoscopy and lumbar puncture, developers have produced a few commercial haptic surgical simulators that are currently available [5,6]. Our intent was to develop a haptic suturing simulator, limited to suturing, that is realistic, simple to operate, economical (runs on a single personal computer), and available for widespread use.

2. Methods & Tools

The development computer is a Windows™ NT workstation with dual 600 mHz pentium processors and the Wildcat™ Open GL graphics accelerator. The Sensable Technologies Phantom™ 1.5 Desktop unit serves as the haptic interface which provides force feedback. A 'Reachin Display'™ unit is used to provide the user with visuo-motor alignment and association. Crystal Eyes™ are used to provide three dimensional stereographic images.

The three dimensional (3D) models of the virtual needle and needle holders were built in 3D Studio Max and stored as 3ds files. The haptics software modules make calls to the General Haptic Software Toolkit (GHOST) development kit from Sensable Technologies. The graphics modules make calls to EAI/Sense8's WorldToolkit API of OpenGL calls.

The skin or soft tissue is modeled as a mesh of mass-springs (dynamic vertices) with a wound texture map wrapped onto the geometry. The system is a physically based particle model utilizing a mass-springs-damper connectivity with an implicit predictor to speed up calculations during each time step. This consists of a set of point masses (nodes) connected to each other with a network of springs and dampers. Internal and external forces act upon the springs. Each vertex in the skin geometry has a mass and is connected to every other vertex with springs and dampers.

Solving mass-springs systems involves repeated application of Newton's first law of motion, $F = ma$. An implicit solver for numerically solving the first order differential equations was developed similar to a technique described by Baraff and Witkin [7] in modeling cloth animation systems. The fundamental problem with implicit solvers is that they need to solve a linear system at each time-step, which is not practical with today's computers. To circumvent this computational expense, an approximate solver based upon the work of Desbrun et. al. [8] that pre-computes the solution to a linear system was incorporated. There are four basic forces (gravity, collision, spring forces and damping) which are manipulated within this system. The gravitational forces accelerate all masses in the y-axis at 10.0 m/s/s. The perfectly elastic collision forces transfer all momentum back to the colliding mass points, for example, prodding the skin with the needle. The springs, which are stretched or compressed away from their initial resting length, are subject to the conventional Hooke's Law restoring force ($F = -kx$). To prevent numerical instabilities due to the approximations, a damping coefficient in which moving masses experience a nominal force opposite to the direction of their movement was calculated.

3. Results

The simulation software calculates contact forces and generates tissue displacements. The resistant force calculations vary depending upon the depth of insertion and the insertion angle of the curved needle. The forces also change when the needle punctures the virtual skin. As the user 'sutures', the software pulls the stitches together utilizing the mass-springs deformation. The user is constrained (force effect) when the needle has penetrated the skin but the forces ease off if the user pulls the needle out in the same path as it was inserted. The user is constrained from sliding the needle along the plane once it has penetrated the skin. The user can, of course, continue penetration of the needle into the soft tissue. Forces are exerted if the user deviates from the natural penetration of the projected needle path and when pulling on the suture or drawing the suture tight (Figure 1).

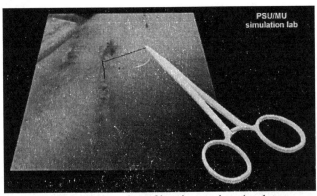

Figure 1: Screen shot of haptic suturing simulator

The software records the positions and orientation of the Phantom encoders and all 3D graphics objects (needle, sutures, needle driver). Therefore, the 3D suturing technique may be replayed showing the user what they did during the training session. Rosen et al [9] developed a model of surgical maneuver states and their transitions which included idle, grasping the needle with the needle driver, puncturing the skin, pushing the needle through the skin, opening the needle driver, closing the needle driver and pulling the needle through the skin. Software analyzing surgical motions, by using a modification of Rosen's finite state model for scoring purposes, is in development.

4. Discussion/Conclusions

Ongoing work is directed toward the development of imbedded instructional materials such as demonstrative video clips, higher fidelity force feedback and a scoring mechanism. Future work includes using a true 6 DOF haptic device to provide more accurate twist constraints and torques. The long-term goal is to measure skills in both haptic virtual surgery and in vivo surgery. The end result is to develop a training system that promotes development of skills in basic suturing techniques are transferable to the real world.

Acknowledgments

This project was funded, in part, by the National Science Foundation under grant numbers DUE-9950742 and DUE-9651237, and a Penn State University College of Medicine Department of Surgery Feasibility Grant, the Eberly Virtual Hospital Project, the Millersville University Neimeyer-Hodgson Grants Program and by the Faculty Grants Committee of Millersville University. Thanks to Cindy Miller for her editorial expertise.

References

1. Bro-Nielsen M, Helfrick D, Glass B, Zeng X, Connacher H. VR simulation of abdominal trauma surgery. Stud Health Technol Inform 1998;50:117-23.
2. Ottensmeyer M, Ben-Ur E, Salisbury K. Input and output for surgical simulation: devices to measure tissue properties in vivo and a haptic interface for laparoscopic simulators. Stud Health Technol Inform 2000;70:236-42.
3. Renig K, Spitzer V, Pelster H, Johnson T, Mahalik T. More real-time visual and haptic interaction with anatomical data. Stud Health Technol Inform 1997;39:155-8.
4. De S, Srinivasan M. Thin walled models for haptic and graphical rendering of soft tissues in surgical simulations. Stud Health Technol Inform 1999;62:94-9.
5. Gorman P, Krummel T, Webster R, Smith M, Hutchens D. A prototype haptic lumbar puncture simulator. Stud Health Technol Inform 2000;70:106-9.
6. Bro-Nielsen M, Tasto J, Cunningham R, Merril G. PreOp endoscopic simulator: a PC-based immersive training system for bronchoscopy. Stud Health Technol Inform 1999;62:76-82.
7. Baraff D, Witkin A. Large steps in cloth animation. Proc Ann ACM SIGGRAPH'98 Conf 1998;33:43-54.
8. Desbrun M, Schroder P, Barr A. Interactive animation of structured deformable objects. Proc Ann Graphics Interface 1999;5:73-7.
9. Rosen J, MacFarlane M, Richards C, Hannaford B, Sinanan M. Surgeon-Tool Force/Torque Signatures - Evaluation of Surgical Skills in Minimally Invasive Surgery. Stud Health Technol Inform 1999;62:290-6.

570

Medicine Meets Virtual Reality 2001
J.D. Westwood et al. (Eds.)
IOS Press, 2001

An efficient method for modelling soft tissue in Virtual Environment training systems

Derek P M Wills and Peter M Chapman

Department of Computer Science, University of Hull, UK

Abstract. Modelling soft tissues in virtual environment training systems is frequently required. The provision of both visually compelling and physically accurate models presents a number of problems for the developer. The Finite element technique presented in this paper, *modal analysis*, can be programmed to allow the user to easily trade-off accuracy of simulation for execution speed. It has been successfully used to produce simulations of the lateral meniscus on low powered portable computer systems.

1 Introduction

The inclusion of soft tissue models in virtual environment medical training systems is frequently required. It is not only important that these models provide an accurate visual simulation but that they also realistically reproduce elastic forces, which can be used for the provision of haptic feedback. Two common methods for modelling soft tissue are the spring-and-dashpot model and the Finite Element Method [1]. The former approach provides a fast method for simulating deformable objects but lacks any physical validity. The Finite Element Method (FEM), however, is based on sound engineering theory but has a tendency to require excessive processing resources. This paper presents a variation on the FEM, called modal analysis, which retains the physical accuracy of the method whilst allowing the user to define a balance between accuracy and execution time. An outline of Modal Analysis is presented together with the results of its application to a model of the lateral meniscus, which is part of the Virtual Environment Knee Arthroscopy System (VEKATS) [2] currently under development at the University of Hull.

2 Method

Finite element analysis is commonly used in engineering to provide a detailed discrete model of continuum mechanics. A body is described by a mesh of finite elements connected at nodes. A system of second order equations (equation 1) is formulated which expresses the motion of the body in response to applied forces.

$$\mathbf{M\ddot{U} + D\dot{U} + KU = R} \qquad \text{Equation 1}$$

where R is the load vector of forces acting upon the nodes, U is the vector of nodal displacement, M is the mass matrix, D the damping matrix and K the stiffness matrix describing the material properties of the object.

Finite element methods have been used for graphics and animation applications [3]. Although the motion equations are physically accurate their solution is computationally expensive, which has prevented their wide spread use for virtual environment applications

There are two classes of solution for the system of finite element equations. In the direct solution the nodal displacements resulting from the application of external forces are calculated directly. Technique such as the central Difference Method or Newark's Method are commonly used for this. The computational expense of these methods is relative to the number of time-steps involved in the simulation, which implies that they are useful if the simulation is short and only involves a relatively few time-steps. However, it may be inferred that the solution is expensive when the amount of time to be simulated increases or for situations when the time-step is very short. To overcome this computational burden several researchers have adapted the solution of the motion equations [4][5][6]. These solutions solve the equations of motion directly to find the displacements of the nodes (or nodal forces) in response to applied forces (displacements). We propose an alternative and more efficient technique which solves the equations indirectly. This method, known as Modal Analysis, is used in the transient dynamic analysis of structures and derived from the mechanics of vibration in structures.

The number of independent co-ordinates required to describe the motion of a system is called the number of degrees of freedom of the system. For example a particle has three degrees of freedom. If a body is described as a mesh of finite elements connected at nodes, and each node has three degrees of freedom, then the finite element representation of the body has $3n$ degrees of freedom for n nodes in the mesh. All bodies with mass and elasticity are capable of vibration. The dynamic properties of the object, the distribution of mass and stiffness across the object, determine the natural frequencies at which the object will vibrate when subject to external forces. For every degree of freedom in a system there is a natural frequency of vibration and a corresponding mode of vibration, where the mode describes the shape of the object when it oscillates at that frequency. Hence a finite element mesh with n nodes has $3n$ modes of vibration.

When an object is subjected to an external force it will deform, and, for a linear system, this deformation can be described as a sum of the individual modes of vibration. The process by which the modes of vibration are calculated and used to compute the response of an object (modal analysis), reduces the complexity of the problem, and thus simplifies the solution of the motion equations.

The derivation of the modal equations is based upon first considering an undamped object, the dynamic equations now becoming

$$\mathbf{M\ddot{U}+KU} = 0 \qquad\qquad \text{Equation 2}$$

The solution to this can be expressed as harmonic motion with the form

$$\mathbf{U} = \phi \sin \omega t \qquad\qquad \text{Equation 3}$$

where φ is a vector representing the amplitudes of the nodal degrees of freedom, t is time and ω is the frequency of vibration of the structure. Substituting equation 3 into equation 2 yields the general eigen problem

$$(\mathbf{K} + \omega^2\mathbf{M})\phi = 0 \qquad\qquad \text{Equation 4}$$

This eigen problem can be solved to provide n eigen solutions (ω_i^2, φ_i) for i = 1, 2, ..., n degrees of freedom in the mesh. φ_i are the modes of vibration corresponding to the frequencies ω_i, where $(0 \leq \omega_1 \leq \omega_2 \leq ... \leq \omega_n)$. Each node φ_i represents the displacement of every node in the body, when the body vibrates with the corresponding frequency ω_i. The matrix Φ is formed from the eigenvectors, and the diagonal matrix Ω^2 is formed from the frequencies of vibration.

$$\Phi = [\phi_1, \phi_2, ..., \phi_n]; \quad \Omega^2 = \begin{bmatrix} \omega_1^2 & & & \\ & \omega_2^2 & & \\ & & \ddots & \\ & & & \omega_n^2 \end{bmatrix} \qquad \text{Equation 5}$$

Since the modes (eigenvectors) are **M**-orthonormal, that is $\phi_i^T M \phi_j = \delta_{ij}$ where δ_{ij} is the Kronecker delta, then:

$$\Phi^T K \Phi = \Omega^2; \qquad \Phi^T M \Phi = I \qquad \text{Equation 6}$$

where **I** is the identity matrix. To change basis from the finite element nodal displacement **U** to normalised modal displacements **q**, the following transformation is used:

$$U(t) = \Phi q(t) \qquad \text{Equation 7}$$

Substituting equation 7 into equation 1, the equilibrium equation corresponding to the modal displacements is

$$\ddot{q} + \Phi^T D \Phi \dot{q} + \Omega^2 q = \Phi^T R \qquad \text{Equation 8}$$

Equation 8 demonstrates that if the damping matrix is not included I the analysis the equations are decoupled, hence instead of n simultaneous equation there are n single equation, which are much simpler to solve.

A damping scheme known as *Rayleigh* or *proportional damping* is used to form the damping matrix **D** as a linear combination of the stiffness and mass matrices.

$$D = \alpha M + \beta K \qquad \text{Equation 9}$$

The mass and stiffness proportional damping factors, α and β, are related to the modal damping factor γ at a frequency ω by

$$\gamma = \frac{1}{2}\left(\frac{\alpha}{\omega} + \beta\omega\right) \qquad \text{Equation 10}$$

When proportional damping is assumed the modal equations are completely decoupled. In this case the damping matrix transform to

$$\phi_i^T D \phi_j = 2\omega_i \gamma_i \delta_{ij} \qquad \text{Equation 11}$$

For an arbitrary disturbing force $r_i(t) = \phi_i^T \mathbf{R}(t)$ the modal displacement becomes

$$\ddot{q}_i(t) + 2\gamma_i\omega_i\,\dot{q}_i(t) + \omega_i^2 q_i(t) = r_i(t) \qquad \text{Equation 12}$$

for each i = 1,2, ..., n degree of freedom. Each equation can be solved by numerical integration or by using the Duhamel Integral Equation.

For the complete response of the object to external loads all n modal displacement equations are solved and displacements of the finite element nodes $\mathbf{U}(t)$ are obtained by summation of the contributions of each mode (equation 13). This summation is known as modal superposition.

$$\mathbf{U}(t) = \sum_{i=1}^{n} \phi_i q_i(t) \qquad \text{Equation 13}$$

In applying the modal approach, the initial eigen solution is an extremely intensive and expensive computation to complete. However, in situations where the modes of vibration can be assumed constant the eigen solutions can be computed once as a pre-processing stage rather than at every time-step of the simulation. The modes of vibration remain the same if the finite element representation remains valid. Therefore the mesh topology must remain constant, that is no cutting or fracturing of the mesh is allowed. Large displacements are also not permitted.

Using the same modes of vibration at each time-step leads to an improvement of performance for modal analysis over direct solutions. However, even greater gains in performance can be gained by inspecting the contribution of each mode to the final displacement. It can be shown that the high frequency modes describe small localised deformations which contribute little to the overall change in object shape.

At the University of Hull a system is under development to aid training in a form of minimally invasive surgery, known as Knee Arthroscopy [7]. The Virtual Environment Knee Arthroscopy Training System (VEKATS) [2] provides a simulated arthroscopic view of a graphical knee model. Using an electromagnetic tracking system to measure the positions of a mock arthroscopic camera and surgical probe, the system displays a view of the knee model based on the current camera position and orientation. Simultaneously the trainee can interact with the models of the deformable tissues of the knee. In addition to the visual display the force data for each object in the environment can be used to drive haptic feedback devices. Transmitting forces through the mock arthroscope and probe will improve the realism of the simulation and broaden the range of skills that can be taught using the simulator.

The current VEKATS implementation does not meet all the requirements for a complete training system. One identified area for improvement is in the provision of a more accurate and efficient model for soft tissue. To this end it was decided to apply the modal analysis method to the dynamic modelling of the lateral meniscus. The lateral and medial menisci are layers of cartilage, which act as cushions to spread the area of contact between two major bones of the knee joint, the femur and the tibia. The realistic simulation of these deformable tissues is essential to teach surgical procedures.

3 Results

To assess the modal algorithm prototype software has been used to develop a dynamic finite element model of the lateral meniscus for simulation. The graphical knee model in

VEKATS is derived from a three-dimensional data set (ViewPoint DataLabs, 1994). The prototype finite element model of the meniscus has also been derived from this data set. To generate a finite element representation the original data was simplified, the curved edges of the shape being approximated by line segments. A commercial finite element package, ANSYS, was then used to generate a suitable mesh topology. To test the relative response error and performance of reduced modal analysis the model of the lateral meniscus was subjected to forces of deformation. To imitate the deformation caused by lifting the meniscus with a surgical probe, forces were applied to nodes on the underside of the meniscus and the resultant behaviour was simulated using modal analysis. The images in figure 1 illustrate examples of the deformation which closely resemble those seen in previously videoed arthroscopies.

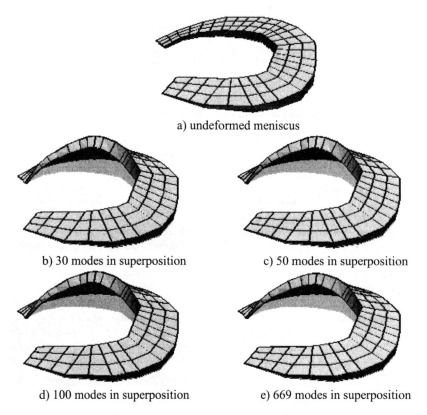

a) undeformed meniscus

b) 30 modes in superposition   c) 50 modes in superposition

d) 100 modes in superposition   e) 669 modes in superposition

Figure 1: Frames from the simulated lifting of the lateral meniscus. a) shows the undeformed mode while b), c), d) and e) illustrate the deformation calculated using different numbers of modes.

A set of simulations was conducted with differing numbers of modes used in the modal superposition. An analysis of the comparative accuracy of the different simulations was conducted by measuring the relative response error using the equation

$$r = \frac{\left\| \mathbf{U}_n(t) - \mathbf{U}_p(t) \right\|}{\left\| \mathbf{U}_n(t) \right\|}$$
         Equation 14

where $\mathbf{U}_n(t)$ is the response at time t when n modes are used and $\mathbf{U}_p(t)$ is the response at time t when p modes.

Essentially the same deformation was seen for simulations involving different numbers of modes of vibration. Figure 2 shows the curve of the relative response error versus the number of nodes in the superposition. The shape of the graph indicates that the error only become significant for simulations involving less than 100 modes of vibration.

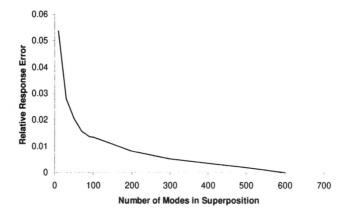

Figure 2: Graph showing the relative response error against the number of modes in superposition when the lateral meniscus is lifted and deformed. Measurements are relative to a 669 mode superposition.

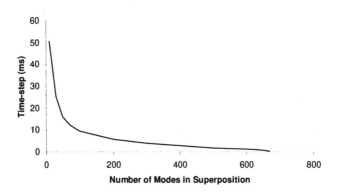

Figure 3: Graph showing the lengths of the time-step corresponding to the number of modes in superposition for the lateral meniscus model.

The performance of the prototype system was also measured. Figure 3 shows the relative length of the time-step for different analyses. The graph indicates an exponential increase in execution time with an increase in the number of modes of vibration used in the analysis. It was also noted that due to the linear nature of the modal solution, the frame rate was found to have a near linear relationship with the number of degrees of freedom in the mesh. Hence a linear increase in the density of the mesh leads to a linear decrease in frame rate.

4 Discussion

From the previous section it can be concluded that the modal algorithm fulfils the requirements of accuracy and interactivity required for the VEKATS training system. Further, the a controlled degradation of the accuracy of the meniscal model is available with the reduction of modes considered in the modal superposition, with this only becoming significant with less than 100 modes of vibration. In addition, a short survey of four orthopaedic surgeons was conducted to assess how the model performed from the perspective of an end user. The surgeons were asked to rate the model in terms of the simulated behaviour of the meniscus and reaction time of the simulation. In general, the results from the users assessment of the model support the experimental finding reported in the last section, although it was noted that more damping and a more detailed description of the internal edge of the meniscus was required.

   In conclusion, the modal method can be used to provide a realistic and interactive model suitable for surgical simulation and training. It retains the physical accuracy of the FEM method whilst allowing the user to define a balance between accuracy and execution time. This method will now be integrated into the next version of VEKATS, currently under development at the University of Hull.

References

[1] M. J. Fagan, Finite Element Analysis. Longman Group, 1st Edition, 1992.

[2] J. W. Ward, D. P. M. Wills, K. P. Sherman and A M M A Mohsen, The Development of an Arthroscopic Surgical Simulator with Haptic Feedback, *Future Generation Computer Systems* **14** (1998) 243-251.

[3] J. P. Gourret, N. M. Thalmann and D. Thalmann, Simulation of Object and Human Skin Deformations in a Grasping Task, *Computer Graphics* **23(3)** (1989) 21-30.

[4] D.T. Chen and D. Zeltzer, Pump It Up: Computer Animation of a Biomechanically Based Model of Muscle Using the Finite Element Method, *Computer Graphics* **26(2)** (1992) 89-98.

[5] M. A. Sagar, D. Bullivant, G. D. Mallinson and P. J. Hunter. A Virtual Environment and Model of the Eye for Surgical Simulation, *Computer Graphics Proceedings, Annual Conference Series*, (1994) 205-212.

[6] M. BroNielsen and S. Cotin, Real-Time Volumetric Deformable Models for Surgery Simulation using Finite Elements and Condensation, *Computer Graphics Forum* **15(3)** (1996) 57-66.

[7] I. P. Logan, D. P. M. Wills, N. J. Avis, A. M. M. A. Mohsen and K. P. Sherman . Virtual Environment Knee Arthroscopy Training System, *Society for Computer Simulation, Simulation Series* **28(4)** (1997) 17-22.

Medicine Meets Virtual Reality 2001
J.D. Westwood et al. (Eds.)
IOS Press, 2001

Immersive Virtual Reality Used as a Platform for Perioperative Training for Surgical Residents

Donald B. Witzke, Ph.D.[1,2], James D. Hoskins, B.S.[1], Michael J. Mastrangelo, Jr., M.D.[1],
Wayne O. Witzke[1], Uyen B. Chu, M.D., S.P.[1], Shirish Pande, M.E.[1],
Adrian E. Park, M.D.[1]

[1]Center for Minimally Invasive Surgery, Department of Surgery
[2]Department of Pathology & Laboratory Medicine
University of Kentucky College of Medicine
Lexington, KY 40536-0293
E-mail dbwitz1@pop.uky.edu
http://www-mis.uky.edu

Abstract. Perioperative preparations such as operating room setup, patient and equipment positioning, and operating port placement are essential to operative success in minimally invasive surgery. We developed an immersive virtual reality-based training system (REMIS) to provide residents (and other health professionals) with training and evaluation in these perioperative skills. Our program uses the qualities of immersive VR that are available today for inclusion in an ongoing training curriculum for surgical residents. The current application consists of a primary platform for patient positioning for a laparoscopic cholecystectomy. Having completed this module we can create many different simulated problems for other procedures. As a part of the simulation, we have devised a computer-driven real-time data collection system to help us in evaluating trainees and providing feedback during the simulation. The REMIS program trains and evaluates surgical residents and obviates the need to use expensive operating room and surgeon time. It also allows residents to train based on their schedule and does not put patients at increased risk. The method is standardized, allows for repetition if needed, evaluates individual performance, provides the possible complications of incorrect choices, provides training in 3-D environment, and has the capability of being used for various scenarios and professions.

1. Introduction

The cost of surgical training is increasing and this is especially true of laparoscopic surgery. There is also an increase in the knowledge and skills surgeons are required to possess while the amount of attending surgeon time and other surgical resources available to train and evaluate residents in surgery is decreasing. Operating room setup, patient positioning and operating port placement are essential to operative success in minimally invasive surgery (MIS).[1] Errors in judgment and/or execution of essential perioperative decisions increase the difficulty of performing MIS procedures and ultimately lead to prolonged operations, conversions to open surgery and increased surgical morbidity.[2][3] A comprehensive perioperative training method is needed to provide residents high quality instruction, practice, and evaluation that is both cost effective and does not increase the risk to patients. While others have investigated the intricate details of surgical simulations (e.g., tissue response, bleeding calculations, completely realistic visuals [4,5,6]), we are exploring an application that bypasses the technological, hardware, and software limitations these methods have encountered.

2. Purpose

We investigated various instructional methods that could help resolve the problems associated with residents' surgical training and decided that immersive virtual reality training satisfied our criteria best. The ultimate goal of our training development effort is to decrease the impact of resident training on health care cost and patient morbidity. In considering solutions to the problems of training, we were sensitive to the need to track and record the decision paths used by the residents. We will use the resulting data to validate the training method and to evaluate residents' performance in a standardized fashion.

3. Methods and Materials

We developed a simulation program that allows residents to learn the proper operating room configuration for MIS procedures and to practice procedure-specific patient, surgeon, and monitor positioning, proper padding and support, and port placement. The simulation operates on a Silicon Graphics Octane workstation connected to the ImmersaDesk (Fakespace Systems, Inc.), which is an immersive three-dimensional projection system.

3.1 Program Design

The CAVE Library (Electronic Visualization Laboratory, University of Illinois at Chicago) was our library of choice because it was capable of fully using the ImmersaDesk and we were already familiar with it. Similarly, the OpenInventor (Silicon Graphics, Inc.) library was chosen because we found it suitable for rapid development of immersive applications using complicated geometric environments, were familiar with it, and knew that we could use it in conjunction with the CAVE Library.

One of the elements that needed to be addressed was that the time required to render the environments that REMIS would incorporate would be relatively large. To compensate for this, other computations must be relatively small, or at the very least temporally contained and infrequent. Our programming staff was able to accomplish this requirement with satisfactory results.

The load time for a surgical environment in the application is approximately twelve seconds, but at no other time does the user of the application have to wait over one second for a frame to update. For the computer that we used to develop the application, the frame rates for the application ranged from twenty-four frames per second to 4 frames per second. There is a linear decay in the frame rate as the complexity of the environment increases during a single training session. Restoration to twenty-four frames per second is achieved once the complicated environment no longer needs to be rendered. While the apparently low frame rate at the end of a training session may seem unacceptable, we found that the low frame rate was not a hindrance to the user and, in many cases, was not noticed.

Interface is one of the most important aspects of any surgical simulation, as the learning curve must be very small, any interaction with objects must be natural, and all interface elements must be both non-intrusive and easy to use. Creating a user interface with a low learning curve was an especially difficult design consideration. The devices that the user would have to work with were limited to the wand, a hand held device that transmits three dimensional coordinates and rotations, three button states, and (x,y) joystick values to the computing platform running the simulation, and the driver's goggles (Crystal Eyes provided by Fakespace Systems Inc.). Goggles worn by the simulation user allow the user to see images displayed by the program stereoscopically and they also send the position and orientation of the users head to the computing platform running the simulation.

We divided the interface into two primary categories. Either the user will be answering questions or the user will be interacting with the environment being displayed by the simulation. This division greatly simplified the issue of interaction. There is no real possibility of using a keyboard with the simulation because the interface is limited to the wand and the driver's goggles. This allows us to group all user decisions that are not interactions with the simulated environment into a menu system. By designing a basic menu system to mimic menus used in most operating systems that use windows, we decrease the learning curve for the user. Implementation of such an interface, however, presented unique design problems for an immersive platform. Although we have been unable to answer completely the questions for all of the design problems that arose, our observations indicate that the system has a small learning curve and is functional. It is also relatively easy to modify the menu and should be easy to incorporate the menu system into other applications.

For the other aspect of the user interface, interaction with elements in the simulated environments, we realized that each instance of interaction would have unique requirements. This would be difficult for the user, who would have to learn a different interface at each interaction. To surmount the difficulty of learning a different interface for each scene, we made the interaction somewhat similar between instances. For example, moving the wand moves the object active in the environment; pressing the joystick rotates the active object in the environment about axes; and pressing the first button finalizes a choice. To further decrease the learning curve, we are developing a method to instruct the user in how to use the primary interface device during each of the instances of interaction. By displaying a model of the wand in the environment, labeled appropriately with the various aspects of the interface, we completely explain the interface to the user in a compact format. Resulting changes in the 3-D models provide an instant visualization of their choices. There are other segments of the simulation where elements of the scene (e.g., operating table adjustments, surgeon and monitor placement) are under the control of the trainee via programmed buttons on the wand-input device.

All aspects of the user interface are designed to make the interface more comfortable to the user, which should help decrease the learning curve. Each section and menu encountered during a training session is appropriately labeled. We have included a rotating numbered wheel that displays how far the user has progressed into the training session and it is our observation that this seems more intuitive for users

The final design consideration was the need to capture every discrete decision that the user made during a training session. Such a record not only provides a means of recording and evaluating the user's performance and progress, but also can indicate where design improvements can be made. Information we capture and associate with each decision includes where it occurs in a menu hierarchy, user name, date, time, procedure, session section, and attempt number. We also capture information regarding what the decision was, the decision's name, the degree of correctness, and any associated floating-point data (e.g., trocar position).

3.2 Modeling

The inanimate models used in the program (e.g., operating table, patient padding, laparoscopic instruments) were created using Rhinoceros 3-D (Robert McNeel and Associates). This application was chosen for its ease-of-use, versatility, and the wide range of file types that can be imported and exported. The patient and surgeon models were authored in Poser 4 (Curious Labs, Inc.). To achieve the accurate patient positions for the procedures, live models were posed in the operating room and photographed using a high-resolution digital camera. These photos were imported as background images into Poser and the patient character was posed using the joint control parameter dials to match the position of the patient in the background. The background was then removed, the figure observed from all possible camera angles to guarantee fidelity, and then exported in 3-D Studio (3DS) format. This intermediary file was then the imported into Rhinoceros 3-D and after being scaled larger by a factor of approximately 100 combined with the remaining OR elements created previously by the program (see Fig. 1).

Color and textures were applied to all of the component elements. Superfluous sides and polygons were removed to reduce the size of the final exported VRML file. Our programmers have written code that allows this VRML file to be used as a scene on the ImmersaDesk and various elements of this scene can be manipulated by direct user control. Examples of these elements include the operating table adjustments, surgeon placement, and trocar positioning. Careful attention was given during each stage of the creation of objects to maintain accurate scaling. We wrote the code to maintain 3-D perspective so that object size was adjusted for distance and angle from the viewer. This allowed the assembled worlds to be authentic in this detail and impart a more realistic feel to the final scene graphs. Fig. 2 provides a pictorial example of trocar placement scene used in our REMIS application.

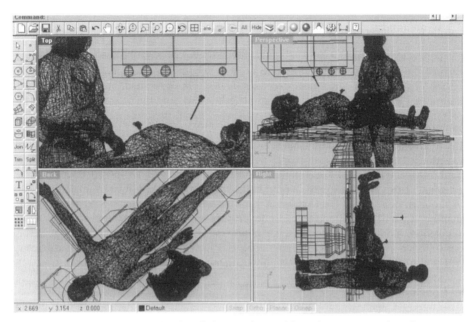

Figure 1. Rhinoceros 3-D example of three orthographic and one perspective view.

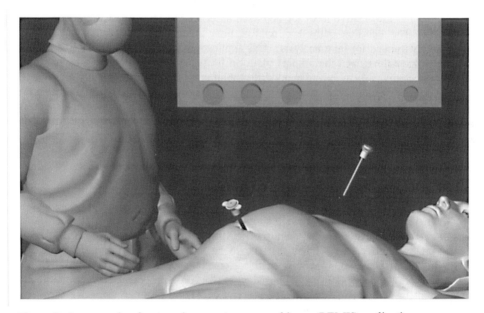

Figure 2. An example of trocar placement scene used in our REMIS application.

3.3 Evaluation

Resident performance data are collected in real-time as the trainee goes through each of the problems. Elapsed time to accurately complete each phase of the training, degree of accuracy in placement decisions, and errors committed, are recorded. Real-time visual and audio feedback is given periodically during the progression through the program. A summation screen of the resident's overall performance is provided at the end of the simulation.

We have planned a multistage evaluation development process for REMIS. First, experienced and expert laparoscopic surgeon faculty will be used to obtain standard performance criteria for the simulation. These values will be incorporated into the program. Next, residents participating in the MIS curriculum will be evaluated in terms of these criteria during the simulation with the results being captured by the program. Finally, we will ask all participants to provide evaluation about the validity of the simulation, along with suggestions for improving it. To date, the surgeons comprising our criterion group indicated that the "look and feel" of the simulation was sufficiently real to allow for comfortable interaction with the scene.

4. Conclusions

We are in the process of developing a comprehensive system to teach and evaluate residents on perioperative aspects of laparoscopic surgery. The REMIS program presents a viable operating room environment where placement decisions can be evaluated and informative feedback delivered based on the course of action taken by the resident. The decision paths and relative time increments between actions can be completely tracked for later analysis. This application is also novel and flexible in that since we have developed the primary platform for patient positioning for a laparoscopic cholecystectomy, we can create many different simulated problems for other procedures. This versatile engine can be a useful training tool and simultaneously a data collection tool to further research on cognitive learning methods and eventually provide a stage for validation of skills transference. We are in the process of conducting a formative evaluation of the program and will begin performance assessment of trainees in the near future to help determine the validity and reliability of the system.

5. Future Directions

This is the first stage of a complete minimally invasive surgery simulation program that will eventually include surgical haptic feedback, visual representation of tissue interaction, distortion and damage. REMIS will also include each of the 10 more common MIS procedures. Items that should be incorporated as future enhancements include "what if scenarios" with adaptable elements such as choice of obese, elderly, juvenile, or pediatric patients. Extension of the program capabilities from trocar-placement to performing of simulated procedures will incorporate using the view that would be seen through the laparoscope. This scene would include haptic feedback returned simultaneously through two input devices that closely mimic the look and feel of the laparoscopic instruments. We will also be able to do data sampling (e.g., tracking navigation) during the instances in which the user is interacting with the simulated environment. The progression to later stages should also include the capability for preprogrammed (or random) complications to gauge the performance of residents under less than ideal conditions.

References

[1] Airan MC.   Patient preperation.In:Scott-Conner C. ed.   *The SAGES manual: fundamentals of laparoscopy and GI endoscopy.* New York, NY, USA: Springer- Verlag: 1999: 12-14.

[2] Berkley J, Weghorst S, Gladstone H, et al. Fast finite element modeling for surgical simulation. In: Westwood JD, Hoffman HM, Robb RA, Stredney D. eds. *Medicine Meets Virtual Reality.* Amsterdam, the Netherlands: IOS Press: 1999: 55-61.

[3] Dubelman A. Complications of laparoscopic surgery: surgical and anesthetic considerations. *Semin Laparosc Surg.* 1994 Dec: 1(4): 219-222.

[4] Wolf JS, Marcovich R, Gill IS, et al. Survey of neuromuscular injuries to the patient and surgeon during urologic laparoscopic surgery. *Urology.* 2000 Jun: 55(6): 831- 836.

[5] Lin W, Robb RA. Dynamic volume texture mapping and model deformation for visually realistic surgical simulation. In: Westwood JD, Hoffman HM, Robb RA,   Stredney D. eds. *Medicine Meets Virtual Reality.* Amsterdam, the Netherlands: IOS   Press: 1999: 198-204.

[6] Çakmak, H.K., Kühnapfel, U. The "Karlsruhe Endoscopic Surgery Trainer" for minimally invasive surgery in gynaecology, *13th Internat. Congress on Computer Assisted Radiology and Surgery (CARS'99),* Paris, F, June 23-26, 1999, p 1050.

Medicine Meets Virtual Reality 2001
J.D. Westwood et al. (Eds.)
IOS Press, 2001

Anatomical Accuracy in Medical 3D Modeling

Wulf J.*, Vitt K.D.***, Gehl H.-B.**, Busch L.C.*

* Institut of Anatomy, Medical University of Lübeck
Ratzeburger Allee 160, 23538 Lübeck, Germany

** Department of Radiology, Medical University of Lübeck
Ratzeburger Allee 160, 23538 Lübeck, Germany

*** Medical Service of the Health Insurances (MDK)
Katharinenstr. 11a, 23554 Lübeck, Germany

joergwulf@yahoo.de

In complex surgery, medical modeling has become an accepted tool for diagnosis, simulation and the planning of surgical interventions [1]. However, the question concerning the accuracy of the model, i.e. the equivalence between the model itself on the one hand and the original anatomical situation on the other hand, remains unanswererd in the current literature.

1. Introduction

The procedure of generating a medical model can be devided into different steps, starting from the computed tomography (CT) scanning via segmentation, 3D visualisation and data processing. The final step is the building of the model itself. The most common technique is called stereolithography. A stereolithograph works as follows: a controler positions a vertical elevator, housed inside a vat filled with a liquide photosensitive resin so that it rests just below the liquid surface. An optical scanning system directs an UV laser which "draws" a shape, one layer at a time, onto the surface of the resin. As the laser strikes the surface, the resin is solidified. The first layer of the model is built. After that, the elevator is lowered, just submerging the solidified layer. The scanning process is repeated and a second layer is built on top of the first one. This process of submerging and laser scanning goes on and on until the entire model is built.

2. Methods

To examine the anatomical accuracy in stereolitographic modeling, a study with unfixed human head and neck cadaver specimens is performed. After CT scanning of the head and neck specimen, its soft tissues will be removed by maceration and the bony structures will be bleached. By means of this CT database after segmentation and data processing, the stereolithographic building can be performed. The result will be a stereolithographic model of the bony structures of the head and neck. Both, the model and its original, will then be measured and compared.

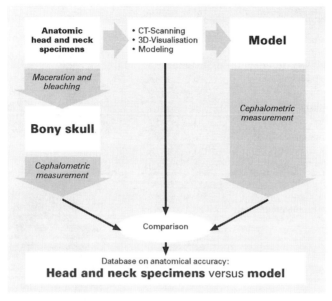

Figure 1: General description

3. Results

The study is currently undergoing validation. We are here presenting the results of the first case.

3.1 Descriptive results

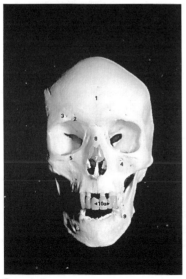

1 Os frontale
2 Incisura frontalis
3 Foramen supraorbitale
4 Foramen infraorbitale
5 Margo infraorbitalis
6 Foramen mentale
7 Septum nasi
8 Os nasale

9 Bony defect, caused
   by a penetrating cyst,
   root dens 36
10a Prosthetic
   reconstruction
10b Artifacts caused
   by prosthetic
   reconstruction

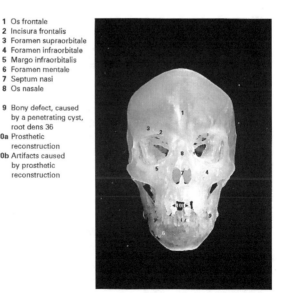

Bony skull

Model of skull

Figure 2: Frontal view

3.2 Morphometric results

Indices	Bony skull	Model
Maximum cranial length (g–op)	177,0	180,0
Length of skull base (n–ba)	104,0	102,0
Maximum cranial breadth (eu–eu) sutura squamosum	138,0	141,0
Least frontal breadth (ft–ft)	103,0	105,0
Maximum frontal breadth (co–co)	124,0	126,0
Basion-porion heigth (ba–po)	140,0	141,0
Auriculo-bregmatic heigth (po–b)	118,0	121,0
Basion-prostion length (ba–pr)	93,8	91,7
Outer biorbital breadth (fmt–fmt)	106,5	108,8
Zygomatic breadth (zy–zy)	131,0	135,0
Bimaxillary breadth (zm–zm)	91,9	95,9
Total facial heigth (n–gn)	124,6	126,7
Nasoalveola heigth (n–pr)	69,2	69,3
Anterior interorbital breadth (mf–mf)	26,2	29,1
Orbital breadth (mf–ek)	35,8	35,9
Greatest heigth of orbit	32,9	33,7
Nasal breadth	21,6	22,5
Nasal heigth (n–s)	53,4	49,9
Internal palatal length (ol–sta)	39,1	33,5
Internal palatal breadth (enm–enm)	32,8	33,5
Palatal heigth	17,0	16,0
Bicondylar breadth (kdl–kdl)	119,3	123,7
Bigonial breadth (go–go)	92,4	95,4
Projective length of the corpus mandibulae	74,0	74,0
Heigth of mandibula symphysis (id–gn)	29,9	30,5
Heigth of ascending ramus	60,0	64,0
Breadth of ramus	27,9	27,9

Figure 3: Measured distances (in millimeters)

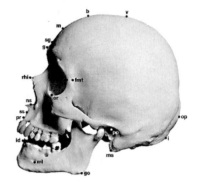

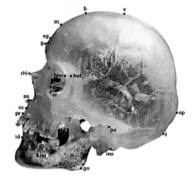

v	Vertex	ss	Subspinale
b	Bregma	ns	Nasospinale
m	Methopion	ms	Mastoideale
sg	Supraglabellare	i	Inion
g	Glabella	op	Opisthocranion
rhi	Rhinion	or	Orbita
go	Gonion	fmt	Frontornalare temporale
ml	Mentale	fmo	Frontornalare orbitale
id	Infradentale	po	Porion
pr	Prostion	fmo	Frontornalare orbitale

Figure 4: Selection of landmarks

4. Conclusion

The aim of this study is to provide and to evaluate a database on the anatomical accuracy of stereo-lithographic modeling, taking into account the overall procedure from CT scanning to model building. In addition to morphometric techniques used in physical anthropology, electronic measurement methods will be applied in our further investigation.

5. Acknowledgements

Model building: Materialise N.V., Technologielaan 15, 3001 Leuven, Belgium
Morphometric measurement in co-operation with: Anthropologische Staatssammlung München (Anthropological State Collection)/ University of Munich (LMU), Karolinenplatz 2a, 80333 München, Germany

Reference

[1] Ericksson DM, et al., An opinion survey of reported benefits from the use of stereotithographic models. J Oral Maxillofac Surg 1999 Sept; 57(9):1040-3

Medicine Meets Virtual Reality 2001
J.D. Westwood et al. (Eds.)
IOS Press, 2001

Reconstructing Hierarchical Tetrahedral Mesh Density Models of Bony Anatomy

Jianhua Yao, Russell Taylor
Computer Science Department, The Johns Hopkins University, Baltimore, MD

Abstract: We proposed an efficient and automatic method to reconstruct hierarchical tetrahedral meshes and build density models for bony anatomy from CT data sets. The mesh is reconstructed from contours extracted in CT images corresponding to the outer bone surfaces and the boundaries between compact bone, spongy bone and medullary cavity. Key problems, such as tiling problem, branching problem, correspondence problem, and constraint problem, have been solved. We then approximated bone density variations by means of continuous density functions in each tetrahedron. The density functions are written as smooth Bernstein polynomial spline expressed in terms of barycentric coordinates associated with each tetrahedron. We further performed the tetrahedral mesh simplification by edge collapsing and built hierarchical structure of multiple resolution meshes. We applied our density model to efficiently generate Digitally Reconstructed Radiographs. This research is part of our effort to build a bone density atlas.

1. Introduction and Background

One of the most critical research problems in the analysis of 3D medical images is the development of methods for storing, approximating and analyzing image data sets efficiently. Many groups are developing electronic atlases as a reference database for consulting and teaching, for deformable registration-assisted segmentation of medical images and for use in surgical planning. Researchers at INRIA have built atlases based on surface models and crest lines [1]. Cutting *et al* [2] have built similar atlases of the skull. These atlases are surface models with some landmarks and crest lines and don't contain any volumetric density information. Chen *et al* [3] have built an average brain atlas based on statistical data of the voxel intensity values. Their atlases only contain intensity information and don't describe the geometrical features of the anatomy.

One goal of our current research is to construct a deformable density atlas for bony anatomy and apply the atlas to various applications. Our intent is to use intensity and shape-based deformable registration methods both in the construction of the atlas and in exploiting it for patient-specific procedure planning and intraoperative guidance. The atlas will provide a basis for representing "generic" information about surgical plans and procedures. The atlas will also provide infrastructure for study of anatomical variation. It may also provide an initial coordinate system for correlating surgical actions with results, as well as an aid in postoperative assessment. The atlas should include: 1) model representations of "normal" 3D CT densities and segmented surface meshes; 2) 3D parameterization of surface shape & volumetric properties; and 3) statistical characterization of variability of parameters.

We adopt a hierarchical tetrahedral mesh model to store volumetric properties for several reasons. The tetrahedral meshes provide the greatest possible degree of flexibility. Furthermore, other mesh can be converted into tetrahedral mesh. Data structure, data traversal, and data rendering for tetrahedral mesh are more involved. And tetrahedral meshes have the ability to better adapt to local features. It is also convenient to assign properties to the vertices and tetrahedra. Computational steps such as interpolation, integration, and differentiation are fast and often can be done in closed form. Finite element analysis is often conveniently performed on tetrahedral meshes. The hierarchical structure of multiple resolution mesh can make the analysis and visualization more efficient.

This paper reports current progress in building hierarchical tetrahedral mesh density models from CT scans. In section 2, we elaborate the method to construct the tetrahedral mesh from bone contours. In section 3, we present the method to assign a density function to the tetrahedron and evaluate the accuracy of the density function. Section 4 describes our method to build a hierarchical structure based on edge collapsing. Then in section 5, we show the results using our density model to efficiently generate Digitally Reconstructed Radiographs (DRRs). Finally section 6 discusses current status and future works.

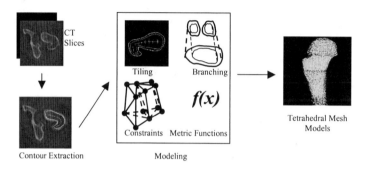

Figure 1. Tetrahedral Mesh Reconstruction from Contours

2. Tetrahedral Mesh Reconstruction from Contours

There are several techniques to construct the tetrahedral meshes. The easiest way first subdivides the 3D space into cubicle voxels that can be divided into five tetrahedra [4]. The drawback of this method is that the mesh generated is too dense and doesn't capture any shape properties. 3D Delaunay triangulation is another method. But this method is time consuming and requires some post-processing since the basic algorithm produces a mesh of the convex hull of the anatomical object. Boissonnat *et al* [5] proposed a method to construct tetrahedral mesh from contours on cross section. They first computed 2D Delaunay triangulation on each section, then tiled tetrahedral mesh between sections. But they didn't consider the intersection and continuity constraints between tetrahedra, and their meshes did not adapt to the anatomy.

Our tetrahedral mesh construction algorithm is derived from those surface mesh reconstruction algorithms [6]. The tetrahedral mesh is constructed slice by slice and layer by layer based on bone contours extracted in a separate algorithm. The running time is *O(n)*, where *n* is the total number of vertices in the model.

We chose a simple data structure to represent the tetrahedral mesh, consisting of a list of vertex coordinates and a list of tetrahedra. Each tetrahedron contains links that reference its four vertices and its four face neighbors. The face neighbors of a tetrahedron are those tetrahedra share a common face with this tetrahedron. Other information such as the density function is also stored in the tetrahedron.

Figure 1 shows the flow chart to reconstruct the tetrahedral mesh from the bone contours extracted in each CT slice.

2.1 Contour Extraction: bones contain two basic types of osseous tissue: compact and spongy bone [7]. Compact bone is dense and looks smooth and homogeneous. Spongy bone is composed of little beams and has a good deal of open space. Figure 2 illustrates the bone structure. We extract both the outer contours and the boundaries between compact bone, spongy bone and Medullary Cavity. In our algorithm, we apply a deformable "snake" contour model to extract the bone contours. Provided the initial value of the contour, the algorithm can automatically converge to the bone contour. The contours are then fitted into smooth B-spline curves and re-sampled at desired resolution for the follow up tiling. We also compute the medial axis of the contour and treat it as the innermost layer.

2.2 Tiling: Tiling is the essential step in constructing the tetrahedral mesh. The idea is to subdivide the space between adjacent slices into tetrahedra, then connect the tetrahedra into a mesh. In previous paper, we proposed a 3D tiling scheme based on the tiling of four ordered contours on two adjacent slices. There are 32 distinct tiling patterns for each single step [8]. It is complex and time consuming to choose the best tiling out of all those patterns. Furthermore, because of the tiling constraints (Section 2.4), the 3D tiling scheme under Greedy strategy may not be able to find a tiling solution in certain steps. In such case, we need to trace back the process and start over again. Due to the disadvantages of the 3D tiling scheme, we propose a new tiling scheme. In this scheme, we separate the complex 3D tiling procedure into two simpler procedures. First we compute the 2D tiling between contours on each slice and the tiling between medial axis. Then the 2D tiling of contours and the tiling of the medial axis can be 'knit' to form a tetrahedral mesh. Hence each tiling step has at most four tiling patterns (by choosing the knit direction). And the constraint problem is much simplified.

2.3 Metric Functions: in order to choose the best pattern for tiling, a metric function must be evaluated on each candidate pattern. The metric function used in our algorithm is a combination of minimizing density error and span length.

2.4 Constraints: in order to form a manifold tetrahedral mesh, some constraints must be imposed. 1) Non-intersection between tetrahedra. This constraint is obvious for a valid spatial subdivision of the volume. When we select a tiling pattern, those newly generated tetrahedra shouldn't intersect with the old tetrahedra already in the mesh. 2) Continuity between slices. A triangle face on one slice should be shared by two tetrahedra in adjacent sections. This constraint is automatically fulfilled in our 2D tiling scheme. 3) Continuity between layers. This constraint is similar to the continuity constraint between slices.

2.5 Contour correspondence between slices: The corresponding problem arises whenever there are multiple contours on one slice. We solved the correspondence problem by simply examining the overlap and distance between contours on adjacent slices.

2.6 Branching problems: There are two kinds of branching problems: branching between layers and branching between slices. The layer branching occurs when the numbers of layers of corresponding contours between adjacent slices are different. The layer branching can be converted to the tiling of three contours, which is a special case of the tiling of four contours. The slice branching occurs when the numbers of contours between adjacent slices are different. One method is to construct a composite contour that connects the adjacent contours at the closest points. This composite contour is then tiled with the single contour from the adjacent slice. Another method is to split the contour into several parts and tile each part with its counterpart on the other slice.

2.7 Tetrahedral mesh models

In manifold tetrahedral mesh, the neighborhood of any face can be continuously deformed to a cone or half cone. In the case of half cone, that face can be defined as a boundary face. The tetrahedral mesh generated by our method is guaranty to be manifold and well behaved because of the constraints we impose during the tiling.

Figure 3 shows wire frame renderings of two tetrahedral mesh models produced by our method. Figure 3.a is a femur model. Figure 3.b is a half pelvis model. Table 1 lists some facts about these two models. Figure 4 shows different layers of the femur model.

Model	Num of Vertices	Num of Tetrahedra	Num of Slices	Total Num of Voxels inside	Avg Num of voxels Per Tetra	Volume (mm^3)	Avg. Vol. Per Tetra (mm^3)
Femur	6163	31537	83	1802978	57.1	312107	9.896
Pelvis	3911	16335	89	456704	27.9	278658	17.1

Table 1. Facts about two tetrahedral model

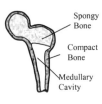

Spongy Bone

Compact Bone

Medullary Cavity

Figure 2. Bone Structure

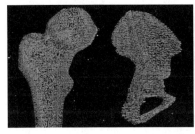

Figure 3. Femur and Pelvis Model

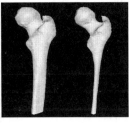

Figure 4. Outer and inner layers of femur model

3   Density Function

We assign an analytical density function to every tetrahedron instead of storing the density value of every voxel in the model. The advantage of such a representation is that it is in explicit form and is a continuous function in 3D space. So it is convenient to integrate, to differentiate, to interpolate, and to deform.

Currently we define the density function as an n-degree Bernstein polynomial in barycentric coordinate. $D(\mu) = \sum_{i+j+k+l=n} C_{i,j,k,l} B^n_{i,j,k,l}(\mu)$, here $C_{i,j,k,l}$ is the polynomial coefficient, and $B^n_{i,j,k,l}(\mu) = \dfrac{n!}{i!\,j!\,k!\,l!} \mu_x^i \mu_y^j \mu_z^k \mu_w^l$ is a barycentric Bernstein basis.

For each tetrahedron, we first get a sample of the voxels inside the tetrahedron, and obtain the voxel density via the CT data set, then fit a Bernstein polynomial function of the density in the barycentric coordinates of those sampled voxels. Once having the density function, we can compute the density at any point inside the tetrahedron by their barycentric coordinate. We use quadratic and cubic polynomials in our initial experiments and they have worked well, although we are considering the use of higher order polynomials in barycentric Bernstein form with adaptively simplified tetrahedral meshes. Table 2 is a comparison of polynomial degree via average density error of the density function. Each tetrahedron may contain hundreds of voxels. Using a density function with few coefficients also shows high storage efficiency (Table 3).

Degree	0	1	2	3	4	5	6	7	8
Coeff Number	1	4	10	20	35	56	84	120	165
Avg. Density Err	3.291	1.583	0.766	0.442	0.298	0.216	0.167	0.149	0.128

Table 2. Degree of Density Function via Accuracy of Density Function

4   Tetrahedral Mesh Simplification and Hierarchical Data Structure

Tetrahedral meshes with multiple resolutions are very desirable for some applications. We can build tetrahedral meshes with different level of details by sampling the contours at different resolution. But there would be no hierarchical connections between different scale of meshes. Our current modeling strategy is as following: first construct a dense model from the pre-segmented contours of bones. Then use a bottom-up approach to produce a hierarchy of tetrahedral mesh, each of which is within a specific error bound of its upper level. Edge collapsing was chose to simplify the mesh. We put all the edges in a priority queue according to their cost functions. And each time we select the edge with smallest cost function for collapsing. The edge collapsing is performed by contracting one of its vertices to the other, while merging all the tetrahedra incident to the diminishing vertex (Figure 5 shows a 2D case of edge collapsing). The hth level of mesh was obtained by simplifying the h-1th level of mesh. This allows one to proceed incrementally, taking advantage of the work done in previous simplifications. It also builds a hierarchical structure in which the vertices at the hth level are a subset of the vertices at the h-1th level.

Our algorithm draws heavily on the work of [4]. Our main contributions are methods for anatomical features preserving and the density preserving during the simplification. We also guarantee that no self-intersections occur in every level of the hierarchy.

4.1 Anatomical Features Preserving: our model is built to adapt to the anatomical features (bone cortical walls). And the mesh is tiled layer by layer (Section 2.2). To preserve the anatomical features, edge collapsing across the layers is prohibited.

4.2 Non-self-Intersection: flipping of a tetrahedron during edge collapsing can cause intersection between tetrahedra. In figure 6, tetrahedron $v_1v_2v_3v_4$ flips and intersects with $v_1v_2v_3v_5$. The normal flipping heuristic can be generalized in order to prevent the flipping of tetrahedra. The method is to analyze the signed volume of involved tetrahedra. If the volume of one of the neighboring tetrahedra changes sign, tetrahedron flipping occurs. Such edge collapsing should be forbidden.

4.3 Density Preserving: the ability to characterize the density property of the tetrahedron after the simplification is very important. As shown in figure 5, after edge collapsing and re-tiling, tetrahedron t_i in h-1th level is replaced by t_j' in h^{th} level. The density function of tetrahedron in h^{th} level is computed from those tetrahedra in h-1th level it intersects with. For instance in figure 5, t_1' in h^{th} level intersects with t_1, t_2, t_3 in h-1th level. Our way to compute new density function for t_j' is as following: first get a sample of voxels in t_j', then for each voxel locate its containing tetrahedron t_i in h-1th level and compute its density, then fit a new Bernstein polynomial for t_j' using the sample. In order to preserve the density function of t_j', we define the error metric of density function as

$$E(t_j') = \oint_{u \in t_j'} \left[D_{t_j'}(u) - D_{t_i}(v) \right]^2 du \text{ , here } v \text{ is the corresponding voxel of } u \text{ in } h\text{-}1^{th} \text{ level, and } t_i$$

is the containing tetrahedron of v. $E(t_j')$ should be smaller than a pre-defined error bound for density preserving. If the error is too big, we can either discard the collapsing or elevate the degree of the density function to improve the accuracy.

Level	Num of Verts	Num of Tetras	Avg Density Diff (Percentage)	Std Dev of Density Diff (Percentage)	Avg Vol. Per Tetra (mm^3)	Avg Num of voxels Per Tetra	Storage in CT image (bytes)	Storage in Tetra model (bytes)
1	6163	31537	2.7%	1.9%	9.896	57	3,605,956	2,344,620
2	2350	12719	4.9%	3.1%	23.4	105	3,605,956	943,968
3	446	2448	8.4%	6.3%	159.9	681	3,605,956	181,608

Table 3 Facts about Hierarchical Femur Model in Figure 7.a

Figure7.a shows a femur model with multiple resolutions, and figure 7.b shows a hierarchical pelvis model. Table 3 lists some facts about the hierarchical femur model and the accuracy and storage efficiency of its density function.

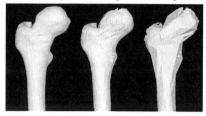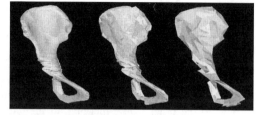

Figure 7. Multiple resolution femur model and pelvis model

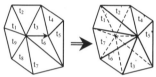

Figure 5 Edge Collapsing in 2D

Figure 6 Tetrahedron Flipping

Figure 8. DRRs from CT data and multiple resolution density models
(a) from CT   (b) from density model with 31537 tetras   (c) from density model with 12719 tetras   (d) from density model with 2448 tetras

5   Computing DRRs from Hierarchical Tetrahedral Mesh Density Model

We can employ a ray-casting algorithm to efficiently generate the DRRs through our tetrahedral mesh density model. When a ray passes through a 3D data set, it may go through hundreds of voxels but only a few tetrahedra. Because the density function is a Bernstein polynomial, its integral along a line can be computed in close form. Furthermore the neighborhood information is stored in the mesh, so it is fast to get next tetrahedron hit by the ray from current hitting tetrahedron. And it is also fast to find the entry point of the casting ray using the neighborhood information. Meanwhile generating DRR from CT data requires computing voxel convolution, which is a time consuming process [9]. So we have an efficient way to generate the DRR from our tetrahedral density model, which is an important technique in 2D-3D intensity-based registration.

	Num of Tetra	Running time	Avg. elems Passed through	Avg Intensity Diff (Percentage)	Std Dev of Intensity Diff (Percentage)
CT Data set	N/A	29.4 s	132.6 voxels	N/A	N/A
Density Model	31537	9.2 s	43.1 tetras	3.2%	2.4%
Density Model	12719	5.6 s	21.8 tetras	7.6%	5.7%
Density Model	2448	1.9 s	7.3 tetras	14.4%	10.3%

Table 4. Comparison of DRRs generated from CT data set and Multiple resolution Density Model

It is obvious that if we generate the DRRs from a lower resolution mesh, the process can be speed up but DRR quality may be sacrificed. There is a tradeoff between speed and quality. Using hierarchical mesh, we can choose the resolution of mesh according to different applications and different situations. Figure 8a is a DRR generated from a CT data using ray casting algorithm. Figure 8b, 8c, 8d are DRRs generated from our density model with different resolution. The image size is 512*512. Table 5 shows the comparison of those DRRs in Figure 8. We used DRR generated from CT (figure 8.a) as the ground truth and compared the pixel intensities of those DRRs in figure 8. The running times are also compared on a Pentium III 400 PC with 256Mb memory.

6   Discussions and Future Work

In this paper we have presented the first phase of our density atlas research. We proposed an efficient and automatic method to construct the tetrahedral mesh from bone contours. We also assigned a density function to the tetrahedron and showed that it is reasonably accurate and efficient in storage. We then simplify the tetrahedral mesh based on edge collapsing scheme and build a hierarchical data structure to represent multiple resolutions of the density model. We also demonstrated the fast generation of DRRs using our density mesh.

We will continue our work on building the density atlas. We will investigate the deformation rule of the tetrahedral mesh. We will build an average density model from a large group of data by incorporating the statistical variation on both shape and density. Ultimately we will apply the density atlas to various application such us 2D-3D registration, surgical planning etc.

Acknowledgements

This work was partially funded by NSF Engineering Research Center grant EEC9731478. We thank Integrated Surgical System for providing the femur data and the Shadyside Hospital for the pelvis data. We specially thank Stephen Pizer, Sandy Wells, Robert VanVorhis, Jerry Prince, and Chengyang Xu for their useful suggestions.

References

[1] G. Subsol, J.-P. Thirion, and N. Ayache, "First Steps Towards Automatic Building of Anatomical Atlas," INRIA, France 2216, March, 1994.

[2] C. B. Cutting, F. L. Bookstein, and R. H. Taylor, "Applications of Simulation, Morphometrics and Robotics in Craniofacial Surgery," in *Computer-Integrated Surgery*, R. H. Taylor, S. Lavallee, G. Burdea, and R. Mosges, Eds. Cambridge, Mass.: MIT Press, 1996, pp. 641-662.

[3] M. Chen, T. Kanade, et al, "3-D Deformable Registration of Medical Images Using a Statistical Atlas," Carnegie Mellon University, Pittsburgh, PA CMU-RI-TR-98-35, December, 1998.

[4] I. J. Trotts, B. Hamann, and K. I. Joy, "Simplification of Tetrahedral Meshes with Error Bounds," *IEEE Transactions On Visualization and Computer Graphics*, vol. 5, pp. 224-237, 1999.

[5] J.-D. Boissonnat and B. Geiger, "Three dimensional reconstruction of complex shapes based on the Delaunay triangulation," INRIA, Le Chesnay, France 1697, May, 1992.

[6] D. Meyers, S. Skinner, and K. Sloan, "Surfaces from Contours," *ACM Transactions on Graphics*, vol. 11, pp. 228-258, 1992.

[7] E. N. Marieb, *Human Anatomy and Physiology*, second edition ed: the Benjamin/Cummings Publishing Company, 1992.

[8] J. Yao, "Tetrahedral Mesh Modeling of Density Data for Anatomical Atlases and Intensity-Based Registration," presented at MICCAI 2000, Pittsburgh, PA, USA, 2000.

[9] P. Lacroute, "Fast Volume Rendering Using a Shear-Warp Factorization of the Viewing Transformation," in *Computer Science*. California: Stanford, 1995.

594

Medicine Meets Virtual Reality 2001
J.D. Westwood et al. (Eds.)
IOS Press, 2001

Anatomic Modeling from Unstructured Samples Using Variational Implicit Surfaces

Terry S. Yoo[1], Bryan Morse[2], K.R. Subramanian[3],
Penny Rheingans[4], Michael J. Ackerman[1]

[1]*National Library of Medicine, National Institutes of Health, Bethesda, MD 20894 USA*
[2] *Dept. of Computer Science, Brigham Young University, Provo UT 84602 USA*
[3] *Dept. of Computer Science, Univ. of North Carolina Charlotte, Charlotte NC 28223 USA*
[4]*Dept. of CSEE, Univ. Maryland Baltimore County, Baltimore MD 21250 USA*

Abstract. We describe the use of variational implicit surfaces (level sets of an embedded generating function modeled using radial basis interpolants) in anatomic modeling. This technique allows the practitioner to employ sparsely and unevenly sampled data to represent complex biological surfaces, including data acquired as a series of non-parallel image slices. The method inherently accommodates interpolation across irregular spans. In addition, shapes with arbitrary topology are easily represented without interpolation or aliasing errors arising from discrete sampling. To demonstrate the medical use of variational implicit surfaces, we present the reconstruction of the inner surfaces of blood vessels from a series of endovascular ultrasound images.

1. Introduction

Medical data analysis and visualization often requires the representation of known segments or objects in an easily processed form. The primitives used for these representations are often either a binary voxel map or a polygonal or polyhedral representation. Each of these modeling primitives has its limitations. As a modeling representation, voxel maps are not invariant with respect to rotation or changes in scale. When arbitrarily rotating or scaling a binary voxel map, grey values will be introduced near the boundary as voxels become partially covered by the rotated or scaled bitmap, making necessary a type change from a binary-valued array to a scalar valued system. The alternative is to enforce a binary mapping of the voxel representation, accepting the subsequent sampling errors.

Surface representations modeled either with polygons (or with volume structuring primitives such as tetrahedra) are invariant with respect to rotation and scale. However, if you create a close-up view of the surface representation, the discretization of the surface into planar primitives becomes apparent, and the viewed surface no longer closely approximates the desired smoothness for the representation of the model. Thus although invariant with respect to changes in scale, polygonal surface models are susceptible to artifacts and errors in the piecewise planar approximation to smooth surfaces when scaled.

What is desired is a smooth representation that is easily captured from a binary segmentation and that is invariant with respect to rotation, translation, and scale. Moreover, it should support resampling of the surface model at any arbitrary sampling rate to support visualization at any level of zoom or scale. We have explored the use of variational implicit surfaces as a modeling primitive for binary anatomical objects. These systems provide the necessary smooth differentiable surface models with the desired properties for robust representation of complex biological structures.

2. Background and History

When viewing the 3D relationships among anatomical structures identified within medical data, researchers often apply direct volume rendering techniques [6]. The generation of surface models from volumetric information is an alternative to direct rendering and is also a common practice in the visualization of anatomy. Reconstruction of piecewise planar polygonal surface models from rectilinear volume data is frequently achieved using computationally efficient methods such as Marching Cubes [7]. However, when either of these techniques is applied to objects that are represented as binary bitmaps, sampling and discretization errors arise leading to terracing and jaggies, a prominent problem in medical imaging.

Recent work in surface fitting has addressed these issues. Gibson extracts smooth surface models treating the existing binary data as a constraining element in an energy-minimizing deformable surface system [4]. The resulting data structure can be used either to create Euclidean distance maps for direct volume rendering or employed directly as a polygonal surface model [5]. Whitaker has modified the constrained deformable surface model to a constrained level-set model, which creates smooth models while bypassing the need for a separate surface representation [14]. However, while these methods generate smooth representations, both the level set model and the surface net remain discretely sampled and retain the problem that they are not zoom invariant. A different modeling primitive is still needed.

Turk and O'Brien adapt earlier work on thin plate splines [1][2] and radial basis interpolants [3][10] to create a new technique in generating implicit surfaces [11]. Their method allows direct specification of a complex surface from sparse, irregular surface samples. The method is quite flexible and has been extended to higher dimensions to support shape interpolation [12]. However, their technique as described cannot be used to model surfaces where large numbers of surface points are included, making it unsuitable for medical applications where range data or tomographic reconstruction often lead to data described by hundreds of thousands of surface points.

3. Methods & Tools

An *implicit surface* is defined by $\{ \bar{x}: f(\bar{x}) = k \}$, $k \in \mathbb{R}$, for some characteristic embedding function $f: \mathbb{R}^3 \rightarrow \mathbb{R}$. Given a set of surface points $C = \{ \bar{c}_1, \bar{c}_2, \bar{c}_3, \dots \bar{c}_n \}$, the variational implicit technique interpolates the smoothest possible scalar function $f(\bar{x})$ whose zero level set, $\{\bar{x}: f(\bar{x}) = 0\}$, passes through all points in C. That is, find the smoothest function f such that $f(\bar{x}_i) = 0$ for each known surface point $\bar{x}_i$, and $f(\bar{y}_i) = 1$ for one or more points $\bar{y}_i$ known to be inside the shape. Following Turk and O'Brien's generalization of the problem, ., given a set of positions $\bar{c}_i$ and corresponding values h_i, solve for an embedding function f such that $f(\bar{c}_i) = h_i$. by employing radial basis interpolating functions $\phi(r)$ in a critically constrained linear system of n equations and n unknowns. Specifically, given a radial basis interpolating function $\phi(r)$ and a series of known points where the desired function f is constrained to be $f(\bar{c}_i) = h_i$, solve the following equation for the unknown weights d_j.

$$f(\bar{c}_i) = \sum_{j=1}^{n} d_j \phi(\|\bar{c}_i - \bar{c}_j\|) + P(\bar{x}) = h_i$$

(1)

Expanding $\bar{c}_i = (c_i^x, c_i^y, c_i^z)$, the entire linear system can be expressed as an $(n+4) \times (n+4)$ matrix M where:

$$\begin{bmatrix} \phi_{11} & \phi_{12} & \cdots & \phi_{1n} & c_1^x & c_1^y & c_1^z & 1 \\ \phi_{21} & \phi_{22} & \cdots & \phi_{2n} & c_2^x & c_2^y & c_2^z & 1 \\ \vdots & & \ddots & \vdots & \vdots & \vdots & \vdots & \vdots \\ \phi_{n1} & \phi_{n2} & \cdots & \phi_{nn} & c_n^x & c_n^y & c_n^z & 1 \\ c_1^x & c_2^x & \cdots & c_n^x & 0 & 0 & 0 & 0 \\ c_1^y & c_2^y & \cdots & c_n^y & 0 & 0 & 0 & 0 \\ c_1^z & c_2^z & \cdots & c_n^z & 0 & 0 & 0 & 0 \\ 1 & 1 & \cdots & 1 & 0 & 0 & 0 & 0 \end{bmatrix} \begin{bmatrix} d_1 \\ d_2 \\ \vdots \\ d_n \\ p^x \\ p^y \\ p^z \\ 1 \end{bmatrix} = \begin{bmatrix} h_1 \\ h_2 \\ \vdots \\ h_n \\ 0 \\ 0 \\ 0 \\ 0 \end{bmatrix}$$

(2)

The resulting matrix is known to be positive semi-definite, and can be solved with a linear decomposition system. Once the weights d_i are found, the embedding function can be written as:

$$f(\bar{x}) = \sum_{i=1}^{n} d_i \phi(\|\bar{x} - \bar{c}_i\|) + P(\bar{x})$$

(3)

Depending on the differentiability of the radial basis function, $\phi(r)$, $f(\bar{x})$ is an implicit surface generating function that can be resampled with arbitrary precision and remains invariant under rotation, translation, and zoom. (For most of this work, we have used the same radial basis function, $\phi(r) = r^3$ for $r \geq 0$, used by Turk and O'Brien from related research on thin-plate splines.) If the constraints $\bar{c}_i$ for $f(\bar{x})$ are abstracted from either a grey-level or a binary bit mask volume sampled volume, the resulting variational implicit surface is a more compact analytical representation of the same data.

4. Results

We have applied this method to the modeling of a bovine aorta from data acquired using an endovascular ultrasound transducer. This particular modality acquires noisy 2D image slices, sampled at uneven intervals with non-parallel orientations. The transducer is drawn slowly through the vessel, acquiring cross-sectional sonographic images (see Figure 1).

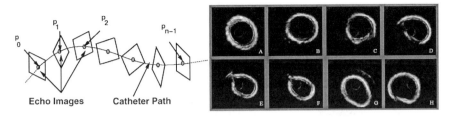

Figure 1. Cross-sectional ultrasound images of an ex-vivo bovine aorta. The slices are acquired at angles perpendicular to the endovascular catheter path. The imaging path is determined by the geometry of the blood vessel.

Each individual slice is then segmented, and the aggregate contours from the tilted slices are processed to form a variational implicit surface. The resulting analytic description can be sampled and rendered using volume rendering approaches, or it can be interrogated and tesselated into a polygonal or parametric surface representation. Figure 2 shows the two views of the interior surface of the bovine aorta from Figure 1 reconstructed as a variational implicit surface. The zero-set of the implicit model has been extracted using a surface tiler, rendering them as polygons at the resolution desired for the magnification shown. If close-up views are desired, the model can easily be reinterrogated and tiled in the surface rendering case or the model simply re-rendered in a direct volume rendering system with arbitrary precision, eliminating aliasing artifacts in the representation of the model.

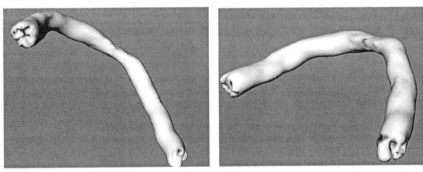

Figure 2. Surface renderings of the interior surfaces of the ex-vivo bovine aorta reconstructed as a variationalimplicit surface from the ultrasound slices in Figure 1. The models are not subject to aliasing artifacts generated by comparable surface or volume. In addition, these models are generated from sparse, non-uniformly sampled non-parallel ultrasound slices.

5. Discussion and Future Work

The radial basis function, $\phi(r) = r^3$ for $r \geq 0$, advocated by Turk and O'Brien is infinite in extent. It has advantages when interpolating across unpredictable spans, making it ideal for morphing and shape interpolation. However, the infinite extent leads to ill-conditioned matrices and increased computational complexity. A naïve approach is easily order $O(n^3)$.

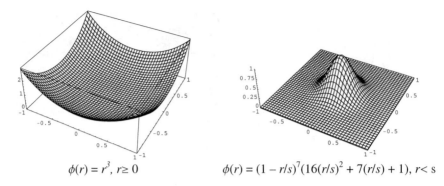

$$\phi(r) = r^3, r \geq 0 \qquad\qquad \phi(r) = (1 - r/s)^7(16(r/s)^2 + 7(r/s) + 1), r < s$$

Figure 3. Two radial basis functions. The left function $\phi(r) = r^3$, $r \geq 0$ has infinite extent. The right function $\phi(r) = (1 - r/s)^7(16(r/s)^2 + 7(r/s) + 1)$ is clamped to zero outside a specified radius of support s, and is proven to be C^4 continuous. The compactly supported function on the right leads to more stable numerics and faster solutions of the variational implicit surface model.

In related work, we address the computational complexity of variational implicit surface modeling. Instead of $\phi(r) = r^3$ as the underlying interpolant, we address select from among a family of radial basis functions presented by Wendland [13] to find a function with the necessary continuity but also with finite, compact local support. Figure 3 shows a comparison of the 3D thin-plate-spline radial basis function and the suggested compactly supported radial basis functions of our current research. The shift from a radial basis function of infinite extent to one that has compact local support has created dramatic gains in memory utilization and computational complexity. Previous work described solutions for systems of equations of order $O(n^3)$ complexity with iterative solutions capable of achieving order $O(n^2)$. The shift to finite interpolants and sparse matrices has shifted the bulk of the computation toward order $O(n)$, depending on the complexity of the model and the uniformity of the density of the surface constraints. We have measured the complexity of the matrix solution for some test cases as $O(n^{1.5})$. For more details, see Morse [8].

The use of compactly supported radial basis functions imposes a restriction on the maximum distance allowed between systems of surface constraints. This trade-off between speed and the granularity of the surface samples is the topic of some of our future research in this area. The infinite radial basis function permits interpolation across wide spans and with arbitrary orientations to the subsets of constraints that comprise the initial surface description. However, the costs of using this system rise with the number of points required to faithfully represent the surface. This trade-off has ramifications in the choice and precision of the segmentation algorithm to be used and the complexity of the objects to be represented.

Future work on this topic includes the development of hybrid representations that incorporate both infinite and compact radial basis functions. In addition, we will explore advanced slice-based segmentation techniques with confidence in our ability to interpolated smoothly between 2D segments. It should be noted that variational implicit surfaces can be generated as the output of segmentation systems; however, as a means of smoothly interpolating between sample slices, they can be used to initialize a deformable contour for segmenting an unknown intermediate slice. The use of variational implicit surfaces to help generate priors for segmentation systems is a current focus for some of our group. Finally, we are investigating algorithms for the automatic generation of variational implicit surface models for the anatomic structures currently identified as part of the Visible Human Project (VHP) [9]. Four hundred thirty-five (435) hand-segmented structures comprise the current segmented thorax database, with each segment modeled using an uncompressed binary bitmask. For example, the bitmask for the heart is over 400 kilobytes, alone. We are seeking a means of automatically generating compact analytical descriptions of these models using the techniques described here.

6. Conclusions

Given a set of surface points $C = \{ \bar{c}_1, \bar{c}_2, \bar{c}_3, \dots \bar{c}_n \}$, the variational implicit technique interpolates the smoothest possible scalar function $f(\bar{x})$ whose zero level set, $\{ \bar{x}: f(\bar{x}) = 0 \}$, passes through all points in C. These surface constraints or points can be generated from a variety of sources including segmentation systems. We show that variational implicit surfaces can be effectively used to model anatomic structures. Earlier limitations of computational and memory efficiency can been solved through a judicious selection of interpolant and improved numerics. Examples including noisy data from modalities generating curvilinear gridded data, such as endovascular ultrasound, demonstrate the utility of this technique.

7. Acknowledgements

This work was performed in large part at the National Library of Medicine under a visiting faculty program supporting both Dr. Morse and Dr. Subramanian. Dr. Rheingans was supported in part by NSF CAREER Grant #9996043. We would like to thank Greg Turk for his useful conversations and for making his code available to us, upon which our implementation is based.

References

[1] Bookstein, F. L. 1991. Morphometric tools for landmark data. Cambridge University Press
[2] Duchon, J. 1977. Splines minimizing rotation–invariant semi-norms in Sobolev spaces, in Constructive theory of functions of several variables, Lecture Notes in Mathematics, edited by A. Dolb and B. Eckmann, Springer-Verlag, 1977, pp. 85–100.
[3] Floater, M. S. and A. Iske. 1996. Multistep scattered data interpolation using compactly supported radial basis functions. J. Comp. Appl. Math. 73, pp 65-78.
[4] Gibson, S. 1998. Constrained elastic surface nets: generating smooth surfaces from binary segmented data, in Proceedings of Medical Image Computing and Computer Assisted Interventions (MICCAI 1998)W. M. Wells, A. Colchester, and S. Delp, *eds.*, Lecture Notes in Computer Science 1496, Springer-Verlag, pp. 888-898.
[5] Gibson, S. 1998. Using distance maps for accurate surface representation in sampled volumes, in Proceedings of the 1998 Symposium on Volume Visualization, ACM SIGGRAPH, pp. 23-30.
[6] Kaufman, A. Volume visualization. IEEE Computer Society Press, Los Alamitos, CA, 1991.
[7] Lorensen, W. and H. Cline. 1987. Marching Cubes: a high-resolution 3D surface construction algorithm. In Proc. SIGGRAPH 87, Computer Graphics, 21(4), pp. 163-169.

[8] Morse, B., T. Yoo, P. Rheingans, D. Chen, and K.R. Subramanian. 2000. Complex Models Using Variational Implicit Surfaces. Submitted to Shape Modeling International 2001.

[9] V. Spitzer, M. J. Ackerman, A. L. Scherzinger, and D. Whitlock. 1996. The Visible Human Male: A Technical Report. J. of the Am. Medical Informatics Assoc. 3(2) 118-130.

[10] Szeliski, R. 1990. Fast surface interpolation using hierarchical basis functions. IEEE Transactions on Pattern Analysis and Machine Intelligence, 12(6):513-528, June 1990.

[11] Turk, G. and J. F. O'Brien. 1999. Variational implicit surfaces, Tech Report GIT-GVU-99-15, Georgia Institute of Technology, May 1999, 9 pages.

[12] Turk, G. and J. F. O Brien. 1999. Shape transformation using variational implicit functions. Computer Graphics Proceedings, Annual Conference Series (SIGGRAPH 99), pp. 335–342.

[13] Wendland, H. 1995. Piecewise polynomial positive definite and compactly supported radial basis functions of minimal degree. AICM 4 (1995), pp. 389-396.

[14] Whitaker, R. 2000. Reducing Aliasing Artifacts in Iso-Surfaces of Binary Volumes. in Volume Visualization and Graphics Symposium 2000, ACM SIGGRAPH, pp. 23-32.

Medicine Meets Virtual Reality 2001
J.D. Westwood et al. (Eds.)
IOS Press, 2001

Intelligent System and Risk of Different Diseases in the General Population

Neda Zarrin-Khameh, Afsaneh Barzi, Sarmad Sadeghi
72270 Fannin St., Suite 200, Houston, TX 77025

Abstract

This is a new approach to define the risk of the general population for a specific disease. We use Bayesian theory to define the risk of the population. Analyzing the major risk factors of a disease, how they affect the incidence and/or prevalence of the disease, and the statistics of each risk factor in the population, along with the power of the Bayes theorem helps us define the risk of that population for that disease. To find out what the risk of the general population for a disease is, prospective epidemiological studies in the population shown are needed. These studies usually lead to the identification of the major risk factors for a disease and their impacts which are quite costly and requires a long time to get to the results. Also a large personnel is needed to perform effectively in the study. The result of the risk of the general population for a first heart attack using our software is in agreement with the result of the Framingham heart study. Large studies like Framingham is not available for other diseases to enable us to evaluate the accuracy of our software precisely. To overcome this shortage we have sought medical experts' evaluation of the predicted risk of the general population for other disease by this software, which needs to be completed.

1. Background

Disease prevention is among the most closely watched and most promising areas in health care today. Prevention is based on decreasing or eliminating the factors that causes diseases. Working on prevention is not only cost effective, but can also save many patients from experiencing the psychological and physical effects of chronic diseases, such as hypertension or diabetes.

Although prevention is mostly categorized as one of physician's responsibilities it is shown that physicians often fail to deliver preventive services. [1,2] This is due to various factors. Different sources have various recommendations, the relative effects of preventive recommendations are usually unclear and it usually can ultimately cause more harm than good; which is hardly acceptable for a healthy person. [3,4] Primary prevention aims to address individual's health practices to eliminate or decrease disease risk factors (e.g. quitting smoking, decrease alcohol consumption). [5] Secondary prevention promotes early detection disease or early stages (e.g. routine cervical papanicolaou screen to detect carcinoma of cervix). Tertiary prevention measures are directed to limit the impact of an established disease (partial mastectomy and adjunctive therapy to remove and control breast cancer). [6] Primary prevention is the most effective and economical of all methods to reduce the incidence and severity of diseases causing morbidity and mortality. Health care providers are advised to take every moment to deliver preventive services. By explaining the benefits and disadvantages of a preventive action the health care provider can increase the efficacy of preventive medicine, empower patients and consult them to change health-related behaviors. [7]

To increase delivery of the preventive medicine measures we have focused on primary and secondary prevention. By increasing the number of internet users having an online risk assessment tools for common diseases like myocardial infarction, diabetes, hypertension and so on we can dramatically increase delivery of preventive health services. Health care consumers should be more involved in decision making for their lifestyle habits. Empowering them with information and assessing their risk for different diseases can be very helpful in this regard.   .

Incidence of heart attack has decreased dramatically in the past two decades but it can still be lowered more. On the contrary, the incidence of many other diseases has increased (e.g. breast cancer incidence in females increased from 88.6 per 100,000 in the early 1970s to 109.8 in the early 1990s, colon/rectal cancer incidence rates increased since 1973 but may have peaked for white males and females, etc). [8] Furthermore, the frequencies of preventable risk factors such as obesity (a major risk factor for myocardial infarction, hypertension, diabetes, colorectal cancer, etc) and sedentary lifestyle (a major risk factor for diabetes, myocardial infarction, hypertension, prostate cancer, osteoporosis, etc) have increased significantly. Education has an important role in taking people into action and reducing these risk factors.

Evaluating a person's risk for various diseases and advising her to work on her preventable risk factors is a practical way to increase participation of people in preventive measures. Reliable risk assessment tools can be useful both for health care providers and consumers.

2. Methods and Tools

To have a proper tool to evaluate the risk of person for a disease it is necessary to study risk factors of a disease. It is essential to determine the extension of risk factors effects and weigh them accordingly to be able to evaluate risk of a disease in an individual. To cover a broader aspect of this evaluation we sought the risk of the general population as the measure. It is more understandable for a person to evaluate her risk and compare it to the risk of the general population. Usually to determine the risk of the general population for a disease, prospective epidemiological studies are conducted. These studies need a long period of time, huge budget and large personnel.

We have been using an intelligent system, based on Bayes theorem to evaluate the risk of a disease in the general population. Risk factors are weighed based on the range of effect of risk factors. In the related tables the frequencies of various risk factors in the general population are entered. The effect of each risk factor on the disease of the scope is defined in the software. The end result shows the risk of the general population for the disease under study. Using this intelligent system the risk of the general population for a first heart attack was defined. Major risk factors for myocardial infarction are age, gender, positive family history, sedentary lifestyle, overweight, diabetes, smoking, total cholesterol, high-density lipoprotein (HDL) and blood pressure. Using medical literature, the effect of each risk factor on the risk of a first myocardial infarction was determined (e.g. smoking increase the risk of myocardial infarction about two times) and weighed accordingly. The prevalence of the risk factors and their effects on the risk of the first myocardial infarction were applied in the software.

3. Results

Risk of a first myocardial infarction in the general population was the end result of the software and it was in close agreement with the result of the Framingham heart study.

4. Conclusion

In 1948, the Framingham Heart Study -- under the direction of the National Heart Institute (now known as the National Heart, Lung, and Blood Institute; NHLBI) -- embarked on an ambitious project in health research. At the time, little was known about the general causes of heart disease and stroke, but the death rates for cardiovascular disease (CVD) had been increasing steadily since the beginning of the century and had become an American epidemic. The objective of the Framingham Heart Study was to identify the common factors or characteristics that contribute to CVD by following its development over a long period of time in a large group of participants who had not yet developed overt symptoms of CVD or suffered a heart attack or stroke.[9]

Because the result of our software for the risk of a first myocardial infarction was in close agreement with the Framingham heart study, we concluded that by using this software we might be able to estimate the risk of other diseases in the general population and use it as the measure for our risk assessment tool. Although there are not large prospective epidemiological studies available for many diseases, using medical experts' opinion can be helpful in evaluating the accuracy of the software.

References

1. National Center for Health Statistics. Healthy People 2000 review, 1993. Hyattsville, MD: Public Health Service, 1994. (DHHS Publication no. (PHS) 94-1232-1.)
2. Montano DE, Phillips WR. Cancer screening by primary care physicians: a comparison of rates obtained from physician self-report, patient survey, and chart audit. Am J Public Health 1995;85:795-800.
3. Battista RN, Lawrence RS, eds. Implementing preventive services. Am J Prev Med 1988;4(4 Suppl):1-194.
4. Frame PS. Health maintenance in clinical practice: strategies and barriers. Am Fam Phys 1992;45:1192-1200.
5. McGinnis JM, Foege WH. Actual causes of death in the United States. JAMA 1993;270:2207-2212.
6. Sox HC Jr. Preventive health services in adults. N Engl J Med. 1994 Jun 2;330(22):1589-95. Review
7. US preventive Task Force: Guide to Clinical Preventive Services, 2nd edition
8. Surveillance, Epidemiology, and End Results (SEER) Program of the National Cancer Institute, National Institutes of Health.
9. Framingham heart study; http://www.nhlbi.nih.gov/about/framingham/

Author Index